Using and Interpreting
Statistics

A Practical Text for the Health, Behavioral, and Social Sciences

Eric W. Corty, PhD

Associate Professor, Clinical Psychology
Penn State Erie, The Behrend College
Erie, Pennsylvania

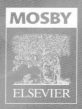

MOSBY
ELSEVIER

11830 Westline Industrial Drive
St. Louis, Missouri 63146

Using and Interpreting Statistics

ISBN-13: 978-0-323-03593-4
ISBN-10:   0-323-03593-0

Copyright © 2007 by Mosby, Inc. an affiliate of Elsevier Inc.

Notice

Neither the Publisher nor the Author assume any responsibility for any loss or injury and/or damage to persons or property arising out of or related to any use of the material contained in this book. It is the responsibility of the treating practitioner, relying on independent expertise and knowledge of the patient, to determine the best treatment and method of application for the patient.

The Publisher

Library of Congress Cataloging-in-Publication Data

Corty, Eric, 1955-
  Using and interpreting statistics: a practical text for the health, behavioral, and social
sciences / Eric W. Corty.
     p. cm.
  Includes index.
  ISBN-13: 978-0-323-03593-4
  ISBN-10: 0-323-03593-0
   1. Mathematical statistics–Textbooks. 2. Statistics–Textbooks. I. Title.

QA276.12.C675 2007
519.5–dc22

2006049400

Acquisitions Editor: Lee Henderson
Developmental Editor: Maureen Ianuzzi
Publishing Services Manager: Jeff Patterson
Project Manager: Amy Rickles
Design Direction: Paula Ruckenbrod

Printed in China

Last digit is the print number: 9 8 7 6 5 4 3 2 1

For my organizing principles, David and Paul.

Preface

To the Instructor

Thanks for choosing my text for your statistics class.

Statistics is a hard class to teach because most students don't want to take it. At the same time, when students "get" the material, or at least end the semester saying, "It wasn't as bad as I feared," it is a rewarding class. To make it more likely that students understand the material, there are a number of techniques I have employed in constructing this book.

First, the book is in full color. This is important because the use of color makes the pages more varied and interesting, making it more likely that students will become engaged in the book and actually read the chapters.

Second, I've tried not to cover too much material. This course is an *introduction* to statistics, so it is important that students get exposed to the broad outlines of the field, not that they learn advanced statistical techniques. Thus, I introduce students to how to summarize and present data, how to transform scores, and how to calculate confidence intervals, Pearson rs, independent-samples t tests, one-way ANOVAs, repeated-measures ANOVAs, and chi-square tests for contingency tables. Interleaved throughout, I teach about the difference between point and interval estimates, effect sizes, power, sample size, and choosing the correct statistical test. This is plenty for a semester.

Third, my focus is on the human side of statistics. Math is certainly involved in this course, but I think it is more important that students learn to do what people, not computers, do best: understand the logic of hypothesis testing and use it to make sense of, to interpret, the results of statistical tests.

Finally, I've used a number of principles from cognitive psychology to help students process the material more deeply and learn it better. Each chapter starts with a "Chapter Roadmap" that points out the upcoming sights so that students will be primed with a framework to which they can fit the material as they encounter it. Review and homework exercises at the end of the chapter are not in the order that material is covered in the chapter, forcing students to think a little bit more about what technique to apply to answer a question. Similarly, the use of examples from a broad array of disciplines both gives students a secure base from which to explore the material and gently pushes them to see broader applications.

Repetition and practice are powerful learning principles, and I give ample opportunity for these to work their magic. Each section in a chapter is followed by group practice problems to reinforce the concepts just covered. I have my students break into small groups and work the problems in class so that I can circulate, check their work, and correct misunderstandings. Though I think that the group aspect—students explaining material to each other—is helpful and recommend it, the problems will still be instructive if students work on them individually and/or out of class. For additional practice there are end-of-chapter review exercises and homework problems for students to work on individually. These use the concepts of distributed practice and cover material from previous chapters as well as the current chapter, again forcing students to process material more deeply.

Deeper processing may facilitate learning, but students also need to have guidelines on how to approach problems: when first learning to cook, it helps to have recipes to follow. Thus, throughout the book I offer "cookbook" approaches, step-by-step procedural guidelines. For example, when I cover the first statistical test I introduce a six-step procedure, along with a mnemonic to remember it, to use when completing a null hypothesis significance test. In every subsequent chapter and for every subsequent statistical test, the same six-step procedure is used. My objective is that by consistently applying this formulaic approach, the students will internalize—and understand—the procedure. Similarly, chapters end with flowcharts that guide the students through the steps of writing an interpretation for a statistical test. My experience is that it is through writing interpretations that students begin to see the big picture of statistics. Writing interpretations is challenging, and students need a procedural guideline so that they can learn how to do it.

Additional teaching and reading resources may be found on the complementary Evolve Learning Resources website (http://evolve.elsevier.com/Corty/statistics/) and the Instructor's Electronic Resources CD-ROM. The resources include the following:

- A 600-item Test Bank
- An Instructor's Resource Manual with answers to the Homework Problems found in this textbook as well as Teaching Strategies and a Quiz for each chapter
- SPSS Tutorials that students may work through online or print out for easy reference
- A *Statistics Quick Reference Chart* of valuable formulae and tables

This is a first edition, and although it has been edited and checked very carefully, it is inevitable that some errors, trivial I hope, have slipped through or crept in. If you find one, please e-mail me (ewc2@psu.edu) so that I can correct it and alert others. At the companion website for this book there is a "Content Updates" link where any errors will be posted. Have your students check it and update their books as needed.

Writing this book was a labor of love for me, and I hope that you and your students get out of it at least a fraction of the joy that I put into it. If you have comments or suggestions about it, don't, as they say in the South, be a stranger now, but please feel free to contact me.

Eric W. Corty
School of Humanities and Social Sciences
Penn State Erie, The Behrend College
5091 Station Road
Erie, PA 16563-1501
ewc2@psu.edu

To the Student

When I teach statistics, I start the semester by putting some quotations up on the board and discussing them with my students so that they will approach the material with the right mind-set. As I was thinking about this preface, it occurred to me that this would be a good introduction to the book as well.

"One does not discover new lands without consenting to lose sight of the shore for a very long time." *Andre Gide*

When adventurers set off to discover new lands they have to have faith that they are headed in the right direction and that the new land will be worth the effort. This faith will sustain them in the long days as their ship plows through empty seas. Similarly, we are heading off on a journey, an intellectual journey to the land of statistics. I am here as your guide: I've been there and have come back alive to tell tales of the riches that await. On our journey there will be times when it seems as if the promised shore will never be reached and mutiny will be appealing. Have faith. I'm a good guide and I know where we are going. The occasional feeling of being lost is just part of the journey.

"The more things are mixed up, the better the solution." *Ms. Frizzle*

OK, so Ms. Frizzle was talking about chemistry in this *Magic School Bus* episode, but I think her statement has a larger application. When we struggle to learn something, when we use our brains to take pieces that don't make sense and—turning them this way and that—finally get the puzzle to fit together, we learn it more deeply than does someone who hasn't engaged in the same effort. Psychologists call this struggle "deep" processing of material, and it is one of the best supported findings in psychology: deep processing leads to better learning. This has several applications in this book. First, you can now label what you are doing when you have lost sight of the shore and are frantically trying to locate it; you can say that you are engaging in deep processing. And, you should be aware that I do a number of things in this book to make you engage in deep processing. For example, the review exercises at the end of the chapter aren't in the same order as the material in the chapter so that there aren't temporal cues about how to answer the question. Through the struggle to resolve the mix-up, your solution—your understanding—will be better.

"The man who carries a cat by the tail learns something that can be learned in no other way." *Mark Twain*

I love this quote. We learn best by experience, and sometimes the best teacher is a mistake. Putting a lot of effort into something and getting it wrong teaches a lesson that is learned deeply. Don't be afraid to try, and don't be afraid of making mistakes. Mistakes are an important part of the learning process.

"There's no education in the second kick of a mule." *Ernest. F. Hollings*

Mistakes are educational only if you learn from them.

"You can no more become a Christian by going to church than you can become an automobile by sleeping in your garage." *Garrison Keillor*

If you want to learn statistics, you have to expend more effort than just showing up for class. You have to interact with the material in regular and meaningful ways—the more you put in, the more you get out.

There are a lot of things you can do to interact with the material. One of the best is reading the book. If you read the chapter before your instructor covers the material, you'll know where he or she is headed. And, if you re-read the chapter after your instructor has covered it, you'll deepen your understanding. If something still doesn't make sense after both I and your instructor have had a whack at explaining it, check out another textbook or check out the World Wide Web. I'm the first to admit that one size doesn't fit all, and someone else may provide an explanation that you find more comprehensible. There are a lot of other good resources out there, so take advantage of them.

"Accidents happen now and again, sometimes just by chance." *Mike O'Donnell & Junior Campbell*

Finally, I want to mention errors, my errors. I've read every chapter in this book multiple times as have reviewers and editors. Still, it is inevitable that there will be some errors in the book. I trust that most will be small and typographic, but there is a chance that something larger, a math error say, has evaded capture. If you find one, either large or small, I want to know about it so that I can correct it; e-mail me at ewc2@psu.edu. There is a companion website for this book at http://evolve.elsevier.com/Corty/statistics/ with a "Content Updates" link where any errors will be posted. Please check this site so that you can make any necessary corrections in your copy.

And now, without further ado, allow me to play Holmes to your Watson. "The game is afoot."

Eric W. Corty
School of Humanities and Social Sciences
Penn State Erie, The Behrend College
5091 Station Road
Erie, PA 16563-1501
ewc2@psu.edu

Acknowledgements

I suspect that most authors spend part of their daydream time thinking about the acknowledgements page. I know I did. Here, in roughly chronological order, are the people who made this book possible.

George M. Diekhoff's *Basic Statistics for the Social and Behavioral Sciences* was published in 1996 and showed me how good an introductory statistics textbook could be. Unfortunately, the publisher, Prentice Hall, chose not to continue it and I was left in textbook limbo. I tried other books, but none measured up, and when I went on sabbatical in 2003, I decided to write my own. My first set of thanks goes to George Diekhoff, Prentice Hall, and whoever invented the sabbatical system.

Linda Workman gave encouragement and advice from beginning to end and introduced me to her editor at Elsevier, Lee Henderson. Linda, thanks for arranging the marriage.

Lee Henderson "got" my book right away and allowed it to develop as I envisioned it, footnotes and all. Maureen Iannuzzi, my editor, used a light touch to make my occasionally more complex than necessary sentences more comprehensible. (Snuck that one by you, Maureen.) Amy Rickles kept me on deadline and nimbly managed all the production details while I kept pressing for last minute changes. Lee, Maureen, and Amy—and the rest of the very professional staff at Elsevier—thanks for making the experience relatively painless.

Bryan Griffin of Georgia Southern University reviewed every chapter and held my feet to the fire on the statistical issues where we disagreed. He forced me to re-think several issues and, thanks to him, the book is better. I am sure that he did not catch all my errors; the remaining ones are, unfortunately, my responsibility.

Richard Lowry had a profound influence on me when I was in college and has graciously allowed me to use some materials from his website. If you ever have difficulty understanding material in my book and wish a fresh perspective, check out his award-winning website: http://faculty.vassar.edu/lowry/webtext.html

Sue Brookhart graciously undertook the task of writing the test bank. Seeing my book mirrored in her words was an enlightening experience and has persuaded me of the value of multiple choice questions.

Derek Mace, a colleague at Penn State Erie, read many chapters and gave constructive criticism. There are a number of other reviewers who read individual chapters and offered feedback and suggestions that improved the book. In alphabetical order, they are: Michele August-Brady, DNSc, RN (Moravian College); Robert Barcikowski, PhD (Ohio University); Gregory A. Bechtel, PhD, MPH, RN (University of North Carolina Wilmington); Susan M. Brookhart, PhD (Duquesne University); Denise Côté-Arsenault, PhD, RNC (Syracuse University); Ruth Davidhizar, DNS, RN, CS, FAAN (Bethel College); Donna El-Din, PhD, PT (Eastern Washington University); Sandra A. Faux, PhD, MN, BSN, RN (Rush University); J. Carolyn Graff, PhD, RN (University of Tennessee); Bryan W. Griffin, PhD (Georgia Southern University); Tamara M. Kear, MSN, RN, CNN (Gwynedd-Mercy College); Sheila Favro Marks, DNS, APRN, BC (Florida Southern University); Barbara Napoli, MBA, BA (Our Lady of the Lake College); Susan K. Steele, DNS, RN, AOCN (Our Lady of the Lake College); Georgianna M. Thomas, EdD, RN (West Suburban College of Nursing); Ann Tritak, EdD, MA, BSN, RN (Fairleigh Dickinson University); and Michael B. Worrell, PhD (Indiana School of Medicine).

Claude & Sue Corty volunteered to proofread chapters and offered the unconditional support that can only come from one's parents. Mom & Dad, you'd make Carl Rogers proud.

My wife, Sara Douglas, is also a statistician (you're probably jealous imagining the late-night conversations that we have about abstruse statistical topics) and was always ready with support and advice. I didn't always take her advice, but I did always need, and appreciate, her love and support. Thanks.

Contents

1

Introduction to Statistics

Purpose, Measurement, Terminology, and Rounding

Learning Objectives

After completing this chapter, you should be able to do the following:

1 Define the purpose of statistics.
2 Describe the three conditions necessary to show cause and effect.
3 Distinguish independent variable, grouping variable, dependent variable, and confounding variable.
4 Define measurement and determine if a variable is being measured on a nominal, ordinal, interval, or ratio scale.
5 Distinguish sample from population, statistic from parameter, descriptive from inferential statistic, and statistical from practical significance.
6 Understand the importance of rounding and apply rules of rounding.

At the start of each chapter you'll find a short section that tells where the chapter is heading so that you'll know what is coming. Think of us as going together on a trip, that we're driving from the east coast to the west. As I am the one with the maps and the guidebooks, I know the route and the sights worth seeing along the way. Thus, each day as we head out, I alert you to what is coming so you won't miss the important sights.*

An important part of the first chapter involves learning the technical language of statistics. I want you to become familiar with the terms used for the measured variables (the independent or grouping variable and the dependent variable), for the subjects studied (a sample from a larger population), and for how to characterize the results of a study (statistically versus practically/clinically significant). In addition, we will talk a lot about measurement. Measurement involves assigning numbers (like 98.6) to attributes that we want to measure (like temperature). There are four different scales of measurement (nominal, ordinal, interval, and ratio) that you'll need to know. The final topic in the chapter is rounding. I want you to learn (and use!) my rules for rounding so that we all end up with the same answers to whatever problems we take on.

OVERVIEW

I may be odd, but I love to teach statistics. As a psychologist, I teach a variety of courses, ranging from abnormal psychology to human sexuality. However, as I tell both my statistics class and my sex class, I'd rather teach statistics than sex.

Why? Because statistics, usually a required course, is more challenging to teach than an elective like sex. Look around your class. How many people would be taking statistics if it weren't required? Which would you rather be taking right now, statistics or sex? It is not hard to take an inherently interesting topic like sex and come up with a class that students like to attend and where they learn things both interesting and useful. Where is the challenge in that?†

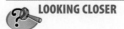 **LOOKING CLOSER**

---

*I'll be honest. When I read textbook chapters, I sometimes skip the introductions and the summaries. That isn't a very good idea. I can assure you that I, as the author, have expended a fair amount of time and pain to write the roadmaps and the summaries. They will help you learn the material if you read them, so take advantage of them.

†Unfortunately, there are also teachers who are skilled at taking interesting topics like sexuality and making them boring. And, since you are reading this footnote, I'll mention that I like footnotes. I put into footnotes little additional facts and things that amuse me. If you skip my footnotes you'll still get an adequate dose of knowledge from the book, but you'll miss some of the fine points. And you won't get to know me as well.

I love the challenge of taking an apparently dry and scary topic like statistics (there's math involved!) and making it into a class students like to attend—one that proves you can master something you fear, teaches you how to apply a useful tool, and changes you by presenting a new logic, a new way of thinking.

Know from the get-go that statistics is not hard to master. Yes, there is math involved. Yes, there is logic involved. And yes, you do need to work at it.* For the most part, though, the concepts are simple. And, nowadays, there are computers around to do the heavy math. (Though I, like most statistics teachers, think it is important to do the math by hand at least once to help you understand the concepts.)

To ease your way through statistics, to give you a glimpse of the framework on which I am going to build my statistical house, let me tell you the basic concept that underlies statistics—comparing the expected to the observed.

Statistics works by making assumptions about some aspect of the world, a model of how we think something should behave if our assumption (or hypothesis) is correct. We call this the expected outcome. However, if the expectation is not met—if the observed outcome is different from what we expected—then we have to ditch our initial assumption and accept an alternate assumption (the alternative hypothesis) about the world.

For example, if your sweetie loves you (your assumption, or hypothesis), then your expectations are that he or she will want to spend time with you, will bring you tokens of affection, and will not be seen chatting up others. As long as you observe what you expect (i.e., your sweetie behaves as you expect), you have no reason to question the assumption that your sweetie loves you. However, if what you observe is different, if he or she doesn't behave as expected, then you'll question your initial assumption and consider accepting the alternate assumption that your sweetie doesn't love you.

Of course statistics is a little more complex than that, but that is the basic idea. For a more statistical example, suppose we assume that boys and girls, on average, are equally smart. To test this we get a group of boys and a group of girls, give all of them IQ tests, and then compare the average score of the boys to the average score of the girls. If the two averages, the observed scores, are very close to each other—if we find an observed difference near the zero difference we expect—then we have no reason to question our assumption that boys and girls are equally smart. However, if we do find a big difference, we'll have to question (or in statistical terminology, reject) our assumption. We will conclude that

---

*One of my father's favorite jokes involves a man with a violin who rushes into a cab in New York City and asks the cabbie, "How do I get to Carnegie Hall?" To which the cabbie replies, "Practice, practice, practice." Ditto for statistics—if you want to get better at it you have to practice it. This means reading (and re-reading) the book, attending the lectures, completing the group practice problems, doing the review exercises, doing the homework, forming a study group, and so on.

LOOKING CLOSER

what had been our alternate assumption, that boys and girls are not equally smart, may be true.

We will spend the rest of this chapter on a number of important introductory tasks. First, I'll tell you why statistics were developed and how they are used. Then, we'll look at how we measure things by assigning numbers to them. And finally I will explain how to round and why it is important to round correctly. Along the way, I'm going to introduce you to the technical language of statistics so that when I use a term, you'll know what it means.

However, please remember, statistics is simply a way to decide whether what you observe is far enough away from what you expected that you have to question your expectations.

STATISTICS: WHY AND WHAT, AND TERMINOLOGY

Statistics was developed as a tool to help scientists answer their questions. Scientists answer questions by using the **empirical method.** This means that scientists find answers by gathering facts *through careful and systematic observation*, not by sitting in their armchairs and speculating.

empirical method

The process by which knowledge is gathered through careful and systematic observation.

Suppose a scientist wants to know whether caffeine consumption affects impulsivity in children. There are a number of different ways that the researcher can address this question. One way is to sit back and speculate. The researcher might think, "I always see that little brat who lives next door drinking a lot of cola, and he's always getting into trouble for doing things without thinking about the consequences. So, caffeine must cause impulsivity." Unfortunately, this is the very weakest sort of evidence, since it involves only a single, unsystematic observation without any formal definition, or measurement, of impulsivity.

operational definition

Defining a variable in terms of the operations (techniques) used to measure it.

A better approach is to develop an **operational definition.** Our scientist's operational definition of impulsivity may be the number of times a child interrupts during a 60-minute quiet period. The researcher can then go to a classroom to measure the impulsivity of each child there.* After the impulsivity data have been collected, the researcher can find out how much caffeine each child consumes and examine the relationship between the two variables—impulsivity and caffeine consumption.

This approach, called a "quasi-experimental research design," is better but still not perfect. The problem is that the researcher is not controlling the one variable (caffeine consumption) that is thought to have an

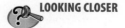
LOOKING CLOSER

*I am using the number of times that a child interrupts during a 60-minute quiet period as the *operation* defining impulsivity. If Buffy speaks 3 times and Skip once, I would conclude that Buffy is more impulsive than Skip. You might say that all that I know is that Buffy interrupts more than Skip, and that it is a large leap of faith to say that this means that Buffy is more impulsive than Skip. That concern is reasonable. Note that it is the openness about the criteria used to measure impulsivity that allows you to think about it critically. This openness is the beauty of an operational definition.

TABLE **1.1** **Number of Impulsive Behaviors Emitted by 80 Children during a 60-Minute Quiet Period**

2	5	4	6	5	6	5	2	6	4	0	2	5	1	5	2	3
1	0	1	3	8	4	3	5	5	2	7	6	0	4	4	2	5
6	1	0	6	7	5	3	5	4	4	3	2	4	6	4	1	4
8	7	5	7	3	5	0	4	3	9	2	1	3	6	5	1	2
2	3	4	6	2	7	4	1	3	4	1	0					

impact on the other (impulsivity), but is simply letting the assumed causative variable vary naturally. As a result there are other variables, called "**confounding variables,**" that may covary with the assumed causative agent. For example, children who consume less caffeine may have parents who are stricter, and it may be the strictness of the parents that affects impulsivity, not caffeine. Or maybe the relationship goes the other way: just as stimulants such as Ritalin are used to treat attention deficit hyperactivity disorder (ADHD), maybe children who are more impulsive are self-medicating with the stimulant caffeine in an attempt to control their impulsivity.

confounding variable

A variable that is uncontrolled or unaccounted for and that may influence the outcome of an experiment.

The solution to this problem is for the researcher to control the presumed causative agent and do what is called a **true experiment.** The researcher can do this by taking a group of children and dividing them into two equal groups. When I say equal, I don't mean that each of the two groups has the same number of children. I mean that they are alike in terms of characteristics. That is, each group should have the same proportion of girls, the same proportion of left-handers, the same proportion of smart kids, the same proportion of children who ate breakfast that morning, and so forth. With the two groups alike in all ways, the researcher then makes them different in one, and only one, way, by giving one group a caffeinated beverage and the other an uncaffeinated beverage. The researcher would then observe how many impulsive behaviors each child emits during the observational period.*

true experiment

An experiment in which the researcher controls the independent variable.

Suppose our scientist does this. She randomly assigns children either to receive a caffeinated or an uncaffeinated beverage and then observes them during a 60-minute quiet period at school where she, according to her operational definition, tallies how many times each child interrupts. Table 1.1 shows the data from the 80 children she observes.

---

*The process by which cases are divided into two equal groups is called random assignment. In addition, as a good scientist the researcher would use something called a double-blind study. This means that neither the researcher nor the children would know who consumed caffeine, so that their expectations could not influence the outcome. And, of course, our researcher has obtained informed consent from both the children and their parents.

LOOKING CLOSER

TABLE **1.2**   **Number, Based upon Whether Caffeine Was Consumed, of Impulsive Acts Committed during a 60-Minute Quiet Period**

NO CAFFEINE

1	5	7	5	2	2	4	0	3	6	5	1	0	1	4	1	3
4	2	8	4	2	4	1	2	2	3	2	1	4	2	3	1	3
0	3	2	1	3	2											

CAFFEINE

3	1	2	4	7	6	5	5	4	3	0	5	6	6	6	8	6
7	5	4	5	7	0	5	7	4	7	9	4	4	3	0	6	4
5	5	4	5	5	6											

TABLE **1.3**   **Number of Impulsive Acts Committed in a 60-Minute Quiet Period, Arrayed in Order Based on Caffeine Consumption**

NO CAFFEINE

0	0	0	1	1	1	1	1	1	1	1	2	2	2	2	2	2
2	2	2	2	3	3	3	3	3	3	3	4	4	4	4	4	4
5	5	5	6	7	8											

CAFFEINE

0	0	0	1	2	3	3	3	4	4	4	4	4	4	4	4	5
5	5	5	5	5	5	5	5	5	6	6	6	6	6	6	6	7
7	7	7	7	8	9											

The task of statistics, as aptly stated by Dodge (2003),* is to bring order to chaos. The numbers in Table 1.1 are uninformative because they are unorganized. As such they don't help us answer whether caffeine has an impact on impulsivity. Just separating these 80 numbers into those associated with whether caffeine was consumed brings some order to the chaos, but it isn't much more informative, as can be seen in Table 1.2.

As our fictitious scientist brings more order to the numbers, both separating them by caffeine consumption and ordering them from lowest to highest, as shown in Table 1.3, we can begin to answer the question.

We can see that there are caffeinated and uncaffeinated children who exhibit very little impulsivity, as well as caffeinated and uncaffeinated children who exhibit a lot of impulsivity. With careful attention to this table we can extract the observation that there are fewer caffeinated than uncaffeinated children with low impulsivity scores, and more caffeinated

LOOKING CLOSER

*Dodge, L. G. (2003). *Dr. Laurie's introduction to statistical methods.* Los Angeles: Pyrczak Publishing.

TABLE **1.4** **Number of Impulsive Acts Committed in a 60-Minute Quiet Period by Children Who Did and Did Not Consume Caffeine**

# of acts	No caffeine	Caffeine
9		x
8	x	x
7	x	xxxxx
6	x	xxxxxxx
5	xxx	xxxxxxxxxx
4	xxxxx	xxxxxxxx
3	xxxxxx	xxx
2	xxxxxxxxxx	x
1	xxxxxxxx	x
0	xxx	xxx

than uncaffeinated children with high impulsivity scores. We have to expend some effort to see this, but it looks like caffeinated children are more impulsive than are uncaffeinated children.*

Organization by itself doesn't complete the task of bringing order to chaos. Statistics bring order to chaos by *reducing* a large mass of data in some meaningful way. As shown in Table 1.4, our scientist can further reduce the data by tallying, side by side, how many caffeinated and uncaffeinated children engage in each level of impulsive behavior. Each "x" in a row in Table 1.4 indicates a child who exhibited that number of impulsive behaviors.

From this meaningfully reduced set of data, the answer to the question becomes clearer—we can see that the caffeinated children exhibited higher levels of impulsivity than did the uncaffeinated. It is possible for us to reduce the set of data even more, to reduce the 40 values for each group to a single value, an average. For the children who received caffeine the average is 4.70, and for the children who did not receive caffeine it is 2.72.[†] Thus, we find that each child who received caffeine commits, on average, about 2 more impulsive acts during the observation period than does each child who received an uncaffeinated beverage. Statistics have helped us see, according to these made-up data, that caffeine consumption causes increased impulsive behavior.[‡]

---

*I just made these data up as an example for this book. Don't go around quoting this as evidence that caffeine leads to impulsivity.

[†]You'll learn in Chapter 4 that this, the mean, is one of three averages that statisticians calculate.

[‡]All studies have limitations, and if this were a real study I'd feel compelled to mention them. For example, this study only addresses the effect of caffeine on children, and it involves only the effect of caffeine on impulsivity that takes place during a quiet period in school. Whether caffeine has any effect on impulsivity in adults or on impulsivity by children in different settings is unknown.

LOOKING CLOSER

INDEPENDENT AND DEPENDENT VARIABLES

Statistics is a way for scientists to reduce a large mass of data that they have collected so that they can more clearly see the answer to the question posed. The questions that scientists ask are usually relationship questions, and sometimes questions of cause and effect.

What is a relationship question? It is a question about how one attribute—let's call it *X*—relates to or affects another attribute, *Y*. For example, many people think that males are more aggressive than females, that there is a difference between the genders.* This could be phrased as a research question: "Is there a relationship between gender and aggression?"

The attributes we examine in relationship questions are called **variables.** A variable is the attribute, characteristic, or dimension being measured or studied. This may be stating the obvious, but these attributes are called variables because they vary.

It is because of this variability that we need to measure variables. If there were no such thing as different genders, then the question of whether there is a relationship between gender and aggression would be non-sensical. Similarly, if everyone in the world exhibited the exact same amount of aggression, then there would be no need to figure out why some people were more aggressive. However, since some people are more aggressive and some are less, we want to know why. Is it due to diet? Gender? Upbringing? To the type or amount of neurotransmitters in the brain? To some other variable?

There are lots and lots of variables that scientists are interested in measuring. To name a few, health researchers may measure blood pressure; psychologists—intelligence; educators—reading levels; sociologists—crime rates; meteorologists—rainfall; economists—gross domestic product; political scientists—voter turnout; chemists—specific gravity; and so forth.

These variables are similar in that scientists measure them, **cases** vary on them, and they are thought to relate to other variables. This examination of the relationship of one variable to another is the basis of science. Examples of relationship questions researchers may ask are the following: what is the relationship between medication level and side effects? between psychotherapy and depression? between nutrition and intelligence? between air quality and asthma? or between books in the home and reading ability?

---

variable

An attribute, characteristic, or dimension being measured or studied.

cases

The objects being studied; also known as subjects or participants.

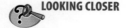 **LOOKING CLOSER**

*I teach a course on human sexuality, and I am aware of the difference between sex and gender, that sex refers to physical status (male as opposed to female) and gender refers to psychological status (masculine vs. feminine). However, there are spots where it gets confusing if I refer to the physical status of cases as "sex," so I'm going to use gender instead.

The questions that scientists ask are about the relationship between two variables and, often, whether there is directionality, or **cause and effect.** I've never heard anyone suggest that being more aggressive causes one to become a male, but a fair number of people wonder whether being a male causes one to be more physically aggressive. Thus, the question about the relationship between gender and aggression can be reframed as a question about cause and effect: does gender cause aggression?* Similarly, we could ask whether higher doses of a drug cause more side effects, whether psychotherapy causes a decrease in depression, whether malnutrition causes retardation, whether poor air quality causes asthma, or whether exposure to books in the home leads to earlier reading.

Let me stress that correlation is not causation: two variables can be related without one causing the other. For example, height and weight in children are related in that, in general, taller children are heavier and heavier children are taller. However, I would be loath to say that height causes weight or that weight causes height. Rather, some third variable, development, causes both height and weight.

Though correlation is not causation, if there is causation there must be correlation. Correlation, or **covariation** as it is sometimes called, is one of three conditions necessary to show cause and effect. If I want to show that caffeine consumption causes impulsivity, then I need to demonstrate (a) covariation, (b) temporal precedence, and (c) absence of plausible alternative explanations. Covariation means that as one variable changes, so does the other, that they vary together, that they "co-vary." For example, by varying the dose of caffeine I give children, I might find that as dose increases, so does impulsivity. Temporal precedence means that one variable, the causative agent, precedes the other in time. In other words, the effect (impulsivity) occurs *after* the cause (caffeine) as we give the caffeine first and then measure the effect. An absence of plausible alternative explanations can only be demonstrated by using random assignment or doing other studies that rule out other explanations for the observed effect. In this case, since we used random assignment to make the two groups similar, I'm hard pressed to think of a confounding variable.†

| **cause and effect** |
| A directional relationship between two variables in which a change in one causes a change in the other. |

| **covariation** |
| The condition in which two variables change together. |

---

*Just because two variables have a relationship does not mean that one causes the other! And knowing that there is a relationship does not tell why the relationship exists. There are many ways that maleness could lead to increased aggression (if that is the case!). It could be something physical, like testosterone level, or it could be something cultural, such as boys' being socialized to be more rough-and-tumble.

†The philosopher David Hume, who generated rules in the eighteenth century by which to judge cause and effect, had a fourth criterion: that the cause always produces the effect and that the effect comes from no other cause. Sometimes called the "necessary and sufficient" clause, this is a bit too strict for most social scientists. It means that without caffeine there will be no impulsivity and there will be no impulsivity without caffeine. My guess it that multiple causes determine whether a child exhibits impulsive behavior, that there is no single cause.

LOOKING CLOSER

independent variable

The variable controlled by the experimenter; the suspected causative agent.

dependent variable

The outcome variable where an effect is measured.

Moving to the question of cause and effect leads us to give different names to the two variables. The variable that we think of as the causative agent is called the **independent variable,** and the variable used to measure the effect, *the outcome variable*, is called the **dependent variable.** These are commonly abbreviated, respectively, as *IV* and *DV.* The dependent variable is called the dependent variable because it is thought that the amount of this attribute a case possesses *depends* on the independent variable. Using my examples from above, does how impulsive a child is depend on how much caffeine he or she consumes, how much physical aggression a person exhibits depend on whether that person is a male or a female, the severity of a person's side effects depend on how much medication he or she receives, how depressed a person is after psychotherapy depend on how much psychotherapy he or she receives, how intelligent a person is depend on the nutrition he or she receives as an infant, whether one develops asthma depend on the air quality to which one is exposed, or does ease of learning to read depend on the presence of books in the home?

In an experiment, the researcher wants to control or manipulate the independent variable. It is with the dependent variable that the researcher measures the outcome, or the effect of the manipulation. Earlier, I introduced an experiment in which a researcher manipulated how much caffeine children received (the independent variable) and measured the impact of this on impulsivity (the dependent variable). Let me offer two other examples. In one, an experimenter might control how much psychotherapy patients receive (the independent variable), with some receiving real psychotherapy and others receiving placebo psychotherapy. The researcher could then measure the effect of this intervention/ manipulation by measuring how depressed the patients are (the dependent variable). Or a researcher might study the effect of two different weight loss programs, the Atkins diet vs. Weight Watchers (the independent variable), on long-term weight loss (the dependent variable) by assigning dieters to use the different diets.*

Though it is helpful to think of the independent variable as the variable controlled by the experimenter, there are some independent variables that we can't manipulate or control. In the effect of gender on aggression study, gender is the independent variable and aggression is the dependent variable. However, we can't manipulate or control gender—I can't take kids and make some of them into boys and others into girls. Similarly, if I were interested in the effects of early nutrition on later intelligence in humans, it would be unethical for me to take some babies and make sure that they get poor early nutrition. So the independent variable is not always manipulated by the researcher.

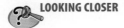 **LOOKING CLOSER**

*Be careful not to think that the diet example has two independent variables. There is only one independent variable, type of diet, but there are two levels of this independent variable. There are experiments with multiple independent variables. For example, a researcher might examine the effect of two variables, such as diet and amount of exercise, on weight loss. It is also possible to have multiple dependent variables; e.g., examining the impact of diet on both weight loss and energy level.

When the independent variable is not controlled or manipulated by the researcher, it is called a **grouping variable** or a subject variable. If I were comparing boys to girls in terms of their level of impulsivity, for example, gender would be a grouping variable, not an independent variable. The difference between independent and grouping variables is an important one, but I will often lump them together and generically refer to the presumed cause as the independent variable.

There is one other important differentiation to make: **predictor variable** versus **criterion variable.** Imagine that I'm examining the relationship between height and weight in children. In general, height and weight are related—kids who are taller are also heavier. However, I could reverse this and say that kids who are heavier are usually taller. In this case, cause and effect is not clear—does height cause weight, does weight cause height, or does some third variable (e.g., nutrition) cause both? And so it is not easy, from the study as described, to categorize the variables as independent and dependent. In these situations, it is easier to talk about what we are trying to predict, height from weight or weight from height, and distinguish between predictor and criterion variables. The predictor variable is the one that we are predicting from and the criterion variable is what is being predicted. Colleges, for example, often try to estimate an incoming student's first year GPA on the basis of his or her SAT score: SAT score is the predictor and GPA is the criterion. The criterion variable is the outcome variable; it is analogous to the dependent variable.

Being able to distinguish the independent (or grouping) variable from the dependent variable, or predictor from criterion, is important for statisticians. The dependent variable, the outcome variable, provides the large mass of numbers that the statistician reduces in a meaningful way. Here are some guidelines to help you figure out which is which:

grouping variable

A variable on which groups differ and which is the suspected causative agent, but is not controlled by the experimenter; also known as "subject variable."

predictor variable

The variable from which another variable is estimated or predicted.

criterion variable

An estimated or predicted variable; the outcome variable.

GUIDELINES FOR DISTINGUISHING INDEPENDENT FROM DEPENDENT VARIABLES

1. Formulate a relationship statement about the two variables under study. (For example, the researcher is studying the relationship between class attendance and exam performance.)
2. Is there temporal contiguity or a logical cause and effect direction? If so, the one that comes first in time or the one viewed as the cause is the independent variable. The variable where the effect of that cause is later measured, the outcome variable, is the dependent variable. (The researcher appears to believe that missing class leads to poorer exam performance, therefore class attendance is the independent variable and exam performance the dependent variable.)*

---

*Be aware that a different person may perceive the direction of the relationship going a different way. That is, it may be possible that poor exam performance leads to a sense of hopelessness that leads to skipping class. Separating variables into independent and dependent depends upon your conceptualization of the relationship. Though if we are measuring performance on the first exam and looking at attendance in subsequent classes, there is clear-cut temporal—and causal—contiguity.

LOOKING CLOSER

3. If you are having difficulty, identify the dependent variable first. Remember, the dependent variable is the outcome variable; it is what is being measured. Once you identify the dependent variable, then the remaining variable is the independent variable. (However, see guideline 6 for a caveat!)

4. As a useful rule of thumb, think of how many "levels" each variable has. (Gender has two levels, male or female. Aggression is called "continuous"; it has a whole range of levels from low to high.) If the variables differ in how many levels they have, the dependent variable, or the outcome variable, is usually the one with more levels. If they don't differ (as class attendance and exam performance, both of which have scores ranging from low to high, don't), think again about cause and effect.

5. If a variable is controlled or manipulated by the experimenter, it is the independent variable. For example, if I give an antidepressant to one group of depressed people and a placebo to the other group, then antidepressant/placebo is the independent variable.

6. Finally, be aware that sometimes the two variables can't be separated into independent variable and dependent variable but are better conceptualized as predictor and criterion variables.

Group Practice 1.1

I've learned that one of the best ways for students to discover that they don't understand something is to try to do it. And, if one student doesn't understand something, often someone sitting quite close to that person does. So, in every chapter I have group-practice assignments.

Answers to the group exercises may be obtained through your instructor. Please give each a serious try.

1. A nurse practitioner is examining the impact of life stress on physical health. She finds two groups of people, one that has had few life stressors in the past year and one that has experienced many life stressors in the past year. (Life stressors are things like divorce, moving away from home, loss of a job, death in the family, etc.) The practitioner measures how many days each person was physically ill in the past year. What is her independent variable? Her dependent variable? Is the independent variable controlled or manipulated by the researcher?

2. A psychologist has a group of young children in his lab and randomly divides them into two groups. To one group he shows an hour of nature films. To the other group he shows an hour of films of altruistic behaviors (things like Boy Scouts doing good deeds, kids picking up toys in a messy room, someone letting someone else "cut" in line). He then takes the kids to a playground and counts, during a 15-minute period, how many helpful behaviors each kid emits. What is the independent variable? The dependent variable? Is the independent variable controlled or manipulated by the researcher?

3. A respiratory therapist wants to see the effect of body position on the amount of oxygen in the blood. She randomly assigns people either to lie on their backs for 15 minutes or to sit upright for 15 minutes, after which she measures their oxygen saturation levels. What is her independent variable? Her dependent variable? Is the independent variable controlled or manipulated by the experimenter?

4. A sociologist measures the physical distress experienced by residents of cities by noting the amount of graffiti in each. Based on this she classifies cities as being high, moderate, or low in terms of physical

Group Practice 1.1—cont'd

distress. The sociologist randomly samples cities in North America until she has 10 cities in each category. Thinking that physical distress leads to social distress, she measures social distress by obtaining the teenage pregnancy rate for each of these cities. What is her independent variable? Her dependent variable? Is the independent variable controlled by the experimenter? Can you think of any plausible confounding variables?

5. A theologian is interested in whether more religious people are more likely to obey traffic laws. He observes people at a stop sign and notes whether drivers come to a complete stop. The theologian then has each driver fill out a scale measuring how often they attend church/ synagogue/mosque/and so on, defining people with more regular attendance as more religious. What is the theologian's independent variable? His dependent variable? Is the independent variable manipulated by the experimenter? Can you think of any plausible confounding variables?

6. An educational researcher is interested in the effects of nutrition on school performance. She classifies students as (a) eaters of breakfast or (b) non-eaters of breakfast. She measures school performance by recording attendance rate for a semester. What is her independent variable? Her dependent variable? Is the independent variable controlled by the experimenter? Can you think of any plausible confounding variables?

MEASUREMENT

I've mentioned measurement several times now. It is the **measurement** of the dependent variable that provides us with the numbers to which we bring order and so it is time to define "measurement." Measurement is the assignment of labels to objects so that the assigned labels *accurately* reflect the underlying attribute being measured. Most commonly, the labels assigned are numbers. For the assigned numbers accurately to reflect the attribute being measured, the numbers must be assigned in a consistent fashion. In other words, there must be some conventions or rules that guide how we assign the numbers.

An example should make this clear. Suppose that I want to measure the heights of the persons in a group. The underlying attribute I am measuring is height, and for me to measure it means that I am going to give each person a number to reflect, *accurately*, his or her height. In this case, accuracy means that if I am shorter than you, then my height number should be lower than yours; if you are shorter than your brother, then your height number should be lower than your brother's.

We have a fair number of conventions that guide us in assigning numbers to measure the underlying attribute of height. Commonly, we have someone take off his or her shoes and stand against a wall while we make a mark on the wall level with the top of his or her head. We then use a tape measure to count the number of inches from the floor to the mark. Since the number of inches accurately reflects a person's height, this is measurement.

If we have people stand against a brick wall and count how many bricks tall they are, that is also measurement. The **metric** has changed, that is, we are measuring in units of bricks, not inches, but it is still an

measurement

The assignment of numbers or labels to objects to accurately reflect an underlying attribute.

metric

A unit of measure.

accurate reflection of the underlying dimension of height since taller people get bigger numbers than short people.

Metric, as I am using it, means a unit of measure. Thus we can measure weight in one metric, pounds, or in another, kilograms, or even make up a new one, such as the number of bales of hay that an object weighs.*

The numbers that are assigned in the process of measurement can represent two different types of attributes: **qualitative** or **quantitative.** For example, we can measure gender, male or female, by assigning the number 1 to males and the number 2 to females. This is qualitative measurement as the numbers reflect the underlying dimension of gender. These numbers reflect a *quality* (maleness or femaleness) and don't provide any *quantitative* information. We can't say that women possess more of the quality of gender than do men because they are given a score of 2 while men are only given a score of 1. *With qualitative measurement the numbers are arbitrary and don't provide any quantitative information such as rank or distance.* If, in measuring gender, we arbitrarily assign the number 37 to men and the number 3.21 to women, we are still performing measurement, since different numbers still accurately reflect the different qualities. The numbers here function as labels.

Commonly, the attributes that we measure are quantitative. This means that the objects we are measuring vary in that some possess *more* of the attribute than do others, and our measure should reflect this *quantitative* difference. Height, which I discussed above, is an example—some people are taller than others and some are, excuse my grammar, "more taller" than others. If Buffy is 64 inches tall, Skip is 67 inches, and Desdemona is 68 inches, accurate measurement of height tells us not just that Skip and Desdemona are taller than Buffy but also that Desdemona possesses more of the attribute of height than does Skip and that Skip possesses more of the attribute than does Buffy.

Many variables that researchers measure, e.g., intelligence, family income, reading level, length of hospital stay, or severity of chest pain, are quantitative. Serum cholesterol level is a good example. The world is not divided into people with cholesterol in their blood and those without. Rather, everyone has some, and we differ in the amount: some of us have very high levels, some of us have very low levels, and most of us are somewhere in the middle. A test has been developed, the lipid panel, that reports total cholesterol level as milligrams of cholesterol per deciliter (mg/dL) of blood. Higher numbers indicate a greater quantity of cholesterol in the bloodstream, so this is a quantitative measure.

It is possible to convert a quantitative measure into a qualitative one. Current guidelines call a total cholesterol level below 200 mg/dL safe, a level between 200 and 240 borderline-high, and a level greater than 240 high. If I labeled cholesterol levels below 200 as "safe" and

---

qualitative

Reflecting the presence of a quality or attribute.

quantitative

Reflecting the amount or extent of an attribute.

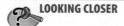 **LOOKING CLOSER**

*If you think my idea of measuring weight in bales of hay is fanciful, you should consider moving to England. There they have the "stone" as an official unit of weight, a stone being equivalent to 14 pounds.

those 200 and above as "unsafe," assigning them, respectively, values of 1 and 2, I would have transformed cholesterol level from a quantitative to a qualitative scale.

However, one can't transform a qualitative measure, a measure of whether a case possesses a quality, into a quantitative one. I can not take my qualitative measure of gender—where 1 = male and 2 = female—and transform it into a quantitative measure, unless I want to do something silly like count the number of X chromosomes that a person has.

LEVEL OF MEASUREMENT

In statistics it is very important to recognize that there are four levels of measurement—*nominal, ordinal, interval,* and *ratio*—and to be able to identify the level of measurement of the numbers to which we are trying to bring order. Why is it important to know whether the numbers you are working with are nominal, ordinal, interval, or ratio? Because different statistical techniques only work with certain levels of measurement. If you apply a statistical technique meant for interval numbers to ordinal numbers, the results may be misleading. Sugar and salt are both white, granular substances, but if you use the wrong one to sweeten your coffee, you won't be happy with the results. The same is true with statistics.

Here are two mnemonics for the levels of measurement: *noir* and *iron*. *Noir* is the French word for black and its four letters represent the four scales of measurement from simplest to most complex: *n*ominal, *o*rdinal, *i*nterval, and *r*atio. *Iron* is an alternative mnemonic because, for practical purposes, there are only three levels of measurement. *I*nterval and *r*atio lump together and are distinct from *o*rdinal which is distinct from *n*ominal; hence, *iron*.

Using NOIR as our guide, let's march through all four levels of measurement in order from simplest to most complex.

Nominal is the simplest level of measurement. Nominal numbers are used to *differentiate* objects from each other, to sort them into categories. The assigned numbers are used as labels in place of verbal names.* Thus, nominal-level measurement represents the measurement of *qualities*. The numbers are used as shorthand names, are entirely arbitrary, and provide no quantitative information. The numbers simply indicate sameness or differentness. Using the example of gender (male = 1 and female = 2): if I am a 1 and you are a 1, then we are of the same gender. If I am a 1 and you are a 2, then we are different genders. Two objects are assigned different numbers if they possess different qualities and the same number if they possess the same quality.

A good example of nominal-level measurement in psychology comes from psychiatric diagnoses. Every decade or so the American Psychiatric

nominal measurement level

Numbers used as labels to differentiate objects or categories; a measurement of a quality. Indicates difference.

---

*The word nominal is derived from *nomen,* the Latin word for name. Nominal measurement involves using numbers as names or labels.

LOOKING CLOSER

Association publishes a listing of all the current psychiatric diagnoses in a book called the *Diagnostic and Statistical Manual*. This book has diagnostic categories like depression, anorexia, paranoid schizophrenia, and sexual dysfunction, and each diagnosis has a number assigned to it. Paranoid schizophrenia, for example, is assigned 295.30 and sexual dysfunction 302.70. These numbers are a nominal level of measurement since they are entirely arbitrary. They are simply shorthand labels for the different diagnostic qualities. Sexual dysfunction has a higher number than does paranoid schizophrenia, but the numbers provide no quantitative information, they tell nothing about the *quantity* of mental illness a person has. Though the number is higher, sexual dysfunction is not a "worse" diagnosis than paranoid schizophrenia. In fact, if I had to choose one, I'd prefer sexual dysfunction to schizophrenia.

Because the numbers are arbitrary and possess no quantitative information, we are limited in what we can do with them. We can tally frequencies or percentages (how many people in your class are female), but that is about it. It doesn't make sense to add or subtract nominal numbers or to calculate averages. Suppose someone has two psychiatric diagnoses—he is a paranoid schizophrenic and has a sexual dysfunction. If you add 295.30 and 302.70 together and divide by two, this person's diagnosis is, on average, 299.00. In the *Diagnostic and Statistical Manual,* 299.00 is the number assigned to autism. Is it reasonable to say that a person with paranoid schizophrenia and a sexual dysfunction is, on average, autistic? Clearly not.

There are statistical tests that can be done with nominal numbers, and we shall learn how to do one of them, the chi square test for contingency tables. But for now, the thing to remember is that if numbers are assigned to objects to measure some underlying attribute, and if two objects receive different numbers, then those numbers reflect a *difference* between the objects. If the numbers also tell the *direction* of the difference, then we have moved to the next level of measurement, the ordinal level.

ordinal measurement level

Scores used to measure the amount of an attribute in a directional manner. Indicates difference and direction.

The **ordinal** level of measurement provides a little bit of quantitative information. For ordinal measurement, we order the objects we are measuring from lowest to highest (or vice versa) in terms of how much of the attribute each possesses, and then we assign numerical ranks. For example, we say the person with the fastest time in a race comes in first place, the next fastest person is in second place, and so on. Thus, ordinal numbers give information about *direction* or order, about which object possesses more or less of the attribute we are measuring. This relative standing information is transitive: if I am faster than you and you are faster than Skip, then I am also faster than Skip. However, the numbers (1, 2, 3, etc.) don't give any information about *how much* difference separates two objects with different ranks. For an example of this, see Table 1.5, which shows the 2003 population of the 10 largest cities in Pennsylvania.

Philadelphia, with the rank of 1, is the largest city in Pennsylvania, followed by Pittsburgh, Allentown, and Erie. In terms of ranks (1, 2, 3), each seems to be very close to the other. The distance from the second to

TABLE **1.5** **Ten Largest Pennsylvania Cities: Population, Rank, and Population Distance from Next Smaller City**

Rank	City	Population	Population Distance from Next Smaller City
1	Philadelphia	1,520,000	1,184,900
2	Pittsburgh	335,100	228,300
3	Allentown	106,800	2900
4	Erie	103,900	22,600
5	Reading	81,300	4800
6	Scranton	76,500	5100
7	Bethlehem	71,400	11,500
8	Lower Merion	59,900	3500
9	Lancaster	56,400	2300
10	Levittown	54,100	4500

the first rank $(2 - 1 = 1)$ is the same as the distance from the fourth to the third rank $(4 - 3 = 1)$. However, by looking at the population distance, we can see that the actual distance from city 1 to city 2 is over a million people, while the actual distance from the third- to the fourth-ranked city is only 2900 people. An examination of the table shows that for the first 10 cities, even though each is ranked next to the other, the ranks represent differences as small as only 2300 people to well over a million.

Rank scores, or ordinal scores, lack something that interval scores have, something called equality of units.* Thus, ordinal numbers give directional information but don't tell the size of the difference. Sometimes the distance between two adjacent objects is small, and sometimes it is large, but ordinal scales are mum on this topic.†

How do ordinal scales deal with tie scores? Well, let's imagine that there are four people running a race and that we have some money to award. The person who wins will get $200, the person in second place will get $100, third place will get $50, and fourth $25. Further, let's imagine that after the first person has finished, two people cross the line at exactly the same time, followed by another person. The person who came in first clearly gets the rank of 1, but what about the others?‡ Is it fair to say that the person who came in last is in third place? Isn't that person behind

---

*Don't worry, I'll explain what equality of units is soon enough.

†One of my students keeps ferrets as pets and tells me that they are the third most popular pet in the United States. I've never checked, but I'd bet that there's quite a jump from the number of households with dogs and cats to the number with ferrets.

‡By the bye, notice that there is no zero point on this scale. This is the case with ordinal *ranks*—people come in first, second, third, and so on, in a race, but no one comes in "zeroth." However, don't let the mere absence of a zero point persuade you that a scale is ordinal—ordinal scales can have zero points.

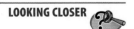
LOOKING CLOSER

TABLE **1.6**   **Ordinal Ranks (with Ties) for Heights of 16 First-Graders**

Number	Height (inches)	Rank
1	48	1
2	47	2
3	46	3.5
4	46	3.5
5	45	5.5
6	45	5.5
7	44	7
8	43	9
9	43	9
10	43	9
11	42	11.5
12	42	11.5
13	41	13
14	40	14
15	39	15
16	38	16

three other people, that is, in fourth place? And how much money should we give to the two people who came in tied for second? Should we flip a coin and give one of them $100 and the other $50? Doesn't it seem more fair to pool the money for second and third places and then divide it equally between them, $75 apiece? That means we classify each of them as coming in at 2.5th place. And this is exactly how ties are dealt with in ordinal scales. The objects are arrayed in order and numbered, and then ranks are assigned so that all objects with ties are assigned the average value of the tied ranks.

Here's another example. Imagine that I measure heights (in inches) of the 16 children in a first-grade classroom and find the following: 39, 43, 48, 38, 45, 46, 47, 41, 42, 43, 45, 44, 43, 42, 46, and 40. In Table 1.6 you see them numbered from 1 to 16 and ordered from tallest to shortest. Following the procedure outlined in the preceding paragraph, I've assigned rank, an ordinal measure, to each child. The number 1 indicates the tallest child and 16 the shortest. Note the ranks I've assigned to the ties.

As with nominal numbers, we are limited as to how much math we can do with ordinal numbers. If there are ties, it makes some sense to tabulate frequencies or percentages. In the height example, shown in Table 1.6, we can say that three of the first-graders (or 18.75%) are the ninth-tallest first-graders. But this is of only limited interest or utility.

As with nominal numbers, we can't add, subtract, or calculate averages for ordinal numbers. My explanation of why this is so is a bit dense, but bear with me. Decibels, a measure of the loudness of sounds, are ordinal-level measures. Decibels are calculated as a *logarithm* of the ratio of the power level of two sounds. You may have forgotten this from your earlier adventures in math, but logarithms (logs) represent the conversion of a number to the exponent expressing the power to which a base number (commonly 10) must be raised to produce that number. For example, the log of 10 is 1 because $10^1 = 10$. The log of 100 is 2 because $10^2 = 100$, and the log of 1000 is 3. Note that the distance from 10 to 100 is 90 units and the distance from 100 to 1000 is 900 units. However, if these numbers are converted to logarithms the distance from 1 to 2 is the same as the distance from 2 to 3. The order is maintained, but the size of the actual distance is now obscured, so logarithms are an ordinal form of measure! The average of the numbers 100 and 1000 is 550. However, if I average 2 and 3, the logarithmic transformations of 100 and 1000, I find an average of 2.5. When I convert the logarithm of 2.5 back to a real number, I get a value of 316.25, far from what it should be (550). Hence, it doesn't make sense to add, subtract, or calculate averages for ordinal numbers.

Nonetheless, there are situations where we do so. There are a number of statistics, commonly with the words "rank order" in their names, that are used with ordinal numbers. We'll learn later about tests like the Spearman rank order correlation coefficient and the Mann Whitney *U*. In the calculations for these, math is done to ordinal numbers, and that is OK.

Before we move on to interval-level numbers, let's review the information given by ordinal-level numbers: ordinal numbers tell us difference and direction of the difference. Looking at the heights in Table 1.6, I know that the person with a rank of 1 is of a different height than the person with a rank of two. I don't know how much distance separates them, but I know that they are different. Similarly, I know that the two people with ranks of 3.5 do not differ in their heights.

Thinking of the people ranked 1 and 2, I know more than just that they are of different heights: I know the direction of the difference, and that is the value added by ordinal numbers. The person ranked 1 is taller than the person ranked 2, and the person ranked 2 is taller than both of the people ranked 3.5. Ordinal numbers provide us with two pieces of information, difference and direction.

Interval is the next level of measurement, and it allows us to talk meaningfully of *distance* as well as difference and direction. We can talk about distance because at the interval level of measurement there is equality of units. Temperature, an interval-level measure, has equality of units. The temperature difference from 32° to 33°, a one-degree distance, is the same as the distance from 111° to 112°. Ordinal measures lack equality of units—the distance between first and second place in a race is not necessarily the same as the distance between second and third place.

Equality of units enables the use of more complex mathematics. With interval-level scales we can sensibly talk about distance, so we can subtract one number from another to see how far apart two objects are on the underlying attribute. If, using the Fahrenheit scale, the high is 80° on a summer day and only 40° on a winter day, then we can say that it was 40 degrees warmer on one day than the other. Interval scales allow us to add, subtract, and calculate averages, but we are still mathematically limited since we can't divide one interval-level measure by another. For example, it is not legitimate to say that the 80° summer day is twice as warm as the 40° winter day.

The reason that one can't divide one level measure by another is that interval-level scales have another hallmark: arbitrary zero points. On an interval-level scale, a value of 0 does not mean the absence of the attribute being measured. For example, if the outside temperature on a winter day is 0° F, it would be silly to say that there is no temperature that day.*

The zero point for temperature is arbitrary and changes when one moves from Fahrenheit to Celsius and, as a result, the ratio changes. If I convert the interval-level Fahrenheit temperatures to another interval-level metric, the Celsius scale, 80° becomes 26.67° and 40° becomes 4.44°. Thus, in Celsius, the summer day is six times hotter than the winter day when in Fahrenheit it is only twice as hot. That doesn't make sense.

With interval-level numbers we can add, subtract, and find averages, but we can't meaningfully divide the numbers by each other. That doesn't limit us very much. Most of the powerful statistics that statisticians use,

interval measurement level

Scores indicating the amount of an attribute, having directionality and equality of units. Indicates difference, direction, and distance.

*This is a personal quirk, but it drives me crazy when someone takes my temperature, finds it normal, and then tells me that I have no temperature. I might not have a fever, but I do have a temperature.

LOOKING CLOSER

things like the *t* test, the Pearson product moment correlation coefficient, analysis of variance, or multiple regression, can be applied to interval-level numbers.

Ratio-level numbers, the final level of measurement, tell us difference, direction, and distance but add a real zero point. This allows us to divide two ratio-level numbers, to turn them into a *ratio*.

What is a real zero point? When a scale has a real zero point, not an arbitrary zero point, a value of 0 means that none of the attribute is present. Most of the time, real zero points exist only for physical variables, not psychological ones. Thus for height, weight, speed, and population, there is a real zero point; but for intelligence, masculinity, and conscientiousness, there is not.*

When a measure has a real zero point, the ratio of two numbers doesn't change as we change from one unit of measure to another. For example, imagine two speeds: 10 miles per hour (mph) and 20 mph. Speed measured in mph has equality of units and a real zero point, so it is legitimate to say that a car traveling 20 mph is going twice as fast as a car traveling 10 mph. If I transform those speeds into kilometers per hour (kph), they become 16.09 kph and 32.18 kph. Note that the ratio is still the same: one is twice the other, even though the metric has changed.†

Real zero points do occur for physical measures like reaction time, heart rate, height, weight, cholesterol level, hospital length of stay, crime rate, or pollution level. Most psychological and subjective variables don't have real zero points unless they are change scores. A change score is calculated over time. For example, I may evaluate a new depression treatment by measuring the depression levels of my participants when they start treatment and again at the end of treatment. If I subtract one score from the other I'll have a change score that indicates whether at the end of treatment the person is less depressed, just as depressed, or more depressed. The zero here is a real zero point: it indicates zero change.

You may find determining whether a real zero point exists confusing. A common sticking point is whether a zero *does* occur in one's data as opposed to whether it *can* occur. Imagine measuring the weights in

---

ratio measurement level

Scores indicating the amount of an attribute, having directionality and equality of units, and a real zero point. Indicates difference, directionality, difference, and proportion.

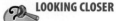 **LOOKING CLOSER**

*For example, why isn't there a real zero point for intelligence? Well, imagine an intelligence test where the lowest score a person could get is zero. A person walks in, picks up the pencil, answers the items on the test, and gets every one wrong, yielding a score of 0. Is it legitimate to say that this person has no intelligence? After all, he or she did walk into the room. Doesn't it take some intelligence to coordinate one's limbs enough to ambulate? Didn't he or she use a pencil to mark down answers? Doesn't holding and using a pencil take some intelligence? Thus a score of 0 means that the person is low on intelligence, lower than the test measures, not that the person lacks it entirely.

†By the bye, there is a measure of temperature, the Kelvin scale, that has a real zero point. Zero degrees Kelvin (K) represents the temperature at which molecules stop moving. It is equivalent to −273.15° Celsius. If we transform the summer and winter temperatures (80° F and 40° F) into Kelvin (299.81° K and 277.58° K) then we can meaningfully talk about the ratio and report that the summer day was 1.08 hotter than the winter day.

pounds of a group of subjects. Is the measure of weight a ratio-level measure? Regularly, students argue, incorrectly, that it is not a ratio level since none of the subjects has a weight of 0. In fact, they argue, no person *ever* has had a weight of 0. If a person has a corporeal existence—that is, has a body—then he or she has a positive, nonzero weight. Although they are right about this fact, they are wrong about the real zero point. The question with a real zero point is whether the *scale* has a real zero point, not whether a subject could ever have a real 0 value.* Weight, even though no human being has a 0 score on it, is a ratio-level variable.

A real zero point is a necessary but not a sufficient condition for a ratio-level measure† as ratio-level measures also must have equality of units. As mentioned at the outset, there is a hierarchy to NOIR. As the levels of measurement increase in complexity, each level has all the qualities of the preceding one. Thus, ordinal-level numbers differentiate as do nominal-level numbers, but they also tell direction. Interval-level numbers differentiate and tell direction, but add meaningful distance with equality of units. Ratio-level numbers differentiate, tell direction, and have meaningful distance, but with a real zero point they also allow meaningful calculation of ratios.

It is possible to scale a measure down but not up. That is, I can take an interval-level measure and turn it into an ordinal one, but I can't take an ordinal-level measure and transform it into an interval-level measure. For example, if the only information I have about a race is who came in first, second, third, and so on, then I can't convert this to an interval level of measurement telling me how much time separates the competitors.

DIFFERENTIATING LEVELS OF MEASUREMENT

I am spending so much time on levels of measurement because the level of measurement of the dependent variable determines what statistics can be used. It is physically possible to calculate a type of average called a

---

LOOKING CLOSER

*Let's return to thinking about a real zero point for psychological variables like intelligence. Clearly physical objects, like a rock, possess 0 intelligence. Similarly, we could say that a dead person has 0 intelligence. So, contrary to what I said a few pages back, it seems that there can be real a zero point for intelligence or for other psychological variables. The difficulty lies in developing a measure to capture this real zero point. Suppose I administer an intelligence test to a dead person and to a very dumb person. The dead person obviously will obtain a 0 on the test and, so it happens, does the dumb person. But earlier I pointed out that a live person who obtains a 0 on a test has some intelligence—he or she walked in, picked up a pencil, read the question, and so on. So these two zeros—one for a live person and one for a dead person—don't represent the same level of intelligence. If the numbers we assign don't faithfully represent the underlying attribute being measured, is this measurement?

†Don't be fooled by the presence of a zero point on a scale. Suppose I am measuring degree of anxiety on a 7-point scale that ranges from 0 = No anxiety to 6 = High anxiety. (And, yes, that is a 7-point scale. Count it off on your fingers.) Just because a person answers "0" on the scale, does the person really have no anxiety?

mean for nominal or ordinal data, but it is wrong to do so.* You must be able to determine what scale of measurement is being used so you can select an appropriate statistic. The simplest way to figure out the scale of measurement is to ask four questions, in order, of the numbers being analyzed. If your answer to question 1 is "yes," go to question 2. If your answer to question 2 is "yes," go to question 3, and so on. Stop when you get a "no" answer. The level of measurement associated with the last "yes" answer tells you the scale of measurement.

Four Questions to Determine Level of Measurement

1. Do the labels indicate difference and sameness? (For example, if one object is assigned the value of 1 and another object is assigned the value of 2, do the two objects differ in terms of the attribute being measured? If two objects are assigned the value of 1, do they both possess the same attribute?) If the answer to this is yes, then the scale of measurement is at least nominal. Depending on the answers to the next questions, it may be more.
2. Do the scores indicate the direction of the difference? (For example, if one object is assigned the value of 1 and another object is assigned the value of 2, does the one with the 2 possess more of the attribute?) If the answer to this is yes, then the scale of measurement is at least ordinal. Depending on the answers to the next questions, it may be more.
3. Do the numbers have equality of units? That is, do they meaningfully indicate the size of the difference? (For example, if I have a score of 1, you have a score of 2, and Buffy has a score of 3, is the distance from 1 to 2 the same size as the distance from 2 to 3?) If the answer to this is yes, then the scale of measurement is at least interval. Depending on the answer to the next question, it may be ratio.
4. Is there a real zero point on the scale measuring the underlying attribute? (If a case is assigned a value of 0, does that indicate that the case truly possesses none of the attribute?) If the answer to all four questions is yes, then the scale of measurement is ratio.

I've presented scales of measurement as black or white: either something is nominal, or it is ordinal, or it is interval, or it is ratio. In actuality, scales of measurement are grey—the level of measurement depends on how you interpret what is being measured. Imagine a 50-item "Nursing Facts" test administered to senior nursing students to measure their level of nursing knowledge. Is this nominal, ordinal, interval, or ratio?

Well, if Buffy gets a 43 on the test and Skip gets a 37, do the two of them differ in how much nursing knowledge they have? Yes they do, so the scale is at least nominal.

LOOKING CLOSER

*I want you to pay attention to levels of measurement throughout this text. So, on occasion I'll challenge you by asking you to use a statistic that is inappropriate for the dependent variable's level of measurement. When this happens, refuse to do the inappropriate calculation and decide whether there is something appropriate that you can do instead.

Does Buffy know more than Skip does? Yes she does, so the scale is at least ordinal.

However, now it gets harder. If Desdemona took the test and scored 49, is the difference between her and Buffy equal to the difference between Buffy and Skip? That is, are the two 6-point intervals, from 37 to 43 and from 43 to 49, the same size, is there equality of units? I don't know. Are all facts on the test equivalent or are some of the 50 questions more important than others? I think a legitimate argument could be made that unless equality of units is demonstrated, then we can't assume that it exists. And so we can be sure that this test is ordinal, but we can't be sure that it is interval.

However, fewer (and less powerful) statistics can be applied to ordinal numbers than to interval numbers and so we put ourselves at a bit of a disadvantage if we stop at ordinal. So, statisticians often take the innocent-until-proven guilty approach and assume equality of units so that they can apply more advanced statistics.* That is a legitimate approach as well. So, if you are willing to assume equality of units, then the nursing facts test measures knowledge of nursing at the interval level.

Let's assume equality of units and explore the fourth question, the existence of a real zero point. In this case it depends on how you conceptualize the measure. Is it a measure of (a) knowledge of the domain of nursing knowledge, or (b) knowledge of these 50 facts? If it is the former, then there is no real zero point, for someone could certainly have knowledge of other aspects of nursing and just not know these particular 50 facts. In this case a score of 0 does not mean the absence of any nursing knowledge. On the other hand, if we conceptualize this measure more narrowly, as just measuring how many of these 50 facts a person knows, then a value of 0 means zero knowledge of these 50 facts and represents a real zero point.

So, at what level of measurement is the nursing facts exam? If you want to be a conservative, Joe Friday type, then you should hold out for ordinal until you can be convinced that equality of units exists. If you're willing to accept equality of units, that a fact is a fact is a fact, then interval is the place for you. Given interval, how do you conceptualize the measure—with or without a real zero point?

Some students find these shades of grey frustrating as, without a clear-cut right answer, there is room for reasonable people to disagree. I'll do my best to make the questions I pose in problems in this text as unambiguous as possible.[†]

*There are even some statisticians (Baker, Hardyck, and Petrinovich, 1966) who offer data suggesting that this is all a tempest in a teapot, that we can apply "strong" statistics to "weak" measures. This means that they believe that it is acceptable to use interval-level statistical techniques on ordinal-level data. (Baker, B. D., Hardyck, C. D., & Petrinovich, L. F. [1966]. Weak measurements vs. strong statistics: an empirical critique of S. S. Stevens' proscriptions on statistics. *Educational and Psychological Measurement, 26*, 291-309.)

[†] At what level of measurement do *I* think the nursing facts exam falls? Interval.

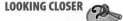
LOOKING CLOSER

Finally, though I want you to be able to tell whether something is nominal, ordinal, interval, or ratio, I also want to be pragmatic and so will tell you that for purposes of statistical analysis you should be more concerned with IRON than NOIR. It is important to differentiate nominal from ordinal, and it is important to differentiate ordinal from interval/ratio. Nevertheless, I am not aware of a single statistic that can be applied to ratio-level data but not to interval-level data. So in practical terms, there are only three levels of measurement, (a) interval/ratio, (b) ordinal, and (c) nominal.*

Group Practice 1.2

1. Here are the names and personal fortunes, according to *Forbes Magazine*, for the 10 wealthiest Americans in 2003. Assign them ranks where lower ranks indicate greater wealth. (That is, the wealthiest person should get a rank of 1.) Bill Gates, $46.0 billion; Warren Buffett, $36.0 billion; Paul Allen, $22.0 billion; Alice Walton, $20.5 billion; Helen Walton, $20.5 billion; John Walton, $20.5 billion; Robson Walton, $20.5 billion; Jim Walton, $20.5 billion; Lawrence Ellison, $18.0 billion; and Michael Dell, $13.0 billion.

2. Patients who have recently had heart attacks are encouraged to exercise regularly, eat a low-sodium, low-fat diet, and take their medications. Based on these three parameters, they are classified as exhibiting (1) poor compliance, (3) moderate compliance, or (2) good compliance. At what level is compliance being measured by these numbers?

3. A dog food manufacturer gets a group of dogs, exposes each to its favorite food for 5 minutes, and measures how many milliliters of saliva each produces during the 5-minute period. Salivation is being measured at what level?

4. Based on these results, the dog food manufacturer classifies dogs as (0) light producers

of saliva, (1) medium producers of saliva, or (2) heavy producers of saliva. Now salivation is being measured at what level?

5. A nurse anesthetist presents information about upcoming surgery to emergency room (ER) patients in two ways. In one condition, he takes them into a quiet room to explain the surgical procedures. In the other condition, he explains the surgical procedures whilst standing in the midst of the busy ER. He wants to know the impact of these different approaches on the patients' presurgical levels of stress. He measures stress level by assessing the level of cortisol, what is sometimes called a stress hormone, in the blood. (Cortisol is measured in mcg/dL, micrograms per deciliter.) At what level of measurement is he measuring stress?

6. A psychologist develops the Neuroticism Inventory (NI) to measure a person's degree of neuroticism. The NI has 25 questions, such as "I am anxious," "I startle easily," and "I am moody." Each question is answered on a scale from 0 to 4. An answer of 0 indicates "This does not describe me at all," and an answer of 4 indicates "This describes me 100%." Each question is weighted equally and the psychologist scales the response options so that there is equality of units. Scores

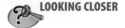
LOOKING CLOSER

*If reading about measurement has piqued your curiosity and you would like to read the original article about NOIR, see Stevens (1946). (Stevens S. S. [1946]. On the theory of scales of measurement, *Science*, 103, 677-680.)

on the NI, then, can range from a low of 0 to a high of 100; higher scores represent greater degrees of neuroticism. The NI measures neuroticism at what level?

7. Having developed the NI, the psychologist wants to find some uses for it. She decides to investigate if dog owners are more or less neurotic than cat owners. She obtains a large sample of people and administers the NI to them. From each person, she also finds out if he or she owns a dog or a cat. Based on these answers she classifies people as "0" if they have no pets, "1" if they have cats, "2" if they have dogs, and "3" if they have both. Pet ownership is being measured at what level?

8. A researcher for the WristWatch Association of America is recording the wrists on which people wear their wristwatches. He observes people in public and codes them as a "1" if a person is wearing a wristwatch on the left wrist and as a "1" if the wristwatch is on the right wrist. He collects no data from people not wearing wristwatches. Which wrist the wristwatch is worn on is being measured at what level of measurement? (There is no typo in this question!)

9. Infants who are being reared by heterosexual couples are observed and classified as (1) being attached to the mother, (2) being attached to the father, (3) being attached to both, or (4) being attached to neither. Attachment is being measured at what level?

10. A kindergarten teacher classifies students as (1) readers, (2) incipient readers, or (3) nonreaders. At what level is reading being measured?

MORE TERMINOLOGY

Having spent a lot of time on measurement, let's spend a little time on terminology before turning to rounding, the final topic for this chapter. I want to address four pairs of terms: (1) population vs. sample, (2) statistic vs. parameter, (3) descriptive vs. inferential statistics, and (4) statistical vs. practical significance.

POPULATION VS. SAMPLE

A **population** is a group of objects that are alike on one or more dimensions as defined by a researcher. In other words, the population is the group being studied. The researcher can define it very broadly (I'm interested in how digestion works in humans) or very narrowly (I'm interested in digestion in 9-year-old girls who live in rural areas of Pennsylvania and whose mothers died during the girls' first year of life.) In the first case there is only one dimension that defines the population, being human, so anyone who fits that criterion—male or female, old or young, living in Asia, Africa, the Americas, Europe, Oceania, or Antarctica, rich or poor—is a member of the population. In the second case, the researcher applies four characteristics (gender, age, location, and maternal loss during a specific time period), and the group that fits these criteria makes up a much smaller population.

population

A group of objects that are alike on one or more dimensions as defined by a researcher.

sample

A group of cases selected from a population.

In either case, a researcher would have a hard time studying the whole population. Even with the more focused population, there is no way that we could find all the 9-year-old girls in rural Pennsylvania who have lost their mothers during the first year of life. Even if we did, we are unlikely to persuade all of them to participate. As a result, researchers almost always conduct their research on a subset of the population, that is, a **sample.** Since a sample is a group of cases selected from the population, it is always smaller than the population.*

The researcher's objective is to gather data from the sample and then *generalize* the results back to the population. The researcher often doesn't care about the sample results per se. The simplest example of this is polling. Every 4 years there is a presidential election in the United States, and pollsters try to figure out whether the Democratic or the Republican candidate is going to win. To do this they call about 2000 registered voters and ask them something like, "If the election were held today, would you vote for X or for Y?" I hate to be blunt, but we don't really care how these 2000 voters will vote. We only care about them for what they tell us about the larger population. And the sample will only have a chance of telling us about the population if the sample is *representative* of the population.†

What makes a sample *representative* of a population? A sample is representative if it contains all the attributes of the population in the same proportion that they occur in the population. If our sample of 2000 registered voters were all male, that clearly would not be representative of the population of registered voters in the United States. If 55% of registered voters in the United States are male, then 55% of our sample should be male. If 10% of registered voters live in California, then 10% of our sample should come from California. If 12% of registered voters are left-handed, then 12% of our sample should be left-handed. The sample should mirror the population on all attributes if it is to be representative!‡ If the sample represents the population, then we can generalize to the population from the sample.

STATISTIC VS. PARAMETER

Statistics, as I mentioned earlier, involves bringing order to chaos by meaningfully reducing a mass of data. Often the reduction is to a single number that characterizes the whole data set as, for example, GPA characterizes a person's whole college career. If this number characterizes

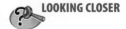
LOOKING CLOSER

*The technical term for a count of the whole population is a census.

†It takes more than a representative sample to guarantee accurate results. The question has to be well phrased and the respondents have to be able and willing to answer truthfully.

‡It should even mirror the population on attributes, like handedness, that may seem irrelevant. After all, an apparently irrelevant attribute may turn out to be important.

a sample, it is called a **statistic.** If it characterizes a population, it is called a **parameter.**

The difference between these two is important, so we use different symbols to refer to a sample or a population. The convention, and I'll follow it, is to use Roman letters to symbolize *sample* statistics and Greek letters to symbolize *population* parameters. For example, there is a measure, called the standard deviation, of how much spread or variability exists in a set of numbers. When one calculates a standard deviation for a *sample* it is a statistic, symbolized by the letter *s*. The standard deviation for a *population* is a parameter, symbolized by the lower-case Greek letter sigma (σ).

DESCRIPTIVE VS. INFERENTIAL STATISTICS

As said, we can draw *inferences* about a population from a sample if the sample is representative of the population. Now let me segue to the difference between descriptive and inferential statistics: Statisticians distinguish between inferential and descriptive statistics, and it is useful to know the difference, but please be aware that the line between the two is not always firm. Sometimes the same number calculated from a sample is treated as a descriptive statistic for one purpose and as an inferential statistic for a different purpose.

A **descriptive statistic** involves reducing a large mass of data to some meaningful value in order to *describe* the characteristics of that group of observations. If I asked for the percentage of your class that is male and you reported 37%, that would be a descriptive statistic. The same goes if I asked how your class did on the first exam and you reported the average grade. Descriptive statistics commonly describes a group of people, but they don't have to. An individual's GPA is an example of a descriptive statistic with data points representing individual courses, not people. Descriptive statistics are handy in that they give an overall view, but please note that it is a simplified view in which we lose details. Your GPA probably gives a fair picture, in general, of your academic performance, but it doesn't show your specific mix of A's, B's, and C's.

An **inferential statistic** also involves reducing a large mass of data to a single meaningful value, but for a different purpose. The goal is not to describe a sample, but rather to make an *inference* about a population. In other words, an inferential statistic allows us to generalize from a sample to a population or to make predictions about the population from the sample.

As an example, I may obtain a representative sample of students at your college, ask how many siblings they have, and calculate the average number of siblings. If I stop there, I have a descriptive statistic and I can make a statement like, "The average number of siblings in the sample of 150 students at the college was 1.75." However, if I generalize to the college it is an inferential statistic, and I can make a statement like, "Students at College X have, on average, 1.75 siblings."

statistic

A number characterizing a sample.

parameter

A number characterizing a population.

descriptive statistic

The reduction of data to a meaningful value in order to describe the characteristics of a group of observations.

inferential statistic

The reduction of data from a sample to some meaningful value in order to make generalizations about a population.

STATISTICAL VS. CLINICAL/PRACTICAL SIGNIFICANCE

In the course of this book we'll explore both statistical and practical significance. Statistical significance has a very specific meaning that is easiest to explain with the example of looking for a difference between two groups, for example, looking for a difference in impulsive behavior between children who do and don't receive caffeine. Finding a **statistically significant difference** between two groups means that we have decided that the difference found between the two groups is large enough to indicate that there is a difference between the populations from which the groups came. One implication of this is that the difference found between the two samples is probably not due to chance: if we took two new samples from the populations, we should find the difference again. In this sense, a statistically significant difference is a consistent difference.

Imagine that we want to know whether there is a difference in the speed with which aspirin and ibuprofen relieve headache pain. We get a large group of people with headaches, randomly divide them into two groups, and give one group aspirin and the other group ibuprofen. We then have each person use a stopwatch and time how long it takes for his or her headache to go away.

Suppose that in the aspirin group the headaches go away in 30 minutes and in the ibuprofen group the headaches go away in 60 minutes. We do the study again, that is, we **replicate** it, and find the same results. We replicate it again, and again, and again, and each time find the same results—aspirin knocks out headaches in half an hour but ibuprofen takes a full hour. This type of result is called statistically significant.

Imagine a different outcome on the first study: we find that the headaches go away for the aspirin group in 45 minutes, while for the ibuprofen group it takes 45.25 minutes. Do you think that if we replicate the study that we will find the same result? Or, is this one quarter of a minute difference so small that chance factors are playing a role and that next time we might find that headaches go away a little faster for the ibuprofen group than for the aspirin group?* If we do the study time and time again and don't get consistent results, then we'll end up concluding that there is not a real difference in the effectiveness of the two medications. We'll end up concluding that the results do not reflect a statistically significant difference.

Of course, we don't usually do studies time after time, after time. We usually do a study once and then examine the difference to see if it is large enough that we can conclude that it reflects a real difference between

statistically significant difference

Concluding that the observed difference between samples is large enough to reflect a difference between populations; the likelihood of obtaining such a difference by chance is low.

replicate

To repeat.

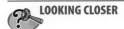 **LOOKING CLOSER**

*What do I mean by chance factors? Chance factors are factors that aren't controlled by the experimenter. In this instance it might be how quickly the pills are swallowed, how much water is used to swallow the pill, what other food was in the stomach, whether a person in one of the groups also had a toothache, how quickly a person presses the button on the stopwatch, and so on.

populations. Think of doing the headache study only once. If we find a 30-second difference, is that big enough to be a consistent difference? 1 minute? 5 minutes? 10? 20? 30? 60? Where do we draw the line and say that the difference is big enough to be a real difference, that it is not due to chance? This is where statistics come in. We shall learn techniques, called significance tests, that help decide where the line should be drawn, at what point we can say that the difference is large enough that we are confident that we would find it again if we did the study again.

Unfortunately, statistically significant differences are not necessarily meaningful differences. Suppose we did the aspirin/ibuprofen study time after time and each time the aspirin group got rid of its headache 1 second faster than the ibuprofen group. Well, that is a consistent difference and therefore reflects a real difference between the two populations. But, although it is statistically significant, it is not a difference that has any *clinical* impact. If you have a really bad headache, the worst headache you've ever had, and you have a choice between aspirin that would get rid of your headache in 30 minutes and ibuprofen that would take 30 minutes and 1 second, would you really care which you took? As my eighth-grade algebra teacher used to say, "Whoopee twang."

So, as well as results being statistically significant, we also care that results be **practically significant** or clinically significant. To be practically significant, a difference has to be big enough to matter. If a difference is practically significant, for example, it affects clinical treatment. As well as learning techniques for determining statistical significance, you'll learn ways to calculate practical significance.*

As noted previously, it is possible to have statistical significance without practical significance. However, it is *not* possible to have practical significance without statistical significance. This takes a moment's reflection, so follow me.

Suppose we do the aspirin/ibuprofen study just once and find a 15-minute advantage for aspirin. We do the statistical test that you'll learn later and the test shows that this difference is NOT statistically significant. In other words, the difference is not large enough for us to conclude that it reflects a real difference. You have a really bad headache and I offer you both aspirin and ibuprofen. Which do you pick?

If you are like most people, you'll pick the aspirin. However, there is no rational reason to do so. The results are not statistically significant, which means that if we do the study again we may get results showing that ibuprofen works faster by 30 minutes. Alternatively, we may find that there is no difference. If the difference is not statistically significant, then it is not one that we can rely on; it is not one that has a consistent clinical impact. You can't have practical significance without statistical significance.

practical significance

Being a meaningful effect, having relevance in practice.

---

*You'll also see that deciding on practical significance is subjective, like deciding if a glass is half full or half empty.

LOOKING CLOSER

Group Practice 1.3

1. A gastroenterologist is interested in studying the effects of alcohol on the lining of the stomach. She gets a sample of medical students in the United States, has them consume different controlled doses of alcohol, and then inserts a tube into their stomachs to observe the stomach lining. Because this is a stressful procedure (have you ever had an endoscopy?), she sedates them with intravenous Valium before inserting the tube. To what population can she generalize her results about the effects of alcohol on the lining of the stomach? Is this a meaningful population to which to generalize?

2. After you've graduated from college (i.e., you are taking no more undergraduate courses), I look up your undergraduate GPA. Is your final GPA a statistic or a parameter?

3. The athletic director at a college is interested in how well female collegiate athletes perform academically. He goes to the women's softball team, finds their average GPA, and reports that the women's softball team has a GPA of 3.37. Is this a descriptive or an inferential statistic? Can you meaningfully turn it into the other?

4. A demographer is interested in the annual incomes of people who live in apartments. From the census bureau she obtains a representative sample of 2500 apartment dwellers from across the United States and finds their annual incomes. She then reports that the average annual income of apartment dwellers in the United States is $29,983. Is this a descriptive or an inferential statistic? Can you meaningfully turn it into the other?

5. A high-school gym teacher collects data on the amount of weight that 10 different samples of 18-year-old boys and girls can lift and finds, each time, that boys can lift about 50 pounds more than girls. Should we conclude that this difference is statistically significant? Is it practically significant?

6. A professor of communications has completed a number of studies in which he measures the amount of talking done by different samples of boys and girls in classroom settings. In some studies he found that boys talk more than girls (up to 3 times as much) and in others he found that girls talk more than boys (up to 4 times as much). He completes one more study and this time finds that the boys talk almost 5 times as much as the girls. Based on all the studies he's done, should we conclude that the difference in talk time between boys and girls is statistically significant? Practically significant?

ROUNDING

The last topic for this first chapter is rounding. Rounding correctly is, unfortunately, not something that most people think much about. I spend time explaining how to round because rounding correctly is important. There are different ways of rounding, and if you round incorrectly, or differently from me, your answers won't be right. They can end up being off by a large amount.*

round

To express a number in a shorter or simpler form.

Rounding means altering a number to make it shorter or simpler so that the rounded number accurately reflects the unrounded number. We round numbers for two reasons: (1) unrounded numbers are unwieldy to work with, and (2) unrounded numbers imply more precision than really exists.

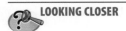 **LOOKING CLOSER**

*Ask NASA what would happen if one were off by just a fraction of a degree when sending a rocket ship off on a mission to a distant target.

Suppose I measure seven people and find their weights (in pounds) to be 108, 121, 145, 175, 198, 100, and 146. Adding the weights I find a total of 993 pounds. I divide this by 7 and find that the average weight of these people is 141.8571428571428571 pounds.

First, that number is unwieldy. If you were to ask me for the average weight of these seven people and I said 141.8571428571428571, well, that would be hard for me to say, and it would cause your eyes to glaze over.

Additionally, it is a lot more precise than it should be. Do you think that the first person weighed exactly 108 pounds? I mean, did he or she weigh 108.0000000000000000 pounds? Might his or her weight not have been 108.2 or 108.37693? So, if the raw data aren't precise, how can we use a final answer that is precise to the sixteenth decimal place?

Finally, do we really need that level of specificity? Unrounded numbers often have more accuracy than we need. If you are driving across a bridge that has a 2-ton limit, do you think that that bridge has exactly a 2-ton limit? Do you think the bridge will collapse if you and your car weigh 4001 pounds? I don't. I think that sign means that it starts to get dangerous after 4000 pounds, not that it will collapse at exactly 4000.01 pounds. Similarly, in statistics we usually don't need every last decimal point of accuracy that comes with an unrounded number.

So let's discuss *how* to round and then I'll give you some rules to live by.

There is a difference between rounding and **truncating.** In truncating, you pick how many digits or decimal places you want and then just truncate, or cut off, the rest. If I truncated the average weight of 141.857128571428571 at two decimal places it would be 141.85.

We're rounding, not truncating, so here is how to go about doing so. Let's work with 141.857142857142857142 and round it to two decimal places. If you don't mind, I'm going to make it a little less unwieldy to work with and shorten it to 141.8571. Next, I'll put a mark after the second decimal place so it is clear where we will be working: 141.85·71. The two options for rounding this to two decimal places are 141.85 (truncating it at the second decimal place) and 141.86 (going one step higher). How do you decide which to pick?

The secret comes from the definition of rounding—the rounded number should *accurately* reflect the unrounded one. One of our options, 141.85, is .0071 units away from the unrounded number, whereas the other option, 141.86, is .0029 units away from the unrounded number. 141.86 is *closer* to 141.8571 and therefore is a more accurate representation of the unrounded number.

Let's do another one for practice. Suppose you need to round 123.7344 to two decimal places. The two options are the truncated version (123.73) and one step higher, 123.74. 123.73 is .0044 units away from the unrounded number, and 123.74 is .0056 units away. 123.73 is closer to the unrounded number and so is the correct answer.

It may help to think of a balance. If you want to round the number 1.228 to two decimal places, the two options are 1.22 and 1.23. Here I

truncate

To cut off a number at a specified decimal place without rounding.

display those two options, and all the places in between, on a number line. I bold the eight, since that is the spot where the unrounded number falls, and I insert a fulcrum at 1.225, because that is the middle of the number line and the scale is balanced at this point. Think of the bolding as adding a little weight to the unrounded number. In what direction would the extra weight cause the scale to tip? Why, in the direction of 1.23. 1.228 is closer to 1.23 and so the scale tips in that direction. 1.228 rounded to two decimal places is 1.23.

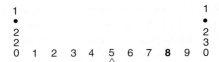

If you're one step ahead, you should be asking the next logical question: what if the unrounded number is 1.225, equidistant between our two rounding options? As you can see below, the scale doesn't tip in either direction but is balanced between 1.22 and 1.23.

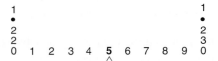

Many years ago you probably learned to round up, and so you are thinking that you should round 1.225 to 1.23. But no, that is not the rule that I want you to use!

My first rule is, "Round to even." Round 1.225 to 1.22 (which ends in an even number), not to 1.23 (which ends in an odd number).

Why should you do this? Because this way, half the time you will round up and half the time you'll round down and, as a result, the little errors that creep into one's answers as a result of rounding should cancel out.*

Thus, rounding to two decimal places, 12.565 becomes 12.56, and 12.575 becomes 12.58. How about, still rounding to two decimal places, 12.8655? This is rounded to 12.87, not 12.86. Why? Because 12.8655 is

---

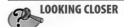 **LOOKING CLOSER**

*Rounding is a powerful technique, as is the concept of errors canceling out. Imagine that you are going to the grocery store and have only a limited amount of cash. As you put items in the cart, you want to keep track of your total. Here are actual prices, in dollars and cents, from one of my recent trips to the store: 4.04, 1.45, 1.79, 3.89, 1.94, 3.29, .80, 3.14, .80, .39, 2.86, and 4.39. You forgot your calculator, so you need to add these in your head. Not very easy, is it? (The answer is $28.78.) Now, let's round each to the nearest dollar: 4, 1, 2, 4, 2, 3, 1, 3, 1, 0, 3, and 4. Isn't that easier to add? When you do so it equals $28. Pretty close to $28.78, no? Some items get rounded up to the next dollar, other items get rounded down to next lower dollar, and the errors cancel each other out, yielding an answer very close to the real answer.

not the midpoint, the balance point, between 12.86 and 12.87. It is closer to 12.87 (.0045 units away) than it is to 12.86 (.0055 units away) and so the scale tips in the direction of 12.87. Don't be fooled into just looking at the final digit of the unrounded number and, if it is a 5, rounding to even. *Think,* and then make sure that the rounded number is an accurate reflection of the unrounded number.

Here is my second rule: round answers to two more decimal places than exist in the original data. The weights I totaled were all integers (i.e., whole numbers with zero decimal places), so my rounded average should have two decimal places: 141.8571428571428571 becomes 141.86.*

The third rule is do not round as you go but save your rounding until the very end. In other words, only round your final answer! Your calculator is happy to carry a lot of decimal places for you: let it do so. If your calculator has a memory, and most do, use it.

Here is my fourth rule: if you do round as you go, even though you shouldn't, then carry two more decimal places than you plan on using. If your raw data are in the form of integers, meaning your final answer will have two decimal places, then your intermediate steps should have at least four decimal places.[†]

Here's a simple example of how failing to follow the fourth rule can lead to an answer that is very wrong. If I take a number, divide it by a second number, and then multiply this by the second number, I should end up back at the first number. Algebraically, $(X \div Y) \times Y = X$.

I'm going to do a problem of this type, and round incorrectly. If I divide 123,456,789 by 987,654,321 and round the answer (.12499999) to two decimal places, I get .12. Now, if I multiply that by 987,654,321, I should end up back at 123,456,789. Unfortunately, because I rounded to only two decimal places, the answer is 118,518,518.52. That answer, even if we round it to 119 million, is almost 5 million away from the real answer of over 123 million. It's not good to be that far off.

Suppose that instead of rounding to two decimal places as you go, you round as you go to two more places than you plan to end up with—that is, to four decimal places. In this case, 123,456,789 divided by 987,654,321 = .12499999 which would round to .1250. When I multiply .1250 by 987,654,321 I get 123,456,790.12. This is only 1.12 away from the correct answer of 123,456,789, not almost 5 million away. Not too shabby.

---

*Clear presentation of results is important and too many decimal places make results hard to read, so use common sense and don't be a slave to my rule. In the next chapter, when I talk about making tables for data, I violate my rule and limit how many decimal places I report. Similarly, if there is a convention—such as reporting prices in cents, not fractions of cents—follow it.

[†] The American Psychological Association (2001) has a style manual that many researchers follow and it recommends that results be reported to two decimal places. Thus, functionally, if you carry four decimal places you will have enough precision to round your final answer to two decimal places. Bottom line: rounding to four decimal places as you go is OK.

LOOKING CLOSER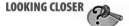

I think my point is clear: carry as many decimal places as you can! However, if you round as you go, carry at least two places more than you'll need at the end.

My final point about rounding: sometimes we'll use the same number two different ways, as an intermediate step and as a final answer. Round those two differently. At the beginning of the section on rounding, I found that the average weight of seven people was 141.8571428… If I were answering the question, "What is the average weight of those seven people?" I would report it to two decimal places, 141.86. In a later chapter we are going to learn about something called a standard deviation. Part of calculating a standard deviation is subtracting the average from each score. In that case, the average is not a final answer but an intermediate number, and so I should use as many decimal places as possible, or at least two more than needed for the final answer. In this instance, then, since I am using the average as a number intermediate to calculating another number, I would use 141.8571, not 141.86.

Lest you think that I am overly concerned about rounding, let me tell you about a recent study where two researchers examined all the papers published during 2001 in two very respected journals, *Nature* and *British Medical Journal*. Garcia-Berthou and Alcaraz* examined all the articles for statistical errors and found that 38% of the articles in *Nature* and 25% in the *British Medical Journal* had at least one statistical error. Stop and think about that. At least a quarter of the papers published in two of the most prestigious journals in the world contain statistical errors. Garcia-Berthou and Alcaraz, without getting access to all of the original data sets, couldn't determine the size of the errors. However, they did conclude that it was likely that a substantial number of the errors were due to incorrect rounding!

I hope this is something that you won't be guilty of. To help you avoid rounding errors, here again is the list of rounding conventions that you should follow.

ROUNDING CONVENTIONS

1. When the unrounded number is equidistant from the two rounding options, round to the even option.
2. Round your *final* answers to two more decimal places than exist in the raw data.
3a. Don't round until the very end.
3b. On the other hand, if you do round as you go, carry two more decimal places than you'll need.
4. Be aware of the difference between a final answer and a number used as a step in other calculations and round these two differently.

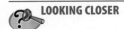 **LOOKING CLOSER**

*Garcia-Berthou, E. & Alcaraz, C. (2004). Incongruence between test statistics and p values in medical papers, *BMC Medical Research Methodology*, 4, 13.

Group Practice 1.4

Round each of the following to the appropriate number of decimal places:

1. $5 \div 3 =$ _____
2. $3 \div 5 =$ _____
3. $.38 \div .37 =$ _____
4. $.380 \div .370 =$ _____
5. Buffy goes to the store and buys seven small items. She spends a total of $6.89. What is the average price per item?

Round each of the following to **two** decimal places:

6. $.03478 =$ _____
7. $18.13878277 =$ _____
8. $.3275 =$ _____
9. $.425789 =$ _____
10. $3.9999 =$ _____
11. $3.991 =$ _____
12. $3.995 =$ _____
13. $3.985 =$ _____
14. $3.9855 =$ _____
15. $3.98500000001 =$ _____
16. $55.01005 =$ _____

SUMMARY

Statistics provide a way to compare the result we observe to the result that we expected. If the observed result is close enough to the expected result, it is reasonable to believe that our hypothesis (the basis of our expectation) is true. Statistics do this by taking the many numbers generated by a researcher's careful and systematic observations and reducing them to a summary number. Statistics bring order to chaos.

The numbers on which statistics are calculated are measured on the outcome variable, or the dependent variable, for a sample of cases. The calculated statistic can be descriptive (describing a sample) or inferential (used to generalize from the sample to a larger population). Inferential statistics are based on the assumption that the sample is representative of the population. (A representative sample contains all the elements of the population in the same proportion in which they occur in the population.)

In addition to the dependent variable, there is another variable, the independent or grouping, variable. The independent variable is the one being investigated for its effect on the dependent variable. Often researchers want to show a cause and effect relationship between the independent and dependent variables. To demonstrate this, a researcher must show three things: (1) that changes in the level of the independent variable lead to changes in the level of the dependent variable, (2) that the changes in the independent variable precede in time the changes in the dependent variable, and (3) that there is no other plausible explanation for the changes in the dependent variable. (Variables that can plausibly account for the changes in the dependent variable are called confounding variables.)

Measurement, assigning numbers to objects so that the number faithfully represents the underlying attribute being measured, is the process by which a researcher measures the degree to which each case possesses the attribute being investigated. (An operational definition explains how the researcher has decided to measure the underlying attribute.) The numbers assigned by measurement can represent either qualities (e.g., male or female) or quantities (e.g., weight). There are also four different scales of measurement (nominal, ordinal, interval, and ratio) that differ in the information (difference, direction, distance, and real zero point) that the number provides.

It is important to differentiate between these terms: statistic vs. parameter and statistical significance vs. practical significance. A statistic is a value that is calculated for a sample, and a parameter is a value calculated for a population; Latin letters are used as abbreviations for statistics and Greek letters for parameters. Calling a difference between two samples *statistically significant* means that we conclude that this difference reflects a real difference between the populations from which the samples came. Just because a result is statistically significant is no guarantee that it is practically significant. For a result to be practically significant, the real-life relationship between the independent variable and the dependent variable has to be strong enough to make a difference.

Finally, rounding improperly can have a devastating impact on your final answer. Follow the rules for rounding: round so that the rounded number faithfully represents the unrounded one, round to two more decimal places than initially existed, don't round until the end, and be aware of the difference between how a final answer and an intermediate step are rounded.

INTRODUCTION TO REVIEW EXERCISES AND HOMEWORK PROBLEMS

This is the first set of review exercises and homework problems, so I want to tell you what to expect. First of all, the review exercises do not follow the order of the chapter! That is, the first problem will not correspond to the first topic covered in the chapter. My reason for this is very simple: when you apply statistics in real life there won't be temporal or spatial cues that tell you what to do—you need to know what technique to apply. The same is true here.

The answers to the review exercises can be found in the book. As you might have gathered by now, I like this stuff and so I am going to spill some ink when I give the answers. If I know of a mistake commonly made by students, I'll point it out. If a question was particularly challenging, I'll tell you how and why.

My questions are often not just rote applications of the material but are intended to push you to have insights, to make connections, to apply the material in new ways. Thus I use the questions (and the answers!) to teach. Sometimes, I include new material in the answers. From my perspective, the material in the answers is part of the text. *To make that clear, the material from the answers at the back of the book is fair game for exams.*

I also revisit material throughout the book. Just because you've left Chapter 1 behind doesn't mean that you can now forget about identifying a dependent variable's level of measurement. The review questions at the end of each chapter will include material from previous chapters.

After the review exercises come homework problems. Like the review questions, they won't follow the order of the chapter. Like the review exercises, you'll find questions from past chapters among the homework questions in future chapters. Like the review exercises, the homework problems should push you to think about the material in new ways. Unlike the review exercises, the answers to the homework problems are not given at the back of the book.

Review Exercises

1. Find the level of measurement for each of the following as indicated in the question:
   a. A meteorologist classifies cities in the United States as having winter weather that is "dreary" (0) or "not dreary" (1). Type of winter weather (0 vs. 1) is measured at what level of measurement?
   b. A neurologist measures how many times per minute a specific neuron in the brain "fires" when a person is in dim light as opposed to when a person is in bright light. She is measuring the neuron firing at what level of measurement?

   c. A social worker obtains the suicide rates for students at colleges in the United States. If the college has a suicide rate that is below average, he classifies it as −1. If the suicide rate is average, the college gets a 0; and if the suicide rate is above average, it gets a +1. Suicide rate (−1, 0, +1) is being measured at what level of measurement?
   d. A person who runs an automobile shipping company classifies cars in terms of size. If a car is a subcompact, she assigns it the value of 1. A compact car gets a 2, a midsize car a 3, and a full-size car a 4. At what level is she measuring car size?

e. The admissions committee at a college does not distinguish between different types of high-school extracurricular activities. As far as they are concerned, being a member of the tiddlywinks club is equivalent to being student council president. On the admission form to the college, applicants are asked to report the number of extracurricular activities they were involved with in high school. The college is measuring extracurricular activities at what level?

f. The same college asks for students to submit their SAT scores, but only on the math subtest. For those who don't know, subtest scores on the SAT range from a low of 200 to a high of 800, with 500 representing an average score. The SAT measures math skills at what level?

2. A college dean wanted to find out which students are smarter, those seeking liberal arts degrees (like English or psychology) or those seeking professional degrees (like nursing, business, or engineering). He obtains a representative sample from each of the two populations from the colleges in the United States, administers IQ tests to everyone, and calculates the average IQ for each sample.

a. Are these two averages statistics or parameters?

b. If he uses the two averages to answer his question, is this an example of inferential statistics or descriptive statistics?

c. Suppose that the dean does this study time and time again, and each time he finds that the same group is, on average, 1 IQ point smarter than the other group. Should we conclude that this is statistically significant? Practically significant?

d. Suppose, instead, the first time he did the study, he found that group A had an IQ of 110 and group B an IQ of 80. Using new samples, the next time he found that group A had an IQ of 101 and group B had an IQ of 99. The third time he did the study, group A had an IQ of 95 and group B of 105. Having done the study multiple times, should we

conclude that there is a statistically significant difference between the two groups? Practically significant?

3. Round these appropriately:

a. $18 \div 17 = $ _____

b. $18.12 \div 17.76 = $ _____

c. $18.1200 \div 17.7600 = $ _____

d. Buffy weighs 126 pounds, Skip weighs 156 pounds, and Desdemona weighs 143 pounds. What is their average weight? _____

Round the following to two decimal places:

e. $55.55 = $ _____

f. $55.0055 = $ _____

g. $55.555 = $ _____

h. $99.995 = $ _____

i. $99.9905 = $ _____

Do each of the next questions three times, each time reporting the final answer to two decimal places. First, carry as many decimal places as your calculator allows, and don't round until the very end. Then, do the calculations again, but round each intermediate step to four decimal places before moving to the next step. Finally, round as you go again, this time rounding each intermediate step to two decimal places.

j. $[(703 \div 503) \times 47.38] \div 4.72 = $ _____

k. $[(123 \div 321) \div .17] \div .27 = $ _____

4. Read each scenario and provide the information requested:

a. The local police department has come to a criminologist for help in evaluating a new type of disposable, plastic handcuffs. They are just as effective as metal handcuffs in terms of immobilizing someone who has been arrested, and they are cheaper than metal handcuffs, but the police are concerned that the plastic ones cause more abrasion to the skin of the wrist. The criminologist gets 20 volunteers, randomly divides them into two groups, cuffs one group with metal handcuffs and the other with plastic handcuffs, and then rides them around in a squad car for 20 minutes. After this, she measures the degree of abrasion on their wrists. The dependent variable is _____.

b. My grandmother, when she had trouble sleeping, used to take an aspirin. Though she swore that it was an effective sleeping pill, I thought that the placebo effect was operating. So, I designed a study in which I measure how long (in minutes) it takes each of 60 people to fall asleep. I randomly divide the 60 people into the following three groups: (1) people who take an aspirin before bedtime, (2) people who take a placebo, which they think is an aspirin, before bedtime, and (3) people who take nothing before bedtime. My independent variable is _____ .

c. Some football players put streaks of black paint under their eyes because they believe that it helps them see better in sunny conditions. An exercise physiologist wants to see if this is correct. So, he gets a group of volunteers and gives each an eye exam while shining bright lights. Each player gets the eye exam twice. Half the group have their eyes examined with the black paint under their eyes the first time, and the second time without. For the other half, the order is reversed. The exercise physiologist's independent variable is _____ .

d. Ever notice that some college students buy all the books for class, complete all the readings, do all the homework, and so on? These students usually end up with better grades. An education professor decides to investigate this to see if these more conscientious students get better grades because they work harder or because they are innately smarter. The professor gets (a) a group of "conscientious" students from a number of different colleges and (b) a group of "non-conscientious" students from the same colleges. He compares the two groups in terms of a standardized IQ test. The dependent variable is _____ .

e. I have noticed that on days when I am less mentally alert, I drink more cups of coffee. Curious as to whether amount of sleep influences my mental alertness, each night I flip a coin. If the coin turns up heads, I set my alarm for 8 hours of sleep; tails, I set my alarm for only 5 hours of sleep. Then, each subsequent day, I note how many cups of coffee I drink. My independent variable is _____ .

5. A group of athletes is arguing about who is in better shape. In order to settle the argument, they have their lung capacities measured. They define lung capacity, forced expiratory volume, as the amount of air (in liters) that is pushed out of the lung, where higher numbers represent greater lung capacity. Below is a list of the athletes and their associated lung capacities. Rank-order them from greatest lung capacity (1) to lowest lung capacity (20).

Anquetil	3.52
Armstrong	3.95
Coppi	3.25
Delgado	3.85
Fignon	3.45
Garin	3.15
Hamilton	3.75
Heras	3.57
Hinault	3.00
Hincapie	3.60
Indurain	3.91
Leipheimer	3.53
Lemond	3.85
McEwen	3.45
Merckx	3.25
Pantani	3.60
Riis	3.25
Roche	3.75
Ullrich	3.94
Zabel	3.89

Homework Problems

1. A researcher gives different amounts of "R" to different subjects and then measures how much "M" each subject produces. She finds that subjects who get more R produce more M, and subjects who get less R produce less M. She also finds no other variable that can account for the different amounts of M that the subjects produce. What conclusion should she draw?
   a. There is a relationship between R and M.
   b. There is a relationship between M and R.
   c. R causes M.
   d. M causes R.
   e. There is not enough information to draw any conclusion.

2. I get a sample of 50-year-old executives and measure how financially successful each has been by measuring the square footage of his or her house. (The larger the house, the more successful the person has been.) House size is which of the following?
   a. A confounding variable for financial success
   b. An operational definition for financial success
   c. A parameter
   d. A way of comparing the expected degree of financial success to the actual degree of financial success

3. Which of the following can't exist?
   a. A result that is practically significant without being statistically significant
   b. A result that is statistically significant without being practically significant
   c. A result that is both practically significant and statistically significant
   d. A result that is neither practically significant nor statistically significant
   e. All of the above can exist.
   f. None of the above can exist.

4. Independent variable is to dependent variable as which of the following?
   a. Grouping variable is to subject variable
   b. Relationship is to cause and effect
   c. Statistic is to parameter
   d. Parameter is to statistic
   e. Generalizability is to representativeness
   f. None of the above

5. If I am assigning numbers to objects so that the number faithfully represents the underlying attribute being measured, then I am using which of the following?
   a. An operational definition
   b. Measurement
   c. A quantitative variable
   d. A descriptive statistic
   e. None of the above

6. Answer each of the following:
   a. Environmentalists have a theory that as smoke-stack and tailpipe emissions have increased over the past centuries, global warming has occurred. According to this theory, what is the dependent variable?
   b. Many parents believe that when their children consume sugar they become more active. A psychologist gets a group of children and randomly assigns them to receive different "doses" of sugar. He then measures how much the children run about on a playground. What is the dependent variable?
   c. A consumer behavior researcher wants to know if how children behave during the year determines how many Christmas presents they receive. She has parents classify their children as naughty or nice for the previous year, and she then calculates how much the parents spent on Christmas presents for the children. What is the independent variable?
   d. A political scientist is curious as to what factors influence voting behavior for school district tax levies. She obtains a sample of voters and divides them, randomly, into three groups. One group serves as the control group—nothing is done to them. To one experimental group she gives information about the tax levy that focuses on positive information: how the levy will improve student performance, make the community more attractive to young families, and so on. To the other experimental group she gives negative information: how much the levy will increase taxes, how it will take funding away from other projects, how wasteful the

school district has been, and so on. She then measures, for each group, the percentage voting in favor of the levy. What is her independent variable?

7. Answer each of the following:
   a. A political pollster calls 2000 registered American voters and finds out whether they plan to vote for the Democratic or the Republican candidate in an upcoming election. From this he predicts the outcome of the election. Is he using the information about the sample as a descriptive or as an inferential statistic?
   b. Every 10 years the United States Census Bureau attempts to collect information from *all* Americans. Assuming that the Census Bureau is successful in this endeavor, would it be a statistic or a parameter if it reported that 12% of Americans are of African descent?
   c. A dean at a college wants to know what the average quantitative SAT is for the first-year class. She calls the registrar, and the registrar accesses the data base for the entire first-year class. When the registrar reports the average to the dean, is this a statistic or a parameter?
   d. Continuing with the previous question, is the average the registrar calculated for a sample or for a population?

8. Answer each of the following in just a few sentences:
   a. Why are the attributes that researchers measure called variables?
   b. What is the empirical method?
   c. "Statistics is about comparing the observed to the expected." What does this mean?
   d. What does it mean to say that a difference is statistically significant?

9. Below are the birth rates, per 1000, for a number of countries. Rank-order them, assigning a 1 to the country with the lowest birth rate.

Australia	12.6
Austria	9.4
Belgium	10.4
Czech Republic	9.0

Denmark	11.5
Finland	10.5
France	12.5
Germany	8.6
Greece	9.8
Hungary	9.3
Ireland	14.6
Israel	18.7
Italy	9.2
Japan	9.6
Luxembourg	11.9
Mauritius	16.1
Netherlands	11.3
New Zealand	14.1
Norway	12.2
Panama	20.8
Poland	10.5
Portugal	11.4
Romania	10.8
Singapore	12.8
Sweden	9.7
Switzerland	9.6
Tunisia	16.5
United Kingdom	11.0
United States	14.1

10. Round the following to two decimal places:
    a. 21.345
    b. 22.467
    c. 22.467800001
    d. 22.467800005
    e. 176.9899
    f. 176.989905
    g. 189.9895
    h. 189.98950000
    i. 15.46566767
    j. 57.1070

11. Answer each of the following:
    a. A medical researcher is examining the influenza rates in different communities. She measures influenza rate as the number of cases per 100,000 people. Influenza rate is being measured at what level?
    b. A nurse researcher is measuring how many minutes it takes before people are seen by the triage nurse after they enter an emergency

room. He's curious to know if waiting time is different on different days of the week. Waiting time is being measured at what level?

c. A political scientist who is investigating voter apathy finds out whether people voted in the last presidential election and in the last off-year election. If a person voted in neither, the political scientist assigns them a value of "0"; voting in the presidential election but not the off-year election receives a "1"; voting in both gets a "2"; voting in the off-year election but not the presidential election gets a "3." At what level is election behavior being measured?

d. A housing developer advertises his houses as being fully carpeted (2), partially carpeted (1), or not carpeted (0). Carpeting is being measured at what level?

2

Tables and Graphs

Sometimes we can summarize a mass of data with a single number in a sentence (the average grade in the class was…), but other times we want to present more information. In those situations, the descriptive statistics of tables and graphs allow us to reduce a large mass of data into a smaller, more organized, more communicative format. In this chapter as we learn how, *and when*, to make tables and graphs, we'll explore two different kinds of numbers: discrete, which answer the question "How many?" and continuous, which answer the question "How much?" Continuous numbers are only as accurate as the measuring instrument used to derive them, and thus we'll see that a continuous number represents a range within which an actual value falls. For example, if you say that you are 22 years old, are you exactly 22 years old, or is your age somewhere in the range from 22 to 23? As we explore graphs, we'll talk about the shapes that data take, both the normal curve (what you may have heard of as the bell-shaped curve) and deviations from it.

TABLES, PART I

Tables are a way to summarize and organize a set of data, and there are two different types of tables that I want you to learn to make: ungrouped frequency distributions and grouped frequency distributions. An **ungrouped frequency distribution** is an intuitive way to organize data. In Chapter 1, we used the example of counting the number of impulsive behaviors emitted during a 60-minute quiet period by children who had received caffeine and children who had not. To bring order to chaos, the data were organized by tallying, from lowest to highest, how many children were at each level of impulsivity.* That was a rudimentary form of an ungrouped frequency distribution.

When making an ungrouped frequency distribution, simply list all the values of the dependent variable, in order from lowest to highest, and count the frequency with which each value occurs. Since we count the *frequency* for *each* value (e.g., each 6, each 7, each 8, each 9, etc.) and

ungrouped frequency distribution

A list of the values of the dependent variable, in order from lowest to highest, with a count of the frequency with which each value occurred.

LOOKING CLOSER

*I haven't mentioned this yet, so let me do so now—the word "data" is a plural noun and so takes a plural verb and is referred to by a plural pronoun. Thus one says, "The data are…," not "The data is…." When referring to data one calls them "them" or "they," not "it." A single data point is a datum, so you could say something like, "That datum was very interesting," if you want to sound like a real statistics nerd.

TABLE 2.1 Number of Impulsive Behaviors Emitted During a 60-Minute Quiet Period by Children Who Did Not Receive Caffeine

0	0	0	1	1	1	1	1	1	1	1	2	2	2	2	2	2
2	2	2	2	3	3	3	3	3	3	3	4	4	4	4	4	4
5	5	5	6	7	8											

not the frequency for *groups* of values (e.g., the number of values from 6 to 10), it is called an *ungrouped* frequency distribution. The word "distribution" is tacked on at the end because the table shows how the values are *distributed* or spread through the range of values.

Table 2.1 shows, in order from low to high, the impulsivity data for the uncaffeinated subjects from Chapter 1. Table 2.2 then shows them organized as an ungrouped frequency distribution.

Note the following points about making ungrouped frequency distributions. First, when ordering the data as in Table 2.1, it is easiest to go from low to high, first listing the low numbers, then the high. Thus, I first listed all the zeros, then the ones, twos, and so on. However, when transforming the data into an ungrouped frequency distribution, the lower numbers go at the *bottom* of the table. The reason for this will be clear shortly, when we add a cumulative frequency column to the table. But for the time being, organize your tables with the higher values at the top.

Second, notice that there are two columns in the ungrouped frequency distribution, one labeled "*X*" and the other "*f*," and that there is a note at the bottom of the table explaining these labels. The *X* column represents the values of the dependent variable and contains a list, in descending order, of its values. Here I've included the value of 9 because it was the highest value obtained by a child who received caffeine, even though no child without caffeine obtained that value. The *f* column contains the frequency with which each of the values occurred. In Table 2.1 you'll note that three uncaffeinated children emitted 0 impulsive behaviors and so the frequency associated with a score of 0 is 3. Similarly, there were eight uncaffeinated children who emitted 1 impulsive act while being observed, so the frequency associated with a score of 1 is 8.

The third thing to note is that the ungrouped frequency distribution has a title. The objective of tables is to communicate, and without a clear title the table may fail at this task. Don't be afraid to spill some ink on the title. The title for this table, "Ungrouped frequency distribution of number of impulsive behaviors emitted during 60-minute quiet period by children who did not receive caffeine," is long, but it is a lot more descriptive than "Impulsivity." Make sure that the title is sufficient so that if someone comes on the table by itself, without any other explanatory information, he or she will know what the table is about.

As I am fond of telling my classes, the three most important words for tables and graphs are "Label, label, label." When you make a table or a

TABLE 2.2 Ungrouped Frequency Distribution of Number of Impulsive Behaviors Emitted during a 60-Minute Quiet Period by Children Who Did Not Receive Caffeine

X	f
9	0
8	1
7	1
6	1
5	3
4	6
3	7
2	10
1	8
0	3

Note: X = value; f = frequency

TABLE **2.3**   **Ungrouped Frequency Distribution of Number of Impulsive Behaviors Emitted during a 60-Minute Quiet Period by Children Who Did Not Receive Caffeine**

X	f	f_c	%	$\%_c$
9	0	40	.00	100.00
8	1	40	2.50	100.00
7	1	39	2.50	97.50
6	1	38	2.50	95.00
5	3	37	7.50	92.50
4	6	34	15.00	85.00
3	7	28	17.50	70.00
2	10	21	25.00	52.50
1	8	11	20.00	27.50
0	3	3	7.50	7.50

Note: X = value; f = frequency; f_c = cumulative frequency; % = percentage; $\%_c$ = cumulative percentage

graph, be sure that you have a clear title, that the column and axes are labeled, and that there is a note explaining the labels if they are not self-evident. It is always better to err on the side of overtitling, overlabeling, and overexplaining.

The ungrouped frequency distribution in Table 2.2 is a perfectly adequate ungrouped frequency distribution. However, it is the entry-level version without any extras or options. Table 2.3 is a top-of-the-line, all-the-options version of an ungrouped frequency distribution table for the uncaffeinated children's data.

Note that I have added three columns, and that my note at the bottom of the table contains brief descriptions of the new columns. The cumulative frequency column, f_c, tells the number of children whose scores were at *or below* each value.* Three children emitted 0 impulsive behaviors while being observed, and eight children emitted 1. Thus there are a total of 11 children who emitted 1 or fewer impulsive acts. Moving up to the next level, 2 impulsive acts, we find a frequency of 10. Add those 10 to the cumulative frequency of 11 for the next lower row, and we have a cumulative frequency of 21 for 2 or fewer acts of impulsive behavior.

The simplest way to calculate cumulative frequency is to start at the bottom row, where the cumulative frequency is the same as the frequency. The cumulative frequency for the next higher row is simply the cumulative frequency of the lower row *plus* the frequency for the next higher row. Proceeding in this stairstep fashion all the way up through the table, you can calculate the rest of the cumulative frequencies.

LOOKING CLOSER   * f_c is pronounced "f sub c."

One important thing to note is that the cumulative frequency for the top row is equal to the total number of cases in the data set. Statisticians commonly abbreviate the number of cases as N, so in this case we say that $N = 40$. The fact that the final cumulative frequency must equal N provides a nice check for a table: if $N \neq f_c$, then you've done something wrong, either in tallying the frequency for at least one category or in totaling the frequencies.

The other two columns, % and $\%_c$, take existing information and transform it to a new and more easily understood metric, percentages. For example, 10 noncaffeinated children emitted 2 acts of impulsive behavior while being observed. Is this a lot of children? Dividing the frequency (10) by N (40) and multiplying this quotient by 100 gives the percentage, 25%. The formula for this is shown in Equation 2.1.

Percentages are more intuitively interpretable than are raw numbers. Which do you think would better communicate these data to a listener: (a) "10 of the children who did not receive caffeine emitted 2 impulsive acts during the 60-minute quiet period" or, (b) "25% of the children who did not receive caffeine emitted 2 impulsive acts during the 60-minute quiet period"? The latter, the one with the percentage, puts the frequency into a context and thus provides more easily understood information.

F O R M U L A

Percentage for a Frequency Distribution

Equation 2.1

$$\% = \frac{f}{N} \times 100$$

Where:

% = the percentage being calculated

f = the frequency with which a score or an interval occurs

N = the total number of cases

The final column, $\%_c$, is simply the cumulative frequency transformed into a percentage; the formula for this is shown in Equation 2.2. All that it involves is dividing a cumulative frequency by the sample size and multiplying this quotient by 100. A look at Table 2.3 shows that a little over 50% (52.5%, to be exact) of the children emitted two or fewer impulsive acts. Again, just as the final cumulative frequncy should equal the sample size, the final cumulative percentage should equal 100%.*

---

*As a practical matter, I don't recommend calculating cumulative percentage by simply adding up the percentages as one goes, because rounding error will creep in. If you do, you may end up with a final cumulative percentage a little above or below 100%.

LOOKING CLOSER

F O R M U L A

Cumulative Percentage for a Frequency Distribution

Equation 2.2

$$\%_c = \frac{f_c}{N} \times 100$$

Where:

$\%_c$ = the cumulative percentage being calculated
f_c = the cumulative frequency for a score or an interval
N = the total number of cases

Not every ungrouped frequency distribution has to have all five of these columns. The objective of a table is communication, and it is your decision what you want to communicate. The first two columns, X and f, are mandatory. After that, you (or your instructor) decide what columns are needed to get across the points you want to make.

Group Practice 2.1

1. An exercise physiologist has people walk up 10 flights of stairs and then measures how many minutes it takes for their heart rates to return to normal. Make an ungrouped frequency distribution that shows frequency, cumulative frequency, percentage, and cumulative percentage for the following data. *Save your table to use in future group practices.*

1, 3, 7, 2, 8, 12, 11, 3, 5, 6, 7, 4, 14, 8, 2, 3, 5, 8, 11, 10, 9, 8, 4, 3, 2, 3, 4, 2, 6, 7, 4, 5, 5, 7, 4, 2, 12, 6, 7, 3, 5, 6, 9, 10, 11, 5, 6, 3, 5, 8, 5, 4, 5, 3, 6, 9, 4, 7, 4, 6, 2, and 5.

GROUPED FREQUENCY DISTRIBUTIONS

Ungrouped frequency distributions work very well as long as there aren't too many values of X. In this case there are 10 values of X (0 through 9) so Table 2.3 is short enough to be visualized and comprehensible. When there are many values of X, you can group them to make a more compact, more comprehensible, table.* Such a table is called, of course, a **grouped frequency distribution.**

For our example of a grouped frequency distribution, let's work with a real set of data. Table 2.4 shows the final accumulated point totals for a random sample of 60 students, taken from the hundreds of students to

grouped frequency distribution

A list of the values of the dependent variable, grouped into ranges, ordered from lowest to highest, with the frequency with which each range of values occurs.

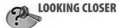 **LOOKING CLOSER**

*You may not like this, but there is no hard and fast number for how many X values are too many for an ungrouped frequency distribution. As a rough rule of thumb, if there are more than 9 or 10 values of X, consider moving to a grouped frequency distribution. However, don't be a slave to this. The objective of a table is to communicate. So, if you have 15 values of X and think an ungrouped frequency distribution will do the best job of telling the story you want to tell, go for it.

TABLE **2.4** **Final, Accumulated Point Totals for a Random Sample of 60 Introductory Statistics Students**

51	47	50	59	66	70	44	58	95	48	46	62
67	58	75	51	63	59	33	58	69	62	48	82
57	83	74	40	58	62	50	69	56	30	61	76
30	45	51	68	34	41	60	55	71	92	75	76
41	51	59	55	65	69	45	57	84	62	28	52

TABLE **2.5** **Ungrouped Frequency Distribution for Final Point Totals for a Random Sample of 60 Introductory Statistics Students**

X	f	X	f	X	f	X	f
95	1	78	0	61	1	44	1
94	0	77	0	60	1	43	0
93	0	76	2	59	3	42	0
92	1	75	2	58	4	41	2
91	0	74	1	57	2	40	1
90	0	73	0	56	1	39	0
89	0	72	0	55	2	38	0
88	0	71	1	54	0	37	0
87	0	70	1	53	0	36	0
86	0	69	3	52	1	35	0
85	0	68	1	51	4	34	1
84	1	67	1	50	2	33	1
83	1	66	1	49	0	32	0
82	1	65	1	48	2	31	0
81	0	64	0	47	1	30	2
80	0	63	1	46	1	29	0
79	0	62	4	45	2	28	1

Note: X = score; f = frequency

whom I have taught introductory statistics. Please be aware that my grading scale is a little unusual: my A range is from 80 to 100, B is from 60 to 79, C from 40 to 59, D from 20 to 39, and F is 19 and below.*

In Table 2.5, I organized the data as an ungrouped frequency distribution. (Note that to make the table fit on one page I used four sets of columns.) This ungrouped frequency distribution does not communicate well in that it does not provide a good overview of how my students have performed.

---

*I use this grading scale because I don't think that the traditional 90/80/70/60 cutoffs yield an interval-level scale since the F range is 60 points wide and each other grade range is 10 points wide.

LOOKING CLOSER

The ungrouped frequency distribution in Table 2.5 gives a picture of all the trees, but gives no overview of the whole forest. By moving to a grouped frequency distribution, where we count the frequency for groups or *intervals* of scores, we'll get an overview of the forest but will lose details about individual trees. Thus there is a tension between moving to the big picture (a grouped frequency distribution) and losing details, as opposed to preserving details (an ungrouped frequency distribution) but missing the overview.

The big question for a grouped frequency distribution is how many intervals to use. My rule of thumb is to aim for five to nine intervals; but again, don't be a slave. The objective is to communicate. If you think fewer than five or more than nine intervals will better communicate your point, that's your decision.

Sometimes there is a logical way to choose the number of intervals. The data in Table 2.4 represent grades in my class and, as I use 20-point intervals for grades, it would be reasonable to use 20-point intervals for the grouped frequency distribution. By the bye, the abbreviation for interval is i and we would use the shorthand $i = 20$ to indicate an interval width of 20.

However, I want more detail in my frequency distribution, so I will use 10-point intervals ($i = 10$). Thus, my intervals will be 90-99, 80-89, 70-79, 60-69, 50-59, 40-49, 30-39, and 20-29. You can assure yourself that the interval width is 10 by counting off on your fingers from 90 to 99. Note that all intervals are the same width. This is important in a grouped frequency distribution: do not make intervals of different widths in the same grouped frequency distribution.*

Also, avoid intervals that have impossible values. Imagine that I made my top interval 86-95 because a score of 95 was the highest score anyone received. And, imagine that I had a student whose final point total was 3. Continuing down from 86-95, the intervals would be spaced such that this student would fall in the interval ranging from −4 to 5. Students can do very well in my class, and they can do very poorly, but it is impossible for a student to score less than 0. To have an interval of −4 to 5, where there are four impossible values (−4, −3, −2, and −1), is wrong.[†]

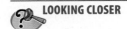

LOOKING CLOSER

*Occasionally different interval widths are unavoidable. Imagine graphing the number of psychiatric hospital admissions by decade from 1950 to the present. The intervals for the 1950s, '60s, '70s, '80s, and '90s are all 10 years wide, but the current decade isn't over yet. The options are to leave the current decade out of the graph, which makes a certain sense as it is hard to compare the rate for a 5-year period to a 10-year period, or to have an interval sized differently than the others.

[†] There are a few questions that logically follow from the material that I present in class that I'm always afraid of being asked by students. Luckily, although I've taught statistics for more than ten years, no one has ever asked me this one. But perhaps the following dilemma has occurred to you: What would I do if I had one student who aced the class and accumulated 100 points and another who absolutely failed every assignment and accumulated 0 points? In that case the range in grades is 101 points and this can't be divided into five or ten equal intervals (unless the interval width is 10.1 or 20.2 or something silly like that). What should I do?   *Continued*

TABLE 2.6   Grouped Frequency Distribution ($i = 10$) for Final Point Totals for a Random Sample of 60 Introductory Statistics Students

X	m	f	f_c	%	$%_c$
90-99	94.50	2	60	3.33	100.00
80-89	84.50	3	58	5.00	96.67
70-79	74.50	7	55	11.67	91.67
60-69	64.50	14	48	23.33	80.00
50-59	54.50	19	34	31.67	56.67
40-49	44.50	10	15	16.67	25.00
30-39	34.50	4	5	6.67	8.33
20-29	24.50	1	1	1.67	1.67

Note: i = interval width; X = scores; M = interval midpoint; f = frequency; f_c = cumulative frequency; % = percentage; $%_c$ = cumulative percentage

Table 2.6 shows the grouped frequency distribution for these data. Compare Table 2.6 to the ungrouped version in Table 2.5. Which does a better job of telling the story of how my students have performed?

I think that Table 2.6 more clearly communicates that most students end up in the range from 40 to 69 with C's and B's. Some students do better (five ended up with A's), and some do worse (five ended up with D's), but nobody had a score lower than 20; nobody failed.

The advantage of a grouped frequency distribution is that it boils the data down so that the big picture is easier to see. Unfortunately, in doing so, we lose information. If all you know about these 60 students is what is contained in Table 2.6, you don't know the actual final scores for the 10 students in the 40-49 range. Are the scores spread across the whole range? Are they all 40s? Are most of them piled up around 45 with some doing better and some doing worse? As I said before, there is a tension between too much and too little information. Table 2.5 contains all the information, but it is hard to interpret. Table 2.6 contains less information but is easier to view.

I don't think Table 2.6 has lost too much information. It does a good job of communicating what I want to communicate, which is how students usually perform in my stats class. For an example of a grouped frequency distribution for these data that is so boiled down that it is useless, see Table 2.7.

TABLE 2.7   A Poor Example of a Grouped Frequency Distribution ($i = 50$) for Final Point Totals for a Random Sample of 60 Introductory Statistics Students

X	f	f_c
50-99	45	60
0-49	15	15

Note: i = interval width; X = scores; f = frequency; f_c = cumulative frequency

(Continued) First, I'd tell the student who asked that question to keep his or her fingers crossed that this situation doesn't happen. It is rare that in a sample one obtains the whole possible range of scores. But, if it occurred, I would violate my rule about equal interval width and would make one of my intervals, either the top or the bottom one, 11 points wide. Thus, the intervals would run something like 90-100, 80-89, 70-79, etc. The only other option would be to make 11 intervals with one of the intervals containing nine impossible values (e.g., 100-109, 90-99, 80-89, etc.) and this seems like a worse option to me. As I said, keep your fingers crossed that this situation doesn't occur.

LOOKING CLOSER

Just as with the ungrouped frequency distribution, one has to decide what columns of information one wants to include in a grouped frequency distribution. If you look at the grouped frequency tables carefully, you will note that there is one new column, labeled "*m*." The new column represents the *m*idpoint, or halfway point, of each interval, and I'll explain what it is in the next section.

Group Practice 2.2

1. Desdemona has a contract to do intelligence testing for a consortium of group homes for the mentally retarded. Here are the IQ scores that she obtained for the residents of the group homes:

30, 31, 32, 34, 30, 33, 45, 47, 56, 65, 42, 75, 56, 72, 60, 55, 48, 59, 69, 35, 42, 53, 66, 52, 38, 39, 47, 60, 55, 54, 49, 38, 31, 33, 56, 65, 64, 63, 53, 49, 51, 52, 45, 39, 74, 37, 55, 53, 47 and 39.

Make a grouped frequency distribution showing *m*, *f*, f_c, %, and $\%_c$ for these data. Use *i* = 5, and start the lowest interval at 30. *Be sure to save the grouped frequency distribution for use in a subsequent in-class group practice problem.* (I give the equation for calculating *m* a little later in the chapter. I'm confident that you can figure out how to do so now, even without the equation. But, if you want to peek, go ahead.)

DISCRETE VS. CONTINUOUS NUMBERS AND REAL VS. APPARENT LIMITS

Now that I've broached the topic of midpoints, it seems the appropriate time to think about numbers from a new perspective: discrete vs. continuous. This will lead us to an exploration of the difference between the real and the apparent limits for intervals.

In Chapter 1, we discussed measurement, assigning numbers to objects so that the number accurately reflects the underlying attribute being measured, and I explained the four levels of measurement: nominal, ordinal, interval, and ratio.

Now we are going to see that numbers can be categorized in another way: discrete and continuous. **Discrete numbers** answer the question "How many," have no in-between values, and are of the frequency or counting type. For example, think of *how many* people are in your family. The answer may be 2, or 3—or 4, or 11—but it can't be fractional, like 3.5 people or 4.67 people.*

Continuous numbers answer the question "How much" and can have fractional, or "in-between" values. If I ask *how much* height you have (OK, most people phrase that as "How tall are you?"), your answer very well may be fractional, like 5 feet, 11½ inches tall.†

discrete numbers

Numbers that have no fractional values and answer the question "How many?"

continuous numbers

Numbers that may have fractional values; their accuracy depends on the precision of the measuring instrument. They address the question "How much?"

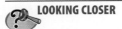 **LOOKING CLOSER**

---

*Discrete numbers aren't fractional and don't have decimal places, but when math is done to discrete numbers, for example when finding the average number of children per family, we can end up with a fractional number.

†See footnote on page 53.

Discrete vs. Continuous Numbers and Real vs. Apparent Limits

53

With continuous numbers, the precision of measurement depends on the accuracy of the measuring instrument. If you measure your height using a ruler marked in inches, then you can report your height only to the nearest inch. If you use a ruler marked to the nearest half inch, then you can report your height to the nearest half inch. Theoretically, there is no limit to how precise a ruler can be, so we can never know your *exact* height. Using a ruler marked to hundredths of an inch, you might measure your height as 67.53 inches, but this doesn't mean that your height is exactly 67.53000000000000000000000 inches. If you had an even more precise ruler, we might discover that your height was really 67.5304 inches.[‡]

With continuous numbers we don't get exact answers to the question of how much, because there can always be a more precise measuring instrument. And much of the data that statisticians analyze is of the "how much" type, such as how much cholesterol a person has, how much intelligence a student has, or how much money a person is willing to invest in the stock market.[§]

Imagine a digital scale that was recently calibrated and is accurate. Skip weighs himself on it. The scale reports that Skip weighs 175 pounds. Buffy comes up next, and the readout says 123 pounds; next, Desdemona weighs in at 145 and then Clothilde at 128. In fact, whenever a person steps on the scale, the readout is an integer value reporting a person's

---

LOOKING CLOSER

(Continued) [†] I'm playing with phrasing here. I could just as easily phrase my question about height as "How many inches tall are you?" which would suggest that inches were a discrete form of numbers. Though "how many" vs. "how much" is a handy way to think about discrete vs. continuous numbers, it can be manipulated for continuous numbers. It can't be manipulated for discrete numbers, i.e., I can't sensibly rephrase the question about how many people are in your family as a how much question.

The bottom-line differentiation between the two comes down to whether the unit of measurement can be subdivided. Inches can be subdivided into fractions of inches, and so inches represent continuous numbers. People, as in how many people are in your family, can't be subdivided into fractional people and so represent discrete numbers.

[‡] If you want a real-life example of increasing accuracy of measurement, look at the Olympic Games. When the modern Olympics started in 1896, timing events to the nearest tenth of a second was adequate. For example, Thomas Burke took first place in the 1896 100-meter run with a time of 12.0 seconds. In 1968, as competition and timing ability improved, events were timed to the nearest hundredth of a second, and Jim Hines came in first place with a time of 9.95 seconds. There are two Olympic events where the competition is so fierce, and the margin of victory so slim, that they are timed to the thousandth of a second: luge and short-track speedskating.

[§] I've been avoiding this issue, but I guess I better deal with it before we move on: what is the relationship between NOIR and continuous/discrete numbers? One can't simply parse one into the other. One can't say, for instance, that all ratio numbers are continuous. Population, for example, is both a ratio number and a discrete number. That said, it is safe to say that nominal level numbers, which measure qualities, are discrete numbers and interval/ratio level numbers are often (but not always!) continuous numbers. Ordinal level numbers are often, but not always, discrete.

weight to the nearest pound. Another way of saying this is to say that the unit of measurement for this scale is 1 pound.

My question for you, then, is how much does Skip *really* weigh? Does he weigh exactly 175 pounds? Don't forget, weight is a continuous variable, and so the precision of the measured value is limited by the precision of the measuring device. If we had a more precise scale, one that measured to the tenth of a pound, might we not learn that Skip weighs 175.3 pounds? And with a more precise scale, could his weight be 175.33 pounds?

It turns out that the best we can do is report the *interval* within which Skip's weight falls. The scale rounds Skip's weight to the nearest full pound. If Skip weighed 174.3, then the scale would report his weight as 174. If Skip weighed 174.8, it would report his weight as 175.

The question is, what are the bounds to the interval? The answer is that the interval falls from half a unit of measurement below the reported value to half a unit of measurement above the reported value. In this case the unit of measurement is 1 pound, so half a unit of measurement is .5 pounds. And, as the reported value for Skip's weight is 175, we can say that Skip's *real* weight falls in the range, or the interval, from 174.5 to 175.5. The formula for this is shown later in Equation 2.3.

The width of the interval depends on the unit of measurement. In Chapter 1 a group-practice exercise involved rank-ordering the 10 wealthiest Americans. The 10, and their personal fortunes, were Bill Gates, $46.0 billion; Warren Buffett, $36.0 billion; Paul Allen, $22.0 billion; Alice Walton, $20.5 billion; Helen Walton, $20.5 billion; John Walton, $20.5 billion; Robson Walton, $20.5 billion;, Jim Walton, $20.5 billion; Lawrence Ellison, $18.0 billion; and Michael Dell, $13.0 billion. How much money did Bill Gates really have in 2003? Was it exactly $46 billion (i.e., $46,000,000,000.00)? I doubt that he had $46 billion to the penny, so what is the interval within which his personal fortune falls?

Well, if you look at the fortunes for these 10 people you'll note that each ends with either a ".0" or a ".5." Apparently the yardstick used by *Forbes* to measure fortunes for the wealthiest Americans measures to the nearest half-billion dollars. In our terminology, then, the unit of measurement is .5 billion. Half of the unit of measurement is .25 billion, so Bill Gates' personal fortune was somewhere between $45.75 and $46.25 billion. (If his personal fortune were higher than $46.25 billion, say $46.27 billion, then Forbes would have reported it as $46.5 billion.)

The idea of an interval within which the "real" value falls can apply to discrete numbers in some situations. Table 1.5 in Chapter 1 listed the populations for the 10 largest cities in Pennsylvania. Population is a discrete number, but if you go back and look at that table, you'll notice something interesting, that the last two integers for each city were always zeroes, i.e., the populations of these cities were measured to the nearest 100 people. Thus, if I report that Erie has 103,900 people, does Erie have exactly 103,900 people? That seems unlikely. Applying the half-unit-of-measurement principle, we can conclude that the true population of Erie lies somewhere in the interval from 103,850 to 103,950.

We have been talking about the interval within which a score really falls when reporting individual scores. But, the concept applies to intervals used in grouped frequency distributions as well. Table 2.6 shows a grouped frequency distribution ($i = 10$) for the final grades for a random sample of 60 introductory statistics students. Let's focus on the bottom interval, which in the table has a lower limit of 20 and an upper limit of 29. These limits are called the **apparent limits,** or the **apparent lower limit** and **apparent upper limit,** because it only *appears* that these values bound the interval. The **real limits** for the interval are 19.5 (the **real lower limit,** or *RLL*) and 29.5 (the **real upper limit,** or *RUL*). Equation 2.3 shows how to calculate the real limits for an interval or for an individual score.

apparent limits

The range of values within which a score appears to fall.

real limits

The range of values within which a score actually falls.

F O R M U L A

Real Limits for an Interval (or for an individual score)

Equation 2.3

$$RLL = ALL - \frac{Unit\ of\ measurement}{2}$$

$$RUL = AUL + \frac{Unit\ of\ measurement}{2}$$

Where:

RLL = the real lower limit for an interval (or for an individual score)

ALL = the apparent lower limit for an interval (or the reported value for a score)

Unit of measurement = the smallest unit of measurement to which scores are reported/measured

RUL = the real upper limit for an interval (or for an individual score)

AUL = the apparent upper limit for an interval (or the reported value for a score)

Let's use Equation 2.3. We already know the apparent limits for the interval, 20 to 29; now we need to figure out the unit of measurement. The unit of measurement for the raw data was 1. How do I know this? Well, I could either go back to Table 2.4 to see the raw data, or I could figure it out from Table 2.6. In Table 2.6, notice that the interval is listed as running from 20 to 29 and the next interval from 30 to 39. The distance from the apparent lower limit of one interval (in this case 30) to the apparent upper limit of the next lower interval (in this case 29) is the unit of measurement: $30 - 29 = 1$. Half of a unit of measurement is .5, and I subtract this from the apparent lower limit and add it to the apparent upper limit to find the real limits of 19.5 to 29.5.

For the interval from 20 to 29 and with a unit of measurement of 1, a value of 20 represents a score that could be as low as 19.5 or as high as 20.5. A value of 29 represents a score in the range from 28.5 to 29.5. Thus, the interval 20 to 29 represents scores that could be as low as 19.5 or as high as 29.5, so the real limits of the interval are 19.5 and 29.5.

The next interval is 30 to 39, and the real lower limit of this interval (29.5) is the same as the real upper limit (29.5) of the interval (20 to 29) below it. I regularly have a small number of students who, having been taught that intervals should not overlap, are bothered that the real upper limit of one interval is the same as the real lower limit of the interval above it. Practically, this is not a problem because of the imprecision of our measuring instruments. Imagine a 100-question multiple-choice test on which each question is weighted equally so that scores on the test can range as integer values from 0% to 100%. Thinking of this as a continuous measure (i.e., it would be possible to design a more precise test) means that the "true" score of a person who scores 75% is really in the range from 74.5% to 75.5%, while the true score of a person who scores 76% is really in the range from 75.5% to 76.5%. Is it a problem that the *RUL* of one interval is the *RLL* of the interval above? No. It is not a problem because we are never faced with the decision of putting a person with a score of 75.5% into one interval or the other. Given the nature of this test—it has 100 questions—it is impossible to obtain a score of 75.5%. One can get a 75% or a 76%, but not a 75.5%. Thus, the point separating two intervals is at a level of specificity that is greater than the precision of the measuring instrument.

Note that when using the real limits, the interval width now makes sense. The interval width, *i*, is 10. When one subtracts 20 (the apparent lower limit) from 29 (the apparent upper limit) one obtains a value of 9, not 10. However, when one subtracts 19.5 from 29.5, the real limits, one obtains a value of 10, which is consistent with $i = 10$. All is right with the world.

We use the real limits to calculate the **midpoint** of an interval. The midpoint, *m*, for the interval 20 to 29 is the halfway point for the interval, 24.5. This is calculated by the following formula, which finds the average of the real limits for an interval:

midpoint

The value halfway between the real limits of an interval.

FORMULA

Midpoint (*m*) of an Interval in a Grouped Frequency Distribution

Equation 2.4

$$m = \frac{RLL + RUL}{2}$$

Where:
  m = the midpoint of the interval
  RLL = the real lower limit for the interval
  RUL = the real upper limit for the interval

Equation 2.4 says to add together the real upper and lower limits and then divide this sum by two. For the 20 to 29 interval, we would calculate $\frac{19.5 + 29.5}{2} = 24.5$. That is the official formula. But, practically, you obtain the same result by substituting the apparent limits for the real limits as in $\frac{20 + 29}{2} = 24.5$.

If you know the midpoint but not the real limits, the midpoint provides an easy way to figure out the real limits for an interval. The real lower limit is the midpoint minus half of the interval width. The real upper limit is the midpoint plus half of the interval width. This is calculated by the following formula:

F O R M U L A

Real Limits of an Interval

Equation 2.5

$$Real\ Limits = m \pm \frac{i}{2}$$

Where:
m = the midpoint of the interval
i = the interval width

Using this formula with the midpoint of 24.5 and an interval width of 10, we would calculate $24.5 \pm \frac{10}{2}$, yielding real limits ranging from 19.5 to 29.5.

Finally, here is another quick way to figure out real limits. If one interval runs from 20 to 29 and the next interval runs from 30 to 39, then the real upper limit of the first interval and the real lower limit of the second interval are halfway between the apparent upper limit of the first and the apparent lower limit of the second. In this case the value is 29.5, which is halfway between 29 and 30. You can then add and subtract the interval width to find the rest of the real limits. In this case, if 29.5 is the real upper limit of the 20 to 29 interval and if $i = 10$, then the real lower limit of the interval is 19.5 (i.e., 29.5 − 10). To calculate the real upper limit of the 30 to 39 interval (remember, we already know the real lower limit is 29.5), simply add i to the lower limit. In this example, that makes the real upper limit of the 30 to 39 interval 39.5.

Why have I spent so much time on real limits and midpoints? For two reasons. First, midpoints are useful. If for some reason we need to assign scores to cases in an interval, the convention is to assign them the value associated with the interval midpoint since doing so minimizes errors. For example, in the 20 to 29 interval there was only one case. If Table 2.6 were all we had to go by, we wouldn't know if that person had a score of 20 or 21 or 22, and so on. So, what score should we consider this person to have? If the person really had a score of 20 and we assign the person a score of 29, we make an 8-point error. By assigning the midpoint, we guarantee that we never make an error of more than half the interval width. In this instance, if the person really has a score of 20 and we assign a score of 24.5, we are in error, but only by 4.5 points, not by 8.

The second reason real limits and midpoints are so important will become apparent when we move to graphs. Some graphs (e.g., histograms) make use of real limits, and others (e.g., frequency polygons) make use of midpoints.

Finally, I want to point out—again—that real limits apply to continuous data. Continuous numbers can always be made more specific by developing a more finely grained measuring instrument, so real limits are always applicable. But, with discrete numbers, numbers without in-between values, real limits don't apply. For example, suppose we count the numbers of people in classrooms and use a unit of measurement of one. People is a discrete number; there is no such thing as a half person. So, if one classroom has 17 people in it, we don't say that the classroom has from 16.5 to 17.5 people. That would be silly.

Group Practice 2.3

1. Listed below are five sets of intervals as might be found in a grouped frequency distribution for continuous data. What are the real upper and lower limits for the last interval (the one in **bold**) in each set?

	RLL	RUL
a. 1-5; **6-10**	___	___
b. .5-.99; **1.00-1.49**	___	___
c. 10-20; **30-40**	___	___
d. .045-.049; **.050-.054**	___	___
e. 0-9000; **10,000-19,000**	___	___

2. For each scenario that follows, decide whether the variable is continuous or discrete:
   a. Temperature of humans, measured in Fahrenheit with an oral thermometer
   b. Number of books on students' desks
   c. Number of pairs of jeans in people's closets
   d. Amount of water, measured in gallons, used by a household, per week, in doing laundry
   e. Number of sheets of 8.5 × 11 paper used in a specific printer in a computer lab, per day
   f. Number of characters (letters and/or numbers) printed on the first page of novels

TABLES, PART II

After our excursion into the intervals within which scores really fall, it is time to finish talking about making tables. So far I haven't addressed the relationship between the level of measurement of the variable and the type of table you choose to make. The two types of tables we've discussed, ungrouped and grouped frequency distributions, are appropriate for use with interval- and ratio-level data.

Nominal-level data present no great problem in making a table. With nominal data there is no numerical order to the data, so it doesn't matter which category comes first. In such an instance, it is reasonable to array the categories in alphabetical order or ascending/descending order, unless there is some other logical approach. For example, suppose a clinical psychologist kept track of the different problems that her clients told her about at their first visit, their presenting problems. She had 32 clients who complained of depression, 34 with anxiety, 31 with marital problems, 28 with alcohol problems, and 47 who fell into the category of "other." The most reasonable thing to do with these data in a table is to report frequency and percentage. It doesn't make sense to report cumulative frequency, since there is no order to the data. Though it would be possible to combine some categories (66 clients had either depression or anxiety) this wouldn't really be a grouped frequency distribution, so the concept of an interval midpoint is meaningless here. Table 2.8 shows how a table would look with these data.*

With ordinal data, the order of categories is relevant, so you can report cumulative frequencies and percentages. For example, the class standing (1 = first year, 2 = sophomore, 3 = junior, 4 = senior) of all the people declared as psychology majors at a school provides ordinal data as displayed in Table 2.9. Note that although cumulative frequencies and percentages make sense and we could combine categories if we chose, the idea of an interval midpoint is nonsensical.

TABLE **2.8** **Frequency Table for Presenting Problems of Clients ($N = 172$) Seen by a Clinical Psychologist**

Problem	f	%
Alcohol	28	16.28
Marital	31	18.02
Depression	32	18.60
Anxiety	34	19.77
Other	47	27.33

Note: N = number; f = frequency; % = percentage

TABLE **2.9** **Class Standing of Psychology Majors**

Class	f	f_c	%	$\%_c$
Senior	43	110	39.09	100.00
Junior	37	67	33.64	60.91
Sophomore	22	30	20.00	27.27
First year	8	8	7.27	7.27

Note: f = frequency; f_c = cumulative frequency; % = percentage; $\%_c$ = cumulative percentage

---

Group Practice 2.4

Save your answers to these questions for use in another group practice.

1. A religion professor at a large and cosmopolitan university in the United States takes a sample of students and asks them their religious faith. He codes Muslims as "M," Buddhists as "B," Hindus as "H," Christians as "C," Jews as "J," other faiths as "O," and atheists as "A." Below are his data. Make a table.

B, C, A, J, J, M, M, J, C, C, O, A, C, C, B, H, J, C, J, C, O, O, J, C, M, C, C, M, B, J, M, O, J, A, M, H, M, C, C, A, O, B, M, O, J, C, C, A, C, M, C, A, J

2. A college administrator conducts an exit survey of students as they are graduating. She asks the students the extent to which they were satisfied with their college experience. She codes their answers as follows: "extremely" as a 1, "considerably" as a 2, "moderately" as a 3, "slightly" as a 4, and "not at all" as a 5. Below are the data. Make a table.

1, 2, 3, 1, 1, 2, 3, 4, 5, 3, 4, 3, 2, 1, 2, 3, 1, 2, 3, 4, 2, 2, 3, 1, 1, 2, 3, 2, 1, 4, 5, 2, 2, 4, 3, 4, 2, 3, 1, 1, 4, 5, 5, 3, 2, 2, 1, 3, 4, 4, 3, 2, 2, 2, 1, 4, 5, 3, 2, 4, 1, 3, 2, 1, 2, 3, 4, 2, 1

---

*Note that, since I have no cumulative frequency column, I include the sample size in the title. It is always a good idea clearly to present information about the number of cases in a table.

LOOKING CLOSER

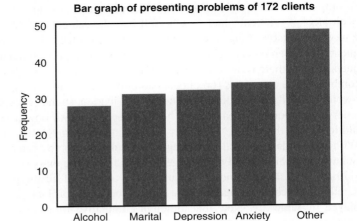

Figure **2.1** Bar graph for nominal data.

FIGURES AND GRAPHS

"One picture is worth a thousand words" is as true in statistics as in other areas. The pictures that statisticians make are called "graphs" or "figures," and we will see how to make a variety of them from the tables we made above.* The advantage of a figure over a table is that information in a figure is often easier to see. Sometimes things that leap out of a figure are not as evident in a table, even though they are present. For example, Table 2.8 shows the distribution of presenting problems for 172 clients seen by a therapist. The same information, in the form of a bar graph, is given in Figure 2.1.

When I see this figure, a few things leap out at me. First of all, the largest category is "other." Though the same information is presented in the table, it is not so apparent there. (At least it isn't to me.) In fact, the first time I saw this figure I went back to the table to see if "other" really was the category with the greatest frequency. The other thing that is apparent in this figure is that the numbers of clients with presenting problems in the other four areas are all very similar. Yes, this information is also evident in the table, but one has to dig a little harder, think a little more, to pull it out.

LOOKING CLOSER

*The American Psychological Association, whose 2001 Publication Manual is the guide for many researchers, differentiates between tables and figures. A table contains only text, whether it is numbers or words, and is typeset. A figure is any type of illustration other than a table and is photographed not typeset. Thus, a figure may be a graph, a drawing, a photograph, or any other non-typeset illustration. "Figure" is a more general term than "graph."

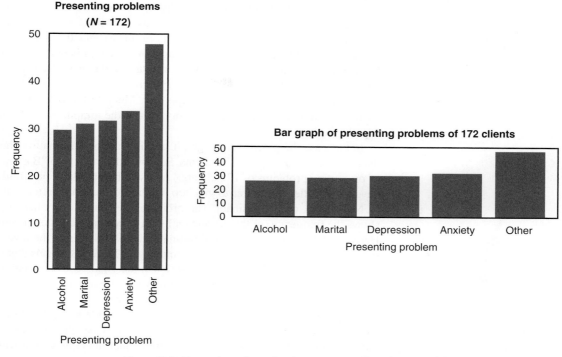

Figure **2.2** Examples of graphs that are too tall and too wide.

The first figure we'll learn to make is the bar graph, which is used for discrete data. We'll then move to the histogram and the frequency polygon for continuous data. Finally, we'll learn about the stem-and-leaf display, an interesting combination of a table and a figure that allows you to see the forest while preserving all the trees. Along the way, we'll discuss the "shape" of a set of data, something that will have a lot of relevance in subsequent chapters.

Bar graphs illustrate discrete data, most commonly nominal and ordinal data. Each bar in the graph represents a different category and the height of the bar represents the frequency with which that category occurs. Because each category is discrete, the bars don't touch each other. (With histograms, for continuous data, the bars touch each other.) In Figure 2.1, for example, the categories are the different presenting problems (e.g., depression and anxiety).

The convention is to make graphs wider than they are tall. There is no official formula for this, but ancient Greek mathematicians considered that certain rectangles, what they called "golden rectangles," had the most pleasing shape. The ratio of width to height for a golden rectangle is approximately 1.6, so aim for that. (A 3 × 5 card, for example, is close to a golden rectangle with a ratio of 1.7, calculated by dividing the width [5] by the height [3].) The graphs in Figure 2.2 violate the golden ratio.

bar graph

A type of graph used to display the frequency distribution for discrete data.

Making a graph is not hard, especially if you work from a table where the tabulation has already been done and use graph (crosshatch) paper. First, draw the lines for the Y axis (the ordinate) and the X axis (the abscissa), remembering to make the graph wider than it is tall. And don't forget the three most important words for figures and tables, "Label, label, label." Be sure to label everything. Everything!

The first label to create is the graph title. Mention the type of graph, clearly communicate what information is in the graph, and tell the sample size.

In this case the graph is a bar graph, and it contains information about the presenting problems of 172 clients. So, I've titled my graph "Bar graph of presenting problems of 172 clients." As I said before, don't be afraid to have a long title. It is better to give too much information than too little.

Next, work on the ordinate. The ordinate, the Y axis, for a bar graph shows the frequency (or the percentage) with which each category occurs. Here, I'll label the bottom of the ordinate, the part that is at the level of the X axis, with the lowest possible frequency, 0. Table 2.8 reveals that the highest frequency is 47. I need to ensure that the Y axis goes high enough to accommodate a frequency of 47 and leave a little room at the top so it looks good. So, I select 50 as my highest frequency.*

Frequencies are marked on the Y axis. It is possible to mark off every single frequency (1, 2, 3, 4, …) but that would make the ordinate too crowded. I chose to divide the ordinate into equal intervals with a width of 10, but that is not mandatory. If you think frequency intervals of two or five or 20 work better, use them. Just don't forget to label your frequency markings.

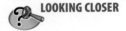 **LOOKING CLOSER**

*It would be possible to select a much higher number, say 1000, for the highest frequency. Do this and note what it does to the bar graph—it makes it very hard to notice any differences in frequency between the five categories, and it makes it look like very few people fit into any of the five categories.

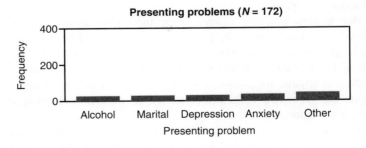

Benjamin Disraeli, an English politician, once said, "There are three kinds of lies: lies, damned lies, and statistics." It is easy to manipulate graphs in order to misdirect the reader. For a good primer on this, I recommend *How to Lie With Statistics,* by Darrell Huff. It came out a year before I was born, has been reprinted ever since, and has sold over a half million copies. Last I checked, its Amazon sales rank was 2600! Get a copy. By knowing what not to do, one learns how to do something correctly.

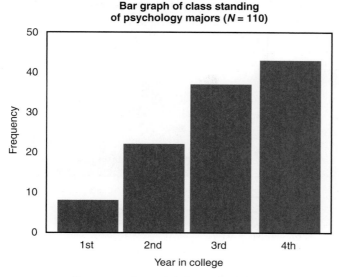

**Bar graph of class standing
of psychology majors (*N* = 110)**

Figure **2.3** Bar graph for ordinal data.

Next turn to the abscissa, the *X* axis. For a bar graph, you need to note the number of different categories (in this case, five) and then divide the *X* axis into that many sections. Remember, this is a bar graph with discrete categories, so the bars should not touch each other since touching implies continuous measurement. Be sure to put the categories in some logical order, perhaps alphabetical or ascending/descending order of frequency. Finally, draw the bars so that the height of each bar represents the frequency for that category. And, once you've labeled the bars, you are done.

As I mentioned, bar graphs display discrete data. Figure 2.3 is an example of a bar graph for the ordinal data of class standing of psychology majors presented in Table 2.9. Note that there is an order to the data (from first-year students to seniors) and that the lowest rank (first-year status) is the initial category.

Our next graph, the **histogram,** is similar to the bar graph but displays continuous data. Functionally, this means that it is commonly used with interval- or ratio-level data. Because the data intervals lie on a continuum, neighboring bars touch each other. For our example, let's use the data about final grades in statistics from Table 2.6. The lowest interval is 20 to 29 and the interval above it is 30-39; the *real* limits for these intervals are 19.5 to 29.5 and 29.5 to 39.5. Two things follow from this and can be seen in Figure 2.4: (1) the two intervals touch at 29.5, so the bars for these two intervals will touch each other; (2) the bars for histograms go up at the real lower limit of the interval and come down at the real upper limit of the interval.

Please note that I followed the graphing rules outlined for the bar graph: I made the graph wider than tall, and I labeled everything. In

histogram

A graph that uses bars to display the frequency distribution for a continuous variable.

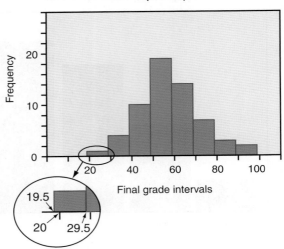

Figure **2.4** Histogram for interval-level data.

Figure 2.4, I marked off the abscissa every 10 points so that it would be clear that the boxes went up and came down at the real limits of the interval, not the apparent limits. There are a couple of other possibilities for labeling the abscissa, either marking it off by intervals or marking the midpoints of the intervals. These are shown in Figure 2.5. Which one you use depends on your aesthetic sense and the clarity with which your choice gets your point across.

The last graph that we are going to learn about is the **frequency polygon,** more commonly known as a line graph. This is another way to display the frequencies of different intervals of values for a continuous variable.

To make a frequency polygon (Figure 2.6), follow the same format as for a histogram or a bar graph. First, construct the axes, and then mark the ordinate for frequencies. On the abscissa, mark the *midpoint* for each interval. Also, be sure to mark one midpoint below the lowest interval and one midpoint above the highest interval. Using the statistics grade data from Table 2.6 as our example, there is a midpoint of 14.5 below the lowest midpoint of 24.5 and a midpoint of 104.5 above the highest midpoint of 94.5. Then, at each midpoint marker put a dot at the correct height to indicate the frequency. At the very lowest (14.5) midpoint and the very highest (104.5) midpoint, put a dot on the abscissa to indicate a frequency of 0. To finish the graph, connect the dots.*

frequency polygon

A graph, commonly referred to as a line graph, that displays the frequency distribution for a continuous variable.

LOOKING CLOSER

*These are the directions for a "classic" frequency polygon. You will frequently see frequency polygons that don't "go to zero" at the midpoints below and above the lowest and the highest midpoints with nonzero frequencies.

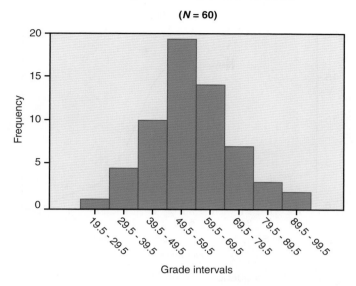

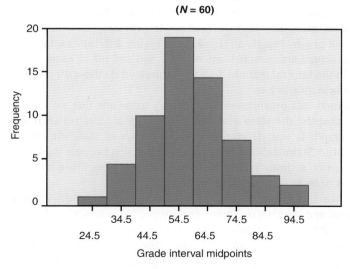

Figure **2.5** Examples of different formats for histogram abscissae.

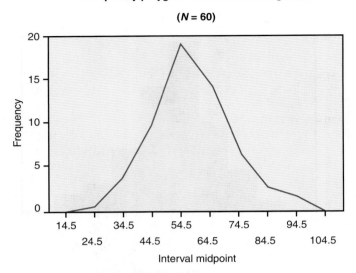

Figure **2.6** Frequency polygon for interval-level data.

stem-and-leaf display

A combination table and graph used to summarize data without losing detail.

A grouped frequency distribution or a graph made from a grouped frequency distribution provides an overview of a set of data. As is often the case, a strength is also a weakness. In providing an overview, these tables and graphs lose detail. Looking at Figure 2.6, for example, we see that the scores are centered around 54.5 and tail off to each side. But, where in the interval that has 54.5 for a midpoint do those 19 people fall? That information is lost.

The final data organization or summary technique that we shall cover in this chapter, the **stem-and-leaf display,** is a cross between a table and a graph. It was developed to reduce a set of data without losing specificity.* Stem-and-leaf displays are called that because they are a bit like a tree or a shrub, having different stems or branches with different numbers of leaves on each stem or branch.

It is harder to describe how to make a stem-and-leaf display than to show one, and showing one gives a pretty good idea how to make one. So, in Figure 2.7 I show a stem-and-leaf display for the statistics grades data.

9	25
8	234
7	0145566
6	01222235678999
5	0011112556778888999
4	0114556788
3	0034
2	8

Figure **2.7** Stem-and-leaf display for final grades in statistics ($N = 60$).

As you can see in Figure 2.7, the stems, which are the bold numbers, are the tens-column digits for the final grades. The leaves are the ones-column digits. For example, the lowest score is a 28, and that is seen in the bottom line. The next line up shows the four people whose final

LOOKING CLOSER

*John W. Tukey introduced stem-and-leaf displays in *Exploratory Data Analysis* (1977).

scores are in the 30s. They are placed in the line in order from low to high, making it apparent that two people have scores of 30, one has a score of 33, and one has a score of 34. Thus, the stem-and-leaf display contains all the details present in the original set of scores back in Table 2.5.

However, this is a condensed version of Table 2.5. In fact, it is similar to Table 2.6, the grouped frequency distribution version of Table 2.5, although in Figure 2.7 it is a graphical display as well as a tabular one. As a graphical display we gain all the advantages of a picture (it is readily apparent that most students get scores from 40 to 69). Yet owing to the use of numbers for leaves rather than Xs, we maintain all the details from the original data set. Stem-and-leaf displays don't require graph paper and are a wonderful way to boil down a data set. They allow you to have your cake and eat it too, so take advantage of them.

Before we turn to the final topic in this chapter, the shapes of frequency distributions, I want to discuss when to use a table and when to use a graph. Edward Tufte,* a graphic designer, recommends using a sentence if one is presenting only one or two numbers, tables when one has more data or wants to present exact numerical values, and graphical figures to give context and interpretation to numbers. Because tables provide more exact information, allowing a person to construct his or her own figure, Tufte* recommends tables over figures. Use figures or graphs, he says, to highlight relationships.

As Tufte (1983, p. 177)* says, visual displays of statistical information "often have a narrative quality, a story to tell about the data." Whether making a table or a figure, be aware that the table or figure may end up standing on its own, separate from whatever text went with it: so make it as self-contained as possible. As I've already stressed, spill some ink on the title and headings—make sure that they convey sufficient information. Finally, don't overwhelm the reader with excessive or obsessive detail. Unless you are making a table to present very exact values, which is sometimes done, use as few decimal places as possible.

Group Practice 2.5

Save these answers for use in another group practice!

1. Take the Desdemona IQ data from the grouped frequency distribution you made in Group Practice 2.2 and make (a) a histogram, (b) a frequency polygon, and (c) a stem-and-leaf display.

2. Make a graph for the religion data from question 1 of Group Practice 2.4.

3. Make a graph for the satisfaction data from question of Group Practice 2.4.

---

*Tufte's 1983 book, *The Visual Display of Quantitative Information* is a gem. One of the reasons that I like Tufte is that he hates pie charts, calling them—and this is a direct quote—"dumb." (Tufte, E. R. [1977]. *The visual display of quantitative information*. Cheshire, CT: Graphics Press.)

LOOKING CLOSER

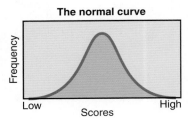

Figure **2.8** Frequency polygon for the normal distribution.

SHAPES OF FREQUENCY DISTRIBUTIONS

The last topic in this chapter involves the shapes of distributions. This is as important as level of measurement and for the same reason: just as it is inappropriate to do interval- or ratio-level analyses on an ordinal-level variable, there are certain statistics that can't be used with certain shapes of distributions.

The normal distribution or normal curve (commonly called the bell-shaped curve) gives the greatest flexibility in terms of the analyses that can be done. This distribution, shown in Figure 2.8, is symmetric and has most scores piled near the middle, with the rest of the scores tailing off to each side. Symmetric means that there is a midpoint to the figure that, if used as a hinge to fold one side over the other, would yield two identical images. In Figure 2.8 you can see that, just as with the statistics grade data shown in Figure 2.6, most cases fall near the middle of the distribution, and the frequencies decrease as the scores get more extreme.*

The normal distribution, as we shall see in Chapter 5 and beyond, has some properties that make it very useful in statistics. However, a lot of frequency distributions of data are not normally distributed. Some of the ways distributions may differ from a normal distribution are in terms of skewness, kurtosis, and modality.

Skewness relates to the symmetry of a frequency distribution. A frequency distribution that tails off to one side is said to be skewed. It is possible for a frequency distribution to tail off to the right (Figure 2.9, *A*), in which case the skewness is called **positive skewness.** A frequency distribution of annual income is an example of positive skew. Most people have annual incomes of a $100,000 or less, but a small number of people have annual incomes in the millions or hundreds of millions

skewness

Relating to the symmetry of a distribution.

positive skewness

The property of a distribution tailing off to the right.

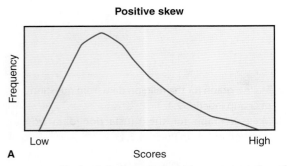

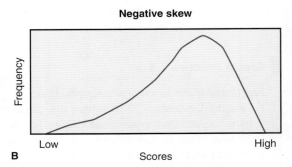

Figure **2.9** Frequency polygon examples of positive skewness (A) and negative skewness (B).

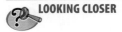 **LOOKING CLOSER**

*In the theoretical normal distribution the scores go on forever, reaching positive and negative infinity, and becoming less and less frequent as they go. This means that the curve goes on and on, never reaching a frequency of 0, never touching the abscissa.

of dollars. Figure 2.9, *B* shows **negative skewness,** a frequency distribution tailing off to the left. As an example of this, think of grades on an easy test. Most people will do well, so the scores will pile up on the high end of the scale. Still, a small number of people will do poorly, skewing the distribution down to the left. The term for scores that are far from the rest of the scores in a distribution of data is **outliers,** as in "these scores lie far out from the rest of the data." Outliers cause skewness.

Skewness can be calculated, and we'll discuss that in Chapter 6. But for now, know that a normal distribution has a skewness of zero, a negatively skewed distribution has skewness below zero, and a positively skewed distribution has a skewness above zero.

Kurtosis refers to how peaked or flat a frequency distribution is, or how much it bulges. There are terms for different types of kurtosis, and I'll mention them here, but I don't really expect you to remember them or use them in conversation. The normal curve is **mesokurtic,** a peaked distribution (Figure 2.10, *A*) is **leptokurtic,** and a flat distribution (Figure 2.10, *B*) is **platykurtic.*** Kurtosis, like skewness, can be measured, and I'll address that in Chapter 6 as well. A normal curve has kurtosis of zero, a distribution that is flatter than normal (a platykurtic distribution) has negative kurtosis, and a distribution more convex than normal (leptokurtic) has positive kurtosis.

Finally, **modality** refers to the number of clearly distinguishable high points or peaks in a distribution. Look at the normal distribution in Figure 2.8, and note that there is only one high point in the graph. This is called

negative skewness

The property of a distribution tailing off to the left.

outlier

A score far removed from the other scores.

kurtosis

Relating to the peakedness or flatness of a distribution.

mesokurtic

Having a kurtosis such as that of a normal distribution.

leptokurtic

Having a peaked distribution.

platykurtic

Having a flat distribution.

modality

Referring to the number of clearly distinguishable peaks in a distribution.

Leptokurtic frequency distribution

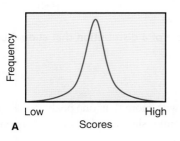

A

Platykurtic frequency distribution

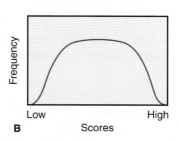

B

Figure **2.10** Frequency polygon examples of a peaked, or leptokurtic, distribution (A) and a flat, or platykurtic, distribution (B).

*Curious about what these odd words mean? "Kurtosis" comes from the Greek word *kyrtos*, meaning convex. "Platykurtic" is a combination of that word with the Greek word *platys*, which means broad or flat. Our word "plate" comes from *platys*. "Leptokurtic" is derived by adding the Greek word for thin, *leptos*, to *kyrtos*. Thus, something that is platykurtic has a broad or flat distribution and something that is leptokurtic has a tall, thin distribution. "Mesokurtic" comes from adding the Greek word *mesos*, which means middle or mean, to *kyrtos*. Thus, a mesokurtic distribution is balanced between the extremes of leptokurtosis and platykurtosis.

LOOKING CLOSER

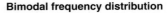

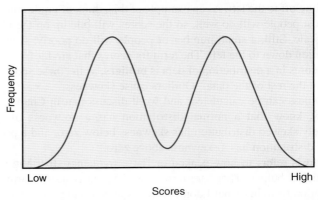

Figure **2.11** Frequency polygon example of a bimodal distribution.

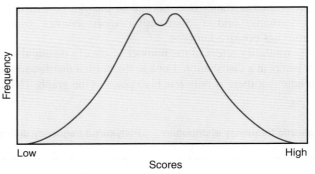

Figure **2.12** Frequency polygon example of a distribution that should be considered unimodal, not bimodal.

unimodal distribution

Having one peak.

multimodal distribution

Having more than one peak.

bimodal distribution

Having two peaks.

a **unimodal** distribution. Distributions with more than one peak are called **multimodal,** a relatively common example, shown in Figure 2.11, is one with two peaks and is called **bimodal.**

My experience with students just starting out in statistics is that they are quick to call a distribution multimodal when it really is unimodal. Please focus on the general shape of a distribution of data, and do not be swayed by a little gap between two neighboring high points. Figure 2.12 is an example of a distribution that, though it technically may be bimodal, is closer to a unimodal distribution.

Finally, before this chapter draws to a close, I want to mention one last fact about the normal distribution, a fact that will come into play in Chapter 5. The normal distribution is symmetric (i.e., is not skewed), is mesokurtic, and is unimodal. However, not all symmetric, mesokurtic, and unimodal distributions are normal distributions!

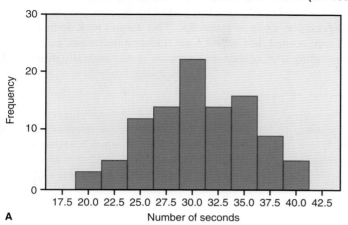

Number of seconds it takes for a match to burn down (*N* = 100)

A

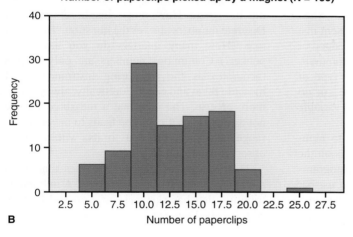

Number of paperclips picked up by a magnet (*N* = 100)

B

Figure **2.13** Histograms for two sets of data.

For now, I want to end the chapter with histograms for two sets of real data,* to make the point that normal distributions don't always look normal—that it can be hard to tell, from a graph, whether a set of data is normally distributed. Figure 2.13, *A* shows the number of seconds it takes for a match to burn and, though it does not look exactly like the theoretical normal distribution seen in Figure 2.8, it is not far off. Thus you will not

*I want to thank two of my students, Melissa Schmidt and Courtney Hopkins, who provided these two data sets.

LOOKING CLOSER

be surprised to learn that these data are normally distributed. Figure 2.13, *B* shows the number of paperclips picked up by a magnet on a string that was dropped into a pile of paperclips. This doesn't look normal to me but it is, in fact, normal. In Chapter 6 we'll learn a technique, more objective than eyeballing a set of data, to determine if it is normally distributed.

Group Practice 2.6

1. Describe the shape of the ungrouped frequency distribution you made in Group Practice 2.1.
2. Describe the shape of the IQ data you graphed in question 1 of Group Practice 2.5.
3. Describe the shape of the religion data you graphed in question 2 of Group Practice 2.5.
4. Describe the shape of the satisfaction data you graphed in question 3 of Group Practice 2.5.

SUMMARY

This chapter introduced ways to summarize a set of data with tables and graphs. Tables are useful when you have more data than is reasonable to present in a sentence. Tables can be constructed as ungrouped or grouped frequency distributions and for nominal-, ordinal-, interval-, or ratio-level data. The type of information presented in a table (f, f_c, %, %$_c$, or m) depends on the level of measurement of the variable and what you wish to communicate.

Figures give context and interpretation to numbers. The type of figure constructed depends on the type of data. For continuous numbers, use histograms and frequency polygons; for discrete numbers, use bar graphs. The stem-and-leaf display is a cross between a table and a figure. It both provides a summary overview and maintains all of the details present in a data set.

Continuous numbers answer the question "How much?" (e.g., How much height do you have?) Discrete numbers answer the question "How many?" (e.g., How many quarters do you have in your pocket?) Continuous numbers are only as precise (accurate) as the measuring instrument used to measure them and can, theoretically, always be made more precise. The idea that a measured number is not as precise as it could be leads to the concept of a range of values, the real limits, within which an observed value actually falls.

Distributions of data take shapes that differ in modality, symmetry, and convexity. A unimodal distribution that has skewness of zero and kurtosis of zero is called a normal distribution.

Review Exercises

1. The college registrar is asked to count the number of usable chairs in different classrooms at her university to determine how many students can be seated in each. At what level of measurement is the number of usable chairs? Is the number of usable chairs a discrete or a continuous variable?
2. These are numbers of usable chairs in the different classrooms:

7, 12, 26, 18, 20, 33, 34, 17, 120, 20, 35, 46, 50, 28, 29, 33, 18, 45, 53, 75, 30, 37, 45, 58, 43, 42, 10, 24, 28, 35, 36, 50, 60, 55, 45, 52, 54, 28, 24, 25, 35, 40, 45, 44, 40, 23, 28, 38, 39, 40, 50, 60,100, 45, 36, 28, 40, 54, 62, 44, 24, 28, 30, 60, 38, 58, and 24.

Make a stem-and-leaf display for these data. Comment on the shape of the data.

3. Make a grouped frequency distribution for the number of usable chairs data from question 2. Use $i = 10$ and start the lowest interval at 5. Be sure to include m, f_c, %, and $\%_c$.

4. Make a graph for the grouped frequency distribution you prepared for question 3. Comment on the shape of the graph. How does this compare to what you observed in the stem-and-leaf display in question 2?

5. What are the real limits of the highest and lowest intervals in the grouped frequency distribution you made for question 3?

6. A member of the National Highway Traffic Safety Administration is examining the relationship between the speed at which cars are traveling when accidents occur and the death rate from accidents. What is the predictor variable? The criterion variable? At what level of measurement is each measured?

7. An epidemiologist whose son is about to attend college is interested in learning more about the alcohol consumption of college students. He obtains a random sample of men from the college his son is planning to attend and measures how often they consume alcohol to excess. Based on these data he classifies the men as nonoverconsumers (0), 1 to 3 times a month overconsumers (1), 4 to 8 times a month overconsumers (2), more than twice a week but less than daily overconsumers (3), or daily overconsumers (4). At what level of measurement is he measuring alcohol consumption? He found 9 zeros, 18 ones, 41 twos, 63 threes, and 7 fours. Make a graph for these data.

8. The epidemiologist realizes that he may have oversimplified the picture of excessive alcohol consumption. Below are the raw data about how many days per month the men consumed alcohol to excess. Make a graph for these data and comment on the shape of the graph.

0, 0, 0, 0, 0, 0, 0, 0, 0, 1, 1, 1, 1, 1, 1, 1, 1, 1, 1, 1, 2, 2, 2, 2, 2, 2, 3, 3, 4, 4, 4, 4, 4, 4, 4, 4, 4, 4, 4, 4, 4, 5, 5, 6, 6, 6, 6, 7, 7, 7, 8, 8, 8, 8, 8, 8, 8, 8, 8, 8, 8, 8, 8, 8, 8, 8, 8, 8, 8, 9, 9, 9, 10, 10, 10, 10, 10, 10, 11, 11, 12, 15, 15, 15, 15, 15, 15, 15, 15, 15, 15, 15, 15, 15, 15, 15, 15, 15, 17, 18, 19, 19, 20, 20, 20, 20, 20, 20, 20, 20, 20, 20, 20, 20, 20, 21, 22, 22, 23, 23, 24, 24, 24, 25, 25, 25, 25, 26, 27, 28, 29, 29, 29, 30, 30, 30, 30, 30, 30, 30.

(Think about what you want your graph to communicate. Do you want to base it on an ungrouped or grouped frequency distribution?)

9. For each scenario, determine the real limits of the interval:

a. If a person's temperature is reported as 100.3, what is the range within which the person's temperature really falls?

b. If a family has seven children, what is the range within which the number of children really falls?

c. If a person's IQ is reported as 115, what is the range within which the person's IQ really falls?

d. If nations' populations are reported to the nearest million and the United States has a population of 300 million, how many people really live in the United States?

e. If a person has three televisions in her house, what is the range within which the number of televisions really falls?

Homework Problems

1. If the real limits and the apparent limits for an interval are the same, then the variable is which of the following?
   a. Continuous
   b. Discrete
   c. Interval
   d. Ratio
   e. Real and apparent limits are never the same.

2. For a row in the middle of a frequency distribution, either ungrouped or grouped, which statement is true?
   a. $f > f_c$
   b. $f_c > f$
   c. $f = f_c$
   d. None of these statements is ever true.

3. I have a grouped frequency distribution with five people in the interval ranging from 50 to 54. What X values should I assign them?
   a. I should use a random number table to select values from 50 to 54.
   b. Since there are five people and there are five integers from 50 through 54, I should assign values of 50, 51, 52, 53, and 54.
   c. 50
   d. 52
   e. 54

4. I have discrete data for which I want to make a figure. What figure should I make?
   a. A histogram
   b. A frequency polygon
   c. A bar graph
   d. An ungrouped frequency distribution
   e. A grouped frequency distribution

5. What is an advantage of a stem-and-leaf display?
   a. It does not require the calculation of mid-points.
   b. It is both visual and tabular.
   c. It shows the forest, not the trees.
   d. It can be used with discrete data.

6. How can the probable distribution of prices of new cars be described?
   a. Normally distributed
   b. Positively skewed
   c. Negatively skewed
   d. Not skewed

7. What scale of measurement do the following represent?
   a. A psychologist measures how physically fearful people are of spiders by measuring how close, in inches, they are willing to get to a very large and ugly (but nonpoisonous!) spider. If they actually touch the spider, the psychologist gives them a score of zero and concludes that they have no physical fear of spiders. Physical fear of spiders is being measured at what level of measurement?
   b. The same psychologist now wishes to develop a fear survey schedule. She makes a list of all the fears she can think of (e.g., spiders, snakes, and heights). When she is done, she has a list of 100 fears. People taking the fear survey can score from 0 (no fears on the list are endorsed) to 100 (all the fears are endorsed). Each fear is treated as equal; that is, a fear of paper cuts is considered equivalent to a fear of snakes. Fear is being measured at what level of measurement?
   c. The psychologist Jean Piaget classified children as being in four different stages of cognitive development. In his theory, a child has to progress through the stages in order. These are four stages (and the approximate ages in years during which a child is in the stage): sensorimotor (0-2), preoperational (2-7), concrete operations (7-11), and formal operations (11 and up). If the numbers 1, 2, 3, and 4 were assigned to the stages sensorimotor, preoperational, concrete operations, and formal operations, respectively, then Piaget's stages would be being measured at what level?

8. I survey a number of western states in the United States to find the rate of left-handedness in each and to see if and how they differ. The percentage of Hawaiians who are left-handed is 12%, Californians 8%, Utahans 3%, Alaskans 10%, Nevadans 7%, Arizonans 6%, and Idahoans 4%. First table and then graph these data. (Note that this question involves making a table that is not a frequency distribution and then making a graph from it. This is different from the material covered in the chapter, but I am confident that you will find a way to communicate what you want to communicate. So before you start, think about the point that you want to make.)

9. A public health researcher finds the number of cases of antibiotic-resistant staph infections reported in the 50 largest metropolitan areas in North America. Here are the numbers:

122, 97, 0, 34, 17, 2, 0, 4, 54, 23, 1, 18, 26, 84, 55, 4, 5, 12, 16, 19, 36, 23, 66, 3, 5, 7, 0, 4, 31, 28, 5, 71, 5, 21, 12, 34, 31, 28, 61, 72, 23, 36, 88, 43, 23, 17, 54, 32, 76, and 44.

Make a grouped frequency distribution for these data using $i = 10$ and starting the first interval at a value of 0. Be sure to report m, f_c, %, and %$_c$.

10. What are the real limits of the highest interval for the grouped frequency distribution you constructed in question 9?

11. A physician has developed a new treatment for people with nausea that lasts for more than 24 hours. He administers the treatment and then measures how many hours it takes before a person feels better. Here are the data he collects:

1, 2, 2, 3, 3, 5, 5, 5, 6, 6, 6, 7, 7, 7, 7, 7, 9, 9, 9, 10, 10, 10, 10, 10, 11, 11, 11, 11, 11, 11, 11, 12, 12, 12, 12, 12, 12, 13, 13, 13, 13, 13, 13, 14, 14, 14, 14, 14, 14, 14, 14, 14, 15, 15, 15, 15, 15, 16, 16, 16, 16, 16, 16, 16, 16, 17, 17, 17, 19, 19, 19, 20, 20, 21, 21, 22, 22, 22, 24, 28, 29, 31, 34, 37, 39, 40, 44, 50, and 56.

Make a graph showing, in 5-hour intervals and starting the lowest interval at 0, how long it takes for his patients to feel the effects of the medication. Comment on the shape of the graph.

12. Is the graph you constructed in question 11 an inferential or a descriptive statistic? Why?

13. Round the following to two decimal places:

a. .9876
b. .1234
c. .1235
d. .1253
e. .1250
f. .125005
g. .125001
h. .455
i. .544

14. A professor of education is curious about students' expectations of academic success. So, she obtains a sample of college students at the start of their college careers and asks what they think their GPAs will be for the first semester. Below are the data she obtains. Make a table using $i = .5$ and an apparent lower limit for the bottom interval of 2.1.

3.9, 4.0, 3.9, 3.0, 3.0, 3.5, 4.0, 4.0, 3.0, 3.5, 3.0, 3.5, 3.5, 3.9, 4.0, 3.0, 3.5, 3.5, 3.0, 3.9, 3.5, 2.5, 3.5, 3.8, 3.9, 3.0, 3.9, 3.5, 3.9, 3.0, 3.5, 3.9, 4.0, 3.5, 3.0, 2.5, 2.5, 3.1, 3.1, 2.9, 2.9, 2.6, 2.7, 3.8, 3.3, 3.4, 3.1, 2.9, 2.6, 3.6, 3.4, 3.3, 3.4, 3.2, 2.8, 2.4, 2.7, 2.6, 3.4, 3.6, 2.5, 3.8, 2.9, 2.6, 2.4, 2.4, 2.6, 2.5, 2.7, 2.7

3

Transformed Scores I

Percentile Ranks

Learning Objectives

After completing this chapter, you should be able to do the following:

1 See the utility of estimating answers before computing them.
2 Transform raw scores into percentile ranks and vice versa.

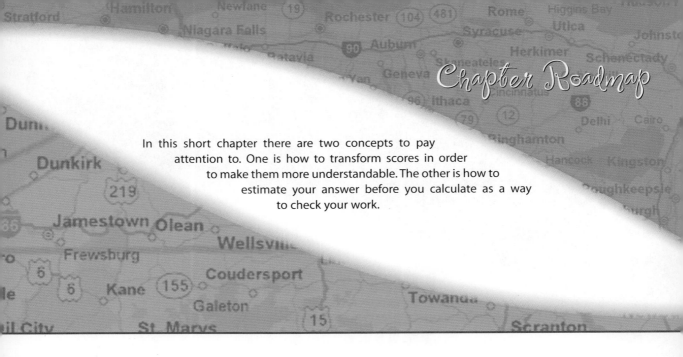

In this short chapter there are two concepts to pay attention to. One is how to transform scores in order to make them more understandable. The other is how to estimate your answer before you calculate as a way to check your work.

TRANSFORMING RAW SCORES

transforming

Changing a set of scores from one metric to another.

In the last chapter we used tables and graphs to describe a set of data. In this chapter we'll continue exploring descriptive statistics, this time **transforming** raw scores to make them easier to understand. Transforming a score from one metric to another may sound foreign to you, but it is something with which you are already familiar. If you are like most people in the United States, you will not have a good idea of what the temperature is outside if I say it is 22° Celsius. However, if I change the temperature from the metric of Celsius to the more familiar metric of Fahrenheit, if I *transform* it, you will discover that it is 72° (Fahrenheit, that is) and you don't need a coat to go outside.

To ease such transformations there are thermometers (see Figure 3.1) that have Fahrenheit on one side and Celsius on the other. Having both scales on one instrument allows us to see at a glance that if it is 50° Fahrenheit it is ≈10° Celsius or if it is 40° Celsius it is ≈100° Fahrenheit. With such a thermometer we can easily transform temperatures from one metric to another.

There are lots of different reasons to transform scores. In the last chapter we learned about the different shapes that sets of data can have, normal or otherwise, and I mentioned that there are advantages to having a data set with a normal distribution. One reason to transform a set of scores, then, is to change the shape of a set of data to make it normal.

Another reason, and the reason we focus on in this chapter, is to free the scores from their original context, to put them into a universal context that is easier to understand or interpret. In this chapter you will learn how to transform raw scores into percentile ranks, and percentile ranks back into raw scores.* In Chapter 5, after you've learned about means and standard deviations, we'll discuss another transformation: raw scores into standard scores.

Percentile ranks are similar to the cumulative percentage calculated for frequency distributions. A **percentile rank** for a score represents the percentage of cases in a specific set of cases scoring *at or below* that score. For example, a percentile rank of 80 represents performance near the top of a distribution of scores. If your score on a test, transformed into a percentile rank (*PR*) is an 80, you are in the top 20% of the people taking the test since your score is equal to or higher than 80% of the people taking the test. Similarly, a person with a *PR* of 10 is performing near the bottom of the distribution since he or she obtained a score equal to or higher than only 10% of the distribution.

Note that the definition of "percentile rank" includes comparison to a specific reference group. Knowing the reference group is very important because it determines how you interpret the percentile rank. In some situations, a percentile rank of 10 is very impressive, and in others it is cause for alarm. If I tell you that my height, in a frequency distribution of NBA basketball players, has a percentile rank of 10, you might conclude that I am a reasonably tall guy. However, if I tell you that my height, as a percentile rank, has a score of 10 in a frequency distribution of elementary school students, you'll conclude that I am quite short. Same percentile ranks, different reference groups, different conclusions: percentile ranks are scores put into a context. To be able to interpret those scores you must pay attention to the context, to the reference group used.

To understand how to convert raw scores to percentile ranks, let's start with a graphic example. In Table 3.1, I bring back the statistics grades data, this time as a grouped frequency distribution with $i = 5$. (I am using $i = 5$, not $i = 10$, because I want to have more detail—more trees—in the table so that my transformations to percentile ranks will be more exact.)

In Figure 3.2, I have taken the data from the final column, the cumulative percentages, and made them into something called a **cumulative percentage polygon.** Note that I have marked the *X* axis of Figure 3.2 with the *real* limits of the intervals and the *Y* axis with the cumulative percentages. At the real upper limit of each interval, I put a dot at the elevation for the cumulative percentage for that interval. Connect the dots and, *voilà*, we have a cumulative percentage polygon. Note that the graph line only stays level or goes up, it never dips down, and it reaches its apex, 100%, at the real upper limit for the final interval. Finally, to make this graph easier to use, I added grid lines, vertical lines at each interval's real limit and horizontal lines every 20 percentage points.

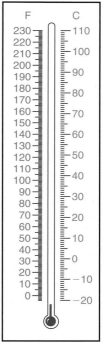

Figure **3.1** A Fahrenheit and Celsius thermometer.

percentile rank

The percentage of cases in a specific set of cases scoring at or below a score.

cumulative percentage polygon

A line graph showing the cumulative percentage ranks for a frequency distribution.

---

*I haven't yet formally defined what a "raw score" is, though by this point you've probably figured it out. A raw score is an untransformed score. If, for example, on a 25-item true/false test you answered 22 items correctly, your raw score is a 22. The score stated as a percentage, 88%, is a transformed score.

LOOKING CLOSER

TABLE **3.1**   **Grouped Frequency Distribution ($i = 5$) for Final Grades for 60 Introductory Statistics Students**

X	f	f_c	$\%_c$
95-99	1	60	100.00
90-94	1	59	98.33
85-89	0	58	96.67
80-84	3	58	96.67
75-79	4	55	91.67
70-74	3	51	85.00
65-69	7	48	80.00
60-64	7	41	68.33
55-59	12	34	56.67
50-54	7	22	36.67
45-49	6	15	25.00
40-44	4	9	15.00
35-39	0	5	8.33
30-34	4	5	8.33
25-29	1	1	1.67

Note: $i =$ interval width; $x =$ interval of scores; $f =$ frequency; $f_c =$ cumulative frequency; $\%_c =$ cumulative percentage

Now, let's go back to Table 3.1. Note that for the 65 to 69 interval, the cumulative frequency is 48 and the cumulative percentage is 80%. That means that by the time we reach the top of that interval (69.5), scores for 48 of the 60 total cases—for 80% of the cases—are encountered. Or, in the terminology of the current chapter, a score of 69.5 has a percentile rank of 80. Look at Figure 3.2 and trace over on the horizontal grid line

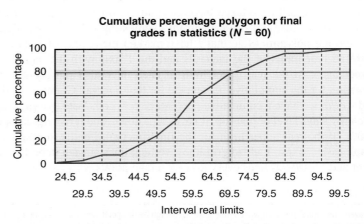

Figure **3.2** Cumulative percentage polygon for final grades for 60 introductory statistics students.

from 80% on the ordinate. You'll find that it intersects the graph line at a vertical line that leads back to a real limit of 69.5 on the abscissa.

Can we take this cumulative percentage polygon and, given a score on the X axis, draw a vertical line up to the graph line and then horizontally to the Y axis? Yes. Would this spot on the Y axis be the percentile rank associated with the score on the X axis? Yes! Just as it is possible to use a cumulative percentage polygon to find a percentile rank for a score, it is possible to reverse the operation and, given a percentile rank, find the score associated with it.

If I asked you to use the graph to find the percentile rank associated with a score of 43, you couldn't reach a very exact answer. Similarly, if I reversed direction and asked for the raw score value associated with a percentile rank, you couldn't find it very exactly. Statisticians like to have answers that are as precise as possible, so we're going to move to formulae for transforming raw scores into percentile ranks and vice versa.

But, before using the formulae, let's think through how to *estimate* the percentile rank for a person whose final score in statistics was a 43. Estimating before calculating is important, and I'd like you to get into the habit. Then, when you do the computation, you can compare the computed answer to the estimate. If the two are close, you can feel confident that your calculated answer is right. If the two aren't close, then either your estimate is wrong or your calculations are off. In either event, you should rethink and recalculate.

ESTIMATING PERCENTILE RANKS

The easiest way to estimate a percentile rank from a raw score is to turn the data into a thermometer where, instead of Fahrenheit and Celsius, the two metrics are X and PR: raw scores and percentile ranks. I've done this in Figure 3.3 for the data from Table 3.1. Note that the X side, the raw score side, is marked off by the real limits of the intervals and the PR side, the percentile rank side, is marked by cumulative percentages. Also note that the intervals are equal on the X side but not on the PR side. The first interval, which is five points wide on the raw score side, is as wide as the second interval on the raw score side, also five points wide. These two intervals are different widths, 1.67 points and 6.66 points, on the percentile rank side.*

To estimate, let's find the interval—we'll call it the **critical interval**—within which the raw score of 43 falls. The thermometer makes it clear that a score of 43 falls in the interval with real limits of 39.5 to 44.5. Looking at the other side of the thermometer, it becomes clear that a raw score of 43 has a percentile rank that falls in the range from PR 8.33 to

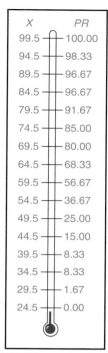

X	PR
99.5	100.00
94.5	98.33
89.5	96.67
84.5	96.67
79.5	91.67
74.5	85.00
69.5	80.00
64.5	68.33
59.5	56.67
54.5	36.67
49.5	25.00
44.5	15.00
39.5	8.33
34.5	8.33
29.5	1.67
24.5	0.00

Figure **3.3** "Thermometer" showing raw scores (X) and percentile rank scores (PR) for 60 introductory statistics students.

critical interval

The interval in which the score being converted falls.

---

*Don't take this as proof that percentile ranks are measured at the ordinal level. Wouldn't it be possible to make a thermometer where the percentile ranks are evenly spaced and the raw scores vary in interval width?

LOOKING CLOSER

PR 15.00. But where in this 6.67 percentile rank unit range does it fall? It turns out that if we assume that the 6.67 percentile rank points are evenly spread throughout the interval, we can do a very good job of estimating.

Here's how. Let's start with the fact that a raw score of 43 is 3.5 points into the five-raw-score-point-wide interval. We know that by subtracting the real lower limit of the interval, 39.5, from the raw score of 43. As another way of thinking about it, we could say that a score of 43 is 70% of the way into the interval as $\frac{3.50}{5.00} \times 100 = 70$. Wouldn't we expect the associated percentile rank score also to be 70% of the way into the interval? So, if we add 70% of the interval width, in percentile rank score units, to the bottom of the interval, also in percentile rank score units, we should find the percentile rank score associated with a raw score of 43.

Since we're estimating, I just want my answer to be in the ballpark and I'll round liberally so that I can do the math in my head. I'll call the interval seven percentile rank points wide instead of the actual 6.67, and I'll round 70% of seven up to five. Adding five points to the bottom of the interval, 8.33, I end up estimating that a raw score of 43 is equivalent to a percentile rank score around 13.33.

The best way to learn the important skill of estimating is by practicing, so here are some problems to help you learn the skill.

Group Practice 3.1

Using Figure 3.3 and the data in Table 3.1, estimate percentile ranks for the following scores:

1. 76   3. 35
2. 58   4. 52

CALCULATING PERCENTILE RANKS

Believe it or not, by estimating we have developed the formula for calculating percentile ranks for frequency distributions. With a grouped frequency distribution we don't know where within an interval the scores really occur. In Table 3.1 for example, there are four scores that fall in the interval 40 to 44. We don't know whether those cases are 40s, 41s, 42s, 43s, or 44s. We learned in Chapter 2 that if we were forced to give them values, we should give all the cases the value of the midpoint (in this case 42) because that minimizes errors. However, for calculating percentile ranks we do something different. As I've already mentioned, we're going to assume that the cases are spread evenly throughout the interval.* Let me explain how that works.

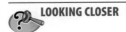 **LOOKING CLOSER**

* The logic of the formula depends on the assumption that the cases are spread evenly. Given the fact that we don't know where the cases actually fall, it seems easier to justify having them spread evenly throughout an interval than to consider them spread unevenly. If they were spread unevenly, which of the many possibilities for an uneven spread would one choose?   *Continued*

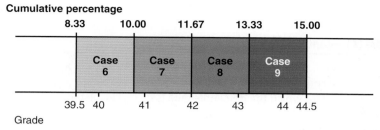

Cumulative percentage

Grade

Figure **3.4** Graphic representation of cases and cumulative percentages (percentile ranks) in the 40 to 44 interval from Table 3.1.

Four cases fall in the interval from 40 to 44 and a total of five cases fall below that interval. Thus, the cases in the critical interval are cases 6, 7, 8, and 9. The interval is five units wide, stretching from the real lower limit of 39.5 to the real upper limit of 44.5. Since there are four cases in an interval that is five units wide, we shall consider that each case takes up 1.25 units of the interval. (5 units ÷ 4 cases = 1.25 units per case.) Thus case 6, as seen graphically in Figure 3.4, spans the distance from 39.5 to 40.75.

We can do the same thing to cumulative percentage/percentile rank. The first five cases are equivalent to a cumulative percentage of 8.33%, and the four cases in the interval add an additional 6.67%. Thus, by the time we get to the top of the critical interval the cumulative percentage is 15.00%. If we take the 6.67% of total cases that fall into the interval and divide that by the number of cases in the interval (4), we find that each case accounts for an additional 1.67%. As shown in Figure 3.4, by the time we reach the end of case 6 (remember, case 6 is now spread throughout the interval), the cumulative percentage totals 10.00%.

If the above makes sense to you, and it should since we used the same logic when estimating, you are ready to calculate the exact percentile rank for a score of 43 using Equation 3.1.

Continued

F O R M U L A

Percentile Rank (*PR*) for a Raw Score (*X*)

Equation 3.1

$$PR = \left(\frac{X - RLL_{CI}}{i} \right) \%_{CI} + \%_{c_B}$$

(Continued) There's an interesting implication of spreading scores evenly throughout an interval—ties don't exist! Imagine a 100-item multiple-choice test. Buffy and Skip take this test and each receives a score of 75. Are they tied? Well, their scores are really in the range from 74.5 to 75.5. If we made a figure like Figure 3.4 for their scores, we would separate them, putting one score in the range from 74.5 to 75.0 and the other in the range from 75.0 to 75.5. As a result, they wouldn't be tied anymore.

LOOKING CLOSER

F O R M U L A

Percentile Rank (*PR*) for a Raw Score (*X*)—cont'd

Equation 3.1	Where:
	PR = the percentile rank being calculated
	X = the score for which the percentile rank is being calculated.
	RLL_{CI} = the real lower limit for the critical interval
	i = the interval width
	$\%_{CI}$ = the percentage of cases in the critical interval
	$\%_{c_B}$ = the cumulative percentage for the interval below the critical interval

Here's the formula in English:

1. Take the X value for which you want a percentile rank, and subtract from it the real lower limit of the critical interval, the interval within which the X value falls.
2. Divide the product of step 1 by the interval width.
3. Multiply the quotient from step 2 by the percentage of cases that fall in the critical interval.
4. Add to the product of step 3 the cumulative percentage for the interval below the critical interval to yield the percentile rank.

Let's apply Equation 3.1 to find the percentile rank for a raw score of 43.*

$$PR = \left(\frac{43.0000 - 39.5000}{5.0000} \right) 6.6667 + 8.3333$$
$$= (.7000)\, 6.6667 + 8.3333$$
$$= 4.6667 + 8.3333$$
$$= 13.0000, \text{ which I'll round to } 13.00$$

The calculated value, 13.00, is close enough to our estimated value, 13.33, that we should feel comfortable we've reached the right answer. What does this value of 13.00 mean? It means that a raw score of 43 is in the bottom 13% of scores; it has a percentile rank of 13, in our introductory statistics class.

We can also go the other way and find a score from a percentile rank. The logic is the same, just reversed.

Suppose that Buffy tells me that she is in the top 10% of students. If this is true, can we predict her final grade in statistics? Being in the top 10% is equivalent to having a percentile rank of 90, so the question becomes, if $PR = 90$, what is X? Let's estimate before using an equation.

Looking at the raw score/percentile rank thermometer we can see that the critical interval that contains a percentile rank of 90 ranges from

LOOKING CLOSER

*Please note that I am following my rules of rounding. As I want to end up with two decimal places for my final answer, I carry two more (four) for my calculations. This means that I've gone back to Table 3.1 and used the raw data to calculate values more exactly.

percentile rank scores of 85.00 to 91.67. The equivalent interval on the other side of the thermometer involves raw scores ranging from 74.5 to 79.5. Since we're estimating, I'll say that the critical interval is ≈ 7 percentile rank points wide, from 85 to 92, and that a score of 90 is $\frac{5}{7}$ of the way through the range. Five-sevenths of a five-raw-score-wide interval is about 3.5 raw score points, so I'll add 3.5 points to the real lower limit of 74.5. As a result, my estimated value of X for a percentile rank of 90 is 78.

Here is the official formula for converting percentile ranks to raw scores:

F O R M U L A

Raw Score (X) for a Percentile Rank (PR)

Equation 3.2

$$X = \left(\frac{\left(\frac{PR}{100} \right) N - f_{c_B}}{f_{CI}} \right) i + RLL_{CI}$$

Where:

X = the raw score you are trying to calculate
PR = the percentile rank for which you want to find X
N = the total number of cases in the data set
f_{c_B} = the cumulative frequency for the interval below the critical interval
f_{CI} = the number of cases in the critical interval
i = the interval width
RLL_{CI} = the real lower limit for the critical interval

In English:

1. Take the specified percentile rank and divide it by 100. Multiply this quotient by the sample size, and subtract from that product the cumulative frequency for the number of cases that are below the critical interval.
2. Divide the result of step 1 by the number of cases in the critical interval.
3. Multiply the quotient from step 2 by the width of the interval.
4. Add the lower real limit of the critical interval to the product from step 3 to yield the raw score.

Using Equation 3.2 to determine the raw score associated with a percentile rank of 90 for our statistics grades data we find:

$$X = \left(\frac{\left(\frac{90.0000}{100} \right) 60 - 51}{4} \right) 5.0000 + 74.5000 = 78.2500 = 78.25$$

Seeing that our answer of 78.25 is close to our estimate of 78, we have confidence that our answer is right. What does this 78.25 mean? A person who has a percentile rank of 90 in this distribution should have a final grade in statistics of 78.25, a grade just a bit below my A range.*

Group Practice 3.2

A nurse practitioner decides to find the "normal" temperature for elementary school children. He takes a random sample of the children who are in school on a given day and assesses each child for illness. If the child is healthy, the nurse practitioner then takes his or her temperature using a carefully calibrated thermometer.

   Use this frequency distribution to answer the next two questions.

F°	f
99.3	2
99.2	3
99.1	4
99.0	8
98.9	17
98.8	16
98.7	14
98.6	20
98.5	19
98.4	17
98.3	16
98.2	12
98.1	9

F°	f
98.1	9
98.0	10
97.9	4
97.8	5
97.7	2

1. If Skip's temperature, measured precisely, is 98.90, what is his temperature as a percentile rank? First estimate, then calculate.
2. Buffy is in the coldest 10%. Estimate her temperature, and then calculate it.
3. Earlier in this chapter we calculated the percentile rank for a score of 43 for the final-grades-in-statistics data in Table 3.1 and found it to be 13.00. My grading scheme, as you may remember, is unusual in that the A range is >80, the B range is from 60 to 79, the C range from 40 to 59, D from 20 to 39, and F <20. Redo Table 3.1 so that it reflects this grading scheme, that is, has 20-point intervals. Then, recalculate the percentile rank for a score of 43. Why is it different? Which do you think is a better representation of the score? Why?

SUMMARY

In this chapter we explored transforming data in order to change the metric in which the data are expressed to one that is easier to understand. A percentile rank is a score expressed as the percentage of cases in a specific set of cases scoring at or below that level. Thus, percentile ranks are similar to the cumulative percentages encountered in Chapter 2. Formulae are given to transform a raw score (X) into a percentile rank (PR) and to transform a PR into an X. Before using those equations to calculate an answer, however, it is important to estimate the answer. If the estimated answer and the calculated answer are close to each other, you can have faith in your calculations. If there is a large discrepancy between the two, then either the estimate or the calculation is in error.

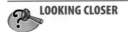 **LOOKING CLOSER**

*By the bye, I've had some students ask me why the denominator in this equation, 4, has no decimal places whereas the denominator in the previous equation, 5.0000, had four decimal places. In this equation the denominator represents a discrete number, a frequency. In the previous equation the denominator represents a continuous number, the width of an interval.

Review Exercises

1. For each of the following, speculate about the shape of the distribution of the data:
   a. A demographer collects data about the age at which women in the United States get married for the first time.
   b. A gambler keeps track of how often the different numbers on the roulette wheel (numbers 1 to 36) show up at a Las Vegas casino.
   c. A radiographer measures the length of the thigh bone in adult men.
   d. The radiographer measures the length of thigh bones in adult men *and* women.
2. The National Weather Service records the temperature in your city every half hour for a 1-week period. That is, they record the temperature at noon, at 12:30 PM, at 1 PM, at 1:30 PM, and so on. If the National Weather Service thinks like a statistician, what is the earliest time that they can take the temperature and still call it the noon temperature?
3. A nutritionist, Dr. Amiama, has a sample of adults keep track of their food consumption. From this she calculates the number of grams of dietary fiber that each person consumes per day and makes the following table:

Average Daily Dietary Fiber Consumption

Grams	Frequency
45-49	9
40-44	11
35-39	19
30-34	21
25-29	24
20-24	38
15-19	44
10-14	59
5-9	28
0-4	11

Buffy eats 38 grams of fiber per day. What is her percentile rank for fiber consumption?
4. The U.S. government recommends consuming 25 grams of dietary fiber per day. How much fiber does the "average" person in Dr. Amiama's data, the person at the 50th percentile, consume per day? How does this compare to the recommended daily consumption?
5. What is the real lower limit for the lowest interval, 0-4 grams of fiber, in Dr. Amiama's data?
6. What is Dr. Amiama's dependent variable? Her independent variable?

Homework Problems

1. Assume that to be handsome is something Skip, a North American male, wants to be. Skip is rated on a 10-point handsomeness scale and is told that his handsomeness score, as a percentile rank in the population of North American males, is 10. If Skip is statistically savvy, which of the following he should feel?
   a. Happy
   b. Sad
   c. Neutral
   d. There is not enough information to draw a conclusion.
2. There is a scale on which scores can range from 0 to 50, and 80 cases are measured on this scale. For the interval in which the twentieth case falls, the apparent limits range from 18 to 19 and the real limits range from 17.5 to 19.5. There are four cases that fall in this interval. What is the score, X, associated with the twentieth case?
   a. 17.5
   b. 18.0
   c. 18.5
   d. 19.0
   e. 19.5
   f. The value can be calculated from the available information, but the exact value is not listed above.
   g. There is not enough information given to calculate this.
3. If there are 50 cases in a distribution and the case with a score of 75 has a cumulative frequency of 25, then the percentile rank for this case is which of the following?
   a. 0
   b. 25
   c. 50
   d. 75
   e. 100

f. The value can be calculated from the available information, but it is not listed above

g. There is not enough information given to calculate this.

4. The first five cases in a distribution fall in an interval with the real limits of zero and one. What is the X score associated with case number 3.5?

a. .35
b. .50
c. .60
d. .70
e. .80
f. None of the above

5. The United States Postal Service has a sample of people record how many catalogs they receive during a calendar year. Below are the results:

# Of Catalogs Received	Frequency
1900-1999	2
1800-1899	8
1700-1799	17
1600-1699	24
1500-1599	47
1400-1499	48
1300-1399	61
1200-1299	75
1100-1199	114
1000-1099	152
900-999	202
800-899	249
700-799	252
600-699	243
500-599	187
400-499	162
300-399	132
200-299	57
100-199	16
0-99	11

What is the percentile rank associated with a person who receives 625 catalogs per year? (Note that these data are discrete, not continuous. This has implications for the real upper and lower limits of the intervals, which has ramifications for calculating a percentile rank.)

6. If a person is in the top 25% in number of catalogs received, how many catalogs does that person receive? The person in the bottom 25%? (Note: don't forget that these data are discrete, not continuous.)

7. How would you describe the shape of the USPS data in Question 5?

8. On what scale of measurement is number of catalogs received being measured? In Review Exercise 3, dietary fiber consumption was measured in grams. Is this a discrete or a continuous measure? What scale of measurement is used for dietary fiber consumption?

9. Round each of the following to two decimal places:

a. 57.999
b. 57.995
c. 56.99
d. 57.445
e. 57.405

10. For each of the following, identify the independent and dependent variables. What scale of measurement is being used for the dependent variable?

a. Dr. Jones is measuring the presence or absence of brain cancer in relation to whether people live (a) close or (b) not close to electric power lines.

b. Dr. Smith does a study in which people are assigned to receive different amounts of nitrous oxide and then listen to the sound of a dental drill. They rate, on a scale ranging from 0 (No anxiety) to 10 (Very, very high anxiety), how much anxiety they feel at the sound of the drill.

c. Dr. Anderson randomly assigns people to receive aspirin, Tylenol, ibuprofen, or a placebo and then measures how much pain they can tolerate. He measures pain tolerance by using the cold pressor test. (The cold pressor test involves timing how long it takes for one to remove his or her arm from the ice water into which a researcher has placed it. Trust me, it is quite painful, and people remove their arms fairly quickly.) In addition, each of the four groups is randomly divided into two; one half of each group is told that they are receiving a pain medicine, and the other half is told that they are receiving a placebo.

4

Descriptive Statistics

Measuring Central Tendency
and Variability

Learning Objectives

After completing this chapter, you should be able to do the following:

1 Recognize the difference between a statistic, a parameter, and an estimated parameter.
2 Choose and calculate the appropriate measure of central tendency (mean, median, or mode) for a data set.
3 Calculate four different measures of variability (range, interquartile range, variance, and standard deviation) for interval- and ratio-level data.

In this chapter we'll focus on describing a set of data in two dimensions: the average score and the variability in scores from case to case. You'll learn to calculate three types of averages (mean, median, and mode) and four measures of variability (range, interquartile range, variance, and standard deviation), and when to use each. In addition, we'll look again at the difference between a statistic (calculated for a sample) and a parameter (calculated for a population). Though we usually want to know population values, we almost always only have information from a sample. Statisticians get around this by "correcting" a sample statistic to estimate a population value, and we'll learn how to do so for two of the measures of variability.

S tatistics bring order to chaos by reducing a large mass of data in a meaningful way. We've already done this using tables and graphs, and we've transformed scores to make them more interpretable. Now we get down to the business of serious data reduction, of taking a large mass of data and transforming it into a *single* number, a *summary* number that provides meaningful information about a whole set of scores.

Statisticians use two different dimensions to describe a set of scores. One is a measure of what statisticians call **central tendency** (what everyone else calls the average), and the other is a measure of variability. Both give us important overviews of a whole set of scores.

The average score, or the *central* area around which scores *tend* to cluster, is important because it provides useful information. If you get a low score on a test, you'll probably feel better if you learn that the class average, the central tendency, on that test was lower than your score. Knowing that Buffy's GPA, the central tendency of her scores, is a 3.5 whereas Skip's is a 2.0 does tell us that there is a difference in their academic performances. We may not be sure why the difference exists—it could be due to brains, or motivation, or alcohol consumption, or a whole host of other potential reasons—but we do know that there is a difference. Based on their measures of central tendency, we can make some reasonably accurate predictions about the two. For example, if both Buffy and Skip apply to medical school, who do you think is more likely to get in?

However, knowing just the average doesn't tell us the whole story. There is almost always **variability** in a set of data. What is variability? Look around your classroom: is everyone the same height? Does everyone have hair that is the same length? Is everyone carrying the same number of books in their backpacks? The answer to all of these questions is no;

central tendency

The value around which scores tend to cluster; the score obtained by a typical case.

variability

The differences among scores within a set.

there is *variability* on all of these dimensions. It is the existence of variability that makes measurement necessary, and it is the reason we call the dimensions we measure *variables*.

Let's think about two more students, Desdemona and Clothilde. Though each has a GPA of 3.0, they are different. Desdemona is a remarkably consistent student; every time she takes a course she receives a B. Clothilde is much more variable; half the time she receives an A and half the time she receives a C. If we just looked at the measure of central tendency we would say that these two students are academically similar, and we would be wrong. By looking at the variability in the scores—Desdemona has no variability and Clothilde has a lot—we get a better picture of the large mass of data being reduced.

And that is our purpose: we want the statistics that we generate to be *simplified but accurate* representations of the large mass of data from which they come.

MEASURES OF CENTRAL TENDENCY

Measures of central tendency are single values that best describe the scores obtained on some variable by a set of cases. They give us some idea of what score is obtained by the typical, or average, case. The set of scores for the cases for which the measure of central tendency is being calculated may be a whole population or a sample.

The term **average** is a generic term for a measure of central tendency. Average is not a precise term since statisticians use three different averages: **mean, median,** and **mode.** Which average you compute depends, in part, upon your type of data. Means can be computed for interval- and ratio-level data; medians for ordinal-, interval-, and ratio-level data; and modes for nominal-, ordinal-, interval-, and ratio-level data. In addition to the variable's level of measurement, you must attend to the shape of the distribution of scores. Means should not be calculated for skewed distributions, and means and medians should not be calculated for multimodal distributions.

The **mean** is what most people have in mind when they talk about an average, and you probably already know how to calculate it: add up all the scores in a set and divide the sum by the number of scores.* We can do this for a sample, abbreviating the mean as M, or for a population, abbreviating the mean as μ (the Greek letter "m," spelled "mu" in Latin characters and pronounced "mew"). Since it is important to differentiate a summary number for a *population* (a parameter) from a summary number for a *sample* (a statistic), statisticians have developed the habit of using Greek letters for parameters and Latin letters for statistics.[†]

average

A generic term for a measure of central tendency.

mean

The average calculated by adding all scores in sample or population and dividing by the number of addends. More specifically called the "arithmetic mean."

---

* Technically, this is the *arithmetic* mean, just one of a variety of means that statisticians calculate. Among the other means are the *geometric* mean and the *harmonic* mean.

[†] When I learned statistics the convention was to abbreviate a sample mean as $\bar{X}$, pronounced "x-bar," and you still will see and hear this.

LOOKING CLOSER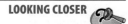

Statisticians use other abbreviations in their formulae, and we've already seen how N is used to represent the number of cases in a set of data. Now, before I show you the formula for calculating a mean, there is one other abbreviation you need to learn: Σ, pronounced "sigma," is the uppercase version of the Greek letter "s," and it means "add them all up."* If my set of Xs has three values (3, 4, and 5), then ΣX means add up all the Xs (i.e., $3 + 4 + 5 = 12$.) Knowing the abbreviations, the formula for the mean in Equation 4.1 should now make sense.

F O R M U L A

Sample Mean (M)

Equation 4.1

$$M = \frac{\Sigma X}{N}$$

Where:

M = sample mean

Σ = summation sign

X = the values of X for the cases in the sample

N = the number of cases in the sample

Note: When calculating μ, the population mean, you add all of the scores in the population and divide this sum by the total number of scores in the population.

---

deviation score

The distance, and direction, a score is from the mean; calculated as $X - M$.

In English, this formula says to add all of the scores in the sample, and divide this sum by the number of scores. Imagine that I select five people and measure their heights, in inches, as 67, 72, 73, 64, and 63. I calculate the sample mean as

$$M = \frac{67 + 72 + 73 + 64 + 63}{5} = \frac{339}{5} = 67.80$$

TABLE **4.1**   **Deviation Scores ($X - M$)**

X	$X - M$
63	−4.80
64	−3.80
67	−.80
72	4.20
73	5.20

This sample mean reflects the average height for these five people.[†] Note that it is OK that no one in the sample has a height that is equal to the mean. The mean, 67.80, can be considerd the *center* of the distribution of scores. To see it as the center, we must calculate each case's **deviation score** by subtracting the mean from each score. Table 4.1 displays the scores ordered from shortest to tallest and shows the deviation score for each case.

LOOKING CLOSER

*If you want to call it something fancier than add-them-all-up, call Σ a summation sign.

[†] Of course, you are now aware that this is just one of the potential averages we could calculate.

Note that three people have negative deviation scores, and two have positive deviation scores. The sign of the deviation score tells whether the person had a score below or above the mean.

Also note that if we add up the deviation scores, they sum to zero:

$$\Sigma(X - M) = -4.80 + (-3.80) + (-.80) + 4.20 + 5.20 = .00$$

As well as being a good way to verify that one calculated the mean correctly, this demonstrates that a mean is the center of the distribution of scores. The mean is the *balancing point* of the *deviation scores*. Even if we don't have the same number of scores above the mean as below, the mean is at the center of the deviation scores. Think of the mean as like a seesaw. If a really heavy person sits on one side of the seesaw, then a number of light people on the other side are needed to balance it. More-over, the closer to the fulcrum that the light people sit, the more of them are needed to balance the heavy person. A large deviation score on one side of the mean can be balanced by lots of small deviation scores on the other side. The absolute value of the sum of the deviations for the scores above the mean is the same as the absolute value of the sum of the deviations for the scores below the mean.*

The **median** is another measure of central tendency. It is a second way to think of the center, or balancing point, for a set of scores. Imagine taking a set of scores and ordering them from lowest to highest. The median is the score separating the bottom 50% of cases from the top 50%. For the data set of heights used above, the median is 67. Again, it may help to think of a seesaw, but in this case how much people weigh is irrelevant. For the median, a case is a case is a case, no matter the weight. A graphic view of this for the median of the five heights is shown in Figure 4.1, where an upcaret (^) indicates the fulcrum of the seesaw. The data are treated at an ordinal level, not an interval one, and the distances between cases don't matter. As you can see, placing the median at the middle score of 67 perfectly balances the seesaw, with half the cases on each side.

With a small number of cases in the data set, you can find the median by ranking the scores and then finding the $\dfrac{N + 1}{2}$ score. With five scores in the height data set, the median is the $\dfrac{5 + 1}{2}$, or third, score. This works easily enough with an odd number of scores, but with an even number of scores the median falls halfway between two scores. If the 7-foot, 7-inch basketball player Manute Bol joined the sample, the sample size would change from five to six and the median would be the "three-and-a-halfth" score. To find the value for this we need to interpolate, to split the distance

median

A measure of central tendency; the average determined by finding the center of the data set with 50% of the cases below and 50% above.

63	64	67	72	73
		^		

Figure **4.1** Seesaw example of median for heights ($N = 5$).

---

*For those who have forgotten, an absolute value is a number reported as a positive value, whether it was positive or negative. Thus, the absolute value of −3.00 is 3.00, and this would be written as $|-3.00| = 3.00$.

LOOKING CLOSER

between the third score (67) and the fourth (72), calculating the median as $\frac{67 + 72}{2}$ or 69.50.

If your data set is large, if you are calculating the median for a grouped frequency distribution, or if the data set includes ties, use a formula to calculate the median. And it turns out that you have already learned the formula! The median is the score at the 50th percentile, the score associated with a percentile rank of 50. Equation 4.2 is a version of Equation 3.2, altered so that it calculates the median. Note that according to this formula the median is the $\frac{N}{2}$ score, not the $\frac{N + 1}{2}$ score as it was when we used the simple counting-off method for finding the median. This change really doesn't make much difference when the sample size is large, but with a small sample size it will lead to different results.

By the bye, there is not as much consistency among statisticians in the abbreviations used for the median as there is for the mean. The abbreviation that I favor is *Mdn,* and so we'll use that.*

FORMULA

Median (*Mdn*)

Equation 4.2

$$Mdn = \left(\frac{\frac{N}{2} - f_{c_B}}{f_{CI}} \right) i + RLL_{CI}$$

Where:

Mdn = the median being calculated

N = the total number of cases in the data set

f_{c_B} = the cumulative frequency for the interval below the critical interval

f_{CI} = the number of cases in the critical interval, the interval that contains the median, the $\frac{N}{2}$ score

i = the interval width

RLL_{CI} = the real lower limit of the critical interval

In English, this formula says:

1. Find the critical interval, the interval that contains the median score, the $\frac{N}{2}$ score.

2. Divide the total number of cases by 2, and subtract from this the cumulative number of cases that are below the critical interval.

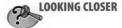 **LOOKING CLOSER**

*Also, there is no abbreviation differentiation between the median for a sample and the median for a population; both are abbreviated *Mdn*. You have to determine from the context which is being used.

TABLE **4.2** **Grouped Frequency Distribution ($i = 10$) for Final, Accumulated Point Totals for a Random Sample of 60 Introductory Statistics Students**

X	f	f_c	%	$%_c$	m
90-99	2	**60**	3.3	100.0	94.5
80-89	3	58	5.0	96.7	84.5
70-79	7	55	11.7	91.7	74.5
60-69	14	48	23.3	80.0	64.5
50-59	**19**	34	31.7	56.7	54.5
40-49	10	**15**	16.7	25.0	44.5
30-39	4	5	6.7	8.3	34.5
20-29	1	1	1.7	1.7	24.5

Note: i = interval width; X = scores; f = frequency; % = percentage; $%_c$ = cumulative percentage; m = interval midpoint; f_c = cumulative frequency

3. Divide step 2 by the number of cases in the critical interval, and multiply this quotient by the interval width.
4. Add this product to the real lower limit of the critical interval.

Let's calculate the median using Equation 4.2 for the statistics grades data, as displayed in Table 4.2. To clarify the sources of the numbers in the calculations, I've shaded the critical interval where the thirtieth case falls and bold-faced the numbers we'll be using.

Plugging the appropriate values into the formula we find:

$$Mdn = \left(\frac{\frac{60}{2} - 15}{19}\right)10.0000 + 49.5000$$
$$= 7.8947 + 49.5000$$
$$= 57.3947 = 57.39$$

The median score, based on a grouped frequency distribution with $i = 10$, is 57.39. This means that half of the students in the class have grades above 57.39, a high C by my grading scheme, and half of the students have grades below this.*

The **mode** is our last measure of central tendency and, you'll be happy to learn, there is no formula for calculating it. The mode is simply the

mode

A measure of central tendency; the score that occurs most frequently.

*In case you are wondering how the median compares to the mean for these data, here's how to calculate a mean for a grouped frequency distribution. As mentioned in Chapter 2, when assigning a score to the cases in an interval for a grouped frequency distribution, we assign each case that interval's midpoint. Thus, to *estimate* a mean for a grouped frequency distribution we multiply, for each interval, the midpoint by its frequency, then add up all of these products and divide by N. The formula looks like this: $M = \dfrac{\Sigma(fm)}{N}$.

For the grouped frequency statistics data, the mean is 58.50. The result of our estimating isn't too shabby: if we had calculated the mean based on the actual scores for the 60 students, we would have found that it was 58.38.

LOOKING CLOSER

score that occurs most frequently. Looking at Table 4.2, the mode is in the 50-59 interval that has a frequency of 19. Since we don't know what the actual scores are for those 19 people, we'll assign all of them the midpoint as mentioned in Chapter 2. Thus we say that the mode is 54.50.

There are some advantages to calculating the mode for a grouped frequency distribution over one for an ungrouped frequency distribution. Table 2.5 displayed these data as an ungrouped frequency distribution. From the data in that table you could conclude that there were three modes for the data: 51, 58, and 62. Identifying three modes probably is not a useful description of the measure of central tendency for these data. This is an example, similar to Figure 2.12, of where a unimodal data set may be mistakenly called multimodal. Because a grouped frequency distribution aggregates values that are near each other, it tends to "smooth out" a data set, clarifying the area around which the mode occurs.

COMPARING MEASURES OF CENTRAL TENDENCY

Before turning to measures of variability, let's compare the three measures of central tendency. How and when do you choose one over the other? What are the pros and cons of each? Remember, the mean can only be calculated for interval and ratio data, the median for ordinal, interval, and ratio data, and the mode for all four levels of measurement. Another way of viewing this is that if your data are at the nominal level of measurement your only option for a measure of central tendency is the mode, reporting which category occurs with the greatest frequency. If your data are at the ordinal level, you can choose to report either a median or a mode as a measure of central tendency. And, if your data are at the interval or ratio level, you can pick any of the three measures of central tendency.

The mean is the most commonly used measure of central tendency. It is the one almost always referred to when people talk about an average. One reason that it is most commonly used is that statisticians prefer to work with interval- or ratio-level data. Why do statisticians prefer interval- and ratio-level data? Because numbers at this level contain more information, information about the size of the difference between values, not just information about which value is most common or the order in which values occur,

Thus, other things being equal, you should pick the most complex measure of central tendency suitable for your data set, the one that takes advantage of more information in the numbers. If you have ordinal-level data, for example, although you can pick either the median or the mode, it is wise to choose the median since that uses more of the information that the numbers contain—information about both difference and direction. Similarly, with interval- or ratio-level data, use the mean if you can, since that takes advantage of information about sizes of differences as well as direction of differences.

There are situations, however, where even though the data are at the interval or ratio level, you should choose to use a median or even a mode to describe central tendency. One such situation occurs when the data set is skewed. Think back to the data set of the heights of five people and what happened when we added the 7'7" Manute Bol to the sample. He's dramatically taller than anyone else in the sample, and so he skews the data set in a positive direction. Without Bol in the sample, the mean is 67.80. When he is added, the mean changes to 71.67, almost 4 inches higher. His one score has dragged the mean 3.87 inches taller, skewing it, and making the mean near the height of the two people (72 inches and 73 inches) who used to be the tallest in the sample. Does this seem like a fair representation of the central tendency of the sample? No.

Earlier, we calculated the median for the five people in my sample as 67.00. With Manute Bol, the median increases to 69.50. This is certainly an increase, but it is less of an increase than was found for the mean. When data are skewed, either positively or negatively, use the median as a measure of central tendency, not the mean, because the median is less influenced by outliers.* In fact, comparing the mean to the median gives us a crude measure of skewness. In a normal distribution the mean and the median are the same. If data are positively skewed, the mean is higher than the median; for a negatively skewed data set, the mean is lower than the median.

With multimodal data sets the mode may be a better choice of a measure of central tendency than either the mean or the median. Imagine that I measure the heights of a random sample of 50 college-age men and a random sample of 50 basketball players. If I make a frequency polygon for the combined data, it will almost certainly be bimodal (Figure 4.2). Both the mean and the median will probably fall between the two humps of the distribution. As they will be in an area where there are relatively few actual scores, this does not seem like a good description of central tendency for this set of scores. It is better to say that the distribution is bimodal and to report the two modes.

Finally, be aware that you can choose your measure of central tendency to make a point. Every few years some professional athletes go on strike, and both the players and the management try to sway public opinion to their side. Both sides report average salary data, but each chooses carefully which measure of central tendency it reports. Let's agree that players' salaries are positively skewed: they all earn a fair amount of money, but some earn amazingly large amounts. The management side will report the *mean* player salary to show how much money these overpaid-and-yet-still-greedy players are demanding. The players will report either the *median* or the *mode* as the average player salary to say,

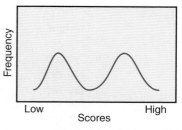

Figure **4.2** Example of a bimodal data set where mean and median are not appropriate measures of central tendency.

---

*In both these instances, for the mean and the median, there was a large change in the measure of central tendency when I added just one case. Such a large change only occurs when the sample size is small. If I had had 100 cases in my sample and added one more, the new case would have to be *extremely* different from the old to have a large impact on the mean. And no matter how different the new case was, it would have a negligible impact on the median, changing it from the fiftieth to the fiftieth-and-a-half case.

LOOKING CLOSER

"Yes, we are well paid, but we are not obscenely well paid." You, as a consumer of statistical information, must ask which average is being reported so that you can evaluate its appropriateness.*

Group Practice 4.1

1. You go grocery shopping at a large grocery store and buy items valued at: $1.97, $2.03, $6.89, $4.17, $7.99, $3.44, and $.79.
   a. Estimate the mean. (Hint: estimate by rounding prices to the nearest dollar.)
   b. Calculate *M*. (It is adequate to report this to two decimal places.)
   c. Calculate the deviation scores for the items, and verify that they add up to zero. If they don't, why? (Don't forget the rules of rounding. When using the mean as a step in calculating another value, carry extra decimal places.)
   d. What can you say about μ for the price of items at this grocery store?

2. Below is a grouped frequency distribution of weights (in pounds) for a sample of students.

Weight	Frequency
210-229	1
190-209	3
170-189	12
150-169	38
130-149	37
110-129	10
90-109	2

   a. In what interval should the median fall?
   b. Estimate the median.

   c. Calculate the median.
   d. What is the mode?
   e. Calculate the mean. (Not sure how to do this? See the footnote on page 95.)
   f. Which measure of central tendency is "best" for this data set?

3. I administer an interval-level depression scale to a large and representative sample of adults in the United States. Scores on the scale can range from a low of 0 to a high of 99. (Higher scores represent greater degrees of depression.) Below are the scores in a grouped frequency distribution. Calculate the appropriate measure of central tendency. Be sure to think before you calculate!

Depression score	Frequency
90-99	0
80-89	1
70-79	3
60-69	11
50-59	28
40-49	37
30-39	54
20-29	78
10-19	195
0-9	238

MEASURES OF VARIABILITY

I said earlier that statisticians use two dimensions to describe a set of data: central tendency and variability. I used the example of two people with the same GPA but different degrees of variability in their scores: Desdemona achieved a GPA of 3.0 by getting B's in every course she ever took, while Clothilde achieved a 3.0 by getting A's in half her courses and C's in

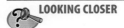
LOOKING CLOSER

*In this situation, the median is the most appropriate measure of central tendency given the skewness present in the data.

half her courses. We agreed that although these two looked the same in terms of a measure of central tendency, they are quite different students, and that the differing degrees of variability are the key to this difference. Now we are going to learn four ways—range, interquartile range, variance, and standard deviation—to calculate a single number that will abstract and quantify the degree of variability.

The **range** is the simplest measure of variability. It is a single value that represents the distance from the highest to the lowest score in a set of scores. To be exact, the range is the distance from the real upper limit of the highest score to the real lower limit of the lowest score. Because it assigns meaning to the distance between scores, the range should only be calculated for interval- or ratio-level measures.

> **range**
>
> A measure of variability, the distance between the highest and lowest scores in a data set.

F O R M U L A

Range

$$Range = RUL_{Highest\ Score} - RLL_{Lowest\ Score}$$

Equation 4.3

Where:

$Range$ = the range being calculated

$RUL_{Highest\ Score}$ = the real upper limit for the highest score in the set of scores

$RLL_{Lowest\ Score}$ = the real lower limit for the lowest score in the set of scores

---

In the height data we were working with earlier, the shortest person was 63 inches tall and the tallest person was 73 inches. The range, therefore, is 11. Why 11 and not 10? Because we use real limits, not apparent limits, and subtract the real lower limit for the shortest person (62.5 inches) from the real upper limit of the tallest person (73.5 inches). Using the real limits to calculate the range yields what is called an "inclusive" range because it *includes* the real limits. The "exclusive" range for these data, which *excludes* the real limits, is 10.

Obviously, with Manute Bol (91 inches tall) added to the mix, the range changes dramatically, from 11 to 29 inches. This is a problem with the range: it is a measure that can fluctuate a lot if a new case with an extreme value, an outlier, is added. In statistics-speak, it is not a robust measure. Adding, or losing, a single score can dramatically alter the range. Further, the range gives no sense of what falls between the two extremes. The range *with* Manute Bol, 29 inches, gives no sense of the 18-inch gap between him and the person who had been the tallest before he was added.

For these reasons the range is not commonly used as a single value to describe variability. You will, however, frequently see the range reported as two numbers, as, for example, "the range of heights, in inches, in the sample was from 63 to 91." Used this way, the apparent limits for the values, not the real limits, are reported. The range reported this way is more useful since it reveals the tallest and the shortest (or oldest and youngest, or heaviest and thinnest, etc.) cases in the sample. If I were doing a study of some variable in college students and, in describing my sample, said that the mean age was 20.35 years with a range from 17 to 32, you would know that there was at least one student in my sample who was older than the traditional 18- to 22-year-old college student. *How many* nontraditional students there were in the sample, however, you would not know.

The fact that an extreme value or two can influence the range has led to the development of the next measure of variability, the **interquartile range.** The interquartile range, or *IQR*, is really a range with the tails of the distribution on each side, the extreme scores, cut off. You can call it a trimmed range, if you wish.*

The interquartile range is calculated as the distance from the value of the score at the 75th percentile to the value of the score at the 25th percentile. Like the range, it measures distance, so you must have an interval- or ratio-level measure to calculate it. It is called the inter*quartile* range because a set of scores can be divided into four quartiles: scores from percentile rank 0 to percentile rank 25 are in the first quartile, those from percentile rank 25 to percentile rank 50 are in the second quartile, and so on. Thus the interquartile range represents the range within which the middle 50% of the scores fall.

---

interquartile range (IQR)

A measure of variability, the difference between the value of the score at the 75th percentile and the score at the 25th percentile.

F O R M U L A

Interquartile Range (*IQR*)

Equation 4.4

$$IQR = PR_{75} - PR_{25}$$

Where:
IQR = percentile range being calculated
PR_{75} = value of the score at the 75th percentile (see Equation 4.5)
PR_{25} = value of the score at the 25th percentile (see Equation 4.5)

You could refer back to Equation 3.2 in the last chapter to figure out the percentile ranks needed for Equation 4.4; to save you a bit of trouble, here are the formulae you need, modified to calculate the specific percentile ranks needed.

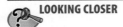 **LOOKING CLOSER**

*There is also a trimmed mean, a mean with a certain percentage of extreme scores on each side trimmed off. This is useful in situations where a few extreme scores can alter the results. Professors like to use trimmed means to examine their student evaluations at the end of the semester because a trimmed mean will remove the really low ratings. It does, of course, also remove the really high ratings. Professors, however, always assume that only one or two people will rate them low while many people will rate them high.

F O R M U L A

Scores Associated with Percentile Ranks of 75 (PR_{75}) and 25 (PR_{25})

Equation 4.5

$$PR_{75} = \left(\frac{.75N - f_{c_B}}{f_{CI}} \right) i + RLL_{CI}$$

$$PR_{25} = \left(\frac{.25N - f_{c_B}}{f_{CI}} \right) i + RLL_{CI}$$

Where:

PR_{75} = value of the score at the 75th percentile
PR_{25} = value of the score at the 25th percentile
N = the total number of cases in the data set
f_{c_B} = the cumulative frequency for the interval below the critical interval
f_{CI} = the number of cases in the critical interval
i = the interval width
RLL_{CI} = the real lower limit of the critical interval

Let's calculate the interquartile range for the statistics grades data set and use the ungrouped frequency distribution found in Table 2.5. You've had experience calculating percentile ranks, both in the last chapter and earlier in this chapter with the median, so I will leave working with Equation 4.5 up to you. If you do the math correctly, you will find values of 68.50 for PR_{75} and 48.50 for PR_{25}. Thus, the $IQR = 20.00$.

Compare this interquartile range of 20.00 to the range for these data. Though we didn't calculate it initially, the range for these data is 68.00. The range tells you that the distance from the highest to the lowest score is 68 points. The interquartile range, which tells you the range within which the middle 50% of the scores fall, is much narrower, just as we would expect, because it is a trimmed value of the whole range.

Technically, the interquartile range, like the range, is a single value. However, I don't find a single value, in this case 20.00, terribly useful. If, on the other hand, one reports the interquartile range as both the 25th and the 75th percentiles, then it is a much more interpretable measure. If I say, for example, that the interquartile range for final grades in my statistics class runs from 48.50 to 68.50, you know that the middle 50% of scores fall in this 20-point range. The interquartile range, reported as a set of scores, provides information *both* about variability and about central tendency, making it a wonderful measure. In fact, you've probably already been using the interquartile range without even knowing it.

Every year *U.S. News and World Report* publishes its guide to colleges. Part of the guide is a compilation of statistics about each college, including the interquartile range for SAT scores. They call it the SAT 25th-75th

TABLE **4.3**   **Interquartile Range for Combined SAT Scores, Selected Colleges**

	IQR*	IQR from
Penn State Erie	200	950 to 1150
Penn State, University Park	210	1080 to 1290
Harvard	170	1410 to 1580

*Note: *IQR* = Interquartile range
Data from "America's Best Colleges," *U.S. News & World Report*, 2002.

percentile and report it as two scores, the first representing the combined SAT score at the 25th percentile for the students at that college and the second the score at the 75th percentile. You probably used these numbers to help decide where to apply for college and now, I hope, you recognize them as an interquartile range.

I teach at Penn State Erie, one of the campuses in the Penn State system. According to the 2002 edition of the *U.S. News'* college guide, the interquartile range for SAT scores at Penn State Erie, as shown in Table 4.3, is 200 points wide, from 950 to 1150. There are several other campuses in the Penn State system, the main one being the University Park campus with over 30,000 undergraduates. (My campus has fewer than 4000.) The interquartile range at University Park is 210 points wide, so there is about as much variability in SAT scores there as there is at Erie. However—and this is the beauty of reporting both scores for an interquartile range—the interquartile range at University Park is from 1080 to 1290. The variability at the two campuses is roughly equal, but the two clearly differ in terms of central tendency. The average student at the main campus of Penn State has more of whatever it is that the SAT measures than the average student at the Erie campus.

Table 4.3 includes one more college, Harvard. The interquartile range for SAT scores at Harvard is from 1410 to 1580, a 170-point range. There is less variability in IQ scores at Harvard than there is at Penn State—it is more homogeneous. In addition, the students there have more of whatever it is that the SAT measures than do the students at Penn State. Based on the interquartile range, I'd bet dollars to donuts that the mean SAT score is higher at Harvard than at Penn State.

The interquartile range is a great measure of both central tendency and variability. It is, unfortunately, underutilized. I would appreciate it if you would aid me in my objective of singing its praises and spreading its use. That said, let's now turn to the most commonly used measures of variability, the variance and its sibling, the standard deviation.

Another way to think of variability is in terms of deviations from the mean. It makes sense, I hope, that if one data set has all its scores clustered tightly around the mean and another has its scores spread further away, that the one with the scores spread further away, the one with bigger deviation scores, has more variability. Wouldn't it make sense, then, to use the average deviation score as a measure of variability? Unfortunately, the sum of deviation scores is zero, so calculating the average deviation score isn't helpful. We get around this problem by squaring the deviation scores before averaging them. The average of the squared deviation scores is called the **variance.**

We will discuss three types of variance, and it is important to keep them all straight. Why are there so many variances? Because it depends on whether we are talking about the variance of a sample or of a population. Once again, we'll use the convention of abbreviating sample statistics with Latin letters and population parameters with Greek ones.

Let's think about the variance of a sample first, what we'll abbreviate as s^2, pronounced "ess squared." Clearly, if we have a sample we can calculate the mean of the sample (M, not μ), and with this we can calculate deviation scores, square them, add them all up, and divide by the number of cases to find the average squared deviation score. The formula for this is shown in Equation 4.6; I'll give the English-language version of the formula in a little bit.*

variance

A measure of variability; the mean of the squared deviations from the mean.

F O R M U L A

Variance of a Sample (s^2)

Equation 4.6

$$s^2 = \frac{\Sigma(X - M)^2}{N}$$

Where:
s^2 = sample variance
X = scores for cases in the sample
M = the sample mean
N = the number of cases in the sample

Similarly, in the rare instances that you have access to all the cases in a population, you can calculate the mean of the population (μ, not M), and go on to calculate deviation scores, square them, and find the average squared deviation score. As an abbreviation for this we'll use σ^2, pronounced "sigma squared," as seen in Equation 4.7.[†]

*Here's a little heads-up for you that will be relevant in later chapters. The numerator in Equation 4.6 has a name: the sum of squares. Why? Because it involves summing a bunch of squared numbers!

[†] Just to make the world confusing, statisticians use an uppercase sigma (Σ) for a summation sign and a lowercase sigma (σ) in the abbreviation for variance. So, if a statistician refers to "sigma," you need to look at the context to know which one is being referred to.

LOOKING CLOSER

F O R M U L A

Variance of a Population (σ^2)

Equation 4.7

$$\sigma^2 = \frac{\Sigma(X - \mu)^2}{N}$$

Where:
σ^2 = population variance
X = scores for cases in the population
μ = the population mean
N = the number of cases in the population

There is a population from which our sample comes, and there is a variance (σ^2) for this population. However, it is unlikely that we will be able to calculate σ^2 since it is rare that we have access to all the cases in the population. Even so, there are occasions where we would like to make use of the population variance. Statisticians have developed a way around this problem, a way to take information from a sample and to modify it, to *correct* it, so that we can estimate a parameter.* Estimated, or corrected, population variance is abbreviated as $\hat{s}^2$, pronounced "ess hat squared"; the formula for it is shown in Equation 4.8.

F O R M U L A

Estimated Population Variance ($\hat{s}^2$)

Equation 4.8

$$\hat{s}^2 = \frac{\Sigma(X - M)^2}{N - 1}$$

Where:
$\hat{s}^2$ = estimated population variance
X = scores for cases in the sample
M = the sample mean
N = the number of cases in the sample

To help all this make sense, let's take a small data set with five cases and calculate the variance. Imagine that we have a sample of five people from the population of the entire world and have measured their IQs as 91, 96, 99, 104, and 110. We calculate the mean (M) for these five IQs as 100.

LOOKING CLOSER   *Did you remember that a parameter is a population value whereas a statistic is a sample value?

We are now ready to calculate the *sample* variance (s^2) by means of Equation 4.6:

1. Subtract the mean from each score to calculate deviation scores.
2. Take all the deviation scores, square them, and then add them all up.
3. Finally, divide this sum by the total number of scores.

Here is what the equation becomes in this case:

$$s^2 = \frac{(-9)^2 + (-4)^2 + (-1)^2 + 4^2 + 10^2}{5} = \frac{81 + 16 + 1 + 16 + 100}{5}$$

$$= \frac{214}{5} = 42.80$$

The variance for this sample of five cases is 42.80. Now, at this moment it is hard to have any sense of what a variance of 42.80 means. Does it reflect a lot of variability in the sample, or little variability? For the moment, just accept that when there is more variability in a sample, the number representing the variance gets larger.

Remember, these five people are a sample from the population of the world. And the world does have a population, right? If we collected data from everyone in the world, we could calculate a population mean and go on to calculate a population variance. Though, theoretically, a population variance (σ^2) exists for intelligence in the world, in actuality we can't calculate it. We may not be able to calculate it, but we can estimate it.

Before going through the mechanics of estimation, let's think. In the sample the lowest IQ is 91; do you think that there are lower IQs in the world? The highest sample IQ is 110; do you think that there are higher IQs in the world? It seems logical that higher and lower IQs exist in the population than are captured in the sample, that there is more variability in the population than there is in the sample. This should be so, though less so, even if the sample is very, very large. So, when statisticians developed a way to estimate population variance from sample variance, they looked for a way to increase the variance. However, they wanted to increase the variance proportionally, to make more of an adjustment when sample sizes were small. In our IQ example, with a very small sample, it is easy to assume that the population variance is much greater. But, if you had a very large sample, you would probably have some people with very high IQs and some people with very low IQs. That is, with a large sample you would come much closer to the full range of the variability that exists in the population.

Statisticians have settled on the correction shown in Equation 4.8; that is, to divide the sum of the squared deviation scores by $N - 1$, not by N.

In this case, it makes the estimated population variance $\frac{214}{5 - 1}$, or 53.50.

Note that 53.50 is greater than 42.80, meaning we estimate there is more variability in the population than in the sample.

The correction for the estimated population variance gets smaller as sample size gets larger. Suppose that the numerator in the variance equation, what is called a sum of squares, is 50 and our sample size is five.

In this case the sample variance is 10.00 and the estimated population variance is 12.50. There is a 25% increase from s^2 to $\hat{s}^2$!

But, what if the sum of squares is 5000 and our sample size is 500. The sample variance is still 10.00, but the estimated population variance is now calculated by dividing 5000 by 499. And this equals 10.02. In this scenario, with a much larger sample size, there is only a .2% increase from sample variance to estimated population variance, not a 25% increase. As sample size increases, there is less need to correct the sample variance to reflect the population variance since we are likely to have captured in our sample more of the whole range of variability that exists in the population.

Let's move on to our final measure of variability, the one most commonly used, the **standard deviation.** One problem with the variance is that even though we have measured our variable in regular score units, we calculate the variance in a new metric, squared score units. That is, we measured IQs, calculated deviation scores, squared them, and then found the average *squared* deviation score of 42.80. Changing metrics is unwieldy and gives us a statistic that is hard to interpret. We can deal with this problem by turning the variance back into the original score units, by taking its square root.

This unsquared measure of variability is called the standard deviation. There are three versions of it: for a sample (s), for a population (σ), and an estimated (or corrected) version for the population ($\hat{s}$). These are called "ess," "sigma," and "ess hat," respectively, and each is calculated by taking the square root of its respective variance. They don't really need formulae, but here they are anyway.

standard deviation

A measure of variability, the square root of the variance, a measure of the average distance by which scores deviate from the mean.

F O R M U L A

Standard Deviations

Equation 4.9 $s = \sqrt{s^2}$

$\sigma = \sqrt{\sigma^2}$

$\hat{s} = \sqrt{\hat{s}^2}$

Where:

s = sample standard deviation
s^2 = sample variance (see Equation 4.6)
σ = population standard deviation
σ^2 = population variance (see Equation 4.7)
$\hat{s}$ = estimated population standard deviation
$\hat{s}^2$ = estimated population variance (see Equation 4.8)

So, for the five IQ scores we have been working with, $s = \sqrt{42.8000}$ or 6.54, and $\hat{s} = \sqrt{53.5000}$ or 7.31.* Again, note that the estimated population value is larger than the sample value.

The standard deviation has advantages over the variance. By taking the square root of what had been squared, we move the number back to the metric with which we started. As a result, the standard deviation is more easily interpreted. It represents the average distance between scores and the mean. The more you use standard deviations, the more easily you'll sense whether the scores in the sample are clustered relatively tightly around the mean (i.e., the standard deviation is small) or are dispersed widely (i.e., the standard deviation is large).

Moving from a sample standard deviation to an estimated population standard deviation is sometimes necessary, so here's a formula for those times when you have been given s but need to know $\hat{s}$.

F O R M U L A

Converting Sample Standard Deviation (s) to Estimated (Corrected) Population Standard Deviation ($\hat{s}$)

Equation 4.10

$$\hat{s} = \sqrt{\frac{(s^2)N}{N-1}}$$

Where:

$\hat{s}$ = estimated (corrected) population standard deviation being calculated
s = sample standard deviation
N = sample size

Finally, remember that the purpose of a measure of variability is to tell how much variability exists in a set of data. If the standard deviation is small, then there is little variability and the scores are relatively tightly clustered about mean. If the standard deviation is large, then scores are more widely scattered. Figure 4.3 shows graphic examples of this.

Also, I should mention that standard deviations and variances can only be calculated for interval- and ratio-level data. This is because calculating them makes use of deviation scores, and deviation scores are only sensible when the distances between scores have meaning. How does one calculate variability for nominal- or ordinal-level data? For nominal data and for some ordinal data you can count the different response options. If, for example, you are studying the variability of religions found at two different schools, you might report that students at one school come from

---

*Remember the rules of rounding! If I were to ask for the variance, you should report it with two more decimal places than were in the original data set, as 42.80. But, when you are using the variance as a step to something else, carry at least two more decimal places than needed at the end.

LOOKING CLOSER

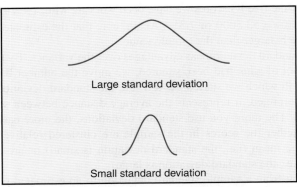

Figure **4.3** Graphs of two distributions of data with the same mean and different standard deviations.

five different religions whereas those at the other school come from seven different religions. The latter school, obviously, has more variability in religion among its students.

Group Practice 4.2

1. Here is a grouped frequency distribution for the final grades in statistics data set.

Grade	Frequency
95-99	1
90-94	1
85-89	0
80-84	3
75-79	4
70-74	3
65-69	7
60-64	7
55-59	12
50-54	7
45-49	6
40-44	4
35-39	0
30-34	4
25-29	1

Answer the questions and fill in the blanks:

a. The _____th score is the score at the 25th percentile.

b. The interval for the score that falls at the 25th percentile has a real lower limit of _____.

c. The _____th score is the score at the 75th percentile.

d. The interval for the score that falls at the 75th percentile has a real lower limit of _____.

e. Calculate the interquartile range.

f. Why is the value calculated in 1e different from the value calculated for the same data in the text? Which provides a better estimate of the actual interquartile range for this data set?

2. Calculate s^2, σ^2, s, and σ for a sample with the following IQ scores: 113, 117, 118, 98, 107, 112, 123, 101, 94, and 109. (Remember, statisticians don't give up easily. If we can't calculate something, we look for a fallback option.)

a. $s^2 =$ _____

b. $\sigma^2 =$ _____

c. $s =$ _____

d. $\sigma =$ _____

3. Below are two sets of scores, each with a mean of 2.00. Which one do you think will have more variability? Calculate the sample variance for each.

Set A: 1, 2, and 3

Set B: 2, 2, and 2

SUMMARY

In descriptive statistics, a set of data can be summarized by describing two important dimensions: central tendency and variability. Statisticians use three different measures—mean, median, and mode—to describe the "average" score in a data set. The mode tells which score is most common and, as it only uses "difference" information, can be used with nominal-level data. The median uses "direction" as well as difference and signifies the point in a data set that evenly divides the top half of scores from the bottom half; the median can be calculated for ordinal-level data. The mean considers "distance" as well as direction and difference and can be used with interval—or ratio—level data. Though the mean is the most commonly calculated average, it is not appropriate for data that are skewed or multimodal.

The amount of variability in a set of data is independent of whether the central tendency of that data set is high or low. There are four measures of variability: range, interquartile range, variance, and standard deviation. Range, which tells the distance from the lowest score to the highest, is the least useful since it is most affected by outliers. The other three measures—interquartile range, variance, and standard deviation—are more robust measures of variability since they are relatively unaffected by outliers. The interquartile range tells the distance from the 25th to the 75th percentile and, when reported as an interval, gives an indication of central tendency as well as variability. The variance tells the average squared deviation score. But the variance is not as easy to interpret as the standard deviation (the square root of variance) because it changes the metric from raw score units to squared raw score units.

A sample value is a statistic; a population value is a parameter. Latin letters are used as abbreviations for statistics and Greek letters for parameters. Thus, we differentiate between the mean for a sample (M) and the mean for a population (μ) and between the variance and standard deviation for a sample (s^2 and s) and for a population (σ^2 and σ). Though we may not *have* population information, we still would like to know population values, so statisticians have developed a way to estimate the population variance and standard deviation, abbreviated as $\hat{s}^2$ and $\hat{s}$, respectively. (In Chapter 6 we'll see a way to estimate, from a sample mean, the range within which we think the population mean falls.)

Review Exercises

1. A meteorologist measured the temperature every 2 hours for a day in January and a day in June. These were the temperatures, in degrees Fahrenheit, for the January day: 23, 22, 21, 21, 23, 27, 28, 31, 32, 32, 30, and 26. These were the temperatures, in degrees Fahrenheit, for the June day: 56, 56, 59, 62, 64, 67, 73, 75, 77, 76, 75, and 74. On which day were the temperatures more variable? Check your expectation by calculating a measure of variability.

2. A phlebotomist (for all you nonmedical people, that's the formal name for the person who draws blood) decides to find out how many times people have blood drawn while they're in the hospital. She takes a random sample of hospital admissions and does a chart audit to find out how many times each person had blood drawn. These are the results: 4, 3, 7, 2, 7, 8, 12, 13, 5, 4, 3, 6, 5, 3, 10, 4, 9, 6, 8, 7, 4, 3, 5, 7, and 5. What is the average for the sample? What is the population to which these results can be generalized? Can you estimate the average for the population?

3. Calculate the median and the interquartile range for the following grouped frequency distribution for an interval level variable.

Interval	Frequency
70-79	12
60-69	14
50-59	18
40-49	16
30-39	11
20-29	8

4. Calculate the mean for the grouped frequency distribution in question 3. (Not sure what to do? See footnote on page 95.)

5. If $s = 12.44$ and $N = 45$, what does $\hat{s}$ equal?

6. These data represent the values of an interval-level variable measured on a sample from a population: 34, 65, 56, 45, 55, 49, 38, and 59. Calculate the following:
   a. $M = $ _____
   b. $s = $ _____
   c. $\hat{s}^2 = $ _____
   d. $\sigma = $ _____
   e. $\Sigma(X - M) = $ _____
   f. The range: _____
   g. The mode: _____

7. Skip was born on January 1, 2000. Rounding like a statistician, and allowing for negative ages, what was his age, in integer years, on each of the following dates:
   a. January 28, 2000
   b. September 15, 2000
   c. December 31, 2000
   d. January 2, 2001
   e. June 1, 2001
   f. July 15, 2001
   g. December 25, 1999
   h. February 14, 1999

Homework Problems

1. Which statement is true?
   a. $\mu > M$
   b. $\mu < M$
   c. $\sigma > s$
   d. $\sigma < s$
   e. a and c
   f. b and d

2. Which of the following is true in a positively skewed distribution?
   a. $M > Mdn$
   b. $M < Mdn$
   c. $M = Mdn$
   d. Skewness does not affect measures of central tendency in any systematic fashion.

3. Which of the following is true of the sum of deviation scores?
   a. When divided by N it equals the mean.
   b. It is always positive.
   c. It is always negative.
   d. It equals zero.
   e. When divided by N it equals the variance.

4. Which of the following measures of variability is most affected by outliers?
   a. The range
   b. The interquartile range
   c. The variance

   d. The standard deviation
   e. They all are equally affected by outliers.

5. An oceanographer is interested in finding the average size (in square miles) of four oceans. She consults an almanac and finds that the Pacific Ocean has a size of 64,186,300 square miles, the Atlantic is 33,420,000 square miles large, the Indian 28,350,500, and the Arctic 5,105,700. What is the mean size of the oceans on earth? Is the mean the appropriate measure of central tendency?

6. She decides to classify any ocean that is more than a standard deviation above the mean as "super-sized" and any ocean that is more than a standard deviation below the mean as "puny." Which oceans, if any, are so classified?

7. What is the range for the size of oceans?

8. If $N = 20$ and $s = 4.34$, what does $\hat{s}$ equal?

9. Here is a table showing, for the 50 U.S. states and the District of Columbia, the percentage of persons living in poverty in the United States. What is the median poverty level for these 51 cases? What is the interquartile range? (Save your answers; you're going to need them for the homework problems in Chapter 5.)

% In Poverty	Frequency
21-22	1
19-20	2
17-18	2
15-16	6
13-14	11
11-12	9
9-10	13
7-8	7

10. A nutritionist is developing a new sugar substitute and has 20 college students taste solutions made of sugar, saccharine, Nutrasweet, and his new substance. The order in which the substances are tasted is changed for each participant. After tasting each substance, the participant rates it on a 10-point scale where $10 =$ "just like sugar" and $0 =$ "not like sugar at all." After each substance is tasted, each participant rinses his or her mouth with water and waits 2 minutes before tasting the next substance. What is the researcher's dependent variable? What is the population to which the researcher probably wishes to generalize his results? Is this the population that the sample represents?

11. A researcher takes a sample from a population. These are the values for the ratio level dependent variable: 45, 67, 34, 55, 87, 56, 60, 51, and 59. Calculate s, $\hat{s}$, and σ.

12. Let's say that $s = 4.00$ and that N is large. Put the following in order from largest to smallest: s, s^2, $\hat{s}$, $\hat{s}^2$. Where would you put σ and σ^2?

5

Transformed Scores II

Standard Scores and the Normal Distribution

Learning Objectives

After completing this chapter, you should be able to do the following:

1 Transform scores back and forth from raw scores to standard scores and percentile ranks.
2 Describe the characteristics of the normal distribution.
3 Estimate and calculate areas under the normal curve.
4 Understand, thanks to the central limit theorem, that a sampling distribution of the mean will be normally distributed even when the parent population is not.

Pay attention to three major sights as we motor through this chapter: standard scores, the normal distribution, and the central limit theorem.

Standard scores, like *z* scores, measure the distance between the mean and a raw score in terms of standard deviation units. Thus, standard scores are a way of transforming scores on different metrics (e.g., an intelligence quotient [IQ] score of 95 and a Scholastic Achievement Test [SAT] Verbal score of 615) so that they can be directly compared.

The normal distribution is a specific bell-shaped curve that is symmetric (so the midpoint is also the mean and the median), where most cases fall at the middle (so the midpoint is also the mode), and where the frequency of cases decreases as one moves away from the midpoint. Each *z* score in a normal distribution is associated with a specific percentage of cases that fall below it, allowing one to transform *z* scores to percentile ranks, and vice versa.

We will spend more time on the central limit theorem in the next chapter, but the concept of the central limit theorem is important enough that it gets a preview in this chapter. Briefly, the central limit theorem says that if we take repeated, random samples from a population and calculate the mean for each sample, then the frequency polygon for the mean—what is called a sampling distribution—will be normally distributed, no matter the shape of the original population. Why will this be important? Because we know a lot about the characteristics of the normal distribution and can use that to make predictions about the sampling distribution. Don't worry if this doesn't seem very clear right now; it will, eventually.

Z SCORES

In this chapter we continue the exploration of transformed scores that we started in Chapter 3 by moving beyond percentile ranks to standard scores and their variations. What are standard scores, and why do we need them? Well, imagine two sixth-graders from different states, each of whom has just taken his or her state's mandated math proficiency exam. By chance they meet and, as kids do, start a game of one-upmanship. Buffy, who took the California exam and obtained a raw score of 75, claims that she is smarter than Skip, who took the New York exam and only obtained a raw score of 50. Did she really do better?

Judging by the raw scores, Buffy does have a higher score than Skip. But comparing scores on two different tests is like comparing apples to oranges. If we knew the means of the two tests, we'd be able to calculate

TABLE **5.1** **Math Proficiency Test Data for Buffy and Skip**

	Raw Score	Test Mean	Test Standard Deviation
Buffy	75	60	15
Skip	50	30	10

deviation scores and get some sense of whether either or both scored above the mean. The mean on Buffy's test is 60; on Skip's, it is 30. Both scored above the mean, but Skip, whose raw score is lower, argues that he is smarter since he scored 20 points above the mean, compared with Buffy's 15 points above the mean. Is it reasonable to conclude that he really is smarter than Buffy?

Knowing means does provide useful comparative information when one case scores above and the other below, but is not very helpful when both cases score on the same side of the mean. Adding information about standard deviations allows us to transform tests with different means to the same metric. The standard deviation for Buffy's test is 15; for Skip's it is 10. Thus Buffy, who scored 15 points above the mean, has a score that is one standard deviation above the mean. Skip, whose score was 20 points above the mean, has a score that is two standard deviations above the mean. Both scores have been converted to a standard metric, number of standard deviations away from the mean, and we can now see that Skip, at two standard deviations above the mean, performed better than Buffy, who scored only one standard deviation above the mean. Table 5.1 summarizes the data for this example.

Believe it or not, you just learned how to calculate *z* **scores,** or *standard* scores. A *z* score is simply a score transformed into how far away, in *standard* deviation units, the score is from the mean. If the score—as a *z* score—is positive, then the score is above the mean. A negative *z* score indicates that the score is below the mean. The bigger the absolute value of the *z* score, the further away from the mean the score is. And, of course, *z* scores of zero indicate scores right at the mean.

As a result of this transformation, any set of scores transformed into *z* scores will end up with a mean of 0 and a standard deviation of 1. For a concrete example of this, let's take a small data set consisting of three scores: 1, 2, and 3. The mean (*M*) for this set of scores is 2.00, and the standard deviation (*s*) is .82. If we transform these scores into *z* scores we get −1.22, .00, and 1.22. Calculating the mean and the standard deviation for these *z* scores gives us values of .00 and 1.00, respectively.

One other thing to know about transforming scores into *z* scores is that it does not change the shape of a distribution of scores. When a set of scores is transformed into *z* scores, the values associated with the scores change, but the shape of the distribution remains the same. Figure 5.1

z score

Also known as standard score, the distance of the score from the mean given in standard deviation units.

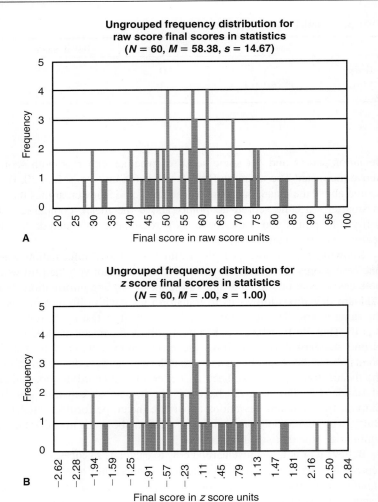

Figure **5.1** Histograms showing how transforming a set of scores from raw scores to z scores does not change the shape of a set of scores.

shows histograms for (a) the ungrouped frequency distribution for the raw score final grades for 60 statistics students and (b) these scores converted into z scores. Note that the two graphs look exactly the same though the metric on the abscissa has changed.

A z score simply uses standard units, standard deviations, to express how far a raw score is above or below the mean. Though I hope that you have an intuitive sense for how to calculate z scores, it probably would help to have an official formula.

F O R M U L A

z Scores (z) from Raw Scores (X)

$$z = \frac{X - M}{s}$$

Equation 5.1

Where:

z = the z score being calculated

X = the raw score for which the z score is being calculated

M = the mean of the raw scores

s = the standard deviation of the raw scores

This formula says that one transforms a raw score (X) into a z score by subtracting the mean from the raw score and dividing the difference by the standard deviation. Buffy's raw score of 75 on the math test becomes, via $\frac{75 - 60}{15}$, a z score of 1.00.

Just as it is important to be able to transform a raw score into a z score, it is also important to be able to reverse directions and transform z scores back to raw scores. This is also intuitive: if a person's z score is 1.5, then you know that his or her score is 1.5 standard deviations above the mean. If you are told that $M = 25$ and $s = 10$, then you know that the person's score is 15 raw score units (10×1.5) above 25, or 40. Here's the official formula for transforming z scores back to raw scores:

F O R M U L A

Raw Scores (X) from z Scores (z)

$$X = zs + M$$

Equation 5.2

Where:

X = the raw score being calculated

z = the z score for which the raw score is being calculated

s = the standard deviation of the raw scores

M = the mean of the raw scores

This formula says to transform a z score into a raw score by finding the product of the z score times the standard deviation and adding this product to the mean. Buffy's z score of 1.00 on the math exam is transformed back, via $(1.00 \times 15) + 60$, to 75.00.

You now know that a positive z score indicates performance above the mean and a negative z score indicates performance below the mean. You also know that the larger the absolute value of the z score, the further the score is from the mean. Thus I find, and I hope you do too, that z scores are easy to interpret. If you know someone's z score you have a good sense of where that person's score places him or her in the distribution of scores. Statisticians, however, fearing that people would have difficulty using/interpreting negative numbers, have developed a number of variations on z scores. With all of them, if you know the key you can easily tell the distance between a case's score and the mean.

In fact, you are already familiar with one of these z-score variations: SAT scores. The SAT has two subtests, a verbal and a quantitative test. The subtest raw scores are transformed to standard scores so that they have a mean of 500 and a standard deviation of 100. In other words, a person whose raw score on the verbal subtest is average obtains a score of 500. If a person's raw score on the performance subtest is half a standard deviation below the mean, then he or she receives a score of 450.

You may be aware that scores on the SAT subtests range from 200 to 800, and this brings up an interesting fact about the normal distribution. In a normal distribution, almost all scores, 99.73% to be exact, fall in the region from three standard deviations below the mean (a z score of -3.00) to three standard deviations above the mean (a z score of $+3.00$). It is so rare that a person scores higher or lower than this (0.27% of the time, to be exact) that ETS (Educational Testing Service, the makers of the SAT) can safely limit scores to the mean ± 3 standard deviations, to a range from 200 to 800.

It is not hard to convert z scores to SAT-style scores and SAT-style scores to z scores or raw scores. Equations 5.3a, 5.3b, and 5.3c do just that.

FORMULAE

Moving Among *z* Scores, SAT-Style Scores, and Raw Scores

Equation 5.3a $SAT = 100z + 500$

Equation 5.3b $z = \dfrac{SAT - 500}{100}$

Equation 5.3c $X = \dfrac{SAT - 500}{100} s + M$

Where:
SAT = SAT-style score
z = z score
X = raw score
s = standard deviation of raw scores
M = mean of raw scores

Another z-score variant is IQ scores, which are commonly transformed so that the mean is 100 and the standard deviation is 15.* Equations 5.3a through 5.3c can be used for IQ scores, by substituting IQ for SAT and replacing the constants of 100 and 500 with 15 and 100.

Before turning to our detailed exploration of the normal distribution, let's practice moving back and forth from raw scores and z scores and into SAT and IQ scores.

Group Practice 5.1

1. There is a math test on which $M = 18$ and $s = 3$. Buffy scores a 14. What is her score as a z score?
2. Skip receives a raw score of 17. What is his score as a z score?
3. Buffy's mom took the same test when she was in school. Though she has forgotten her raw score, she remembers that her z score was .53. Calculate her raw score. (It is OK if the score you calculate is not an integer.)
4. Skip's dad recalls that his score on that test, as a z score, was $-.73$. What was his raw score?
5. Based on Skip's performance on this math test, estimate what his score will be on the SAT quantitative subtest.
6. Desdemona took a standard IQ test ($M = 100$ and $s = 15$) and scored 137. What is her score as a z? If I developed a new IQ test that had $M = 60$ and $s = 7$, what would Desdemona's score be on this test?

THE NORMAL DISTRIBUTION

I trust that you remember from Chapter 2 that a frequency polygon is a graphic display of a frequency distribution. In a frequency polygon, the values that a variable can have are listed on the X axis, the abscissa. The frequency with which these values occur are marked on the Y axis, the ordinate. I mention this because our next topic is a specific frequency polygon called the normal distribution, or the normal curve. The normal curve, shown in Figure 5.2, is often called the bell-shaped curve because it does look a bit like a bell in profile.[†]

The normal curve has a number of important characteristics. First, it is symmetric, which means that if it were folded over at the midpoint the left half (the lower scores) would perfectly overlap the right half (the higher scores). As a result of this—and a little thought should convince you—the midpoint is the median and the mean.

Second, the greatest frequency on the normal curve is at the midpoint. As one moves away from the midpoint, either to the left or the right, the frequencies get smaller and smaller. Therefore the midpoint is the mode, as well as the median and the mean.

---

*Just to confuse things, some IQ tests use a standard deviation of 16, not 15. For this text, though, whenever I refer to an IQ score, s will always equal 15.

[†] FYI, real statistics nerds refer to the normal distribution as the Gaussian distribution.

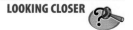

LOOKING CLOSER

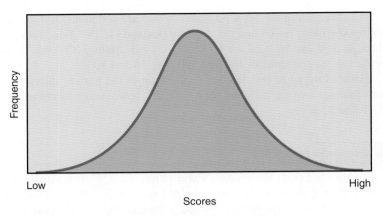

Figure **5.2** The normal distribution.

Third, the normal curve has an infinitely large sample size, and the X values, which are continuous, range from infinitely small to infinitely large. This means that in the normal curve, at least in the normal curve that *theoretically* exists (the one based on an infinitely large sample size and a variable that extends to positive and negative infinity), the curve extends forever, never touching the abscissa.* In reality, the populations and the sample sizes we work with are not infinitely large, and our variables have a finite range, so we only approximate the normal curve with these variables.

A number of bell-shaped curves fit the characteristics outlined above, but not all bell-shaped curves are normal curves. The normal curve is a specific bell-shaped curve that is defined by the percentage of cases (or observations) that fall in specified regions of the curve. This is important, so let me repeat it: *Not all bell-shaped curves are normal curves!* The normal curve is a specific bell-shaped curve, one that is described by the percentages of cases that fall in specified regions of it.[†]

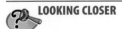 **LOOKING CLOSER**

*There's a gap here between theory and practice. In theory, if a variable like height is normally distributed, there should be a very small number of people who are very, very tall and a very small number of people who are very, very short. And, ad infinitum, there would be even smaller numbers of people who were even taller and shorter. In reality, however, there are limits on how tall—or short—people can be. Remember: although theoretically, z scores of ± 10 or even ± 100 can exist, functionally, it is rare in the social sciences for a z score to be greater than ± 3. In situations where the cost of an error is high—for example, for bridges that need to stay up and nuclear power plants that had better not leak—specifications for components are five or more standard deviations from the mean.

[†]Another way to distinguish the normal curve is by skewness and kurtosis. For a normal curve, both skewness and kurtosis equal zero. I mentioned this back in Chapter 2, and we'll come to make use of it in Chapter 6.

Before we see the percentages, let me explain why the normal curve is a useful thing. Many of the variables that researchers care to measure are, they assume, normally distributed. That is, we think that things like intelligence, aggression, heart rate, cholesterol level, daily caloric intake, reading ability, amount of rain per day, number of ants per square yard, and so on are normally distributed.* Thus if we took a large and random sample of people from the world, measured their IQs, and made a frequency polygon, we would expect to find a bell-shaped distribution on which most people scored near the midpoint (*aka* the mean, the median, and the mode).

In addition, though our sample should be bunched near the mean, cases will be spread, symmetrically, above and below it. We should find a large number of people who are somewhat smart (a bit above the mean) and an equally large number of people who are somewhat dumb (a bit below the mean). As we move away, either to the right or the left, there should be fewer and fewer people further and further above or below average. This distribution should occur for many variables that we care about: most observations bunch near the mean, and there are fewer and fewer cases as one moves further and further away.

We've seen what the theoretical normal distribution looks like (Figure 5.2), and I've told you that we assume that many of the variables that we care to measure are normally distributed. Now it is time for the rubber to meet the road. Let's see if we can generate a normal distribution, if this curve really exists. And, to make it harder, I'm going to try to approximate it with a sample that is not too large and with a variable that is not continuous.

Get 9 pennies, toss them, and count the number of heads. Do this a few times. You probably got 4 or 5 heads, maybe 3 or 6. Still, you might have obtained as few as 0 heads or as many as 9 heads, so there are 10 options for the number of heads you can obtain when you toss 9 coins. Leading a relatively quiet and boring life, I sought excitement one afternoon by tossing 9 coins 300 times. Figure 5.3 is a bar graph showing my results.

I think you'll agree that this is a fairly symmetric distribution, that most observations fall near the middle, and that there are fewer and fewer observations as one moves away from the midpoint. This looks more than a little bit like a normal distribution![†] In fact, if I kept on tossing 9 coins and counting heads an infinite number of times, I would end up with a very good approximation of a normal distribution, as seen in Figure 5.4. And, remember, this is for a discrete (noncontinuous) variable with a restricted range.

---

*The normal distribution was termed the "normal" distribution by Sir Francis Galton because he believed it was almost universal, that it expressed the natural order of nature.

[†] I can't resist getting a little ahead of myself and making one more point. On each of the tosses of the nine coins, whether they landed heads or tails was determined by chance, by a random process. Please note that it was a random process that generated this normal distribution!

LOOKING CLOSER

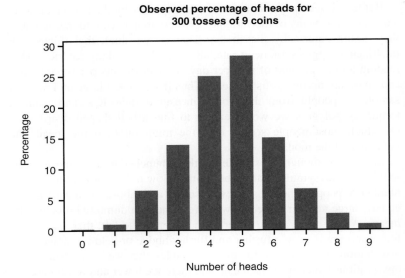

Figure **5.3** Approximation to the normal distribution for a discrete variable of restricted range in a small sample.

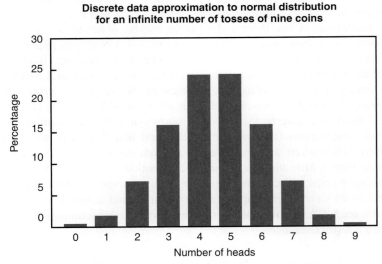

Figure **5.4** Approximation to the normal distribution for a discrete variable of restricted range in an infinitely large sample.

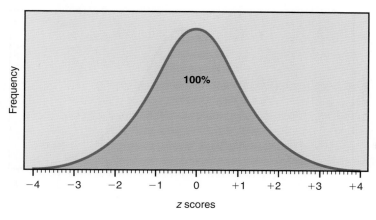

Figure **5.5** Area under the normal curve.

Having some sense of why the normal distribution is useful—we assume that many variables we wish to measure are normally distributed—and having seen one instance in which a variable is normally distributed, let me now show you a way that we can use z scores and the normal curve to transform scores and calculate probabilities.*

Suppose that I have a set of scores for some variable—X—that is normally distributed, and I plot the frequency polygon for these scores. It should be normally distributed, right? I could then take all my X values, transform them into z scores, and make a frequency polygon for the z scores. Since transforming scores into z scores doesn't change the shape of a distribution, the frequency polygon for the z scores will also have a normal shape. Since the normal distribution has a specific shape and all normal distributions have exactly the same shape, the convention is to describe them by z scores rather than by raw scores. So, let's draw a normal distribution and, finally, talk about the area under the curve.

Figure 5.5 shows a frequency polygon for a normal distribution with the z scores marked on the abscissa. As a result, the middle of the normal distribution—the spot that is the mean, the median, and the mode of the distribution—has a value of zero. Scores that are above the mean, that are off to the right of the mean, have positive values; scores that are below the mean, that are off to the left of the mean, have negative values. I've extended the abscissa from −4.0 to +4.0, but the line, theoretically at least, extends from −∞ to +∞. And, under the curve, I've written "100%" to

---

*Maybe variables we care about aren't normally distributed. Gladwell (2006) offers a number of instances—violence by officers in the LA Police Department, length of time that people remain homeless—that are not normally distributed. (Gladwell, M. [2006, February 13 & 20]. Million Dollar Murray: Why problems like homelessness may be easier to solve than manage. *The New Yorker, 82,* 96–107.)

LOOKING CLOSER

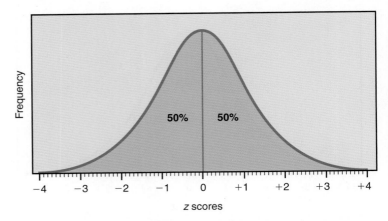

Figure **5.6** Area on each side of midpoint for the normal curve.

indicate that 100% of the cases fall in the area under the curve. This is simple but important, so let me restate it: *this curve bounds, or captures, all the possible observations for all the cases for this infinitely large, normally distributed data set.* *

In Figure 5.6, I've taken the normal distribution and drawn a line at the midpoint. Since the midpoint is the median, the spot that separates the top 50% of the cases from the bottom 50%, I've written 50% in each of the two halves to indicate that the area under the curve for each half of the normal distribution contains 50% of the cases.

So far, these percentages are true for any symmetric distribution: all the cases fall under the curve and half are above the median. But now, in Table 5.2 and Figure 5.7, we see the percentages that are unique to the

TABLE **5.2**   **Percentage of the Area under the Normal Curve That Falls in Each Standard Deviation as One Moves Away from the Mean**

From	To	Area
Mean	$1s$	34.1345%
$1s$	$2s$	13.5905%
$2s$	$3s$	2.1400%
$3s$	$4s$	.1318%
$4s$	$5s$	.0031%
$5s$	∞	.000029%

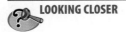

LOOKING CLOSER

*Whenever I restate something that seems clear to begin with I am reminded of a professor I had for a Russian novel class in college. Speaking of Dostoevsky's *Notes from the Underground,* he said (and I am not making this up), "The underground, clearly, to me, suggests that which is below the surface."

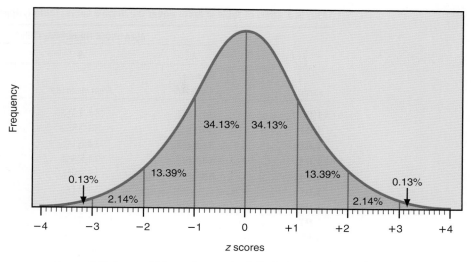

Figure **5.7** Area within each standard deviation for the normal curve.

normal distribution. In Figure 5.7 I've marked each standard deviation as we move away from the mean and noted the percentage of cases that fall in each bounded area. Since the normal distribution is symmetric, the percentage of cases that fall from the mean to one standard deviation above the mean, 34.13%, is the same as the percentage that fall from the mean to one standard deviation below.

If you add up the areas in the first three standard deviations on each side of the mean, the area from a *z* of −3.00 to a *z* of +3.00 (and if you allow for the rounding error that crept in when I rounded the areas to two decimal places), you'll see that 99.73% of the cases in a normal distribution fall *within* three standard deviations of the mean. Or, phrased another way, 0.135% of the observations fall more than three standard deviations *above* the mean, and 0.135% of the observations fall more than three standard deviations *below* the mean.

It is possible to cut *z* scores into smaller intervals than integers, and so we can calculate the area under the normal curve more finely. For example, 3.98% of the cases fall from the mean to one tenth of a standard deviation above it. Remember, there are fewer and fewer cases as we move away from the mean in a normal distribution. Thus we should predict that a smaller percentage of cases falls in the next tenth of a standard deviation under the normal curve; and, as the answer is 3.94%, we are right.

There are formulae for calculating the area under the curve in a normal distribution for any *z* score, but the convention is to use a table that has already done the work. Table 1 in the Appendix is a *z* score table that reports the area under the normal curve in percentage format and, to explain it, I've put a section of it here in Table 5.3.

TABLE **5.3**   **Part of Table of Areas under the Normal Curve (Table 1, Appendix A)**

	AREA UNDER THE NORMAL CURVE		
	A	B	C
z score	*Below +z* *Above −z*	*From mean to z*	*Above +z* *Below −z*
1.00	84.13%	34.13%	15.87%
1.01	84.38%	34.38%	15.62%
1.02	84.61%	34.61%	15.39%
1.03	84.85%	34.85%	15.15%
1.04	85.08%	35.08%	14.92%
1.05	85.31%	35.31%	14.69%
1.06	85.54%	35.54%	14.46%
1.07	85.77%	35.77%	14.23%
1.08	85.99%	35.99%	14.01%
1.09	86.21%	36.21%	13.79%

To make this table as user-friendly as possible, I've used percentages, not proportions.* First, note that the bold numbers indicate z scores, and they increase by hundredths. Then, note that there are three columns (A, B, and C) that report the areas under the curve. Column A reports the area that falls below a given positive z score (or, symmetrically, above a negative z score), Column B reports the area that falls from the mean to a z score (either a positive z score or a negative z score), and Column C reports the area that falls above a positive z score (or, symmetrically, below a negative z score.).

Figure 5.8 shows a normal curve with the area below $z = 1.0$ shaded in. The area below the mean is marked with 50%, as half of the area under the curve falls below the mean. You'll see also that 34.13% of the area under the normal curve falls in the region from the mean to one deviation above. Note that 50% plus 34.13% equals 84.13%, the area listed in Table 5.3's Column A for $z = 1.00$. Note also that the area listed in Column B, 34.13%, is already in the figure as the area from the mean to the z score. A little math should tell us that if the total area under the curve is 100% and we have already accounted for 84.13% of the area as falling below our specified z score, then 15.87% (that's 100.00 minus 84.13) falls above our specified z score. And this is the information presented in Column C. Thus, for all the z scores listed in the table, you

LOOKING CLOSER

*Percentages and proportions are just transformations of each other. For a proportion, the entire area under the curve is 1.00, not 100%. Thus, the proportion of the area under the normal curve that falls below the mean is .50, not 50%. It is easy to move from one to another: a proportion times 100 equals a percentage, and a percentage divided by 100 equals a proportion.

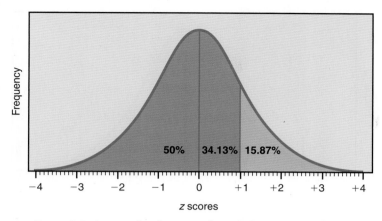

Figure **5.8** Area under the normal curve for a *z* score of 1.00.

know the area that falls under them, the area from the mean to them, and the area above them.

You may have noticed that the *z* score table contains only positive scores. What do you do with a negative *z* score? Well, statisticians hate to be redundant, and since the normal distribution is symmetric, we can also use this table with negative *z* scores. First, realize that Column B doesn't change. If 34.13% of the cases fall from the mean to a *z* of 1.00, then 34.13% of cases fall from the mean to a *z* of −1.00. Figure 5.9 shows this, as well as the areas below and above the specified *z* score. Then note the dual labels for Columns A and C. Column A tells the area under the curve that falls *below* a *positive z* score, which is the same as the area

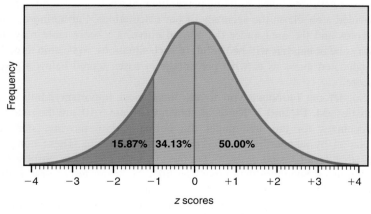

Figure **5.9** Area under the normal curve for a *z* score of −1.00.

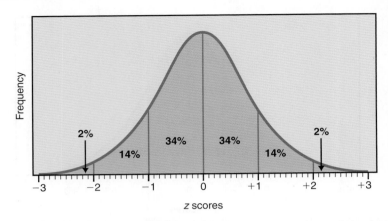

Figure **5.10** Good-enough-for-purposes-of-estimation values of the area under the curve for the normal distribution.

that falls *above* a *negative z* score; Column C tells the area that falls *above* a *positive z* score, which is the same as the area that falls *below* a *negative z* score.

I've said that statisticians hate to be redundant and, if you are on the ball, you're calling me a poor statistician right about now because my table of the area under the normal curve is as redundant as can be: Columns A, B, and C all contain the same information. If you know the Column A value, 84.13% for a *z* score of 1.00, then you can quickly calculate the Column B value (34.13%) by subtracting 50% from Column A's. Similarly, you can calculate Column C's value (15.87%) by subtracting Column A's from 100%.

With this table, it should be fairly easy to find the *exact* area from the mean to a given *z* score and the area above or below that *z* score. But, again, I would like you to estimate before you calculate. Back in Chapter 3 we saw that estimating percentile ranks before calculating them provided a check on the accuracy of our calculations. Furthermore, with *z* scores and the area under the normal curve, a *z* score table may not always be at hand; it will be useful, in such situations, to be able to make an educated guess as to what percentage of cases scored below a given *z* score.

So, let me introduce you to the three most important numbers in statistics: **34, 14, and 2.** These, as shown in Figure 5.10, are the rounded percentages for the area under the normal curve, moving, standard deviation by standard deviation, away from the mean. These numbers are what I call "good-enough" numbers: good enough for purposes of estimating areas under the curve. The first, 34, is our easy-to-remember approximation of the 34.13% of observations that fall from the mean to one standard deviation above (or below) it. The second, 14, approximates the 13.59% of cases that fall from a *z* of 1.0 to a *z* of 2.0 (or from −1.0 to

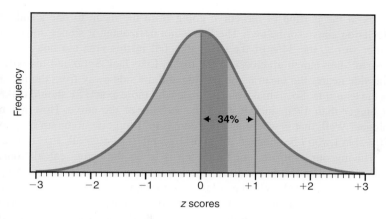

Figure **5.11** Estimating the area under the normal curve from z = .00 to z = .50.

−2.0). And the third, 2, approximates the 2.14% of cases that fall from a z of 2.0 to a z of 3.0 (or from −2.0 to −3.0). The three numbers added together equal 50, telling us that half the observations fall on either side of the mean. With the good-enough-for-estimating numbers, we are not going to worry about the minuscule number of observations that fall more than three standard deviations away from the mean. For all practical purposes in the social sciences, all observations fall within three standard deviations of the mean.*

Now that we know the three most important numbers in statistics, let's use them to find the percentage of observations falling between the mean and half a standard deviation above. We'll follow a three-step procedure: (1) draw; (2) estimate; and finally, (3) calculate.

The first step is to draw a picture of the area being sought, as shown in Figure 5.11. Note that I've shaded the area I want to calculate.[†]

Now, for step b, let's use a little logic and estimate the answer. We know that the area from the mean to one standard deviation above is 34%, so the percentage we're seeking has to be less than 34. The question is, how much less. One reasonable place to start is to say 17%, as that is half of 34% and .5 is halfway to 1.0. That is not a bad estimate, but we can do a little better if we note something about the normal curve: it is not flat!

---

*As I said before in a footnote, in situations where the cost of failure is high we do need to be concerned with the area beyond the third standard deviation. Would you want to drive over a bridge that had a .135% chance of failure? Wouldn't you feel better if it were built so that the chance of failure was beyond the fifth standard deviation (.000029%) or beyond the sixth standard deviation (.00000010%)?

[†] You might complain that I skipped a step. How did I know that half a standard deviation above the mean was a z score of .50? Remember, we use z scores or standard scores to describe the normal distribution. z Scores have a standard deviation of 1.00, so half a standard deviation would equal .50.

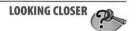

LOOKING CLOSER

Look at the portion of the curve going from the mean to one standard deviation above (or below). The line is not horizontal; it slopes down. In other words, the 34% of the cases that fall in this area are not evenly spread; they bunch up closer to the mean. Like Jack Sprat and his wife, the side nearer the mean is the fat side and the side away from the mean is the lean side. So, to make our estimate a bit more exact, we should make it bigger than 17% since it is on the fat side of the curve. How much bigger? Well, that is where practice comes in. I'm going to bump it up to 20%, but I won't be shocked if I'm off by a bit. It is, after all, an estimate.

Having our estimate, our third step is to do the actual calculations, using Table 1 in the Appendix. Is the information you want answered by column A, B, or C? Well, the columns are redundant so any can be used, but Column B, the area from the mean to a z score, provides the most direct route. So, head down the z scores (in bold) until you find 0.50 and then look at column B, the area from the mean to the z, where we find the answer of 19.15%. This is greater than 17%, as we expected, and pretty close to our estimate of 20%, so I am confident that the calculation is correct: 19.15% of the area under the normal curve falls between the mean and one half of a standard deviation above.

Let's do one more together before I turn you loose. What percentage of cases under the normal curve fall at least one-and-two-thirds standard deviations below the mean? Translating the question, it should be apparent that I want the percentage of cases that fall at or *below* a z score of −1.67.

The area is shown in Figure 5.12. Here's a spot for you to make your own estimate: _____

Here's how I would estimate it. The estimate has to be higher than 2% because 2% of the cases fall below $z = -2.00$. Another 14% of the cases fall in the next standard deviation up, and I only need the bottom third of that standard deviation. One third of 14 is about 5 (hey, I'm just

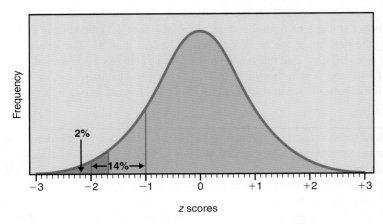

Figure **5.12** Estimating the area under the normal curve below $z = -1.67$.

estimating), but don't forget that I'm on the side away from the mean; I'm on the lean side of the curve. Looking at the curve, it looks that I am in fact on the *very* lean side, so I drop that rough estimate of 5% back to 3%. So, my final estimate is 2% plus 3%, or 5%. I estimate that 5% of the area under the normal distribution falls more than 1.67 standard deviations below the mean.

Let's go to Appendix Table 1 and see how we did. First of all, remember that the z scores are symmetric, so don't be concerned that there are no negative z scores in the table. We can use a z of 1.67 for −1.67 and look in Column C, which tells us the area below a negative z score. Looking at that column, we find that the answer is 4.75%. Again, as this is close to the estimate of 5%, I feel confident that I used the table correctly. Our conclusion is that 4.75% of the observations in a normal distribution fall more than 1.67 standard deviations below the mean.

I think it is time for you to do a little practice with estimating and calculating areas under the normal curve. Also, I think that you can use the Group Practice to learn some more advanced ways to use the z score table.

Group Practice 5.2

Draw, estimate, and then calculate the area under the normal curve for each of the following:

1. The area two or more standard deviations below the mean
2. The area from the mean to 1.50 standard deviations above
3. The area from the mean to .33 standard deviations below
4. The area at least 1.25 standard deviations above the mean
5. The area less than or equal to 2.25 standard deviations above the mean
6. The area at or above 1.10 standard deviations below the mean

The next set of problems asks you to apply the material in ways we haven't covered yet. I'm confi-dent that you can do it, but you can always look at the answers if you get stuck. Don't forget to draw and estimate before you calculate.

7. The area *within* one standard deviation of the mean. (Think about what "within" means!)
8. The area *within* 1.50 standard deviations of the mean
9. The area from .75 standard deviations below the mean to .25 standard deviations above the mean
10. The area from .80 standard deviations below the mean to 1.20 standard deviations above the mean
11. The area from .50 standard deviations above the mean to 1.00 standard deviations above the mean
12. The area from 1.50 standard deviations below the mean to 2.50 standard deviations below the mean

---

I trust that you figured out how to calculate the area under the normal curve from a z score below the mean to a z score above the mean as in questions 7 to 10. It may have taken a little more thought to calculate the area between two z scores on the same side of the mean in questions 11 and 12, but you had the answers at the back of the book to fall back on.

Now, knowing how to calculate areas below, above, and between z scores, let's move on to using the z score table in reverse: figuring out z scores or even raw scores for areas under the curve.

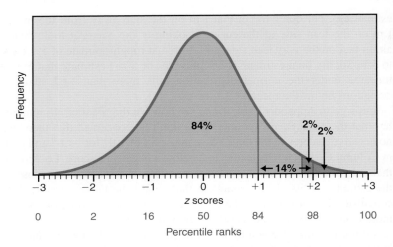

Figure **5.13** Estimating the *z* score for *PR* 96.

Suppose Buffy claims that she took a normally distributed IQ test and scored in the top 4%.* With the help of a *z* score table we should be able to find her actual score. Back in Chapter 3, we learned about percentile ranks, so we know that we can say Buffy's score, as a percentile rank, is 96. We interpret this by saying that she did better than 96% of the people taking the test and, if we had a frequency distribution we could apply Equation 3.2 to find her score. However, we don't have a frequency distribution. Is there anything we can do to figure out her score?

Of course there is. Statisticians never give up! To start, let's draw a normal curve and estimate Buffy's score. If Buffy had scored one standard deviation above the mean, what would her percentile rank score be? Well, if 50% of the people fall below the mean, and ≈34% of the people fall from the mean to one standard deviation above, then ≈84% fall below one standard deviation—and Buffy's score, as a percentile rank, would have been about 84. Similar logic and math lead to the realization that if Buffy had scored two standard deviations above the mean, her percentile rank score would be around 98. As Buffy's percentile rank score was a 96, her score is somewhere between one and two standard deviations above the mean. Figure 5.13 shows a normal distribution with the abscissa marked both with *z* scores and percentile ranks.

We have 2% of the area under the normal curve that falls two or more standard deviations above the mean and, as shown in Figure 5.13, we need to add another 2% to that area to total 4%.

By our approximation of the area under the curve (34, 14, and 2), we know that about 14% of the area under the curve falls from one to two

LOOKING CLOSER

*Remember, when I say IQ test you should immediately think $\mu = 100$ and $\sigma = 15$.

standard deviations above the mean. We need 2 of those 14 percentage points, or about 15% of it (that is, 15% of that 14%). The interval is 1 standard deviation wide, and 15% of 1 is .15. However, and here is where drawing it out really helps, we are moving .15 down from the top, from a z score of 2.00, so our estimated z score is 1.85. We're almost done, but I have one finishing touch to add. Are we on the fat side or the lean side of the interval from a z of +1.00 to a z of +2.00? The lean side! I'm afraid that just moving in .15 standard deviations won't give us the 2% we need, so let's adjust the interval up a bit, making it .20, not .15. Our estimate is that Buffy's score on the IQ test, as a z score, is 1.80.

Now that we've estimated, let's calculate it using the z score table in the Appendix. Again, we could use any column to figure this out, but let's choose the column that has already done the work for us, Column A. For a positive z score, Column A tells us the percentage of the area under the normal curve that is below a given z score. Here we are looking for the number closest to 96.00%. Since we estimate our score to be about 1.80, let's start there and move up or down as necessary. Looking at the table, we see that 96.41% of the area under the normal curve falls below a z score of 1.80. Move down, closer to a z of 0, and stop at 1.75: that is the z score with the Column A area, 95.99%, that is closest to 96.00. Thus, Buffy's score on the IQ test, as a z score, was a 1.75.*

But, we are not done yet. A z score of 1.75 fails what I call the parent test. Would Buffy's parents, two reasonably intelligent people who have never had a statistics course in their lives, have any sense of what this score means? So, let's turn this back into an IQ score via Equation 5.2. As our IQ test has a mean of 100 and a standard deviation of 15, we end up calculating as follows:

$$X = (1.75 \times 15.00) + 100 = 126.25$$

Buffy's score on the IQ test was 126.25.[†] She is one smart lady. (Though, as z scores are now transparent to you, you already knew that.)

Rounding can be a problem when using the z score table backwards, as we are doing. Suppose that Buffy's score had been in the top 5%, not the top 4%. In this case, we would be stuck deciding between a z score of 1.64, with 5.05% of the area under the normal curve above it, and a z of 1.65, with 4.95% of the normal curve above it. Neither of these is closer to the value we want (5.00%), so what do we do? I have three solutions. The first is to use logic. Buffy is in the top 5%, not in the top 4.95%. Thus,

---

*Column C would have led you to the same conclusion, but you would have used 4.00%, not the 96.00% we used. Or, you could have used Column B and looked for 46.00%. As I've said, the table is filled with redundant information.

[†] If you want to say that her score is *at least* 126.25, that would be fine by me. After all, I said that she had scored in the top 4%, so it is possible that she could have done better than 126.25. And, don't be bothered by the fact that even though IQs are measured and reported as integers, I am reporting the answer to two decimal places. That's just the way it is done when scores are transformed.

LOOKING CLOSER

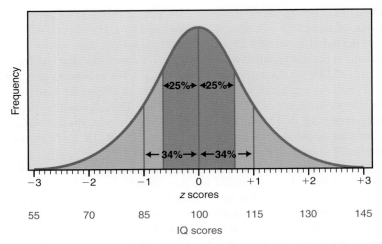

Figure **5.14** Estimating IQ scores associated with the middle 50% of the area under the normal curve.

it is possible that a *z* score of 1.65 would not capture Buffy, so we should use the value 1.64, which does capture the top 5% plus an additional .05%. Another option is interpolation, that is, to split the difference and say that the *z* score is 1.645.* Finally, one can always hunt up a more detailed *z* score table. When I consult a table[†] that goes to three decimal places, the answer turns out to be 1.645.[‡]

The area under the normal curve can also be used to assess percentages or probabilities for sets of events. For example, imagine that I wanted to know the IQ scores within which the *middle* 50% of people fall.[§] By a middle percentage, I mean an area symmetric about the mean. In this case, as shown in Figure 5.14, that means 25% above the mean and 25% below the mean.

Note that Figure 5.14 shows IQ scores on the abscissa as well as *z* scores. I estimate that a *z* score of about 0.70 should capture the first 25% of the area under the normal curve, as one moves away from the

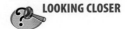 **LOOKING CLOSER**

*I hope that you remember that the area under the normal curve is not spread evenly, that there is a fat side and a lean side in any section between two points. Thus, one shouldn't interpolate between two points by just splitting the area. However, at this level of specificity, the third decimal place, I'm not going to worry about it.

[†]One of the best I've found is by Laurencelle & Dupuis (2000). (Laurencelle, L., & Dupuis, F-A. (2000). Statistical tables, explained and applied. River Edge, NJ: World Scientific.)

[‡] Actually, there's a fourth way as well. Spreadsheets such as Lotus and Excel allow you to calculate the area under the normal curve for any *z* value. Using Lotus, I calculated a more exact *z* score value of 1.64485. Rounded to three decimal places, this is 1.645. I guess interpolation works.

[§] Isn't this the same as the interquartile range?

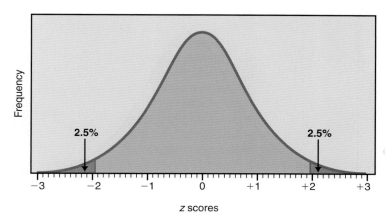

Figure **5.15** *z Scores associated with the extreme 5% of scores in a normal distribution.*

mean. Using Column B of the *z* score table in the Appendix reveals that a *z* score of .67 is the *z* score closest to 25.00%. Thus the middle 50% of scores in the normal distribution fall from a *z* score of −.67 to .67. Converting that back to IQ scores, via Equation 5.3a, I conclude that the middle 50% of IQ scores should fall from a score of 89.95 to 110.05.

I could use the same logic to figure out where in a normal curve the *extreme* 5% of scores fall. There are two ways a score could be extreme—extremely high or extremely low. Thus, when I talk about the extreme 5%, I mean 5% total (that is, the highest 2.5% and the lowest 2.5%). In terminology that statisticians use, I am talking about the *two tails* of the distribution. (The inverse of the extreme 5% is the middle 95%. And, if I were talking about only the highest scores, the extreme highest 5%, then I would be focusing on *one tail* of the distribution.)

A moment's reflection on the three most important numbers in statistics should tell you that the *z* scores associated with the extreme 5% of scores are just on the inside, the mean side, of *z* scores of ±2.00 (see Figure 5.15). Consulting the table of area under the normal curve, the exact *z* scores that separate the middle 95% from the extreme 5% are ±1.96. In fact these numbers, **−1.96** and **+1.96,** are two very important numbers in statistics. We'll encounter them again and again in subsequent chapters. In the next chapter, when we calculate something called a 95% confidence interval, these numbers will make their first return appearance. So when you see them, don't forget where they came from!

Let's do one more example, this one involving probabilities, before you do some on your own. Imagine a large and random sample of people taking a test that measures a normally distributed attribute—say, how long it takes to metabolize 1 ounce of alcohol. What is the probability that a person chosen from the sample at random is a very fast metabolizer of alcohol, defining a fast metabolizer as someone whose metabolic rate is at

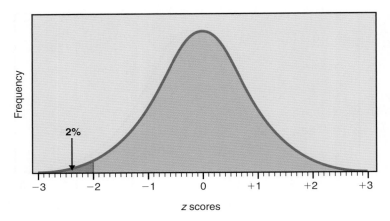

Figure **5.16** Estimating the probability of a case drawn at random being more than two standard deviations below the mean.

least two standard deviations below the mean? To rephrase that, what is the probability that a person selected at random has a score that is less than or equal to two standard deviations below the mean?

The area of interest is a darker shade of green in Figure 5.16. I trust that by now you recognize that there is about a 2% chance of a score falling in this area. Turning to the *z* score table, we find that the exact percentage is 2.28. There is a 2.28% chance, or a probability of .0228, that a person selected at random would be a fast metabolizer of alcohol. It is not very likely, if I drew someone at random from the sample, that he or she would be a rapid metabolizer of alcohol.

Group Practice 5.3

1. Skip took the quantitative subtest of the SAT and scored in the top 12.51%. (Remember, SAT sub-tests have a mean of 500 and a standard deviation of 100.) In *z* score format, what is the lowest score he could have had? In SAT format?

2. Buffy scored in the bottom 7.50% on the quantitative subtest of the SAT. In *z* score format, what is the highest score she could have earned? In SAT format?

3. If Clothilde took the SAT quantitative subtest and scored 647, what is her score as a percentile rank?

4. Desdemona's score on the SAT quantitative subtest, as a percentile rank, is a 67. What is her score as a *z* score?

5. How far apart, in *z* score units, are percentile ranks 80 and 85? How far apart, in *z* score units, are per-centile ranks 60 and 65? Why does this discrepancy exist?

6. What are the *z* scores associated with the *extreme* 1% of the scores in a normal distribution?

7. Your college decides to shoot for excellence and now will only admit people whose math score on the SAT is in the top 20%. What is their cut-off score for admission on the SAT quantitative test? They are considering using a new math test that has a mean of 15 and a standard deviation of 3.75. What would the cut-off score be on this test?

8. I consider a person a genius if his or her IQ is higher than 140. If I pick a person at random from the population of the world, what is the probability that he or she is a genius?

THE *REAL* REASON WHY THE NORMAL CURVE IS SO IMPORTANT...

I said before that the normal curve is important because we assume that many of the variables that we want to measure are normally distributed. Now, as a way to close out this chapter and as a preview of what is coming in the next chapter, let me explain the real reason why the normal curve is so important. For the real reason to make sense, however, you must understand the concept of a sampling distribution.

At the college where I teach, there are about 3800 students. Imagine that I draw a random sample, with replacement,* of 30 students from this population and with this sample of size $N = 30$ I calculate the mean height, M. Obviously, more than one sample of size $N = 30$ can be drawn from this population; in fact, there are thousands of them. So, if I do this time after time, if I engage in repeated, random sampling until I have all possible samples of size $N = 30$, I will have several thousand Ms for height. All these Ms would make up a sampling distribution, technically a sampling distribution of the mean.†

And here is an amazing fact. According to something called the central limit theorem, which we'll learn about in more detail in the next chapter, if the N for our repeated, random samples is large enough,‡ the shape of the sampling distribution will approach a normal distribution, *no matter the shape of the original population*. In other words, the original population can be skewed to the left or to the right. It can be multimodal. It can be leptokurtic or platykurtic. It can be any possible combination of those things. Still, if the size of the samples that comprise the repeated, random samples is large enough, the sampling distribution of the mean will approach a normal distribution. And this is useful because we know a lot about the normal distribution.

The central limit theorem tells us that as long as our sample size is large enough, the sampling distribution of the mean will approach normality no matter the shape of the parent population. Why take this on faith? I can demonstrate it with a clever example from George M. Diekhoff, whose

---

*I haven't talked about this yet, but there are two types of sampling, with and without replacement. With replacement means that when a case has been drawn from the population and placed into the sample, it is thrown back into the population, replaced, and it has a chance of being drawn again. Thus, in this scenario it is possible (though very unlikely) that my sample would consist of the same person sampled thirty times. Sampling without replacement means that each case can be in the sample only once.

†If you want a more formal definition of a sampling distribution, here it is: A sampling distribution is the set of values of some statistic (like a mean) that has been calculated for all possible samples of size N that have been drawn, with replacement, from some population. Sampling distributions, like the normal distribution, are theoretical. Could we really calculate the sampling distribution of height for all samples of size 25 from the population of 300 million Americans?

‡How large is a large enough sample? I've seen some authors say ≥ 25, others ≥ 35, and others ≥ 50. Me, I'm a conservative guy, so I like ≥ 50.

LOOKING CLOSER

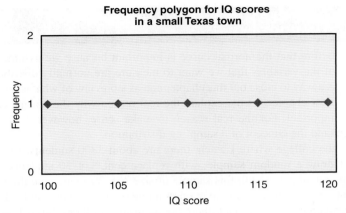

Figure **5.17** Flat, nonnormal distribution of IQ scores for a small Texas town.

text, *Basic Statistics for the Social and Behavioral Sciences*,* is, unfortunately, no longer published.[†] Diekhoff talks about a small town in Texas that has a *population* of five. Imagine that he has measured the IQs of everyone in this town and found that person A had a score of 100; person B, 105; C, 110; D, 115; and E, 120. As shown in Figure 5.17, the distribution of scores for this population is clearly non-normal. In fact it is what is called, for the obvious reason, a "flat" distribution.

Now, I am going to construct a sampling distribution of the mean based on repeated, random samples of size two. (I have to warn you that there are a lot of *N*s that I am throwing around here, and it can get confusing. So, pay attention to whether I mean the *N* for the number of cases in the population, the *N* for the number of cases in each sample, or the *N* for the number of samples.)

That is, I will pick one person at random from the town, record the IQ, put him or her back into the town (I'm sampling with replacement), sample another person, record the IQ, find the mean IQ for these two people, and do the process over again until I have obtained all possible samples. It turns out that there are 15 possible, *unique* samples that I could obtain in this situation where the population is five and my sample size is two.

Table 5.4, *a*, displays the 15 possible samples, such as person A twice, or persons A and B, or A and C, and so on. (Order is not important, so I don't list a sample consisting of person B and person A, as that would be

![icon] **LOOKING CLOSER**

*Diekhoff, G. M. (1996). *Basic statistics for the social and behavioral sciences.* Upper Saddle River, NJ: Prentice Hall.

[†]Of course, if his text were still around there wouldn't have been a need to write mine. So, depending on what you think of my text, maybe every dark cloud does have a silver lining.

TABLE **5.4**　**Sampling Distribution in a Small Texas Town**

A: POSSIBLE SAMPLES

A, A	A, B	A, C	A, D	A, E
B, B	B, C	B, D	B, E	
C, C	C, D	C, E		
D, D	D, E			
E, E				

B: IQS FOR MEMBERS OF SAMPLES

100, 100	100, 105	100, 110	100, 115	100, 120
105, 105	105, 110	105, 115	105, 120	
110, 110	110, 115	110, 120		
115, 115	115, 120			
120, 120				

C: MEAN IQS FOR SAMPLES

100	102.5	105	107.5	110
105	107.5	110	112.5	
110	112.5	115		
115	117.5			
120				

redundant with my sample of person A and person B.) Table 5.4 also displays the pairs of IQs for each of the 15 samples (Table 5.4, *b*) and the mean IQs for the pairs (Table 5.4, *c*).

If I now take the mean IQs from Table 5.4, *c,* and make a frequency polygon for them, I'll end up with the shape seen in Figure 5.18. Though the central limit theorem "works" when the sample size is "large," you can

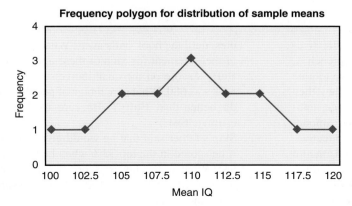

Figure **5.18** Frequency polygon for sampling distribution of the mean for IQs in a small Texas town.

see in Figure 5.18 that the sampling distribution approximates a normal shape even when the sample size is small. How and why this is useful in statistics will become clear in the next two chapters. But, for now, just remember the normal distribution and standard scores. And, of course, never forget the three most important numbers in statistics!

SUMMARY

A raw score can be transformed to a z score, which is a metric expressing the distance, in standard deviation units, between a raw score and the mean. z Scores are a linear transformation of raw scores, so the shape of the distribution of z scores is the same as the shape of the distribution of raw scores. A set of z scores has a mean of zero and a standard deviation of one; positive z scores are above the mean and negative z scores are below the mean. z Scores are just one example of standard scores; others are IQ scores or SAT scores.

The normal curve is important because a lot of the variables that researchers measure are assumed to be normally distributed. The normal curve is a specific symmetric distribution where most scores fall near the mean and the frequency with which scores occur tails off as they get further away from the mean. A lot of symmetric distributions meet these criteria, so the normal curve is defined by the percentage of cases that fall in each standard deviation as one moves away from the mean. The "good-enough-for-estimating" percentage of the area under the normal curve that fall from the mean to one standard deviation above is 34%; about 14% of cases fall from one to standard deviations above the mean; and about 2% of cases fall in the next standard deviation above the mean. If you need more exact percentages, you can consult a table of areas under the normal curve.

Knowing the specific amounts of area that fall within specified regions of the normal curve allows you to move back and forth among raw scores, z scores, and percentile ranks. For example, an IQ score of 115 is equivalent to a z score of 1 or a percentile rank score of ≈ 84.

An application of the normal curve occurs with the central limit theorem, which posits that any set of data, even one that is not normally distributed, will yield a sampling distribution of the mean that is normally distributed as long as the sample size is large enough. (A sampling distribution is the distribution of the values for some statistic, such as a mean, that have been calculated for repeated, random samples drawn from a population.) Because the sampling distribution is normally distributed, we can apply what we know about the characteristics of the normal curve to it. As we shall see in future chapters, this has useful ramifications.

Review Exercises

1. An adhesive company measures the effectiveness of new adhesives two ways. In approach A, they use a specified amount of adhesive to glue a hook to the ceiling of a test room. They then add weight to the hook, ounce by ounce, until the hook falls from the ceiling. The amount of weight applied is the measure of effectiveness. In approach B, they use a specified amount of adhesive to glue the hook to the ceiling, then apply a 25-pound weight to the hook. They measure the length of time, in seconds and minutes, until the hook pulls away. What is the level of measurement for each of these approaches?

2. Buffy's score on the quantitative subtest of the SAT was 680. What percentage of people should do better than Buffy? (Be sure to draw and estimate first!)

3. Skip's father said that he would give Skip $100 if he scored in the top 33% when he took an IQ test. What is the lowest score that Skip could have in order to get the $100? (Again, be sure to draw and estimate first.)

4. This is one of my favorite questions! A researcher has developed a course that he guarantees will add an additional 1 percent of the normal distribution to one's score on the quantitative subtest of the SAT. The course costs $1000. Clothilde and Desdemona disagree about whether they should spend the $1000 on the course. Clothilde's quantitative score was 520, and Desdemona's was 720. For which one does it make sense to spend the money on the course and why?

5. Draw, then estimate, the percentage of scores that should fall between z scores of $-.50$ and $+.25$. Calculate the exact percentage. Draw, estimate, and then calculate the percentage of scores falling between z scores of 1.80 and 2.20.

6. Marilyn vos Savant claims that her IQ was once measured at 228 and that she is the smartest person in the world. (I'm not making this up. She's a real person and has a weekly column in *Parade* magazine.) Let's assume that she took a standard IQ test. How credible is her claim that her IQ is 228?

7. A radiographer has developed a new imaging technique that she claims is more sensitive than existing techniques in finding small tumors. She claims that existing techniques fail to find tumors that are more than 3 standard deviations smaller than the mean size of tumors. She says that her technique can find tumors that are up to 3.70 standard deviations smaller than the mean. If the technique works as she claims, how many more tumors will it find? And what percentage of tumors will remain unfound?

8. Here's a small data set: 12, 23, 18, 22, 19, 7, 15, 16, 14, and 16. Using the mean and standard deviation from this data set, calculate the score that is 3.5 standard deviations above the mean.

9. What are the z scores associated with the middle 75% of scores?

10. What are the z scores associated with the extreme 1% of scores?

Homework Problems

1. Answer this without consulting a table of area under the normal curve. Under the normal curve, does a higher percentage of scores fall between z scores of 1.1 and 1.2 or between z scores of 2.1 and 2.2?
   a. 1.1 and 1.2
   b. 2.1 and 2.2
   c. The two percentages are the same.
   d. This can't be answered without consulting a table of areas under the normal curve.

2. I have obtained a population of scores and have made a frequency polygon for the distribution. The distribution of scores is symmetric, has the highest percentage of scores occurring at the midpoint, and has the frequency of scores decreasing as it moves away from the midpoint. The distribution is which of the following:
   a. Normally distributed
   b. Not normally distributed
   c. May be normally distributed
   d. Not enough information to tell

3. In a normal curve, the area above a positive z score is _____ the area below that same z score as a negative z score. Which of the following options best fills in the blank?
   a. the same as
   b. greater than
   c. less than
   d. None of the above; there's not enough information to tell

4. The extreme 12% of scores means which of the following?
   a. The highest 12%
   b. The lowest 12%
   c. The highest 12% plus the lowest 12%
   d. The highest 6% plus the lowest 6%
   e. None of the above

5. Let's assume that annual income in the United States is positively skewed. I take thousands of random samples of 50 people, with replacement, from the U.S. population, and each time I find the mean income for the sample. Describe

how the sampling distribution of the mean incomes *should* be distributed.
a. Positively skewed
b. Negatively skewed
c. Normally distributed
d. There's no way to know what shape it will take.

6. In one of the Homework Problems for Chapter 4, you calculated the interquartile range for the percentage of people living in poverty for the 51 states and the District of Columbia in the United States. Here's the table on which you based your *IQR*:

% Living in Poverty	Frequency
21-22	1
19-20	2
17-18	2
15-16	6
13-14	11
11-12	9
9-10	13
7-8	7

Using the raw scores for these 51 cases, I calculated the mean as 11.9309 and the standard deviation as 3.1711. Using this mean and standard deviation, calculate the *IQR* by using z scores. (HINT: what is the z score associated with percentile ranks, or *PRs*, of 25 and of 75?) Compare the two *IQR*s. Why do they differ? Which do you think is more accurate?

7. Draw, estimate, and then calculate the percentage of cases in the normal distribution that fall between z scores of 1.33 and 1.67.

8. Would the percentage of cases that fall between the z scores of 1.33 and 1.67 decrease, stay the same, or increase if the distribution were positively skewed? Explain your answer.

9. During flu season a public health researcher has obtained a sample of people from across the United States in order to find out how many are planning to obtain a flu shot next flu season.

This information is being obtained in order better to plan how much flu vaccine to produce. Is the percentage in the sample planning to obtain a flu vaccine next year being used as a descriptive or an inferential statistic?

10. What are the z scores associated with the extreme .5% of scores in the normal distribution?

11. T scores have a mean of 50 and a standard deviation of 10. Skip's IQ score, as a percentile rank, was 12.3. What is his score as a T score?

12. Your college has decided to advertise itself as the school for regular people. That is, it doesn't want people too smart or too dumb to seek admission. Rather, it wants people in the middle 33% of SAT quantitative scores to attend. What is the range of SAT-Q scores that should seek admission?

13. In the normal distribution, what percentage of scores fall in each of the following areas?
a. At or above a z score of 1.34
b. At or below a z score of 2.34
c. At or below a z score of −.85
d. At or above a z score of −2.57
e. From a z score of −.57 to the mean

14. In a survey of college students about their e-mail preferences, 389 report that they use their college/university e-mail address as their primary mail address, 87 report that they use AOL, 57 used Hotmail, 93 use MSN, and 122 use "other" e-mail servers. Make a graph for the results of the survey.

15. A psychologist has developed a new treatment for depression that has some potentially serious side effects. She has agreed to limit this treatment to the most severely depressed people, those with scores on a depression inventory in the highest 3%. If the depression inventory has a mean of 18 and a standard deviation of 3, what score must a person have to be eligible to receive this new treatment? (Higher scores on the depression inventory mean higher levels of depression.)

6

Sampling and Confidence Intervals

Learning Objectives

After completing this chapter, you should be able to do the following:

1 Define representative sample, random sample, sampling with and without replacement, and sampling distribution.

2 Use a random number table to draw a sample and explain the role of sampling error in generating samples that are not exact replicas of populations.

3 Describe three facts about the central limit theorem and explain how the variability of a sampling distribution depends on the variability in the parent population and the size of the repeated, random samples drawn.

4 Define confidence interval, be able to calculate a confidence interval for the mean, and be able to use confidence intervals both as a descriptive and an inferential statistic.

(Continued)

5 Explain why a more narrow confidence interval is better, know how to make a confidence interval narrower, and be able to calculate the sample size needed for a confidence interval.

6 Explain the probabilistic nature of conclusions based on statistics.

7 Explain why it is advantageous for a dependent variable to be normally distributed, and be able to use confidence intervals to determine if it is likely that a variable is normally distributed.

Chapter Roadmap

Though we care about populations (Who is going to win the upcoming election?…), because of their large size we usually have to base our understanding of them on a sample (…and based on a poll of 2000 registered voters, the incumbent holds a slim lead…). In this chapter we begin our journey into inferential statistics. We will learn that the best way to gather a sample from a population is by a process called **random sampling** and that, in general, larger samples are better than smaller samples. However, even when random sampling is used to gather a sample, it is unlikely—due to **sampling error**—that the sample will be an exact replica of the population. There is nothing malicious about sampling error, it just occurs, and it makes it hard for us to picture a population exactly. Fortunately, the **central limit theorem** comes to our aid and allows us to generate, from a sample, a range within which we think a population value falls. For example, if we know the mean (*M*) of a sample, we are able to predict the range within which we think the mean of the population (μ) falls. This range is called a **confidence interval**, because we have a degree of confidence that the population value actually falls in that range. As we'll see, narrower confidence intervals are better because there is a smaller range for the predicted population value. We'll learn how to make confidence intervals narrower.

Confidence intervals can be used to describe population values or to make inferences about population. As an **inferential statistic**, a confidence interval can be used for **hypothesis testing**, to see if what we predict about the population value is likely true. Though we may be confident that we've captured the population value in a confidence interval, we aren't 100% certain. In fact, we might be making an error—drawing the wrong conclusion—without knowing it. So, in this chapter we'll start to understand the **probabilistic** nature of statistics, that our conclusions are *probably* true but not *certainly* true.

Finally, we'll learn that many statistical tests only work on data that are **normally distributed**, and we'll see how confidence intervals for **skewness** and **kurtosis** can help us judge whether a variable is normally distributed.

Y ou may remember from Chapter 1 that statistics are divided into two types: descriptive and inferential. Descriptive statistics, things like tables and graphs, means and standard deviations, are used to *describe* a set of data. Inferential statistics have a different purpose—they are used to take information from a sample and make *inferences* about the population from which the sample comes. For example, I might take a sample of students from your school, measure some characteristic such as the number of times in the past month the members of this sample drank alcohol to excess, and then use these data—inferentially—to discuss alcohol consumption among students at your school *in general*.

SAMPLES AND POPULATIONS

A population is a group of elements (or cases) that are alike on one or more characteristics as defined by a researcher. A population is defined by a researcher for a particular purpose, and all elements that meet the criteria are part of the population. Thus, if a researcher were interested in studying igneous rocks found in glacial fields, then any and all igneous rocks that are found in glacial fields would be this researcher's "population" of study.

Populations are usually large—glaciers have existed all over the planet and have pushed a lot of rocks around—so it is usually impractical to study an entire population. Researchers, therefore, almost always select some objects from the population for study; these selected objects comprise a sample.

How one obtains a sample is important. If our geologist gathered his or her sample only from glacial fields in Switzerland, you would probably question how meaningful his or her results could be. Is it not possible that the igneous rocks found in glacial fields in Canada or China have different qualities than those found in Switzerland? Therefore we want the sample to be a "good" one, what is called, technically, **representative.** A representative sample contains all of the attributes of the population in the same proportion that they exist in the population. This allows one to *generalize* from the sample to the population, to make *inferences* from the sample to the population.

Unfortunately, a logical problem exists in knowing that our sample is representative of the population: we can't be sure that it is. Think back to the sample of students asked how many times they drank alcohol to excess in the past month. To be representative, we must have the same percentage of teetotalers in the sample as exist in the population, the same percentage who drank to excess on only one occasion in the sample as is found in the population, the same percentage with two occasions, and so on. Here's the problem: if we knew the percentages in the population so we could compare them to the sample, there would be no need to have a sample because we would already have the answer from the population. But, for reasons of practicality, we can't get the answer from the population. We are left going in a circle, like a dog chasing its tail.

representative

In a sample, containing all the attributes of the population in the same proportion.

How do we resolve this problem of getting a good sample, of drawing a sample that is representative of the population? The approach is to gather a sample by a methodology, a procedure, that should yield a representative sample and then to trust that, since we applied the correct procedure, we'll get the correct result. We are acting on faith and have to be accepting of the fact that we can't be sure that our sample will be representative of the population. In other words, you can do everything right but still end up at the wrong place. And, to add insult to injury, you won't know that you ended up at the wrong place. It's like driving from Los Angeles to New York and ending up in Boston, but not knowing you're in Boston.

RANDOM SAMPLING

What is the method that is thought to lead to a representative sample? It is officially called **simple random sampling,** though most just call it random sampling. Simple random sampling means that every object in the population has an *equal chance* of being selected, or drawn, for inclusion in the sample. When lottery numbers are placed in a barrel, the barrel is shaken up, and a blindfolded person reaches in and picks out a winner—that's simple random sampling. The easiest way to explain random sampling is by giving an example of what is not random sampling.

Imagine that I want to find the average height in a class of 40 people and decide to do this by finding the average height of half the class. I divide the class in two by having everyone in the class count off by twos: person A says, "1," person B says, "2," person C says, "1," person D says, "2," and so on. I then take all the "2s" as my sample. This does not produce a random sample! The reason is simple: once person A has been passed by, he or she no longer has an equal chance—or any chance—of being in the sample.

Contrast this "every-N[th]-person" approach with the use of something called a random numbers table (Appendix Table 2). A little piece of that table is reproduced here in Table 6.1. A random number table is a list of numbers in random order—in the long run, a 1 in the table is as likely to be followed by a 2 as it is by a 3 or a 4 or any other number.

In this table the numbers are broken into groups of four, the columns are labeled with letters, and the rows with numbers. The four numbers in

simple random sampling

Selecting a sample so that every object in a population has an equal chance of being selected.

TABLE **6.1   Part of random numbers table, Appendix Table 2**

	A	B	C	D	E	F
1	4963	4775	6746	1453	6349	3103
2	3538	8169	4029	8333	6806	4925
3	9475	6997	8843	5435	2479	3814
4	4783	3087	6777	8001	9582	9193
5	6985	7743	5185	7611	2279	2830

cell A1—4963—could be considered to be a 4-digit number (4963) or two 2-digit numbers (49 and 63) or four 1-digit numbers (4, 9, 6, and 3), or, combined with the numbers in cell B1, as an 8-digit number (49634775). The number of ways of breaking these numbers up or of combining them is limited only by your imagination.

If I wanted to use this random number table to obtain a sample that consists of half of the 40-person class, there are a number of ways to do so. One simple way would be to take each person in class and assign him or her the next random number in the table. Thus, the first person would be assigned "4," the next, "9," the next, "6," the next, "3," the next, "4," the next, "7," and so on. I could then declare that anyone assigned an odd number is in my sample. Note: this means that each person has an equal chance of being in the sample, even if the person before him or her were even. In fact, if you look at cell B1 you'll note that three people in a row (7, 7, and 5) would end up in my sample.*

Another way to obtain a random sample is to have the class count off sequentially from 1 to 40. To end up with 20 people in the sample, I'd pull 2-digit numbers from the random numbers table. In the first cell, I don't find anyone for my sample since the numbers—49 and 63—don't correspond to the numbers assigned. In cell D1 I find the first person for my sample, Person #14, and in cell F1 I find two more people (Persons #31 and #03).

SAMPLING WITH AND WITHOUT REPLACEMENT

This brings us to another aspect of sampling, sampling with or without replacement. I mentioned this in the last chapter when we discussed taking repeated, random samples for sampling distributions. In **sampling with replacement,** a case that has been sampled is put back into the population and has a possibility of being sampled again, of being in the sample multiple times. In **sampling without replacement,** a sampled case can be in the sample just once; once it has been sampled it is *not* placed back into the population, and so it cannot be in the sample more than once.

In the present scenario, sampling with or without replacement becomes an issue when we reach cell D3 with number 35. Person number 35 was included in our sample back in cell A2. What should we do, have him or her in the sample once or twice?

Intuitively, almost no one likes sampling with replacement. The idea of having person #35 in the sample twice (or even more often!) seems somehow not right, even un-American. However, sampling with replacement is the statistically correct way to go.

Why? Because random sampling, where each case has an equal chance of being selected, leads to a representative sample when the chance of a

---

sampling with replacement

A case that has been sampled is put back into the population and has a possibility of being sampled again.

sampling without replacement

A sampled case can be in the sample just once.

---

*Random sampling does not guarantee even sample sizes. By selecting the odd numbers for the sample, 23 people out of the 40 in the class will be in the sample.

LOOKING CLOSER

case possessing a certain attribute being selected for the sample is equivalent to the *probability with which that case exists in the population.* If the class of 40 people is half male and half female, then the chance of drawing a male from the class is 50% the first time a person is selected for the sample. Let's say that the first person I draw, #14, is a male, and I don't replace him. Now there are 39 people left in my sample, 19 males and 20 females. The percentage of males eligible for the sample has dropped from 50% to 48.72%. Since the percentage of males in the reduced population now is not an exact reflection of the percentage of males in the population, I am less likely to draw a male than would be true based on population values.

Sampling with or without replacement is only an issue for small populations. With large populations the likelihood of sampling the same case twice is infinitesimally small. Imagine drawing a sample, with replacement, of 2000 people from the entire population of the approximately 300,000,000 people in the United States. Since each person has only one chance in 300 *million* to be in the sample, the chance of one person being in the sample twice is so low as to be functionally zero.* With a large population, sampling without replacement and removing people from the potential sample pool once they've been sampled has little impact on the representativeness of the sample. If our 300,000,000 Americans are evenly split between men and women, and the first person I draw for my sample is a man, the percentage of men in the population has now dropped from 50.00% to 49.999,999,833% and I am not particularly less likely to sample a man the next time I draw a case for my sample.[†]

Before moving to a discussion of sampling error, I have a few final points to make about drawing samples. First: other things being equal, a larger sample provides a better representation of a population than does a smaller sample. If I draw a random sample of two people from a statistics class and find the mean height for those two people, would you be comfortable that this is a good representation of the average height of the whole class? Wouldn't you be more comfortable if the sample were a random sample of 10 people? And yet, size isn't everything. How the sample is gathered is important! A smaller sample that is randomly gathered is better than a larger sample that is gathered by some biased method.[‡]

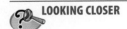

LOOKING CLOSER

*Do you want to know the actual likelihood? A U.S. citizen who is sampled once would be sampled a second time 0.0000000000000001% of the time.

[†]Survey researchers have developed something called the finite population correction, a way to account for an adjustment that needs to be made to a sample size if one is sampling without replacement. As the size of the population gets larger, the amount of adjustment gets smaller.

[‡]"Biased" has a specific meaning here. A sample is biased if it is gathered in such a way that some systematic error has entered into the process. My favorite way to think of it is target shooting. If, aiming carefully, you fire 10 shots at the bull's-eye, and all the shots cluster together in a tight circle a foot away from the bull's-eye, then there was some systematic error that crept in and biased your shooting.

Although sampling with replacement is the correct way to gather a sample that is representative of a population, sampling without replacement is much more common in actual practice. Most statistical tests require that the cases in a sample are independent of each other and should not have the same case in the sample more than once.

SAMPLING ERROR

Unfortunately, no matter how large the sample and no matter how it was gathered, it is unlikely to be a perfect representation of the population. The term for this is **sampling error,** or **random error.** Just as gravity explains why objects fall to the ground when dropped, sampling error explains why a large sample that is randomly drawn from a population may not be a very good representation of the population.

For an example of this, consider the single serving–size bags of M&M's® sold at checkout counters. Every day the Mars Company makes about 400,000,000 M&M's and pours them into bags of different sizes. The classic M&M colors are red, orange, yellow, green, blue, and brown, but let's simplify the world and divide M&M's into red and not-red. Every day, 80,000,000 of the 400,000,000 M&M's made, or 20%, are red.* This 20%, as it is the value for the population, is a parameter.

I've never visited the Mars factory, but I have a vision of how their bagging machine works: six different chutes, one for each color; feed M&M's into a large mixing vat in which a paddle swirls them around— mixes them together—until they proceed, in their randomly mixed color state, to the bagging machine. As a result, every bag of M&M's is a random sample from the population of M&M's.

Here is my question for you: if you bought a bag of M&M's and calculated the percentage of red in your bag, would you be surprised if it were not exactly 20%? My guess is that you would not be surprised to find that your bag deviated from the expected 20% red, that it contained 18% red or 23% red, or maybe even 25% or 30% red. Further, I guess that you would not ascribe anything malicious to this deviation. You would probably say that the deviation was just due to the random fluctuations that occur with random mixing, that random sampling has presented you with a sample that is not a perfect representation of the population. Let's take this question to a logical extreme: would it be possible—*not likely but possible*—to get a bag that contained no red or a bag that was 100%

sampling error

The random error that occurs in a sample and that results in a sample statistic being different from a population parameter.

---

*For those who are interested, the percentages are: red (20%), orange (10%), yellow (20%), green (10%), blue (10%), and brown (30%). Also, by my calculations, a path of 400,000,000 M&M's would stretch 3294 miles—more than enough to cross the United States from the Atlantic to the Pacific. In the course of a year the Mars Company makes 1.2 million miles of M&M's, enough to go around the equator 48 times! (Since I collected my data on M&M's, the Mars Company has changed the percentages. The new percentages are: red [13%], orange [20%], yellow [13%], green [16%], blue [24%], and brown [13%].)

LOOKING CLOSER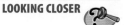

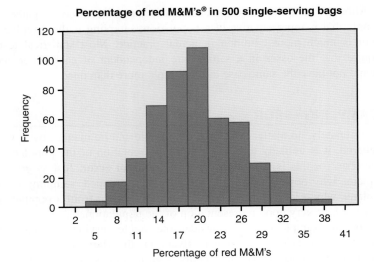

Figure **6.1** Histogram showing percent red M&M's in 500 single serving–size bags.

red? Yes, this occurrence is possible, but not likely. And if this occurred, wouldn't you still have to hold that it was random error—sampling error—that resulted in this unusual situation? As Aristotle said, "It is the nature of probability that improbable things will happen."

To move from speculation to the empirical method, I, along with my students, family, and friends, have opened and counted colors in 500 of these single serving–size bags of M&M's. Though I have never found one that was entirely without red M&M's or one that contained nothing but red M&M's, I've found one that had only 3.57% red and another that was 38.89% red. (These values, 3.57 and 38.89, because they are calculated from samples, are statistics. Don't forget: a parameter is a value calculated for a population, and a statistic is a value calculated for a sample.) Figure 6.1 is a histogram showing the percentages of red M&M's for these 500 single serving–size bags. (Remember, the expected value is 20% red.)

There are several things worth noting about the results and this figure. First, though only a small number of the 500 bags contained exactly 20% red (3% of them, to be exact), the distribution of all 500 bags is centered around the interval that contains the expected value of 20%. In fact, the mean of all 500 means is very close to 20.00% at 19.81%. Second, there is spread, or variability, on each side of the mean but—like the normal distribution—the scores tend to pile up near the midpoint and become more scarce as they move further away. And, again like the normal distribution, the distribution is relatively symmetric.

M&M's, which come in bags of different sizes, provide a nice way to demonstrate something I mentioned earlier: other things being equal, larger samples provide better representations of the population than do

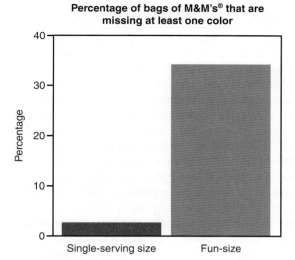

Percentage of bags of M&M's® that are missing at least one color

Figure **6.2** Bar graph showing percentage of bags of M&M's that are missing at least one color.

smaller samples. Not only have I recorded data from 500 single serving–size bags of M&M's, but I also collected data from 500 "fun-size" bags of M&M's. Fun-size bags are the size that are handed out as Halloween treats and contain about 24 M&M's per bag, a little less than half the size of the single serving–size bags, which contain about 56 M&M's per bag. The fun-size bags represent smaller samples from the population of M&M's.

Remember, for a sample to be representative of a population it must contain all the characteristics of the population in the same proportion that they exist in the population. A random sample of U.S. citizens that does not contain anyone of African descent is not representative of the United States. Similarly, a bag of M&M's that is missing one color is not representative of the population of M&M's. As you can see in Figure 6.2, more than one third of the fun-size bags of M&M's were missing at least one color and therefore were not representative samples. The rate of a bag missing a color was 11 times *lower* in the larger, single serving–size bags! The larger samples were more likely to be representative of the population from which they came (although they occasionally—and entirely as a result of sampling error—provided samples that were *not* representative). This is concrete evidence that, other things being equal, larger samples are better because they are more likely to be representative of the population.

I'm going to get ahead of myself for a bit, but I want to raise a concern and have you ponder it. Imagine that you have never had any experience with M&M's. I give you a bag, you open it, and it contains only orange, yellow, green, blue, and brown M&M's: no red. This one sample constitutes your entire experience with M&M's. How can a person tell, from a single sample, that the sample is not representative of the population?

THE CENTRAL LIMIT THEOREM, AGAIN

Chapter 5 ended with the real reason the normal curve is so important to statistics: according to the central limit theorem, even when the underlying distribution from which our sample is being drawn is not normally distributed, the sampling distribution of the sample mean will approach a normal distribution *if the sample size is large enough.*[*] (Remember, a sampling distribution is the set of values of some statistic— here, the mean—that has been calculated for all possible samples of size *N* that have been drawn, with replacement, from some population.) Because I find Diekhoff's (1996)[†] example of a small town in Texas with a population of five people so helpful, I am repeating it here in Figure 6.3. It shows that even though the population distribution of IQ scores in the town was not normal, the sampling distribution of the mean for the 15 possible samples of $N = 2$ was starting to approximate a normal distribution.

I hope that with this refresher on sampling distribution, you will recognize that the histogram of the percentages of red M&M's in 500 bags (Figure 6.1) is a sampling distribution of the mean,[‡] since I took repeated, random samples (albeit without replacement) and calculated a statistic (*M*) for each one.[§] So, let's use the M&M's data to explore three facts that derive from the central limit theorem.

Fact 1: the central limit theorem holds that the sampling distribution, as long as the sample size is large enough, will approach normality. We've already seen, in Figure 6.3, that this holds true even when *N* isn't very large. Now, looking back at Figure 6.1, we can see that the sampling

---

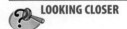

LOOKING CLOSER

[*] As I've noted before, there is no globally accepted definition of a "large enough" sample size. I've seen it defined as low as 25 and as high as 50. Let's be on the conservative side and consider a sample size of >50 as "large enough."

[†] Diekhoff, G. M. (1996). *Basic statistics for the social and behavioral sciences*. Upper Saddle River, NJ: Prentice Hall.

[‡] This could be called a sampling distribution of a proportion (as in, the proportion of M&M's that are red), but it is also a sampling distribution of the mean. In Chapters 1 and 4 I made a big deal of telling you that you can't calculate a mean for nominal data. Well, I simplified things. You *can* calculate a mean for nominal data when the data are dichotomous (i.e., there are only two options, here "red" and "not red") and they are scored as 0 and 1. If I have 10 M&M's, 7 non-red and 3 red, then 30% of them are red. If I assign a value of 1 to the red M&M's and a value of 0 to the non-red, then the mean value for these 10 M&M's is .30. Isn't .30 just 30% expressed as a proportion? So, in this instance one can calculate a mean for nominal data. Similarly, one can meaningfully calculate the variance and standard deviation in this scenario.

[§] Yes, the official definition of a sampling distribution makes reference to *all* samples of size *N* comprising the sampling distribution. Clearly, it is impossible to obtain all samples of $N = 56$ for the billions and billions of M&M's that have been produced in the past decades. I'm willing to accept my 500 samples as a reasonable (and pragmatic) approximation to a sampling distribution.

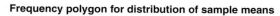

Frequency polygon for IQ scores in a small Texas town

Frequency polygon for distribution of sample means

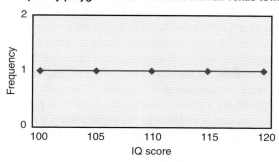

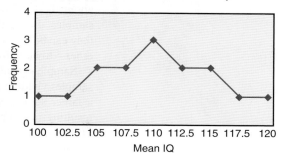

Figure **6.3** Distribution of IQ scores and sampling distribution of the mean for small Texas town.

distribution for the percentage of red M&M's approximates a normal distribution when we have "large enough" samples, as *N* for the single serving–size bags is greater than 50.

Fact 2: the mean of the sampling distribution is the same as the mean of the population. In the Texas IQ example, where we have all possible samples from the population in the sampling distribution, it works perfectly, and the mean of the sampling distribution (110) equals the population mean. In the M&M's example the mean of the 500 samples is 19.81, which is close to the population value of 20.00. Since I'm a trusting soul and believe the Mars Company when it says that 20% of their M&M's are red, I'm confident that if we had all possible samples from the population of M&M's the mean of those samples would be spot on 20.00.

VARIABILITY IN A SAMPLING DISTRIBUTION

Fact 3 involves variability. Thanks to random sampling error, no sample presented a perfect mirror of the population in either the Texas IQ example or the M&M's example. Thus the samples don't all have the same mean. This results in variability in the samples, as can be seen in Figures 6.1 and 6.3. Given this variability, we can calculate a measure of variability, like a standard deviation, for a sampling distribution. Unfortunately, when a standard deviation is calculated for a sampling distribution, statisticians have seen fit to call it something else. The **standard error of the mean,** abbreviated σ_M (pronounced "sigma sub em"), is the standard deviation of the sampling distribution of the mean. You'll also, occasionally, see the standard error of the mean abbreviated as *SEM* or SE_M.

The amount of variability in a sampling distribution, the size of the standard error, is influenced by two things: (1) the amount of variability in the original population, and (2) the size of the repeated, random

standard error of the mean

The standard deviation of the sampling distribution of the mean.

samples that are drawn from it. Both of these make sense when you think about them. If a population has a lot of variability, if σ is large, then samples drawn from that population have a larger range from which they can be drawn. As a result, samples are more likely to differ from each other—to be more variable—yielding a larger standard error of the mean.

Sample size also influences the standard error of the mean, with larger samples yielding a smaller standard error of the mean. This occurs because a larger sample size provides a more accurate estimate of a parameter, resulting in sample means that are closer to the population mean. When Ms are closer to μ, they are also closer to each other, and there is less variability. Figure 6.4 demonstrates the increased variability in a sampling distribution when sample size is smaller. Compare M&M's sampling distributions for the larger bags (the single serving–size bags) to the smaller bags (the fun-size bags). Note that for the fun-size bags the range for percent red is from 0% to 56%, while for the single serving–size bags it is narrower, from 5% to 38%. There is less variability and the standard error of the mean will be smaller when the sample size is larger.

With both the Texas IQ data and the M&M's data, it is possible to calculate the standard errors of the mean for the 15 cases and the 500 cases, respectively, that make up the sampling distributions. In real life, however, we usually don't have repeated samples from a population. Thus, researchers use the formula in Equation 6.1 to estimate the standard error of the mean from just one sample. This formula, which grows out of the central limit theorem, is useful because it allows us to calculate the standard error of the mean when we have only a single sample from a population.

One point that I made in that last paragraph is particularly important, so let me stress it: Though statistics depends upon the concept of a sampling distribution, we almost never have an actual sampling distribution to work with. So, we extrapolate the characteristics of the sampling distribution from the sample(s) that we do have.

FORMULA

Standard Error of the Mean (σ_M), the Standard Deviation of the Sampling Distribution of the Mean

Equation 6.1	$$\sigma_M \frac{\sigma}{\sqrt{N}}$$

Where:

σ_M = the standard error of the mean being calculated

σ = the standard deviation of the population

N = the number of cases in the sample

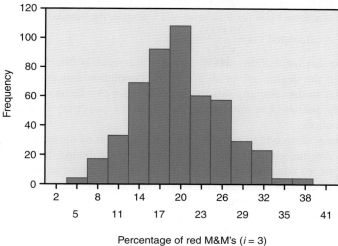

N for single serving–size bags ≈ 56
N for fun-size bags ≈ 24
i = interval width

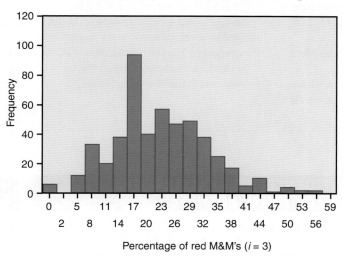

Figure **6.4** Histograms comparing amount of variability in sampling distributions as a function of size of samples.

Equation 6.1 says to find the standard error of the mean by dividing the population standard deviation by the square root of the sample size. Thus, if one has found IQs for a sample of 25 people, the standard error of the mean is calculated via $\dfrac{15.0000}{\sqrt{25}} = 3.00$.

You can see that the standard error of the mean is determined by two factors: the degree of variability in the population and the size of the samples in the sampling distribution. These are two factors that we have already discussed as influencing the degree of variability in a sampling distribution.

It may seem odd to calculate the standard error of the mean when we have only one sample rather than a sampling distribution, but as you are about to see when we venture into the world of confidence intervals, the standard error of the mean is a very useful number. Knowing the shape (normal) and the standard deviation of the sampling distribution (the standard error of the mean) will allow us to do a lot.

Group Practice 6.1

1. If samples of size $N = 8$ are taken from a population with $\sigma = 4.8923$, what is σ_M? What is σ_M if the samples are of size $N = 73$? What should the shapes of the sampling distributions of the means be in these two instances?

2. a. Without doing any calculations, which will have a smaller standard error of the mean? $\sigma = 2.00$, $N = 12$ or $\sigma = 2.00$, $N = 144$.

   b. Other things being held equal, what is the effect of N on σ_M?

   c. Without doing any calculations, which will have a smaller standard error of the mean? $\sigma = 5.78$, $N = 50$ or $\sigma = 7.58$, $N = 50$.

   d. Other things being held equal, what is the effect of σ on σ_M?

3. The entire population of this year's *summa cum laude* graduates at a small college consisted of seven students. If you took repeated, random samples, with replacement, of size $N = 2$ from this population, how many possible samples could you have?

4. Design three different ways to obtain a *random* sample of 10 people from a class of 60. At least one procedure must make use of the table of random numbers in the Appendix (Table 2).

CONFIDENCE INTERVALS, ERRORS, AND TESTING HYPOTHESES

To understand where we are now heading, remember the difference between a parameter and a statistic. A parameter is a value calculated for a population, and a statistic is a value calculated for a sample. In Chapter 4 we learned that though populations have variances, it was very rare to be able to calculate σ^2. However, because knowing the population variance is useful, statisticians developed a way to estimate σ^2 from a sample by calculating $\hat{s}^2$.

Well, just as populations have variances, they also have means. And, just as it is rare to know σ^2, it is rare to know μ. Similarly, just as there are times that we would like to know the population variance, there are times that we would like to know the population mean. For example, even if I found out how many of a sample of 2000 registered voters planned to vote for the incumbent in the next election, wouldn't I really rather know about registered voters in general, about the whole population? We are about to use both the central limit theorem and the normal distribution to calculate a range, called a **confidence interval,** within which we think it is likely that a population mean falls. Put most simply, given M we are going to estimate where μ falls.

Most often, our only information about a population comes from a sample—a single sample—and samples, as we know, are imperfect representations of populations. Thus, when we draw a *random** sample from a population and calculate M, we do not expect, because of random error, that M will exactly equal μ.[†]

We are going to work with a single sample to make a prediction about the population. With this sample, we are going to use the central limit theorem and the properties of the area under the curve in a normal distribution to make some inferences about the population mean.

Thanks to the central limit theorem, we know (a) that a sampling distribution is normally distributed, (b) that the mean of the sampling distribution is equal to the mean of the population, and (c) that the standard deviation of the sampling distribution, what we call the standard error of the mean, is calculated by Equation 6.1. Thanks to the z score tables we covered in Chapter 5, we also know that in a normal distribution 95% of the area under the curve falls from 1.96 standard deviations below the mean to 1.96 standard deviations above the mean.[‡]

If we put what we know about z scores together with what we know from the central limit theorem, we can reason that 95% of the time the sample mean (M) will fall within 1.96 standard errors of the mean of the midpoint of the sampling distribution of the mean, which is μ. This is an important concept to grasp, so stop and think about it for a moment: 95% of the time, a sample mean in a sampling distribution of means will fall within 1.96 σ_M of μ. Figure 6.5 demonstrates this graphically.

This is so important to grasp, that I want to give a concrete example using the single serving–size bags of M&M's. Earlier we looked at the

confidence interval

The range, calculated from a sample statistic, within which a population parameter likely falls.

---

*I have to stress how important it is that this sample is a random sample. The whole logic of confidence intervals is based on the sample being a random sample.

[†] I'm reminded of a psychologist, David Funder, who has formulated some "laws," one of which says that there are only two kinds of data in the world: (a) flawed, imperfect data, and, (b) no data.

[‡] Do you remember that in Chapter 5 I had asked you to remember the z score 1.96 and that I had said that we'd be seeing it again?

LOOKING CLOSER

Sampling distribution of the mean

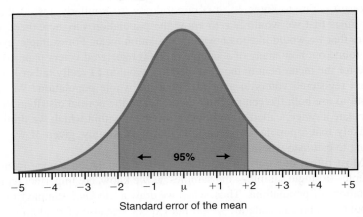

Standard error of the mean

Figure **6.5** Showing the area within which a sample mean (*M*) should fall 95% of the time in a sampling distribution of the mean.

sampling distribution of the percentage of red M&M's for the 500 single serving–size bags, and I mentioned that the mean percent red, based on all 500 bags, was 19.81. The standard deviation for this sampling distribution of 500 bags is 6.28.* Thus, the range within which 95% of the sample means in the sampling distribution should fall is from 7.50 to 32.12.[†] Figure 6.6 displays the sampling distribution for the M&M data with vertical lines marking off the region from 7.50 to 32.12. Remarkably, exactly 475 of the bags of M&M's, or 95%, fall inside this region.

Now, suppose that we draw a random sample from the population and, purely due to random error, the sample has a mean (*M*) that is a full standard deviation above the population mean (μ). If we drew vertical lines that were 1.96 standard errors of the mean above and below the sample mean, would the population mean fall within those lines? Looking at Figure 6.7, you should see that the answer is yes.

Let's draw another random sample from the population but this time— and again as a result of nothing but random error—let's get a sample where *M* is three standard deviations below μ. Again, let's draw vertical lines that are $\pm 1.96\sigma_M$ from *M*. And again, let's see if μ falls within those lines. Looking at Figure 6.8, you can see that this time the answer is no.

If you think about this for a few minutes, I think you'll agree that as long as the sample mean is within 1.96 standard errors of the mean of the

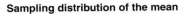

LOOKING CLOSER

*This standard error of the mean that I am calculating here is based on the 500 samples, not a population, and so I would abbreviate it as s_M not σ_M.

[†]Want to see the calculations that led to that? $19.81 \pm 1.96(6.28) = 19.81 \pm 12.31$.

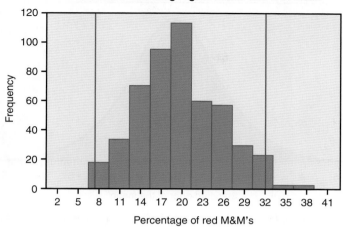

Figure **6.6** Sampling distribution of percent red M&M's in 500 single serving–size bags with vertical lines indicating region within 1.96 standard deviations of the mean.

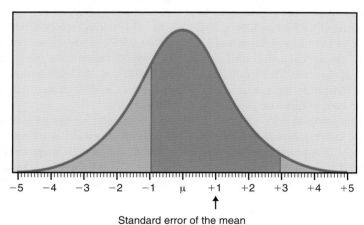

Figure **6.7** Sampling distribution of the mean indicating region falling within 1.96 standard errors of the mean for $M = 1.00$.

Sampling distribution of the mean

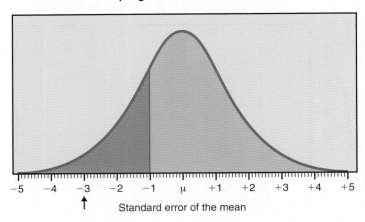

Standard error of the mean

Figure **6.8** Sampling distribution of the mean indicating region falling within 1.96 standard errors of the mean for *M* = –3.00.

population mean (see the shaded region in Figure 6.5), the region from $M - 1.96\sigma_M$ to $M + 1.96\sigma_M$ will capture μ. How often will *M* fall within $1.96\sigma_M$ of μ? Since the sampling distribution is normally distributed, the answer is 95% of the time.

We've just learned how to calculate a 95% confidence interval for a population mean! This 95% confidence interval gives us a range that should capture the population parameter, μ. It is unlikely, or implausible, that the parameter μ falls outside of the confidence interval. The official meaning of a 95% confidence interval is that if you took repeated, random samples from a population and calculated the 95% confidence interval for each, the calculated confidence interval would capture the parameter 95% of the time. That's quite a mouthful, and if you just want to think of it as indicating the range within which there is a 95% chance that the parameter, in this case μ, falls, that's fine by me.*

I'm going to give you two formulae for calculating the 95% confidence interval. Equation 6.2a, which we've been informally working with already, is appropriate when *N* is large, and Equation 6.2b is appropriate when *N* is not large. What is large enough for *N*? I'll follow the standards I used for the central limit theorem and say that an *N* that is at least 50 is large enough.

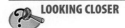 **LOOKING CLOSER**

*That simple interpretation is also fine by others. Cumming and Finch (2005), in an article on interpreting confidence intervals, offer that as one of the acceptable interpretations of a confidence interval. (Cumming, G., & Finch, S. (2005). Inference by eye: Confidence intervals and how to read pictures of data. *American Psychologist, 60*, 170-180.)

95% Confidence Interval for a Population Mean (μ) When N Is Large

$95\% \ CI = M \pm 1.96\sigma_M$ **Equation 6.2a**

Where:

$95\% \ CI$ = the 95% confidence interval being calculated

M = the sample mean

σ_M = the standard error of the mean (see Equation 6.1)

NOTE: Please report the 95% confidence as a range, from the lower number $(M - 1.96\sigma_M)$ to the higher number $(M + 1.96\sigma_M)$.

As we discussed above, this formula says that in order to calculate a 95% confidence interval for the population mean one takes the sample mean and both subtracts from it and adds to it 1.96 standard errors of the mean.

The second formula, Equation 6.2b, is used when N is not large, when it is less than 50. Why do we need this second formula? Because when our sample size is not large, the sampling distribution is less likely to approach normality. As a result, we need to make the confidence interval larger to maintain our desired level of confidence that the parameter falls within the calculated interval. It turns out that the degree of correction is greater, the smaller the sample size. First I'll show you the formula, and then I'll explain how it works.

95% Confidence Interval for a Population Mean When N is Not Large

$95\% \ CI = M \pm t\sigma_M$ **Equation 6.2b**

Where:

$95\% \ CI$ = the 95% confidence interval being calculated

M = the sample mean

t = critical value of t with $N-1$ degrees of freedom (Appendix Table 3)

σ_M = the standard error of the mean (see Equation 6.1)

NOTE: Report the 95% confidence interval as a range from the lower number to the higher number.

In Equation 6.2b, the value of 1.96 that was a constant in Equation 6.2a is replaced by a value, called a t value, that depends on the number of cases in the sample. t Values vary depending on something called the degrees of

TABLE **6.2**   **Section of Appendix Table 3: Critical Values of t for 95% Confidence Intervals**

df	t
1	12.7062
2	4.3027
3	3.1824
4	2.7764
5	2.5706
50	2.0086
infinity	1.9600

freedom; for calculating a confidence interval for the mean, the degrees of freedom is calculated as $N - 1$. Critical values of t for different degrees of freedom are shown in Appendix Table 3, and a section of it is shown here in Table 6.2.

To find the correct t value, called the critical value, convert N into degrees of freedom, abbreviated as df, by subtracting 1 from the sample size. If N were 5, then df would be 4. Then go down the df column until you find the appropriate degrees of freedom, and look in the next column for the critical value of t. If $df = 4$, the critical value of t for a 95% confidence interval is 2.7764. Note that as the degrees of freedom increase—that is, as N increases—the critical value of t decreases until, with an infinitely large sample size, the distribution of t becomes the same as the distribution of z and $t = 1.96$. Thus, the correction decreases as sample size increases.

If you have a sample of size five from a population where $\sigma_M = 3.00$ and you find that $M = 12.00$, then you would calculate the 95% confidence interval as ranging from $12.00 \pm 2.7764(3.00)$ rather than as $12.00 \pm 1.96(3.00)$. Thus, with the correction afforded by the t value to take into account the small sample size, the 95% confidence interval would range from 3.67 to 20.33, not from 6.12 to 17.88.

Though I only mandate using this correction when N is small, less than 50, if one wants to be a stickler one can use it with larger Ns as well. Appendix Table 3 provides t values for individual degrees of freedom up to 100 and then skips by tens, twenties, and so on, up to 5000. If the exact degrees of freedom that you need aren't in the table, then use the next smaller degrees of freedom. For example, the critical value of t for 265 degrees of freedom would be 1.9691, not 1.9688, and not an interpolated value.

Group Practice 6.2

1. Imagine a sample in which $N = 7$, $M = 10.00$, and $\sigma = 2$. Which confidence interval will be wider, one calculated via Equation 6.2a or one calculated via Equation 6.2b? First answer this by thinking about it, then check your answer by doing the calculations. Which confidence interval is the "right" one?

2. Someone from overseas is coming for a June vacation in the United States. During that month he is planning on driving all around the country. He wants to know what clothes to bring. To help him plan, I've taken a *sample* of 50 cities from the 48 contiguous states and have consulted an atlas to find their "normal" temperature, to the nearest degree in Fahrenheit, during June. I calculated $M = 69.9500$ and $\hat{s} = 7.5705$. What should I tell this visitor about what the population value is for the average normal temperature in the United States during June?

NARROWING THE CONFIDENCE INTERVAL

As we would like to nail down the neighborhood in which the population value lives, having a narrower (or tighter) confidence interval is a good thing. If I told you that I am 100% certain that the average GPA at my university falls somewhere between .00 and 4.00, that would not give you any meaningful information. A tighter confidence interval, say that the average GPA falls in the range from 2.90 to 3.10, would be more helpful. There are a couple of different ways that we can have a narrower confidence interval: (1) being less certain, and (2) having a larger sample size.

Let's look at being less certain first. The most common confidence interval, the standard, is the 95% confidence interval. Someone, many years ago, arbitrarily set the standard that we're willing to make an error 5% of the time (which is the flip side of the 95% confidence interval), and that has become the convention. However, by changing the z score from the 1.96 used in the equation, you can calculate an alternative confidence interval. Two common confidence intervals are 90% (using a z score of 1.65 instead of 1.96) and 99% (using a z score of 2.58).

Let's use these three common options to calculate confidence intervals for a single serving–size bag of M&M's that contains 8 red M&M's and 49 non-red M&M's. First, we must calculate a mean for this sample. Though I've said before that one shouldn't calculate a mean for nominal data (and red vs. non-red is nominal), this is the one instance that we can. When dichotomously scored nominal data (i.e., data with only two options) are scored as 0 and 1, then the mean is the same as the proportion. In this instance, you can say that 14.04% of the M&M's are red, or, if you score red M&M's as 1s and non-red M&M's as 0s, you can say that the mean of this sample is .1404.

We have the mean; now we need σ_M. For this, according to Equation 6.1 we need N and σ. We know that $N = 57$. We don't know σ, but we can estimate it by finding $\hat{s}$.* So, let's plug our values into the equation and find $\hat{s}_M$.[†]

$$\hat{s}_M = \frac{\hat{s}}{\sqrt{N}} = \frac{.3505}{\sqrt{57}} = .0464$$

Then, by Equation 6.2a, we can calculate the 95% confidence interval:

$$95\% \, CI = M \pm 1.96\sigma_M = .1404 \pm 1.96(.0464) = .1404 \pm .0909$$

This should be reported as a range, from the low of .0495 to the high of .2313. Putting this back into percentage format and based on our sample, there is a 95% chance that the percentage of red M&M's in the population falls in the interval from 4.95% to 23.13%. Note that the 20% value claimed by the Mars Company does fall in this range.

---

*Want to know a shortcut for calculating variability for dichotomous data scored as 0s and 1s? In this case the proportion red, call that p, is .1404, which means that the proportion non-red, which we'll call q, is .8596. The variance is then calculated as pq, which makes the standard deviation equal $\sqrt{pq}$. Back at the end of Chapter 4 there was an equation (Equation 4.10) for converting s into $\hat{s}$, and applying that here turns .3474 into .3505.

[†]Note that here I am abbreviating the standard error of the mean as $\hat{s}_M$ since it is based on a *sample* standard deviation, not a *population* standard deviation.

LOOKING CLOSER

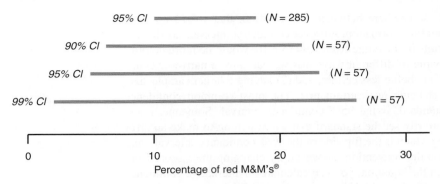

Figure **6.9** Visual representation of 90%, 95%, and 99% confidence intervals (*CI*s) for percent of red M&M's around observed percent = 14.04 for a sample where *N* = 57, and of the 95% confidence interval for a sample where *N* = 285.

That interval, about 18 percentage points, is a wide interval. One way to make the interval narrower is to be less certain that the interval will capture μ. This makes sense when you think back to my example of GPA: I may be 100% certain that the average GPA at my college falls in the interval from .00 to 4.00, but, as the interval gets narrower, I have to be less confident that it contains the population value.

Thus the 90% confidence interval for the bag of M&M's should be narrower, and the 99% confidence interval should be wider. This turns out to be true. The 90% confidence interval is about 15 percentage points wide, ranging from 6.38% to 21.70%, and the 99% confidence interval is about 24 percentage points wide, ranging from 2.07% to 26.01%.* All three confidence intervals are displayed visually in Figure 6.9.

Changing the width of the confidence interval by changing one's level of confidence involves a trade-off; you can't have your cake and eat it too. You can either be more confident that the interval contains the population mean, or you can have a narrower, more exact, more meaningful interval.

SAMPLE SIZE AND CONFIDENCE INTERVALS

However, you can have your cake and eat it too if you take advantage of the other way of narrowing a confidence interval: increasing the sample size. The width of the confidence interval is determined by the size of the standard error of the mean. If the standard error of the mean is smaller, then the confidence interval will be narrower. As discussed with the introduction of Equation 6.1, the standard error of the mean is determined both by the population standard deviation and the sample size. There is

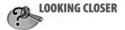 **LOOKING CLOSER**

*Remember, to calculate the 90% confidence interval, substitute 1.65 for 1.96 in Equation 6.2. To calculate the 99% confidence interval, substitute 2.58 for 1.96.

not much that we can do to change σ, the standard deviation of a population, but often we can control N, how large a sample we obtain.

Let's again calculate a 95% confidence interval for a bag of M&M's that contains 14.04% red, but this time let's use a bag that contains 285 M&M's instead of 57. For our 57-M&M bag, the 95% confidence interval was based on $s_M = .0464$; it turned out to be about 18 percentage points wide, ranging from 4.95 to 23.13. Here are the numbers for a 285-M&M bag (also with 14.04% red): $\hat{s} = .3480$, $\hat{s}_M = .0206$, and the 95% confidence interval is about 8 percentage points wide, ranging from 10.00% to 18.08%.* You can see this confidence interval at the top of Figure 6.9 and note that it is by far the narrowest. Increasing N is an effective way to narrow a confidence interval.

If you think algebraically, you should realize that we can make a confidence interval any width desired by manipulating the sample size. Suppose, for example, that we want a 95% confidence interval to be a total of 5 points wide, or $M \pm 2.5$. Since the 95% confidence interval is calculated from $M \pm 1.96\ \sigma_M$, we solve for $1.96\ \sigma_M = 2.5$. For the $N = 57$ bag of M&M's where $\hat{s} = .3505$, this becomes

$$1.96\ \frac{.3505}{\sqrt{N}} = .0250$$

Therefore, $N = 756.^\dagger$ That is, to calculate a 95% confidence interval that is a total of 5 percentage points wide, we need a sample of more than 750 M&M's.

To make life easy, here's an equation to calculate the sample size necessary to achieve a confidence interval of any width.

F O R M U L A

Sample Size Necessary to Achieve a 95% Confidence Interval of a Desired Width

$$N = \left(\frac{\sigma}{\frac{width}{1.96}} \right)^2$$

Equation 6.3

Where:

    N = the sample size being calculated (round *up* to an integer)
    σ = the population standard deviation (use $\hat{s}$ if σ is not available)
  Width = the width of *one side* of the confidence interval (i.e., half of the
        total width of the confidence interval)

---

*Note: Even though the proportion of red is the same for the two bags of M&M's, the standard deviations are different. Why? Because I am using $\hat{s}$, and $\hat{s}$ is "corrected" for the sample size.

†The actual answer, calculated with Equation 6.3, is 755.11, but since it is hard to have fractional cases the convention for sample sizes is to round up—yes *up*, no matter what—to the next integer value.

LOOKING CLOSER

This equation says that to find the sample size for a confidence interval one takes the standard deviation of the population and divides it by the quotient of the width of one side of the confidence interval divided by 1.96. This overall quotient is then squared to yield the sample size. For the M&M example I've been working with where $\hat{s} = .3505$ and I want a confidence interval of ±2.5%, the first thing I would do is convert the width of the confidence interval, ±2.5%, into a proportion, ±.025. I'd then substitute into the equation, finding:

$$\left(\frac{.3505}{\frac{.025}{1.96}} \right)^2 = \left(\frac{.3505}{.0127551} \right)^2 = 27.4792044^2 = 755.11 = 756$$

MAKING ERRORS: WHEN BAD THINGS HAPPEN TO GOOD PEOPLE

As I said earlier, you can think of a confidence interval as measuring your confidence that the reported interval captures the population value. Thus, based on the bag of 57 M&M's, we are more certain that the interval from 2.07% to 26.01%—the 99% confidence interval—contains the population percentage of red M&M's than we are that the interval from 6.38% to 21.70%—the 90% confidence interval—contains it. However, this "degree-of-confidence" interpretation is not the *technical* definition of a confidence interval. The technical definition of a confidence interval, say a 95% confidence interval, is that if you drew repeated, random samples from the population and each time calculated the 95% confidence interval, 95% of the time the confidence interval would contain the population value. That's a lot to ponder, so let me explain it using my M&M's.

The 95% confidence intervals for my 500 samples of single serving–size M&M's are arranged in order in Figure 6.10. Any confidence interval that does not cross the horizontal line marking a proportion of .20 red (i.e., 20% red) has failed to capture the population proportion of red as reported by the Mars Company. Note that there are some confidence intervals on the left side of the graph that don't capture .20 because they don't go high enough, and there are some on the right-hand side that don't capture .20 because they don't go low enough.

According to the technical definition of confidence intervals, only 25 of the 500 intervals (5%) should fail to capture μ. Here we have exceeded that, since 49 of the intervals (9.8%) don't capture the known population value. There are three possible explanations for this. Let me dispose of one right away—that I've given you an incorrect definition of a confidence interval—by assuring you that I haven't done so. Let's then use the other two—(a) we have a bad sample and (b) we are wrong about the population value—to inaugurate our exploration of using inferential statistics to test theories or hypotheses.

The "bad sample" explanation allows that the proportion of red M&M's in the population is indeed .20, but that we have, purely by

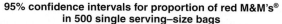

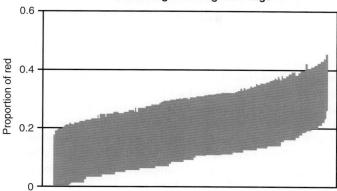

Figure **6.10** 95% confidence intervals for proportion of red M&M's in 500 single serving–size bags of M&M's.

chance, obtained more than the expected number of random samples that, entirely as a result of random error, are not reflective of the population. In other words, we expect a certain percentage of the time—and with a 95% confidence interval that is 5% of the time—to obtain samples that are not reflective of the population. We just had the bad luck to get more of these nonrepresentative samples in our 500 samples than we budgeted for.

The "we-were-wrong-about-the-population" explanation takes the other tack. It says no, our samples were fine, we followed all the appropriate procedures in gathering them, and there is no reason to question their representativeness. Instead, it is our basic assumption that is called into question: if we did everything right and we didn't get the results we should have based on our assumption that 20% of M&M's are red, then our assumption is not true. In other words, this explanation leads us to conclude that the Mars Company is lying when they report that 20% of the M&M's made are red, since we found more than twice as many confidence intervals as expected that did not capture 20%.

Both of these explanations are plausible. Inferential statistics are useful because they provide a procedure for deciding which explanation to believe.

As mentioned earlier, it is rare to have a sampling distribution of values for a statistic; we almost always have just a single sample from a population. So, let's take a single sample from a population and see how these two options play out in that scenario.

Suppose that we want to know the average weight of American men. A random sample of 157 men gives a mean weight (*M*) of 183.54 pounds with a standard deviation (*s*) of 19.52. What is the 95% confidence interval for these data?

To calculate a 95% confidence interval we need M, σ, and N. We have M and N, but not σ. Absent σ, we can use $\hat{s}$ to approximate it. Using

Equation 4.10 to convert s to $\hat{s}$, I find that $\hat{s} = 19.5825$. Then, substituting $\hat{s}$ for σ in Equation 6.1, I find that $\hat{s}_M = 1.5629$. Using Equation 6.2a, the 95% confidence interval for the average weight of American men ranges from 180.48 to 186.60 pounds. (Take a break here to do the math yourself.)

Suppose I proclaim that the average weight of American men falls in the range from 180.48 to 186.60 pounds. There are two possibilities about my proclamation: I could be right or I could be wrong. I'd be right if my sample were a "good" one, and I'd be wrong if my sample were "bad."

Now, the odds are in favor of my being right. There's a 95% chance that μ falls in the interval and only a 5% chance that it doesn't, so the odds are 19 to 1. If I offered you a gambling game where the odds predicted that you would win 19 times for every time that I won, you'd be a fool not to take me up on it. If we wagered a dollar every time and played the game 100 times, you'd win \$95 and I'd have won only \$5. Doesn't seem very fair to me.

But the gambling game we're playing with the confidence interval is a little different. Suppose we're playing our gambling game and the only information you have about the odds is that I won the first time. What does that win mean? That you have a 95% chance of winning and this was just one of those rare times that I won, so you should continue playing? Or, that the odds are really in my favor, that any win you get will be a fluke, and that you should quit before you lose more money?

The bottom line answer is that with a single sample—and we almost always only have a single sample!—we don't know for sure. There is a reasonable probability, a 95% chance, that we are right, that our confidence interval contains μ. But, we also know, thanks to the concept of sampling error, we will occasionally get an odd sample even if we follow all the correct sample-gathering rules.

Statisticians are hedgy people. A statistician would never say that he or she is *sure* that the average weight of the American male falls in the interval from 180.48 to 186.60 pounds; rather, he or she would only admit certainty to a degree. That is, a statistician would only say that it is *probably* true, that there is a 95% chance that the average weight of American males is in the range from 180.48 to 186.60 pounds. "And," the statistician would go on to say, "there is also a 5% chance that I made the wrong decision. Although I don't know if that mistake happened or not, it is more likely that I am right than that I am wrong."

And, that's the kicker: we never know if our conclusion is correct or in error, if an accident happened or not.

Errors—accidents—happen in statistics just as they do in the rest of life. The advantage of car crashes, over erroneous confidence intervals, is that you know when you've been in one. Erroneous confidence intervals are more like carbon monoxide poisoning—it's not something you're planning on doing, and you're usually not aware that you've been inhaling carbon monoxide until it's too late.

replication

Repetition of an experiment.

The resolution to this problem is something called **replication,** gathering another random sample and calculating the confidence interval again. If the two confidence intervals overlap—that is, if the hypothesized population value is captured by both—you should be more certain that you are not in error. Though of course, there is a chance that this is one of those rare instances where you got two bad samples in a row. Maybe a third sample is called for. But, ultimately, no matter how many samples one has, one can never be sure.*

TESTING HYPOTHESES, MAKING DECISIONS

How can we use confidence intervals to make decisions, to decide if a theory about the world, a hypothesis, is true? Suppose Buffy and Skip argue about whether Americans are really fatter now than they were a generation ago. Buffy digs up some data that say that the average weight of adult Americans was 155.00 pounds in the 1970s. Skip gathers a contemporary random sample of 102 adult Americans and finds an average weight of 159.50 pounds with a standard deviation (s) of 22.98. He states that a change of less than 5 pounds in 30 years doesn't sound like very much, that 159.50 is so close to the old mean of 155 that sampling error can account for the variability, and, therefore, he doesn't think that Americans have gotten heavier. Buffy maintains that a 4.5-pound weight gain indicates that Americans are heavier now. Who is right?

A confidence interval can be used in a situation like this to provide some objective standard by which to make this decision, as well as to quantify the likelihood that a conclusion is wrong. If the confidence interval around Skip's sample mean of 159.50 contains the 1970s population mean of 155.00, then it seems reasonable to conclude that it is possible that a sample with this mean ($M = 159.50$) could have come from a population where $\mu = 155.00$. Phrased differently, we conclude that M is close enough to μ that sampling error can account for the distance. If, however, the confidence interval around the sample mean does not contain the 1970s population mean, then even though it is *possible* that this sample came from that population, it doesn't seem *likely*. Something other than sampling error—such as the sample being drawn from a different (and now fatter) population—should be invoked to explain the observed difference.

Transforming s into $\hat{s}$ and calculating the 95% confidence interval yields an interval from 155.02 to 163.98.[†] As the 1970s population mean of 155.00 falls outside the interval, we should conclude that it is likely that our current sample comes from a different population than the one with a mean of 155.00: in other words, that Americans are probably heavier than they were 30 years ago. However, we need to be aware that we are

---

*This reminds me of one of my favorite jokes… There was a nervous airplane pilot who was afraid that there might be a bomb on his plane. He approached a statistician who told him that the odds were 1 in a 1000 of there being a bomb on a plane. The odds were even lower, 1 in a million, of there being two bombs on a plane, the statistician told him. So, the pilot always brought his own bomb.

[†]If you want to do the math, and I suggest that you do for practice, you should calculate $\hat{s} = 23.0935$, $\hat{s}_M = 2.2866$, and the 95% confidence interval $= 159.50 \pm 4.4817$.

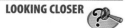
LOOKING CLOSER

only *probably* correct in our conclusion. There is a 5% chance that our conclusion is wrong and that sampling error is a legitimate explanation of the observed difference from a population mean of 155.00.

Some readers may be grumbling at this point about a different matter, that the old population mean was 155.00 and our confidence interval started just .02 pounds above, at 155.02. Isn't the confidence interval close enough to the old population value—just a fraction of a pound away—that we are splitting hairs when we say that the confidence interval did not capture μ? It's so close: can't we just say that sampling error explains the observed difference?

No! Statistics is like pregnancy, not horseshoes. With horseshoes, getting close can be good enough; with pregnancy and statistics, either you are or you aren't. Statisticians set the rules in advance—I'm going to make a 95% confidence interval and will conclude that μ falls within it— and then play strictly by the rules, living with the outcome.

Group Practice 6.3

1. The American Nurses Association wants to find out what percentage of first-year nursing students are male. They plan to find the genders of a random sample of first-year students and then calculate the 95% confidence interval for the percentage of male students in the population. Coding men as "1" and women as "0," they estimate that σ is .4330. They want the confidence interval to be fairly narrow with a *total* width of 3%. Using their estimate of σ, how many subjects will they need in their sample? What is the impact on sample size if they decide to have a confidence interval with a total width of 5%?

2. I have a friend who claims that the students at her college are of significantly above-average intelligence. By this she means that the average IQ at her college is greater than or equal to 130. I've been to her college, and the students there are very nice—and they are even smart—but they are not all Einsteins. So, I obtain a random sample of 65 students and find that $M = 127.00$. With this mean I argue that the average IQ at her college is less than 130. Is this a reasonable conclusion? Support your reasoning with a 95% confidence interval. Might the conclusion based on the confidence interval be wrong? (Don't forget that on standard IQ tests $\sigma = 15$.)

APPLYING CONFIDENCE INTERVALS TO QUESTIONS OF NORMALITY

As I've mentioned before, many statistical techniques should only be used with variables that are normally distributed.* We can tell if a variable is normally distributed by observing the skewness and kurtosis for the variable and seeing if they are near the expected values of zero. (Do you remember from Chapter 2 that in a normal distribution both skewness (symmetricity) and kurtosis (peakedness) equal zero?) There are two ways of assessing skewness and kurtosis—logic and calculation.

LOOKING CLOSER

*When we talk about a variable being normally distributed, we mean that it is normally distributed in the population.

I don't advocate using logic to determine if a variable is normally distributed, but I think it is an occasionally useful way to conclude that a variable is *not* normally distributed. For example, use your logic and knowledge of the world to think about the variable of age in college students: is age in college students normally distributed? Most college students are 18 to 22 years old, and the proportions at these ages are relatively equal—making a flat distribution, not a normal one. Further, the manner in which age is distributed in the tails of the distribution is not symmetrical. On the low end, there is probably a reasonable number of 17-year-old college students but very few 16-year-olds, and almost no students aged 15 or younger. But, think about the high end, where there are students who are 23, 24, 25, even 35, 45, and 55 years old, and beyond. Doesn't the distribution tail off in this direction, isn't it positively skewed? As Figure 6.11 shows, it is reasonable to conclude, just by thinking about it, that this variable is not normally distributed.

To decide if something *is* normally distributed, on the other hand, takes more than thought: it takes the calculation of confidence intervals for skewness and kurtosis.

What we shall do is very simple: first calculate skewness and kurtosis for the *sample*, and then calculate the 95% confidence intervals for these two values. If the confidence intervals *for both* capture the value of zero, then it is reasonable to conclude, with a 95% chance of being correct, that our sample came from a *population* where the values for this variable are zero. That is, even though the observed sample values of skewness and kurtosis may differ from zero, it is reasonable to conclude that sampling error could account for getting a sample that is this asymmetric or convex from a normally distributed population. However, if either the confidence interval for skewness *or* the confidence interval for kurtosis does not capture zero, then we should conclude that it is likely that the variable is not normally distributed *in the population*.

All we need to do, then, is calculate skewness and kurtosis and build the 95% confidence intervals around them. Skewness and kurtosis are examples of something called moments about the mean and they are, respectively, the third and fourth moments about the mean. And even though you've not yet been aware of it, we already calculated the first and second moments about the mean when we calculated means and variances. Moments about the mean are averages of z scores raised to different powers. The first moment about the mean is the average of z scores raised to the first power, the second moment about the mean is the average of z scores raised to the second power, the third moment about the mean is the average of z scores raised to the third power, and so on. The first moment about the mean, $\frac{\Sigma z^1}{N}$, equals .00 (the mean of

mean of the z scores) and the second, $\frac{\Sigma z^2}{N}$, equals 1.00, the variance of the

z scores. The first two moments, then, are the mean and the variance and the third is skewness and the fourth is kurtosis. The formulae for skewness and kurtosis are listed as Equations 6.4a and 6.4.b.

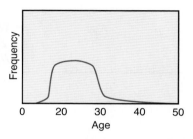

Figure **6.11** Expected non-normal distribution of ages of college students.

FORMULAE

Skewness and Kurtosis

Equation 6.4a	$Skewness = \dfrac{\Sigma z^3}{N}$
Equation 6.4b	$Kurtosis = \dfrac{\Sigma z^4}{N} - 3$

Where:
$z = z$ scores
N = number of scores

I'll be honest. I rarely calculate skewness and kurtosis by hand, since the process is tedious and computer-based spreadsheet and statistical programs are happy to churn them out.* Computer-based statistical programs also calculate standard errors for skewness and kurtosis so that you can calculate confidence intervals. Still, you might like to know how to calculate these standard errors on your own. Snedecor and Cochran (1980)[†] present simple formulae for *estimating* the standard errors for skewness and kurtosis, formulae that work well when the sample size is "large enough." I present these formulae in Equations 6.5a and 6.5b.[‡]

FORMULAE

Estimating Standard Errors for Skewness and Kurtosis

Equation 6.5a	$SE_{Skewness} = \sqrt{\dfrac{6}{N}}$
Equation 6.5b	$SE_{Kurtosis} = \sqrt{\dfrac{24}{N}}$

Where:
$SE_{Skewness}$ = the standard error for skewness being calculated
$SE_{Kurtosis}$ = the standard error for kurtosis being calculated
N = sample size

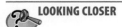

LOOKING CLOSER

*The formulae that statistical programs like SPSS or Excel use to calculate skewness and kurtosis are a little more complex and have some correction factors built in so that they generate estimated population values, not sample values.

[†]Snedecor, G., & Cochran, G. (1980). *Statistical methods,* (7th ed.). Ames, IA: Iowa State University Press.

[‡]See footnote on page 173.

Continued

Let's apply Equations 6.4a, 6.4b, 6.5a, and 6.5b to the final-grade-in-statistics data set to see if it is reasonable to conclude that grades in my statistics class are normally distributed. First, let me remind you that this data set consists of a random sample of 60 people from the hundreds to whom I have taught introductory statistics over the years. Thus, the question that we are addressing is not whether this variable is normally distributed in this *sample*, but whether final grades are normally distributed in the *population* of people to whom I have taught statistics.

I'm going to save you having to calculate skewness and kurtosis and just tell you that, by the formulae above, skewness for these data equals .1465 and kurtosis equals −.0720. If the data were normally distributed, both of these should equal 0. Are .1465 and −.0720 far enough away from 0 that we should worry that the sample, if it is representative of the population from which it came, came from a "non-normally" distributed population?

The way to determine this is to calculate the 95% confidence interval for both skewness and kurtosis. If both confidence intervals capture zero, then it is reasonable to conclude that the sample probably came from a population that is normally distributed.

Via Equations 6.5a and 6.5b, we can calculate the standard error of skewness:

$$\sqrt{\frac{6}{N}} = \sqrt{\frac{6}{60}} = .3162,$$

and the standard error of kurtosis:

$$\sqrt{\frac{24}{N}} = \sqrt{\frac{24}{60}} = .6325$$

From these, we calculate the 95% confidence intervals for skewness and kurtosis by bounding the values for skewness (.1465) and kurtosis (−.0720) with 1.96 of their respective standard errors. As a result, the 95% confidence interval for skewness runs from −.47 to .77, and the 95% confidence interval for kurtosis runs from −1.31 to 1.17. (The formulae for calculating 95% confidence intervals for skewness and kurtosis are given in the following material.)

Both of these confidence intervals capture zero, allowing us to conclude that the variable, final grade in statistics, is probably normally

---

(Continued) [†]These formulae are right, but I find them very odd. You'll note that the standard errors are entirely dependent upon *N*. For example if you have an *N* of 75, the standard error for skewness will always be .28 whether the data are normally distributed, skewed to the left, or skewed to the right.

LOOKING CLOSER

distributed in the population.* Are we certain that the variable is normally distributed in the population? No! As we calculated a 95% confidence interval, there is a 5% chance that we obtained an aberrant sample from a non-normally distributed population, a sample that was more normal than its population. In other words, there is a 5% chance that we are in error—and don't know it—when we conclude that final grades are normally distributed.

As Aristotle said, it is the nature of probability that improbable things can happen. With inferential statistics we probably make the right decision, but we recognize that we are never sure; in other words, that an improbable thing *may* have happened.

F O R M U L A E

95% Confidence Intervals for Skewness and Kurtosis

Equation 6.6a	$95\% \ CI_{Skewness} = Skewness \pm 1.96SE_{Skewness}$
Equation 6.6b	$95\% \ CI_{Kurtosis} = Kurtosis \pm 1.96SE_{Kurtosis}$

Where:

$95\% \ CI_{Skewness}$ = the 95% confidence interval for skewness being calculated

$Skewness$ = the skewness calculated for the sample, by Equation 6.4a or from a statistical program

$SE_{Skewness}$ = the standard error for skewness, by Equation 6.5a or from a statistical program

$95\% \ CI_{Kurtosis}$ = the 95% confidence interval for skewness being calculated

$Kurtosis$ = the kurtosis calculated for the sample, by Equation 6.4b or from a statistical program

$SE_{Kurtosis}$ = the standard error for kurtosis, by Equation 6.5b or from a statistical program

NOTE: Be aware that statistical programs like SPSS and Excel use a different formula to calculate skewness and kurtosis.

There is one final point to make about assessing normality of a distribution. Though calculating the confidence intervals for skewness and

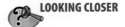

LOOKING CLOSER

*My experience has been that students initially have trouble understanding what confidence intervals for skewness and kurtosis tell them, so let me go over it one more time. In this scenario the only information I have about my population comes from my sample. I calculate the skewness and kurtosis for my sample and find that each is nonzero. Are the observed deviations from zero so great that I should be concerned that the variable is not normally distributed in the population?

I answer this question by coming up with an estimate of the ranges within which the population values of skewness and kurtosis likely fall. Since the likely ranges for the population values—the confidence intervals—include zero (remember that in a normal distribution skewness = 0 and kurtosis = 0), I conclude that this variable has a reasonable probability of being normally distributed in the population.

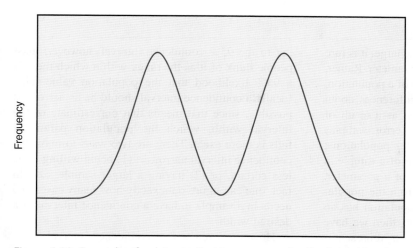

Figure **6.12** Example of a data set that is not normally distributed but has normal skewness and kurtosis.

kurtosis is a good thing to do, it is no substitute for actually visualizing your data set and using common sense. Figure 6.12 shows a frequency distribution that clearly is not normally distributed since it is bimodal. Yet, the calculated confidence intervals for skewness and kurtosis of these data do capture zero. Actually looking at—and thinking about—your data is always a good idea.

This chapter is almost over, and I want to reiterate that, in general, narrower confidence intervals are better because they are more exact—they provide a smaller estimate of the range within which we believe the population value falls. Size of confidence intervals depends heavily upon sample size and, usually, getting a larger sample takes more effort. How large should a sample be? As a practical rule of thumb, you don't want to calculate a confidence interval if you have fewer than 12 cases (VanBelle, 2002*). So, be very wary of interpreting a confidence interval if your sample size is smaller than 12.

Group Practice 6.4

1. I have a sample of 73 fourth-grade students on whom I have measured, using an interval scale, their reading level halfway through the school year. (A 4.0 on this scale indicates beginning fourth-grade level, 5.0 = fifth-grade level, 4.5 = halfway through fourth grade, etc.) I calculated $M = 4.63$, $\hat{s} = 1.25$, skewness = .75, and kurtosis = −1.06. Is the mean an appropriate measure of central tendency for these data?

---

*VanBelle, G. (2002). *Statistical rules of thumb*. New York: John Wiley & Sons.

LOOKING CLOSER

SUMMARY

Because populations are usually quite large, it is rare that we know a population value, a parameter. Rather, we have to rely on studying a subset of a population, a sample, and using that to make inferences about the larger population. Unfortunately, as a result of the random process called sampling error, samples are not exact replicas of their parent populations; so we cannot be sure that a measure of a sample, a statistic, is a faithful representation of a parameter. If a sample is randomly gathered from the population, that is, if every case in the population has an equal chance of being in the sample, then we have the greatest likelihood of having a representative sample. In addition, other things being equal, a larger sample will provide a better representation of the population than will a smaller sample.

Even a large, random sample, however, does not guarantee that a sample statistic is a faithful representation of a population parameter. Thus we use the concept of a sampling distribution (a frequency distribution of a sample statistic calculated for all repeated, random samples of size N from a population) and the derivations of the central limit theorem to learn how to calculate a range—a confidence interval—within which we have a reasonable degree of certainty that the population parameter falls. Though such intervals can be constructed for any degree of confidence, the most common is the 95% confidence interval. There is a technical meaning to the 95% confidence interval; however, most people think of it as the range within which there is a 95% likelihood that the population value falls. Ideally a confidence interval should be as narrow as possible, since that means that our estimate of the interval within which the population parameter falls is more exact. There are two ways to make the confidence interval narrower: (1) being willing to be less certain, or (2) having a larger sample size. In fact, one can figure out exactly how many cases one needs in a sample to have a confidence interval of a desired width.

However, even with a confidence interval, there is a chance that the population parameter does not fall within the confidence interval. With a 95% confidence interval, there is a 5% chance of having obtained a sample that is not representative of the population and, as a result, having a confidence interval that does not capture the population parameter. Unfortunately, when this "accident" occurs, there is no twisted metal lying about or other evidence that it happened. Thus it is possible that one will proclaim that the population parameter falls within a calculated confidence interval and, unknowingly, be wrong. The best way to increase one's faith that the confidence interval has captured the population value is by replication, by gathering a new sample from the population and calculating a second confidence interval.

Review Exercises

1. Here is a small data set that is a sample from a population: 7, 12, 9, 16, 8, 8, 10, and 9. What should we conclude about whether the *population* is normally distributed? (HINT: Think—and calculate—skewness and kurtosis.)

2. Only two candidates ran in a recent election. Candidate W, the winning candidate, received 50,100 votes and Candidate L, the loser, received 49,900 votes. In other words, the proportion of the vote that W got was 0.501, and the proportion that L got was 0.499. Candidate L claims that given the margin of error based on a standard deviation of 0.5000 (and this is a reasonable standard deviation to use), she has a legitimate claim to be the winner. What do you think? (WARNING: This question is quite tricky. If you understand that confidence intervals are used to estimate *population* values from sample values, then you can answer it without doing any calculations.)

3. Buffy draws a sample of 50 people, and Skip draws a sample of 70 people, from a population where $\sigma = 12.34$. Buffy's sample has a mean of 112.72, and Skip's has a mean of 110.23. If both of them calculate 95% confidence intervals, whose is wider?

4. Buffy draws a sample of 50 people from a population where $\sigma = 8.00$ and calculates a 90% confidence interval for her sample. Skip draws a sample of 80 people from a population where $\sigma = 9.50$ and calculates a 95% confidence interval. Whose confidence interval is wider?

5. A pollster for a national ballot initiative on which people can only vote "Yes" or "No" wants to have a 95% confidence interval for his poll with a margin of error of plus or minus two percentage points. Assuming that $\sigma = .5000$, how large must his sample size be?

6. Not to be outdone by Diekhoff, I've found a small town in Ohio that has a population of six. I take repeated, random samples of size $N = 2$ and for each person measure his or her blood pressure. The systolic blood pressures (that's the top number for you nonmedical types) for each person were 108, 132, 120, 116, 120, and 124.

   Part I: Graph the systolic blood pressure for the population and for the sampling distribution, and note their differences. Comment on the normality of the two distributions.

Part II: Calculate s, the standard deviation for the sampling distribution, and, via Equation 6.1, calculate σ_M. What do s and σ_M represent? Are the two values different? Which do you think is a more accurate reflection of the standard deviation of the sampling distribution? Why?

7. An unmanned space probe goes to Mars, gathers a sample of 63 Martians, and brings them back to Earth. These 63 Martians provide our only view of Martian life. How can we know that the conclusions we make about Martians based on these 63 are accurate?

8. Both N and σ determine σ_M. Why is it a good thing to have a smaller standard error of the mean?

9. I draw a sample of size $N = 66$ from a population and find skewness $= -1.4546$ and kurtosis $= .9873$. Is it appropriate to conclude that $\approx 84\%$ of the cases *in the population* fall below a z score of 1? (HINT: Base your answer on confidence intervals for skewness and kurtosis.)

10. If $M = 45.00$ and $\sigma_M = 4.00$, estimate the 68% confidence interval.

11. Calculate a 95% confidence interval for the following sample: $N = 17$, $M = 15.00$, and $\sigma = 1.50$.

Homework Problems

1. Buffy and Skip both draw samples of size 55 from a population with a known standard deviation (σ). Buffy's sample has a mean of 36.23 and Skip's a mean of 37.84. Each calculates a 95% confidence interval for μ. Which of the following is true?
   a. Buffy's confidence interval is wider.
   b. Skip's confidence interval is wider.
   c. The two confidence intervals are equally wide.
   d. There is not enough information provided to tell.

2. According to the central limit theorem, a sampling distribution of the mean will be approach a normal distribution as long as which of the following is true?
   a. At least 50 random, repeated samples are drawn.
   b. The population has at least 50 cases in it.
   c. Each repeated, random sample has at least 50 cases in it.

   d. σ, not $\hat{s}$, is used to calculate the standard error of the mean.

3. I obtain a random sample of 150 students from your university, find out each person's weight, and calculate M. Why will this not exactly equal μ?
   a. Because the sample is random
   b. Because the sample size is >50
   c. Because of sampling error
   d. Because $\hat{s}$ is used to calculate the standard error of the mean
   e. M will equal μ.

4. I take a sample from a population, calculate $\hat{s}$ and M, and then plan to calculate a confidence interval within which μ should fall. Which confidence interval for the mean will be the widest?
   a. 99%
   b. 95%
   c. 90%
   d. Not enough information to tell

5. I want to be sure that my confidence interval captures the mean. Which confidence interval makes this more likely?
   a. 99%
   b. 95%
   c. 90%
   d. Not enough information to tell

6. Imagine that I know μ and σ for a population. I draw a random sample from the population, calculate the 95% confidence interval for the mean, and discover that the confidence interval does NOT capture μ. Why did this occur?
   a. My sample was a random one.
   b. My sample was not representative.
   c. My population value was wrong.
   d. The central limit theorem does not apply when μ is known.

7. A school librarian hypothesizes that the average reading level of books in her elementary school library is at the third-grade level. She obtains a random sample of books from the library, has a reading specialist classify each book's reading level (1 = first grade, 2 = second grade, etc.) on an interval-level scale, and finds the mean reading level of the books in the sample. From this she calculates the 95% confidence interval and finds that it ranges from 2.85 to 3.46. What does she conclude, based on this?
   a. Her hypothesis is probably right.
   b. Her hypothesis is certainly right.
   c. Her hypothesis is probably wrong.
   d. Her hypothesis is certainly wrong.

8. You draw a sample from a population and use the sample to determine if the population is normally distributed. Which of the following is not possible for the population?
   a. Normal skewness and normal kurtosis
   b. Normal skewness and abnormal kurtosis
   c. Abnormal skewness and normal kurtosis
   d. Abnormal skewness and abnormal kurtosis
   e. All of the above can occur.

9. You draw a sample of 120 people from the population, measure each person's systolic blood pressure, and find $M = 129.7511$ and $s = 15.4515$. If you wanted to calculate a 95% confidence interval for systolic blood pressure that is ± 1.0000 units wide, how many subjects would you need?

10. A kinesiologist has measured the resting heart rates of 27 elite athletes and found $M = 41.8900$ and $s = 9.6706$. He claims that elite athletes have resting heart rates that are significantly lower than the general population. He consults the scientific literature and learns that the mean resting heart rate for the general population is 76 beats per minute. Is he justified in his conclusion that elite athletes have lower resting heart rates?

11. I draw a sample of size $N = 43$ from a population and measure a variable, X, on each case. I calculate $M = 4.8933$, $s = 1.7286$, skewness = .6527, and kurtosis = .7472 for this variable. What should I conclude about whether this variable is normally distributed in the population?

12. A physical therapist does a study in which he measures range of motion (how far a person can bend a limb) in elderly people both before and after a water aerobics class. What is his independent variable? His dependent variable?

13. Suppose that I have collected oral temperatures from a large and representative sample of adults, have calculated a 95% confidence interval, and have concluded that μ falls somewhere between 98.48° F and 98.76° F. Assuming that I have done the math right, is my conclusion correct? Why or why not?

14. A large World Health Organization initiative, the Monica Project, collected data relevant to cardiovascular disease in 21 countries. For adults in the United States, the researchers found that the mean systolic blood pressure was 124 with a standard deviation of 16. If blood pressure is normally distributed, and a systolic blood pressure 140 or above is considered hypertension, what percentage of adults in the United States has hypertension?

7

Relationship Tests and Hypothesis Testing

The Pearson Product Moment Correlation Coefficient

Learning Objectives

After completing this chapter, you should be able to do the following:

1 Differentiate relationship tests from difference tests and state a research question as a formal question.
2 Select the appropriate statistical test to answer a relationship question and determine which variable is the predictor and which is the predicted (criterion).
3 Follow a six-step procedure for completing a null hypothesis significance test.
4 Describe the role that assumptions play in statistical tests, determine whether the assumptions for a Pearson product moment correlation coefficient have been violated, and decide whether a Pearson correlation can be calculated.

(Continued)

5 Determine the population to which the results of a statistical test can be generalized.
6 State the null and the alternative hypotheses for a Pearson product moment correlation in symbolic notation and in English.
7 Explain how the null hypothesis is tested by comparing the observed value of a test statistic to the expected sampling distribution of the test statistic.
8 Explain: (a) the two correct decisions that can be made in null hypothesis significance tests, (b) the difference between Type I and Type II error, and (c) the consequences of each error.
9 Explain when a one-tailed and when a two-tailed statistical test should be used, explain the impact of alpha level and sample size on the critical value of r, state the decision rule for a Pearson product moment correlation coefficient, and graph the "common" and "rare" zones in a sampling distribution of r.
10 Calculate a Pearson product moment correlation coefficient and report it in APA format.

Chapter Roadmap

This chapter is long, but it is also one of the most important in the book. If you understand the concepts in this chapter, you should have no problem with the material in the rest of the book. (And, if you don't follow everything in this chapter, don't fret too much since the material will recur in future chapters. You'll have a second (and a third) chance to bite the apple.) So, here are some of the things to watch out for as we travel through this chapter.

We start out by learning how to differentiate a relationship test from a difference test and how, since this chapter focuses on relationship tests, to pick the correct relationship test based on whether the variables are continuous or categorical and their level of measurement. I then introduce my mnemonic ("Tom and Harry despise crabby infants") for a six-step procedure to complete statistical tests. This procedure will lead you through (1) deciding what **t**est to do, (2) evaluating the **a**ssumptions that must be met for the test to be completed, (3) understanding the **h**ypotheses that the test will help you decide between, (4) formulating the **d**ecision rule that will be used to decide whether the null hypothesis can be rejected, (5) **c**alculating the test statistic, and (6) **i**nterpreting, in English, the results of the test.

We'll explore the first five steps of this procedure in this chapter and learn about a lot of new concepts. Pay close attention, in particular, as we drive by (a) the null hypothesis and the alternative hypothesis, (b) Type I and Type II error, (c) the decision rule for the Pearson product moment correlation coefficient, and (d) how to calculate and report the Pearson product moment correlation coefficient.

In the last chapter we saw how confidence intervals could be used as inferential statistics, using *sample* descriptive statistics to make inferences about *population* parameters. We also used confidence intervals to see if there was support for a theory, a hypothesis, about a population parameter. Though confidence intervals can be used for testing a hypothesis, they weren't developed for that. In this and subsequent chapters we will learn about some of the tools in the statistician's tool chest that have been specifically designed as inferential statistics for hypothesis testing.

Inferential statistics are commonly dichotomized into two categories: relationship tests and difference tests. In **relationship tests** we have *one* group of cases, and for each case we measure its standing on *two* variables. Then we do some calculations to yield a single number, called a *correlation coefficient,* that tells us the degree to which those two variables covary. For example, I might get a group of kids of different ages and measure each one's height and foot size. I'd then calculate a correlation coefficient that would tell me whether taller kids have bigger feet, shorter kids have bigger feet, or if there is no relationship between height and foot size.

In **difference tests** we have *two (or more)* groups of cases that differ on some independent variable. For each subject, we measure its standing on *one* variable, the dependent variable. Then we do some calculations that yield a single number that tells us if the groups differ in terms of how much of the dependent variable they possess. For example, I might get a group of adults, give half of them a placebo and half of them an aspirin, and see how long they can keep their hands immersed in a bucket of ice water as a measure of how much pain they can tolerate. (Try it sometime; it hurts.) I'll find the average time for the placebo cases and the average time for the aspirin cases and then compare the two means using something called a *t* test to see if an analgesic (aspirin) helps, hinders, or has no impact on pain tolerance.

Note that with difference tests, we have independent variables and dependent variables. In the example just cited, the independent variable is the presence or absence of the analgesic and the dependent variable is the subject's pain tolerance.* Relationship tests need not involve a differentiation between independent and dependent variables, though there are some instances where it is appropriate to label them as such. These instances usually involve a chronological direction, where the independent variable precedes the dependent variable in time. For example, imagine a group of adults for whom we have information about their fat consumption as teenagers, as well as their body mass index

relationship test

A statistical test determining whether two variables covary, or are related.

difference test

A statistical test used to determine if groups differ in terms of how much of the dependent variable they possess.

---

*For those who need a refresher, the independent variable (IV) is what the experimenter controls or manipulates and the dependent variable (DV) is where the outcome of the study is measured. When the independent variable in a difference test is not controlled or manipulated by the experimenter, as when comparing boys to girls, it is called a grouping variable.

LOOKING CLOSER

(BMI) levels as adults. Suppose we find that those who consumed more fatty foods as teenagers have higher BMI levels as adults. It seems reasonable to consider teenage fat consumption as the independent variable that had some influence on the dependent variable of adult BMI levels. Conversely, it seems silly to think of adult BMI levels as the independent variable that influenced the dependent variable of teenage eating habits.*

Though we may talk about independent and dependent variables in connection with relationship tests, more commonly we talk about *predictor* and *predicted* variables, or predictor and *criterion* variables. If there is a relationship between two variables, then knowing something about a subject's standing on one variable, the predictor, gives us information about the subject's standing on the second variable, the criterion or predicted. If a relationship exists between height and foot size such that taller people have longer feet, then if I know your foot size I should be able to make an educated guess, a *prediction* or an estimate, about your height. In this case I would be using foot size as the predictor variable and height as the criterion variable.

However, correlation coefficients are ambidextrous. If there were a relationship between height and foot size, I could just as easily (and just as accurately!) use height as the predictor variable and foot size as the criterion variable. Because of this dexterity it is important, when one starts to calculate a correlation coefficient, to think about which way the prediction should go. The tradition is to label the two variables that are used in calculating a correlation coefficient as X and Y and to use X as the predictor variable and Y as the criterion, or predicted, variable.[†]

I have one final point to make before we move on to a detailed study of correlation coefficients: I have, once again, simplified the world. I said earlier that we divide inferential statistics into two different types of tests, relationship tests and difference tests. That is an oversimplification and a bit of a false dichotomy.

Why? Because difference tests can easily be construed as relationship tests. Back in Chapter 1 I gave the example of measuring the amount of impulsive behavior exhibited by children who did and did not receive caffeine and presented fictional data showing that caffeinated children were more impulsive than uncaffeinated ones. This certainly sounds like a difference test scenario: children who receive caffeine differ in level of impulsive behavior from those who don't receive caffeine. But, this can

---

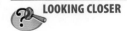 **LOOKING CLOSER**

*Don't forget the four most important words in statistics: "Correlation is not causation." Just because two things are correlated does not mean that one causes the other! Note that I was careful to say that teenage fat consumption *influenced* adult BMI level, *not* that it *caused* adult BMI levels. It is likely that some third variable, probably some genetic factor, causes both fat consumption and body size.

[†] When we use a correlation coefficient to estimate a Y value from an X value, the estimated Y value is called Y', pronounced "Y prime."

easily be construed as a relationship test if I phrase my results differently, such as, there is a *relationship* between caffeine consumption and impulsivity. Partly for this reason, correlations are considered one of the basic units of statistics; and so we start with them.*

CORRELATION COEFFICIENTS

To calculate a correlation coefficient, three conditions must be met: (a) there must be at least three cases; (b) there must be two variables, X and Y, that are measured for each case; and (c) there must be variability both on X and on Y.

Why do we need at least three cases? Well, one case alone cannot reveal a relationship between two variables. I am 5′7″ tall, and my foot is 10″ long. From this, as shown in Figure 7.1, *A*, can you tell if there is a relationship between foot size and height? No! With only a single point in this scatterplot,† you can't tell if taller people have longer feet, taller people have shorter feet, or if there is no relationship between height and foot size.

In Figure 7.1, *B*, I've added my wife, who at 5′4″ tall has a foot that is 9″ long. As you can see, there is a relationship between foot size and height: taller people have longer feet. The problem is that there are only two cases; and with two cases, since we can always draw a straight line between two points, we are destined to find a relationship. It is only when a third case is added, in this instance my eight-year-old son at 4′3″ tall with a 7″ foot, that there is a chance of *not* finding a relationship between the two variables. Figure 7.1, *C*, shows the relationship between foot size and height that exists for these three people. It certainly appears to confirm the notion that taller people have longer feet since all the cases fall on a reasonably straight, diagonal line. If my son's foot size had been different, say 9.5″ instead of 7″, then the scatterplot would have looked like Figure 7.1, *D*, and there would appear to be little relationship between height and foot size, since the cases don't fall on a straight, diagonal line. By adding a third point we have the potential to move away from the straight line that can be drawn between any two points and thus have the potential to find that there is no relationship between the two variables.

---

*Yes, you can take a relationship test and rephrase it as a difference test, but I find it awkward. For example, if there were a relationship between height and foot size such that taller people had longer feet, I could construe this as a difference test. It would probably be true that if I took two groups of people, one tall and the other short, that I would find a difference in foot size between the two groups.

†This type of graph is called scatterplot, or scattergram, and was not discussed in Chapter 2. In scatterplots, dots placed at the intersections of X and Y for each case show the relationship between two variables. When the dots are scattered in an amorphous blob, there is little linear relationship; the more the cases fall along a straight, diagonal line, the stronger the linear relationship between X and Y.

LOOKING CLOSER

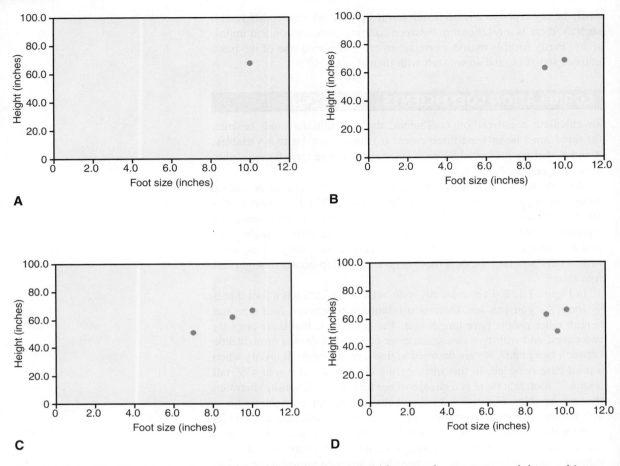

Figure **7.1** Scatterplots showing the relationship between height and foot size for one, two, and three subjects.

Thus, an *N* of three is the minimum condition for calculating a correlation. And, for all the reasons I've mentioned in previous chapters, a larger sample size is more desirable.*

We've seen that we need three or more cases to decide whether a relationship exists, but why do we need two variables, *X* and *Y*, for these three or more cases? Because that's what correlations do: they look at the relationship between *two* variables. If I have a group of cases and only

---

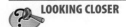 **LOOKING CLOSER**   *The difference between relationship tests and difference tests is really a difference in how the results are interpreted.

know their heights, not their foot sizes, I can't correlate height because there is nothing to correlate it with.*

Finally, why do I need variability on each variable? The easiest way to explain this is to use a difference test example—say, comparing boys to girls in terms of their physical aggressiveness on the playground. Imagine that we get a group of boys, measure physical aggressiveness on the playground, and find variability: some exhibit a lot of physical aggressiveness, some exhibit very little physical aggressiveness, and most are somewhere in the middle. Having measured all the boys, we ask whether boys are more aggressive than girls. The answer is that we don't know yet. We can't answer this question since we haven't collected any information about the physical aggressiveness of girls. That is, we have no variability on the variable of gender, and without such variability—without a comparison group—it is impossible to do a difference test. Similarly, if one of the variables in a relationship test, either X or Y, has no variability—if it is a constant—we can't do a relationship test.

Though we will learn to calculate only one in this chapter, there are three relationship tests that you should know about. Each one measures whether a relationship exists between two variables, but they differ in terms of the level of measurement of the variables.

If both variables are measured at the interval or ratio level, as with height and foot size, then the correlation of first choice is the **Pearson product moment correlation coefficient,** commonly called the Pearson r. Because this is the most commonly calculated correlation coefficient, it is often just referred to as r, though to distinguish it from other correlation coefficients it is better to call it r_p (that's "r sub p," as in "p" for "Pearson").†

If both variables are ordinal, or one is ordinal and the other interval or ratio, then the correlation of first choice is the **Spearman rank order correlation coefficient,** commonly called the Spearman, Spearman's r, or r_s (pronounced "r sub s," the "s" standing for "Spearman"). As an example, Spearman's r would be used to examine the relationship between order of finish in a footrace (an ordinal measure) and length of stride (a ratio-level measure).

If both variables are nominal, for example to examine the relationship between gender (male vs. female) and hand preference (right vs. left), then the correlation of first choice is the **chi-square test of association,** commonly called chi-square and abbreviated with the Greek letter chi as χ^2. Chi, by the way, is pronounced "kai" to rhyme with "pie."

Pearson product moment correlation coefficient

A relationship test used when both variables are measured at the interval or ratio level.

Spearman rank order correlation coefficient

A relationship test used when both measures are measured at the ordinal level, or when one variable is ordinal and the other is interval- or ratio-level.

---

chi-square test of association

A relationship test used when both variables are measured at the nominal level.

---

*SPSS® (Statistical Package for the Social Sciences) calls the correlation coefficients that I am talking about "bivariate" correlations because they involve two variables.

†Wonder why the abbreviation "r" is used? Officially the r stands for regression, but if you want to think of it as short for relationship, that's fine by me.

LOOKING CLOSER

	X is interval/ratio	X is ordinal	X is nominal
Y is interval/ratio	r_p	r_s	Difference test
Y is ordinal	r_s	r_s	Difference test
Y is nominal	Difference test	Difference test	χ^2

Note: r_p = Pearson product moment correlation coefficient

r_s = Spearman rank order correlation coefficient

χ^2 = Chi-square test of association

Figure **7.2** Deciding what test when for correlation coefficients (relationship tests).

categorical variable

A variable used to classify cases into groups or categories.

So far I've differentiated variables as nominal, ordinal, interval, or ratio and in earlier chapters as discrete or continuous. Now I have one last way for you to think of some variables: as categorical. A **categorical variable** is one that classifies cases into categories as, for example, gender categorizes people as male or female. Categorical variables are almost always used as independent variables, though when cases can't be randomly assigned to groups the more appropriate term is "grouping variable." Categorical variables are almost always nominal level, though it is possible for them to be ordinal as, for example, if we categorized people receiving a drug as being in high-, medium-, or low-dose groups.

If, when completing a relationship test, one variable is categorical (e.g., gender) and the other variable is ordinal, interval, or ratio (e.g., weight), then the appropriate test for a relationship question (e.g., Is there a relationship between a person's gender and his or her weight?) is a difference test, and the question could be reconstrued as a difference question (e.g., Is there a difference in weight between men and women?).*

Though we will calculate only r_p in this chapter, I still expect you to know which test to use in which situation, what I call the "what-test-when" question. The matrix in Figure 7.2 summarizes what test should be chosen depending on the level of measurement for both X and Y.

Just to make the what-test-when question a little harder, you should be aware of one more thing. You might have noted that I introduced each correlation coefficient as the correlation "of first choice" if the level-of-measurement conditions are met. But, as we shall soon see, all

LOOKING CLOSER

*The difference between relationship tests and difference tests is really a difference in how the results are interpreted.

statistical tests have assumptions that must be met in order to use them. We may *want* to correlate two ratio-level variables, but if one of the other assumptions for the Pearson r is not met, then we *shouldn't* calculate r_p. Statisticians hate to quit, so they have fallback options. If the assumptions for the Pearson r are not met, they'll scale the variables back to the ordinal level and see if they can do the Spearman r instead. And, if it turns out that the assumptions for the Spearman r are not met, they'll scale the variable back even further to the nominal level and try the chi-square test of association. And if the assumptions for the chi-square aren't met? Well, there are other tricks that they'll try. So, the what-test-when question will involve paying attention not only to the level of measurement, but also to the other assumptions!

TOM, HARRY, AND THE PEARSON PRODUCT MOMENT CORRELATION COEFFICIENT

It is time to calculate a correlation coefficient, specifically the Pearson product moment correlation coefficient. For this to be reasonable, let's start with a small data set—height and foot size. I've taken a random sample ($N = 6$) from the population of students at my college and measured these variables to see if there is a relationship between foot size and height. And, given that I want you to get into the habit of thinking in advance about which variable is X and which is Y, the question is: Can you predict a person's height from his or her foot size? So, in the data set in Table 7.1, foot size is X and height is Y.

Though you are probably chomping at the bit to get down to some actual calculations, that is not the first step in conducting a statistical test. I have a six-step procedure for every statistical test we do. It goes by the mnemonic "Tom and Harry despise crabby infants." The first letters of those six words refer to the six steps to be followed for all statistical tests, outlined in Table 7.2.

Using this mnemonic will guide you through all the steps that need to be followed and decisions that need to be made when conducting a statistical test. First you need to figure out what statistical test should

TABLE **7.1** **Data set ($N = 6$) of Foot Size (X) in Inches and Height (Y) in Inches**

X	Y
9.00	64.00
9.00	67.00
10.00	67.00
8.00	62.00
10.00	72.00
8.00	64.00

TABLE **7.2**   *Tom and Harry Despise Crabby Infants: A Six-Step Procedure for Hypothesis Testing*

1. **Test**	:	What statistical **T**est is being chosen and why?
2. **Assumptions**	:	What are the **A**ssumptions for the test? Can the test be completed?
3. **Hypotheses**	:	What are the null and alternative **H**ypotheses?
4. **Decision rule**	:	What is the **D**ecision rule? Is the sample size adequate?
5. **Calculation**	:	**C**alculate the test statistic.
6. **Interpretation**	:	**I**nterpret the results.

be done. Then you need to determine if the conditions for the test have been met and it is OK to proceed. After this you need to clarify what the two hypotheses are that the test is testing. Once that is clear, you need to spell out your decision rule so that when you actually calculate the value of the test statistic you'll know which hypothesis to believe. Only then can you calculate the test statistic, here the Pearson r, and apply the decision rule. Then, finally, you need to make sense of—interpret—the results.

Step 1: Tom

The first step involves picking the correct statistical *test* to be applied to the data to answer the question being asked. There are two broad paths that lead to statistical tests: the relationship path and the difference path. The simplest way to choose a path is to phrase the question—as a question, complete with question mark—using either the word "relationship" or the word "difference." The way the question trips off your tongue more easily (i.e., "Is there a relationship between…" vs. "Is there a difference between…") helps determine which path to follow. Here, I would phrase the question as, "Is there a relationship between height and foot size in adults?"—which suggests a relationship test. Now we must choose among the tests listed in Figure 7.2.

Figure 7.2 shows three correlation coefficients and the unspecified category of "difference test" that could be used, depending on the level of measurement of the variables. So, the next thing to consider is the level of measurement of the variables. Here both variables, height in inches and foot size in inches, are ratio-level measures. So, referring to Figure 7.2, the appropriate correlation coefficient is the Pearson r.

Thus, the answer to Step 1—what statistical test are we choosing and why—is the Pearson r, because we are examining the relationship between two ratio-level variables.

The first set of group practice problems in this chapter involves choosing a test—a relationship test or a difference test. Because a relationship test can be interpreted as a difference test and vice versa, the distinction between the two is not always black and white.

The difference between relationship and difference test is in the interpretation of the statistical test, not in the type of test used. If I were comparing boys to girls to see which has longer hair, you could construe that either as a relationship test (Is there are relationship between gender and hair length?) or a difference test (Is there a difference in hair length between boys and girls?). Though this situation can be construed as either *type* of test, there actually is a correct statistical test to choose in this situation, a specific difference test called an independent samples *t* test. I could *interpret* the results of the *t* test as indicating either a relationship or a significant difference, but in either event I would calculate a *t* value. So, how do I decide what test to do?

The simplest thing to do is to pay attention to whether the *independent variable* is continuous or categorical and/or to see how many values it has. If the variable is continuous, think *correlation coefficient*; if discrete, especially when it has only a small number of values, think *difference test*. In the example that I have been using, the independent variable is gender, and the dependent variable is hair length. Gender is a categorical variable with only a limited number of values (1 = boy, 2 = girl). This question should be answered with a difference test.

For a different example, imagine examining the relationship between height and hair length and treating height as the predictor variable. Height is a continuous variable and, with a reasonably large sample, you will probably have cases with all different heights, from less than 5 feet tall to well over 6 feet tall. In this case, the test of choice is a correlation coefficient, like Pearson *r*.

With some juggling, we could make this hair length-height test into a difference test and compare the hair length of short people to that of medium-height people to that of tall people. And this is where the proviso to pay attention to the number of values for the independent variable comes into play: if there are a small number of values for an independent or grouping variable, consider a difference test even if the variable is continuous. Suppose, for example, that we compare the effectiveness of three different doses of a medicine, 0 mg, 10 mg, and 20 mg. Milligrams is a continuous measure, but since we are using only three of the multitude of values here, a difference test makes more sense. For now, you only have to worry about whether the research question calls for a Pearson *r*, Spearman's *r*, a chi-square, or a difference test. With practice, you will feel comfortable making these decisions.

Group Practice 7.1

For each of the first three scenarios, (a) phrase the research question as a question, and (b) tell if the study calls for a relationship test or a difference test.

1. An education researcher wants to compare interval level reading performance scores for sixth graders from three different types of school districts: urban, suburban, and rural. He gets a sample of children from urban schools, a sample from suburban schools, and a sample from rural schools and, looking for differences, finds the average reading level for each sample.

2. A developmental psychologist is investigating the impact of sugar consumption on children's activity level. She measures how many grams of sugar each child in a group consumes during an 8-hour period, then measures how many calories each child expends on a playground during a subsequent 30-minute play period.

3. A public health researcher is interested in the impact of public service announcements (PSAs) on behavior. He obtains a sample of 30 comparably-sized cities and for each one measures the number of broadcast PSAs that stressed the need for children to wear helmets while riding bikes. He then goes to each city and observes, near playgrounds, the percentage of children who wear helmets while riding bikes.

Continued

Group Practice 7.1—cont'd

For the next three scenarios, (a) tell which relationship test would be the appropriate one to use, and (b) tell which variable is the predictor (*X*) and which is the criterion (*Y*).

4. A nurse is investigating the impact of predischarge patient education on postdischarge compliance with medication use. She obtains the names of 100 recently discharged patients and searches their hospital charts to see if it is documented that before they were discharged a nurse explained to them how they should continue to take their medications after their discharge. If it is documented in the chart, the researching nurse considers that predischarge patient education occurred; if it is not documented, she considers that it did not occur. A month after discharge, she visits each patient and determines if he or she has been compliant (yes) or not (no) with use of postdischarge medications. What statistical test should she use to see if there is a relationship between

predischarge patient education and postdischarge compliance?

5. An anthropologist has rated, on an interval scale, 150 societies in terms of the degree to which they honor and respect mothers and women. He believes that respect for women and mothers leads to greater societal peacefulness. For each society he calculates the per capita rate of violent crime as his measure of peacefulness. He wants to correlate these two variables to see if they are related. What correlation should he choose?

6. A teacher suspected that the speed with which students completed a test influenced how well they did on the test. On a 100-item multiple choice test where each item was worth 1 point, he kept track of the order in which the tests were completed. That is, the first student who handed in the test received a rank of 1, the second student a 2, and so on. What statistical test should the teacher use to see if there is a relationship between grade on the test and test completion speed?

Step 2: And

The second step involves examining the *assumptions* for the statistical test, determining if any have been violated, and then deciding if it is OK to proceed with the planned statistical test. Although the Pearson *r* may be appropriate for the level of measurement, it may not be the test we will use. We have to see if we meet the assumptions that underlie the use of the test.*

What are assumptions? Well, every statistical test has certain conditions that must be met before it can *meaningfully* be conducted. Why did I italicize meaningfully? Because if the assumptions haven't been met, if they have been violated, you can still physically go ahead and do the test, you just won't know the meaning of what you have calculated.

For example, one of the assumptions that professors have when they give tests is that a student's work on the test is his or her own, in other

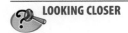
LOOKING CLOSER

*To be technical, we care about assumptions when we are conducting hypothesis tests for inferential statistics. If you are calculating a correlation coefficient for purely descriptive reasons, just to describe the degree of linear relationship between two variables, then you don't need to worry about most of the assumptions.

words that the student didn't cheat. If a student violates that assumption (and doesn't get caught), the professor will grade the test and use that grade to make inferences about how well the student knows the material. But does that grade mean anything? Does it represent the student's real degree of knowledge of the material? We can physically assign a grade, but it isn't meaningful and shouldn't be interpreted.

Similarly, when assumptions for a statistical test have been violated, we don't know what the results of a statistical test mean. Perhaps the same results would have occurred if the assumptions hadn't been violated, and perhaps not. We don't know. To help understand this, imagine that the presidents of Harvard and Yale get together and after a few beers start arguing about which school has students who are more physically fit. Being empirically minded sorts, they agree to a test in which random samples of students from the two schools will be compared in terms of the number of push-ups they can do. The president of Yale, however, starts to fear that if his students lose, he'll be the laughing stock of the Ivy League. So, he decides to cheat by packing his "random" sample with members of the Yale athletic teams. As a result, Yale wins the contest. Knowing that the assumption that each sample was representative of its respective school was violated, what do the results tell us about the relative physical fitness of Yale and Harvard students? Absolutely nothing. It is possible that Yale students are more physically fit than Harvard students, and it is possible that Harvard students are more fit than Yale students, just as it is possible that the two schools have equally fit students. The push-up test, because an assumption was violated, sheds no light on the original question.

Statistical tests are *robust* to violations of some assumptions and *not robust* to violations of other assumptions. Robustness refers to how serious it is to violate an assumption If a test is robust to violations of an assumption, there is probably not too much impact on the test results if the assumption is violated. If Yale's president had only snuck a few members of Yale's ping-pong team into his "random" sample, it probably would not have altered the results very much. Statistical tests are not robust to violations of other assumptions—which means that violating them is so serious that if you do, you shouldn't proceed with the test.

I think of robustness like physical health. If you are in good physical health, if you are robust, then you probably eat right, get 8 hours of sleep a night, exercise regularly, and don't often drink alcohol to excess. Now, imagine that a woman with a cold walks by and, just as she is passing you, she sneezes right in your face, causing you to inhale a large bolus of cold germs. Because you are in good health, because you are robust, it is unlikely that this challenge to your system will cause you to get sick.

Contrast that with a guy whose health is not robust: someone who never gets enough sleep, who regularly drinks alcohol to excess, who doesn't exercise, and who eats only junk food. If someone with a cold sneezes in this immunocompromised person's face, he is more likely to get sick.

Robustness is a good thing in an assumption, but it doesn't make it bulletproof. Assumptions are robust to a point, but they can be pushed beyond the breaking point. Imagine that you are in robust health and that you experience a number of challenges, a number of violations to your system: a person with a cold sneezes in your face, you shake hands with a person who has the flu, by mistake you use your sick roommate's toothbrush, and your significant other who spent the weekend with you calls to report having been diagnosed with mononucleosis. Even though you are in robust health, there are enough threats to your system that you are likely to fall ill. So it is with robust assumptions for statistical tests. You can violate them to some degree, but they do have limits beyond which they won't stretch.

With all that lead-in, here are the five assumptions for the Pearson r:

1. The sample is a random sample from the population (robust).
2. Both X and Y are interval- or ratio-level variables (not robust).
3. Both X and Y are normally distributed (robust if N is large enough).
4. The relationship between X and Y is linear (not robust).
5. The variables display homoscedasticity* (robust if N is large enough).

Assumption 1

The first assumption is that the sample for which we are calculating the correlation coefficient is randomly chosen from its parent population. This is an important assumption. Inferential statistics compare the statistic calculated from a sample, the *observed statistic*, to the *expected distribution* of the sampling distribution for that statistic. And how do we get a sampling distribution? By drawing repeated, *random* samples from the population. If the observed value of the test statistic is obtained one way, not by random sampling, and we compare it to a distribution obtained another way, by random sampling—well, isn't that like comparing an apple to oranges? And the problem with comparing an apple to oranges is that it is not a meaningful comparison as long as we think we are comparing an orange to oranges.[†]

The Pearson product moment correlation coefficient, like all null hypothesis significance tests,[‡] is built on comparing the test statistic observed in

---

![LOOKING CLOSER icon]

LOOKING CLOSER

*Cool word, no? Don't worry, I'll tell you what it means soon enough.

[†] It doesn't make sense to compare an apple to oranges *if* I think it is an orange. Comparing an apple to an orange and concluding, "This orange has skin that is much thinner than the other oranges" isn't very useful. However, if I were aware that the fruit I was comparing to oranges was an apple, then a statement like, "This apple has a skin that is thinner than the skin of the oranges" would be useful.

[‡] I'm getting a little ahead of myself here, but this is such a common term that I can't avoid it any longer. Tests, like the Pearson r, in which we are testing whether something called the null hypothesis is likely true, are called null hypothesis significance tests, or NHST for short. This will make sense in a few more pages when we learn what a null hypothesis is, but I was getting tired of the awkwardness of avoiding the use of this term.

one random sample to the distribution of the test statistic found in a sampling distribution of repeated, random samples. But this assumption is almost always violated since it is rare that we have a random sample from the population of interest. Luckily, the Pearson r is robust to violations of this assumption. You can violate this assumption and still meaningfully calculate a Pearson r. However, violating this assumption has ramifications for the final step of Tom-and-Harry, how you interpret the results.

I'm a psychologist and it is easiest for me to draw on an example from that discipline to make this point, but I'm sure you can apply this to your discipline as well. Most studies in psychology use college students as participants. College students are not a random sample from the general population, and clearly they differ from the general population in a number of dimensions, notably age, intelligence, and socioeconomic status. Thus, the results from a study of college students can't be taken as applying to humanity in general.

Further, most psychology experiments draw on students who are part of a subject pool as a result of taking an introductory psychology class, and this additionally limited subset of college students further limits the applicability of results. What is more, most psychology experiments are conducted at only one college at one point in time, further limiting generalizability. Even if we limited the population to which we wished to generalize our results to introductory psychology students at University A who are taking intro psych in year B, it is hard to imagine how it would be possible to get a random sample of that population. After all, we can't force people to participate in experiments against their will.*

So why, if we don't have a random sample from the desired population, can we still go ahead and do a statistical test? Because we couldn't do very much science if we limited ourselves only to doing studies that have random samples from the relevant populations.† So pragmatically, we forge ahead and hope that other people doing similar research in other nonrandom samples will find similar results, and that the accretion of results over time will be persuasive enough. In doing so, though, we have to keep in mind that since the sample we are examining is not a random sample from the relevant population, it is possible that it is odd in some way and cannot meaningfully be compared to the sampling distribution. This limitation is something that we'll need to bear in mind when we get to the last Tom-and-Harry step, the interpretation.

Assumption 2

The Pearson r is not robust to violations of the second assumption, that both X and Y are measured at the interval or ratio level. This assumption means that if either of the two variables on which the Pearson r is being

---

*And if we did get a random sample, is this very limited population one that we care about? I think not.
† Though it probably wouldn't be a bad thing if researchers completed fewer, but better, studies.

LOOKING CLOSER

calculated is being measured at the ordinal or nominal level, then the Pearson r shouldn't be calculated. This isn't much of a problem, since there are fallback tests that can be performed if it is violated.*

Assumption 3

The third assumption, which says that both variables, X and Y, are normally distributed *in the population*, is a "robust if" assumption and is called the *normality* assumption for short. Please note: This assumption refers to normality *in the population*, not the sample. That is, if we examined the relationship between height and foot size in a sample of college students, we would be concerned with whether height were normally distributed in the *population* of college students and if foot size were normally distributed in the *population* of college students—and not how they were distributed in our sample. How can we know if they are normally distributed in the population? By applying the concepts discussed in Chapter 6—making confidence intervals around a *sample's* skewness and kurtosis in order to make inferences about the population values.

If we determine that either of the variables is not normally distributed, we may be able to make use of the "robust if" provision for this assumption. The Pearson r is robust to violations of this assumption if the N, the number of cases in the sample, is large enough. What is large enough? Well, I've seen some statisticians say that the Pearson r is robust to violations of normality if $N \geq 25$, others say N should be ≥ 35, and others say ≥ 50. I'm conservative and don't worry about violating the normality assumption when $N \geq 50$. I would like you to be conservative as well. To state this more clearly, consider the normality assumption robust if the number of cases is greater than or equal to 50. (Though, also remember that robustness does not protect against extreme violations, even if the sample size is greater than 50.)

What do we do if N is less than 50 and either X or Y is not normally distributed? Go to a fallback test! One option is to treat the data as ordinal, not interval/ratio, and turn to Spearman's r. If that doesn't work, we can fall back further to the χ^2 test.

Assumption 4

This is called the linearity assumption for short, and it says that r_p should only be calculated if the relationship between X and Y is a linear one. The Pearson r is not robust to violations of this assumption, so if the relationship between X and Y is a nonlinear one, then the Pearson r should not be calculated.

What do I mean by a linear relationship or a nonlinear relationship? A linear relationship is one that can be described by a straight line, and a

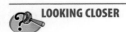
LOOKING CLOSER

*I'm being hardcore here in calling the Pearson r not robust to violations of this assumption. As we'll see in the next chapter, there is a special form of the Pearson r that can be calculated for nominal data.

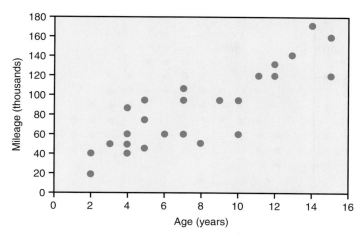

Figure **7.3** Scatterplot showing linear relationship between age of used cars and number of miles driven.

nonlinear relationship is one that is described by a curved line. For an example of a linear relationship, see Figure 7.3, which shows the scatterplot for age (in years) of used cars and their mileage (in thousands). As you might expect, older cars have, in general, been driven for more miles. And you can see in Figure 7.3, the data points fall roughly along a straight line that is sloped up and to the right.*

The linearity assumption exists because the math behind r_p is meant to capture a linear relationship. If you apply it to a nonlinear relationship, there may appear to be no relationship even if a relationship really exists. The data displayed in Figure 7.4 show a nonlinear relationship between the IQs of college students and how many hours they report studying for an easy test: less bright and more bright students spend less time studying than do students of average intelligence.[†] The scatterplot shows a relationship between intelligence and time spent studying, but the relationship does not take the form of a straight line. If one calculated a Pearson *r* for these data, it would show that there is no *linear* relationship between these two variables. If the word "linear" is omitted from an interpretation, as it often (and erroneously) is, one would conclude that there is no relationship between the two variables. And that conclusion would be wrong since there is a relationship, just not a linear one. The

---

*Slope refers to the angle of a line, how much the values for *Y* rise (or fall) as values on *X* increase. If the line is moving up and to the right, it has a positive slope. If it is moving down and to the right, it has a negative slope.

[†]In case you haven't figured it out yet, I just made these data up. My actual experience is that the rich get richer—bright students study more and as a result do better on tests.

LOOKING CLOSER

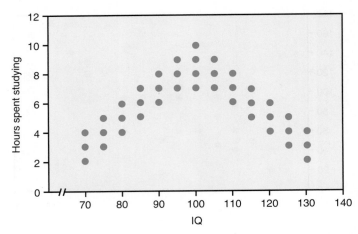

Figure **7.4** Scatterplot showing a nonlinear relationship between intelligence and hours spent studying for an easy test.

Pearson product moment correlation is not meant to assess nonlinear relationships!

To evaluate whether the assumption of linearity has been violated, construct a scatterplot and eyeball the data set for linearity or nonlinearity.* It is rare that you will get a scatterplot that is as obvious as my examples in Figure 7.3 and 7.4, so what you are looking for is a clear, nonlinear relationship. If the data don't show a clear, nonlinear relationship as in Figure 7.5, for example, don't fret—go ahead with the Pearson *r*. Only consider the linearity assumption violated if you can see a well-defined curve in the data set. Oh yes, if you have violated the linearity assumption, proceed to the fallback test, to Spearman's *r*.

Assumption 5

The last of the five assumptions for a Pearson *r* is called the homoscedasticity assumption and also relies on a scatterplot for assessment. Scedasticity refers to the spread of a variable around another, the spread of *X* around *Y and* of *Y* around *X*. It is possible for the spread of one variable around the other to be equal at all levels of the other variable, which is what we want in order to proceed with r_p, and which we call homoscedasticity. If the spread of one variable around the other variable varies depending on the level of the other variable (called heteroscedasticity), then we should consider not proceeding with r_p.

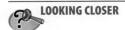
LOOKING CLOSER

*If, like one of my old stats professors, you want to make it sound more scientific than "eyeballing" the data, you can say that you applied the "interocular test."

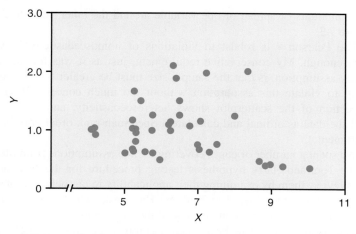

Figure **7.5** Example of a scatterplot that shows neither a clear-cut linear nor a clear-cut nonlinear relationship between *X* and *Y*.

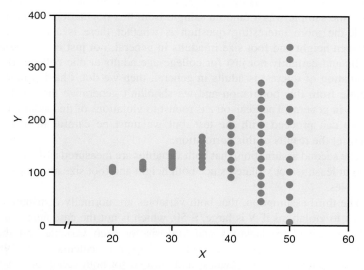

Figure **7.6** Scatterplot of a heteroscedastic data set that violates the assumption of homoscedasticity.

This sounds more complex than it is. Figure 7.6 shows a data set that is heteroscedastic, violating the assumption of homoscedasticity. Note that as the values of *X* increase, the variability in *Y* scores around the *X*s increases. This differing variability in one variable at different levels of the other is heteroscedasticity. For a picture of homoscedasticity, roughly equal amounts of spread of one variable around the other, refer back to Figure 7.3.

The Pearson r is robust to violations of homoscedasticity if N is large enough. My conservative requirement, just as it was for the normality assumption, is that the sample size must be greater than or equal to 50 to violate this assumption without too much concern. If visual inspection of the scatterplot shows heteroscedasticity, and N is <50, treat the data as ordinal and calculate a Spearman rank order correlation coefficient.

We spent a number of pages covering all five assumptions from Step 2 of the Tom-and-Harry hypothesis testing procedure for the Pearson r. Let's review them by examining their applicability to our height–foot size data set. Remember, Step 2 of Tom-and-Harry asks whether we can proceed with the test after having evaluated the assumptions.*

The assumptions for the Pearson product moment correlation coefficient are (1) random samples, (2) interval or ratio data, (3) normality, (4) linearity, and (5) homoscedasticity. The first assumption, that the sample is a random sample from the population, may or may not have been violated, depending on the population of interest. If the population of interest is the students at my college, then the assumption was not violated since the sample was a random sample from this population. However, I think the more interesting question is whether there is a relationship between height and foot size in adults in general, not just in college-age adults and certainly not just for college-age adults at one college. If the population of interest is adults in general, then we don't have a random sample from this population and we shouldn't generalize the results to adults in general. The Pearson r is robust to violations of this assumption, so we can proceed with the test, but we must be careful in how we interpret the results of this correlation.

The second assumption, that both variables are measured at the interval level at least, is not violated since both height and foot size are ratio-level variables.

The third assumption, that both variables are normally distributed, is robust to violations if N is large, ≥ 50, which is not the case here. I used SPSS to calculate skewness and kurtosis for each variable and then, following the procedures outlined in Chapter 6, calculated the 95% confidence intervals for skewness and kurtosis for both variables.[†] As the confidence intervals captured zero, it seems reasonable to conclude that

---

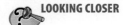

LOOKING CLOSER

*If you decide that it is inappropriate to proceed with the planned test, then suggest the appropriate fallback test. Ideally, you should go on to check the assumptions for the fallback test and, if they are met, complete it. If the assumptions for the fallback test aren't met, then suggest an appropriate fallback test for the fallback test.

[†]Why use SPSS rather than the skewness and kurtosis formulae from Chapter 6? Because SPSS gives corrected estimates of skewness and kurtosis, values that are estimates of the population values. Since our concern is with the population, not the sample, it makes more sense to use corrected values.

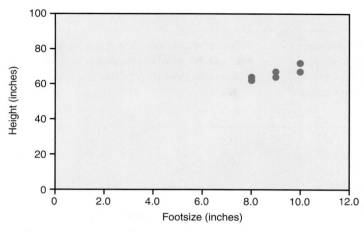

Figure **7.7** Scatterplot of relation between height and foot size for height–foot size data set.

both height and foot size are normally distributed in the population.* Assumption 3, normality, is not violated.

The next two assumptions, linearity and homoscedasticity, are assessed by viewing a scatterplot of the data. Inspection of the scatterplot (Figure 7.7) shows both that it looks like there is a linear relationship between the two variables and that there do not appear to be differing degrees of variability in one variable as a function of the level of the other variable. Thus, neither of these two assumptions seems to be violated.

The only assumption violated was that the sample is a random sample from the population of adults. As the Pearson r is robust to violations of this assumption, it seems reasonable to proceed with calculating the correlation coefficient. And so, after some group practice on what we've covered so far, we'll move on to Step 3, Harry, of the Tom-and-Harry procedure.

Group Practice 7.2

For each of the scenarios on p. 200, do the following:

(a) Determine which variable is X and which is Y.

(b) Evaluate all five assumptions for the Pearson r (this includes calculating confidence intervals for skewness and kurtosis).

(c) Decide whether to proceed with the test.

(d) Whether you proceed with the test or not, describe the population to which the results can be generalized.

Continued

---

*It is always good to practice calculating confidence intervals. According to SPSS, skewness and kurtosis for height are .948 and .970; for foot size they are .000 and −1.875. The standard errors for skewness and kurtosis are .845 and 1.741. Thus the two confidence intervals for height are from −.71 to 2.60 (skewness) and from −2.44 to 4.38 (kurtosis); for foot size they are, respectively, from −1.66 to 1.66 and −5.29 to 1.54.

LOOKING CLOSER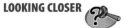

Group Practice 7.2—cont'd

1. A pharmaceutical company researcher investigates the relationship between the dose of a new sleep aid medication and the number of minutes to sleep onset after ingestion. He had a large group of cases, but has now selected a subset (women over age 70) in whom he wants to examine the relationship. Here are his data:

Case#	1	2	3	4	5	6	7	8	9	10
Dose	0	5	10	15	15	15	20	20	25	30
Min	45	38	29	31	27	26	24	10	25	22

Here are descriptive statistics for these data:

	M	*s*	**Skewness (*SE*)**	**Kurtosis (*SE*)**
Dose	15.5000	8.5000	−.185 (.687)	−.141 (1.334)
Min	27.7000	8.8775	.085 (.687)	1.365 (1.334)

2. An oceanographer is examining the relationship between sand temperature and the percentage of sea turtle eggs that hatch as males. She observes six sea turtle nests from a beach in Dolphin Cay, Florida, and records the average temperature, in degrees Celsius, in the sand near the nests during the middle third of the approximately 2-month incubation period. Here are her data:

Nest #	1	2	3	4	5	6
Av. temp	23	25	28	30	32	34
% males	83	72	55	48	41	32

Here are descriptive statistics for these data:

	M	*s*	**Skewness (*SE*)**	**Kurtosis (*SE*)**
Temperature	28.6667	3.8152	−.166 (.845)	−1.322 (1.741)
% males	55.1667	17.5444	.452 (.845)	−1.061 (1.741)

Step 3: *Harry*

The third step in the six-step Tom-and-Harry procedure is to state the *hypotheses* that are being investigated. This introduces us to some new terminology, specifically the null hypothesis and the alternative hypothesis, the hypotheses that are tested in null hypothesis significance testing. These hypotheses are theories about how the world is set up, and they are written to be all-inclusive and mutually exclusive.

What does all-inclusive and mutually exclusive mean? "All-inclusive" means that the two hypotheses cover all the possible options. "Mutually exclusive" means that only one of them can be true. For example, if you and I were looking at a paint chip and trying to determine the color, I might think it is black and you might think that it is white; and those two hypotheses would not be all-inclusive since it is possible that the paint chip could be navy blue, or ecru, or any of hundreds of other colors. But, if I said it was black and you said it was "not black," then our hypotheses would be all-inclusive. In addition, they would be mutually exclusive since both cannot be true. In fact, if one is false, the other has to be true.

Let's get back to statistics. The first hypothesis, what is called the **null hypothesis,** is abbreviated as H_0 (pronounced "H sub oh") and the second, what is called the **alternative hypothesis** is abbreviated either as H_1 (pronounced "H sub one") or as H_A (pronounced "H sub A").* Thanks to the rule that our hypotheses are all-inclusive and mutually exclusive, if H_0 is true, H_1 can't be true; similarly, if H_1 is true, H_0 can't be true.

This stuff is a little confusing, so stick with me on faith for a while. The alternative hypothesis (H_1 or H_A, though I prefer, and will use, H_1) usually represents the way we think the world is set up—our true belief or the prediction made by a theory.[†] In the height–foot size example that we've been working with, my belief is that there is a relationship between height and foot size, that height and foot size are correlated. So, I would assign H_1 to that hypothesis. And the statistician's way of saying that is to write:

$$H_1: \rho xy \neq 0$$

Now, what is ρ_{xy} and why are we saying that it is not equal to zero? Just as we use M to refer to a sample mean and μ to refer to a population mean, we use r to refer to a correlation coefficient for a *sample* and the Greek letter ρ (the Greek equivalent of r, spelled "rho," and pronounced "row" as in "row, row, row your boat") to refer to a correlation coefficient for a *population*. And we add the subscript "*xy*" to indicate that we are talking about the *population* value for the correlation between the two variables, *X* and *Y*. So, the alternative hypothesis is that we believe the relationship between the two variables in the population is different from zero. It doesn't say how different from zero, it just says that ρ_{xy} is not exactly zero.

We haven't talked yet about the values that a Pearson r can take, and it is time to do so. When we calculate a Pearson r, we end up with a single number that represents the degree of linear relationship between two variables. This single number, the Pearson r coefficient we calculate, is a summary number. It has the objective of capturing the *overall* degree of

---

*You might have guessed this from the context, but the "oh" in H_0 is the number zero, not the letter o.

[†]It is true more often than not that the alternative hypothesis reflects our true belief. But, there are occasions where a researcher wants to support the null hypothesis. For example, rather than doing a difference test to show that two groups have different means, a researcher may want to show that two groups don't differ in order to make the point that they are equivalent. In such a situation, these tests are called equivalence tests. If you want to learn more, see Cribbie, Gruman, and Arpin-Cribbie (2004). (Cribbie, R.A., Gruman, J.A., & Arpin-Cribbie, C.A. [2004]. Recommendations for applying tests of equivalence. *Journal of Clinical Psychology*, 60(1), 1-10.)

LOOKING CLOSER

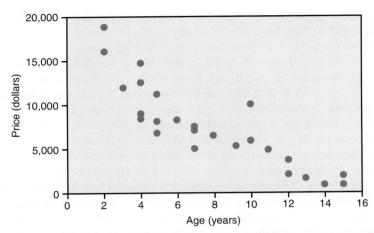

Figure **7.8** Example of an inverse (or negative) relationship between age of cars and price of cars.

linear relationship between the two variables. As a summary number the Pearson r will almost certainly only imperfectly capture the linear relationship, just as your GPA, a summary number, captures your academic performance by smoothing out details.

If there is no linear relationship between the variables, then r is zero. Let me say that again: an r of zero indicates that there is no linear relationship, no correlation, between two variables. If there is a *direct* linear relationship, which means that bigger values of X are associated with bigger values of Y, then the value of r is positive. An example of a direct or a positive relationship was shown in Figure 7.3 where, *in general*, as the age of a car increased, so did the mileage. If there is an *inverse* linear relationship, which means that bigger values of X are associated with smaller values of r, then the value of r is negative. An example of an inverse or negative relationship is shown in Figure 7.8; *in general*, as the age of a car increases, its value decreases. Note that the data points in Figure 7.8 roughly form a straight line as they did in Figure 7.3, but the slope of the line is different. Inverse relationships are sloped down and to the right, whereas direct relationships have a slope that is up and to the right.

The values that r can take may be positive or negative, but they are constrained: r can only range from -1.00 to $+1.00$. The further r moves from zero, in either a positive or a negative direction, the stronger the linear relationship between X and Y. A value of $+1.00$ indicates a perfect, direct, linear relationship between X and Y. If you graph $r = 1.00$ on a scatterplot, it will show as a straight line moving up and to the right at a 45-degree angle. This is called a **perfect linear relationship** because, as

---

perfect linear relationship

A relationship which, when graphed as a scatterplot, falls along a straight line ascending or descending to the right at a 45-degree angle; values of Y can be exactly predicted from values of X.

all points fall on a straight line, if a case's score on one axis (X or Y) is known, then the score on the other axis (Y or X) can be exactly—perfectly—predicted. A value of −1.00 indicates a perfect, inverse, linear relationship, and all points fall on a straight, diagonal line moving down and to the right.

The closer $|r|$ is to zero, the weaker the linear relationship between the two variables.* An r value of zero indicates that there is no linear relationship between the scores on the two variables. This means that knowing a case's standing on one variable gives us no information about its standing on the other variable. So, when for H_1 we say that $\rho_{xy} \neq 0$, we mean that we believe that the population value of the correlation is different from zero, that there is some linear relationship between X and Y.

I said earlier that the null and the alternative hypotheses have to be all-inclusive and mutually exclusive. So if the alternative hypothesis says that there is some linear relationship between X and Y, then the null hypothesis has to say that there is no linear relationship. Since the value of a correlation coefficient is zero when there is no linear relationship between two variables, this is how we phrase the null hypothesis: H_0: $\rho_{xy} = 0$.[†]

Now, it may seem odd that the alternative hypothesis is what we really believe. And it will probably seem odder when I mention that we generate the null hypothesis just so that we will have a chance to knock it down. Because we make the hypotheses mutually exclusive, if we show that one isn't likely true, then it is likely that the other is true. If we show that the null hypothesis is not tenable, we'll be forced to accept the alternative as more likely true. If we disprove what we don't really believe, we'll be forced to accept what we really believe as the truth.

To understand this, it helps to think about Martians. Suppose that I believe Martians exist and are walking around on the earth right now. Let's call my belief that Martians exist a "hypothesis" and, since it's really what I believe, let's call it the "alternative hypothesis." Since the null hypothesis has to be mutually exclusive of the alternative, the null hypothesis is that Martians do not exist. When statisticians write hypotheses they put the null first, so our hypotheses look like this:

H_0: No Martians exist

H_1: Martians exist

I'm going to assume that you are a rational, intelligent person and you believe the null hypothesis, that there is no such thing as a Martian. Unfortunately, there is no way to prove that.

---

*I trust you haven't forgotten that those upright bars bracketing a value indicate the absolute value, the positive value, of a number. Hence, $|-3| = 3$ and $|4| = 4$.

[†]And, yes, this means that ρ_{xy} is exactly equal to zero. If $\rho_{xy} = 0.000001$ then the null hypothesis, technically, is not true.

LOOKING CLOSER

Philosophers and logicians point out that it is impossible to prove a negative, to prove the absence of something. No matter how much you tell me that you've looked for Martians and been unable to find one, I'll tell you that they exist, that you just haven't been looking for them in the right places. All the evidence you present ("I found no Martians in New Haven, New Rochelle, New York, New Delhi, or New Zealand") might *support* the null, but it won't prove it, since I'll retort that you've neglected to look in New Jersey, New Mexico, or Papua New Guinea.

Though a negative can't be proved, it *can* be disproved. And it can be disproved by a single instance. Suppose that one day I walk in carrying a Martian, wouldn't that serve to disprove the null hypothesis that no Martians exist? The null and the alternative are mutually exclusive, and we agreed earlier that if one isn't true, then the other must be. So, if we have made the null hypothesis untenable—or as statisticians say, *rejected* it—then we must accept the alternative. In this case, rejecting the null means accepting the alternative and concluding that Martians do exist.

Understanding that one can't prove a negative is important, so let me give you a real-life example. When a pregnant woman has an ultrasound to determine the gender of her fetus, the ultrasonographer looks for something very specific, a penis. Armed with the fact that boys have penises and girls don't, the ultrasonographer uses hypothesis testing to determine the fetus' gender. Specifically, the null hypothesis is that there is no penis (i.e., fetus is a girl), and the alternative is that there is a penis (i.e., the fetus is a boy):

H_0: No penis present (girl)
H_1: Penis present (male)

So, if the ultrasonographer sees a penis, it disproves the null hypothesis. As a result, the ultrasonographer rejects the null hypothesis and informs the parents-to-be that the fetus is a boy. But, what conclusion does the ultrasonographer draw if he or she does not see a penis? Does that prove that there was no penis, that the fetus is a girl? Remember, we can't prove a negative, we can't prove the absence of a penis. Thus, it is possible that the fetus is a boy but had his limbs arranged in such a way that his penis wasn't visible. It's also possible that the fetus is a girl and thus has no penis to be seen. The absence of a penis is not conclusive. It does not call into question the null hypothesis that the fetus is a girl, but neither does it prove it. Thus, if no penis is visualized, the ultrasonographer tells the parents-to-be that the fetus *may* be a girl, but that he or she isn't sure. Do not confuse a failure to reject the null hypothesis with proving the null hypothesis!*

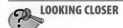 **LOOKING CLOSER**

*By the bye, isn't it possible that what appears to be a penis, on ultrasound, actually isn't? Might not a female fetus have her limbs arranged in some awkward way so that it looks like a penis is there? In such an instance, the ultrasonographer would conclude that a penis had been visualized, would reject the null hypothesis, and would inform the parents-to-be that they are having a boy. And that would be the wrong conclusion. So, be aware that the null can be incorrectly rejected, leading to an erroneous conclusion.

Let's move from gender back to statistics and think about the hypotheses for our correlation:

$$H_0: \rho_{xy} = 0$$
$$H_1: \rho_{xy} \neq 0$$

Our null hypothesis is a negative, that there is no relationship; and we just saw that one can't prove a negative. However, a negative can be disproved! (Or at least we can find evidence inconsistent with it.) If we manage to call into question the null then we are forced to conclude, as we really believed all along, that the alternative hypothesis is probably true, that there is a relationship between the two variables. If we fail to reject the null hypothesis, however, we can't say that we have proved the null. The best we can say is that there is not sufficient evidence for it to be rejected.

To understand this, let's think about the American legal system and a defendant who has been accused of some crime. The prosecution tries to prove that the defendant is guilty, and then the jury deliberates and returns a verdict of either "guilty" or "not guilty." Note that the verdict choices are not "guilty" vs. "*innocent,*" but "guilty" vs. "*not guilty.*" If the prosecution has not done an adequate job of proving guilt beyond a reasonable doubt, then they have failed, and the defendant is found not guilty. This does not mean that the defendant is innocent, only that the prosecution did not do a sufficient job of proving guilt. We might *interpret* this not-guilty verdict as meaning that the defendant is innocent, but that was not the verdict.* The difference between the results and our interpretation of the results is subtle, but important.

So, in statistics, how do we decide which of the two hypotheses we think is true? By assuming that the null hypothesis is true and using a sampling distribution!

Let's go back to our height–foot size example and think this through. The null hypothesis, $\rho_{xy} = 0$, says that in the population of college students there is no relationship between height and foot size. If this is true, and we draw a random sample from the population, what should we expect to find as our r for the sample? We would expect to find r_{xy}, a correlation for the sample, to be near zero. Would we expect it to be exactly zero? No. Why? Just as we found random samples of M&M's that had a larger or smaller percentage of reds than the expected value of 20%, we would expect that random sampling error could easily lead us to having obtained a sample in which $r_{xy} \neq 0$. It should be *close to* zero, but we won't be surprised if it is not *exactly* zero.

Suppose that H_0 were true, and we drew random sample after random sample from the population. Each time we drew a sample we calculated r_{xy} for that sample. What we would be generating, then, is a sampling distribution of r_{xy}s. We would expect that this sampling distribution

---

*Want examples of not guilty verdicts that many people didn't believe indicated innocence? Think OJ Simpson and Michael Jackson.

LOOKING CLOSER

should be centered around the value of zero, and, if the N for each sample were large enough, we would expect the sampling distribution to be normally distributed.* We could also calculate the standard deviation of the sampling distribution, what is called a standard error. And, assuming that the sampling distribution is normally distributed, we should expect that 95% of the correlations in the sampling distribution would fall within 1.96 standard errors of the center of the sampling distribution, that is within 1.96 standard errors of the hypothesized mean of zero.

This should be putting you in mind of how we used confidence intervals for hypothesis testing in the last chapter. Suppose we had a sampling distribution centered around the presumed population value of $\rho = 0$. If we could compare the observed correlation between X and Y for our actual cases—$r_{observed}$—to the sampling distribution of r_{xy}, we would find either that the observed correlation fell within the confines of the 95% interval around zero, or it didn't. If $r_{observed}$ fell within the 95% interval around zero, there would be no reason to question the null hypothesis that $\rho_{xy} = 0$. That is, if the null hypothesis were true, then sampling error would be a credible explanation for why our observed correlation fell as far away from the hypothesized value of zero as it did. But, if r_{xy} didn't fall within the confines of the 95% interval around the mean for the sampling distribution, then we would say, as we did earlier with confidence intervals, that we don't think it likely that this observed statistic came from the population that generated the sampling distribution. Thus, if $|r_{xy}|$ is at or beyond 1.96 standard errors away from the hypothesized mean correlation of zero, we will decide to reject the null hypothesis and be forced to conclude that the alternative hypothesis ($\rho_{xy} \neq 0$) is probably true.[†]

We will use this logic time and time again in null hypothesis significance testing. Over years and years of teaching statistics I've managed to boil it down to 23 words:

> *If something happens that could happen, but should happen only rarely if the null hypothesis is true, then we reject the null hypothesis.*

To help this make sense, here's a concrete example. Imagine a population of 1,500 cases with a random value for X and a random value for Y assigned to each case.[‡] Since both X and Y are random values, knowing a case's score on X gives no information about the case's score on Y. In other words, in this population X and Y are uncorrelated, so $\rho_{xy} = 0$.

Figure 7.9 shows the scatterplot of the values of X and Y for all 1,500 cases in the population. Note the square shape of this graph, indicating

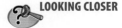
LOOKING CLOSER

*In the example we are working with here our sample size is six and this is not large enough for us to count on a normal distribution.

[†] Note the word "probably."

[‡] The random values assigned have four decimal places and range from .0000 to 1.0000.

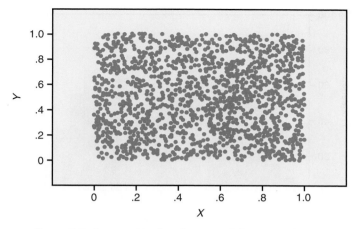

Figure **7.9** Scatterplot showing $\rho_{xy} = 0$ for a population.

that there is no relation between X and Y.* Since for any given X (or Y), the Y (or X) values range over the whole gamut of available options, knowing a case's X value gives no information about its Y value and knowing a case's Y value gives no information about its X value. Hence $\rho_{xy} = 0$.

Don't worry that you don't know how to calculate Pearson r yet; I do. So, 1,000 times I've drawn a random sample of six cases from this population, and each time I've calculated r_{xy}. We would expect that the distribution of these r_{xy}s will be centered around the population value of ρ_{xy} (.00) and will spread out both above and below this value. (Remember, values for the Pearson r can range from -1.00 to $+1.00$.) Figure 7.10 illustrates the sampling distribution for these 1,000 r_{xy}s.

Note several things about this distribution of Pearson rs. First, as expected it is centered around a value of zero. (In fact the mean of the 1,000 r_{xy}s is .0150, very close to zero.) Second, though the size of each sample is six, which is not large, this distribution does have a vaguely normal shape. Finally, let's notice one more thing: even though $\rho_{xy} = 0$, most of the calculated r_{xy}s are not zero. In fact they range from $-.98$ to $+.97$, with quite a few of them very far away from zero. Random error—sampling error—has led to a distribution of r_{xy}s where many of them are not zero, even though each sample comes from a population where $\rho_{xy} = 0$. How can we use this to decide between our two hypotheses?

---

*Most statisticians describe the scatterplot for a zero correlation as having the shape of a circle and they are right if both variables are normally distributed. But, I've always liked a rectangle as a descriptor for the shape of the scatterplot for a zero correlation since they clearly show the lack of prediction that is seen when $\rho = 0$.

LOOKING CLOSER

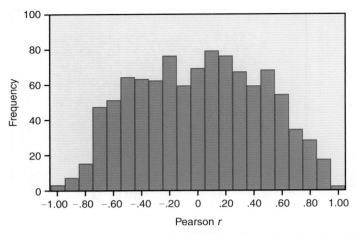

Figure **7.10** Sampling distribution of Pearson *rs* calculated for 1,000 samples of size *N* = 6 from a population in which $\rho_{xy} = 0$.

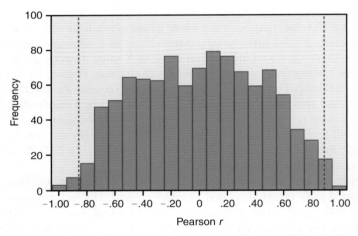

Figure **7.11** 95% confidence interval constructed for sampling distribution of Pearson *rs* calculated for 1,000 samples of size *N* = 6 from a population in which $\rho_{xy} = 0$.

If the null hypothesis ($\rho_{xy} = 0$) were true, as it is here, then we would find a sampling distribution like we did in Figure 7.10. This sampling distribution has a mean (.0150) and a standard deviation (.4475) that we could use to construct a 95% interval. If we did so, it would range from −.86 to .89, and if we drew vertical lines to demarcate it, the 95% interval would look like what is shown in Figure 7.11.*

LOOKING CLOSER

*The confidence interval is not symmetric around zero because the mean was not exactly zero.

If the observed value of the statistic, r, falls within the limits of the interval centered around the hypothesized value of the statistic based on the null hypothesis, then there is no reason to question that it could have come from a random sample drawn from the population that generated the sampling distribution. That last sentence is important (and dense), so read it again. Then, carefully read the next paragraph where I apply the idea.

Following that logic in the present scenario, if I draw a sample of size six, calculate the Pearson r for it, and find that it falls in the interval from $-.86$ to $.89$, there is no reason for me to doubt that $\rho_{xy} = 0$. However, what if I find the correlation for a sample to be, for example, $.93$? That falls beyond the critical values of the 95% confidence interval, and thus it appears unlikely that the sample that generated this r came from a population where $\rho_{xy} = 0$.

There have been a lot of threads that I've been playing out, so let me gather them all together and try to weave them into a coherent explanation of how we use the two mutually exclusive hypotheses to decide if there is a relationship between two variables.

Remember, our real belief is that there is a relationship between X and Y, and we would like to show this. However, we assume the opposite is true: the null hypothesis is true and there is no relationship—in short, that $\rho_{xy} = 0$. Then we make a model of the world that would be true if the null hypothesis *were* true, the *expected* distribution of r_{xy} (see Figure 7.10), and we compare the *observed* correlation, $r_{observed}$, to this expected distribution. If the observed correlation falls in the range where we think it should fall if the null hypothesis is true, then there is no reason to question the null hypothesis. But, if the observed correlation is a result that we think unlikely to occur if the null hypothesis is true—if it falls outside the interval—then we question, *or reject*, the null hypothesis and are forced to conclude that the alternative hypothesis is more likely true.*

This stuff is tricky, so let me use a new example both to help you think about it and to lead us into some new territory. Suppose I pull a coin from my pocket, show you that it has both a "head" and a "tail," and ask you to decide whether it is a fair coin.†

You must decide whether the coin is fair based solely on information from flipping the coin. So, I flip the coin once, and it turns up heads. I turn to you and ask whether the coin is fair. How do you decide? By using hypothesis testing, of course: by comparing what you observe to what you would expect if the coin were fair.

---

*At the same time, of course, we are aware that we may be in error in rejecting the null hypothesis, because sometimes random sampling generates an odd sample.

†A fair coin is defined as one where there is an equal chance, when it is flipped, of turning up heads or tails. In other words the probability of it landing heads equals the probability of landing tails. Statisticians would write this as $p(\text{heads}) = p(\text{tails}) = .50$, where p stands for probability. Thus, every time I toss the coin it has a 50% chance of turning up heads, and it has a 100% chance of turning up either heads or tails.

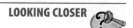

LOOKING CLOSER

What is our null hypothesis here? It is that the coin is fair. Because the alternative hypothesis has to be mutually exclusive, the alternative hypothesis is that the coin is not fair.* The two hypotheses are:

$$H_0: \text{Coin} = \text{fair (or } p(\text{heads}) = .50)$$
$$H_1: \text{Coin} \neq \text{fair (or } p(\text{heads}) \neq .50)$$

We will proceed by flipping the coin time after time, and after each flip we'll stop, tally up the number of heads that have occurred, and compare it to the number that we would expect if the coin were fair. If the observed result is consistent with the expected result, we'll have no reason to reject the null hypothesis. As statisticians say in this situation, we'll have failed to reject the null.[†] However, if the observed results are inconsistent with the expected results, we'll have reason to reject the null hypothesis and to conclude that the coin is not fair. Got it? (Remember the first chapter, where I said that statistics was about comparing the observed to the expected!)

The coin is flipped once and turns up heads. Is it possible for a fair coin, if tossed once, to turn up heads? Absolutely! In fact, we would expect a fair coin to turn up heads half of the time. And thus, so far, we are getting results that are consistent with our expected results based on the null hypothesis being true.

I flip it again and it turns up heads again. My guess is that you think it perfectly likely that a fair coin would turn up heads twice in a row, that so far there is no reason to question this coin's fairness. And, I would agree with you. However, statisticians like to be a bit more exact, and like to calculate the probability of an outcome occurring.

In this situation there are four possible outcomes for a fair coin that has been tossed twice, and these are shown in Table 7.3. One of these four possible outcomes is two heads in a row, so the probability of two heads in a row is one out of four or .25. There's a 25% chance that a fair coin will turn up heads twice in a row. (There is also a 25% chance of two tails in a row and a 50% chance of one heads and one tails.)

I toss the coin a third time, and once again it turns up heads. Are you starting to get a little suspicious about this coin? Table 7.4 shows that it is possible for a fair coin to turn up heads 3 times in a row. In fact, this should occur once in every 8 times that a fair coin is tossed. Or, as a

TABLE **7.3**   **Potential Outcomes for Two Tosses of a Fair Coin**

First Toss	Second Toss
H	**H**
H	T
T	H
T	T

TABLE **7.4**   **Potential Outcomes for Three Tosses of a Fair Coin**

First Toss	Second Toss	Third Toss
H	**H**	**H**
H	H	T
H	T	H
H	T	T
T	H	H
T	H	T
T	T	H
T	T	T

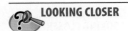

LOOKING CLOSER

*Why is our null hypothesis the proposition that the coin is fair? Well, a fair coin leads to a clear belief about the probability of heads, $p(\text{heads}) = .50$. The hypothesis that the coin is not fair leads to a whole slew of possibilities for the probability of heads. Maybe $p(\text{heads}) = .49$, or maybe .48, or .47 or .46 or .51 or .52 or— well, you get the idea. Since we will use the null hypothesis to make a model of the world, to derive expected results if it is true, we prefer a null hypothesis that yields only one model.

[†] Remember, failing to reject the null is not the same as proving the null.

statistician would say, the probability of three heads in a row is .125.* Is this a result that is unexpected enough for us to reject the null hypothesis?

How rare must an observed event be for us to say it is rare enough that we don't think sampling error could account for it? That's a topic for the next step in Tom-and-Harry, but I'll give you the short answer here. Statisticians most commonly use the 5% rule: if something happens that should happen less than 5% of the time if the null hypothesis is true, then they call it a "rare event" and reject the null hypothesis.

Given that, even if I toss the coin a fourth time and it turns up heads yet again, it wouldn't be considered an unusual observed outcome because that outcome could happen 6.25% of the time with a fair coin. However, if my coin turns up heads again on the fifth toss, then we've stepped over the line into what I call the "rare zone" since this event happens with a fair coin only 3.125% of the time, less than 5% of the time.

So, if I toss a coin 5 times and each time it turns up heads, you should, thinking like a statistician, conclude that the coin is not fair: something happened that should happen only rarely if the coin were fair.

But, and here is a problem, there is no guarantee that this is the correct decision. Isn't it *possible*, not probable but possible, that a fair coin could turn up heads 5 times in a row? We know that this happens a little more often than 3% of the time. So, if we conclude that the coin is unfair we might be in error.[†]

And, there is no way ever to be sure that we have made the right decision, even if we toss the coin time after time after time and it turns up heads every one of those times. Because isn't it *possible*, not very likely but possible, for a fair coin to turn up heads 10, 20, or even 30 times in a row?[‡]

So, let's think about the ways that we might make a right decision and ways that we might make a wrong decision. In this example there are two options for reality: either the coin is fair, or it is unfair. And, there are two options for the decision that we make about the coin: either we conclude it is fair, or we conclude that it is unfair. The matrix in Table 7.5 shows the four ways that reality and our decision can intersect.

---

*This type of probability is called a conjunctional probability as in the conjunction, or co-occurrence, of several events. This case is the conjunction of a heads on the first toss with a heads on the second toss, with a heads on the third toss. Conjunctional probabilities are calculated by multiplying together the probabilities of the individual events; in this case, .5 × .5 × .5 = .125. If you want to know more about probability I have a great book to recommend: *The Architecture of Chance*, by Richard Lowry. He was a professor of mine when I was an undergraduate. (Lowry, R. [1989]. *The architecture of chance: an introduction to the logic and arithmetic of probability*. New York: Oxford University Press.)

[†]Remember Aristotle: It is the nature of probability that improbable things happen.

[‡]A fair coin should turn up heads 10 times in a row .10% of the time, 20 times in a row .0001% of the time, and 30 times in a row .0000001% of the time. Not *likely* outcomes, but *possible* outcomes. (If all 7 billion people in the world tossed coins 30 times in a row, seven of them should get 30 heads in a row.)

LOOKING CLOSER

TABLE **7.5**   **Reality Options vs. Conclusion Options for Coin Toss Example**

	Coin really is fair	Coin really is unfair
	A	B
We conclude coin is fair	Correct decision	Incorrect decision
	C	D
We conclude coin is unfair	Incorrect decision	Correct decision

There are two ways that we can make a correct decision. If the coin really is a fair coin, and we toss it several times yielding the expected mix of heads and tails, then we'll end up making the correct decision that the coin is fair (Cell A). Similarly, if the coin really is unfair, we toss it several times, and it comes up with too many heads or too many tails, we'll end up—correctly—concluding that the coin is unfair (Cell D).

However, there are also two ways that sampling error can lead us to an erroneous decision. Let's start with the one we've been talking about: the coin really is fair, we toss it several times and, owing to sampling error, we get a bad sample, a sample that has more heads (or tails) than we would expect for a fair coin. We obtain a rare outcome and then, incorrectly, conclude that the coin is unfair (Cell C). That's one way we can make an incorrect decision.

The other way also relies on obtaining a bad sample. Imagine that the coin is unfair, that it is weighted so that it turns up heads about 75% of the time. We toss the coin several times and get a nonrepresentative sample, one that has a more even split between heads and tails than the coin was weighted to give. As a result we observe an outcome similar to what we'd expect for a fair coin, and we conclude, erroneously, that the coin is fair (Cell B).

Let's move from this specific example of a coin toss back to a more general example involving the null and alternative hypotheses, and let's give the two errors names. Statisticians, cleverly, have named the two errors "Type I" and "Type II."

Table 7.6 shows how Type I and Type II errors relate to our decision about the null hypothesis. **Type I error** occurs when the null hypothesis is really true (e.g., there is no relationship between height and foot size, or the coin is fair) and we conclude that it is not true. The name that statisticians give to the probability that Type I error will occur is "alpha," and they use the lowercase version of the Greek letter alpha, α, to symbolize it. As we shall shortly see, statisticians "set" α; that is, they decide in advance of doing the statistical test how willing they are to make the mistake of erroneously rejecting the null hypothesis.

The probability of making a **Type II error** is called "beta" and is symbolized by a lowercase version of the Greek letter beta, β. A Type II error occurs when the null hypothesis is really false (there is a relationship

TABLE 7.6   **Reality Options vs. Conclusion Options for Null Hypothesis Significance Testing**

	H_0 really is true	H_0 really is false
We conclude H_0 is probably true	**A** We correctly fail to reject H_0	**B** *Type II error* We accept H_0 when we should reject it $(p = \beta)$
We conclude H_0 is probably false	**C** *Type I error* We reject H_0 when we should fail to reject it $(p = \alpha)$	**D** We correctly reject H_0

between height and footsize or the coin is unfair) but we conclude that it is true. This has changed in the past few years, but for many years statisticians were less concerned about making a Type II error than they were about making a Type I error. The probability of a Type II error wasn't set in advance, as is done with alpha, but was calculated after the fact. Nowadays, it has become more common to set beta in advance.

When you do a statistical test it is possible to make only one of these errors. If you reject the null hypothesis, you must be concerned that you may have made a Type I error. If you fail to reject the null, you must be concerned that you may have made a Type II error.

Either of these errors can have serious ramifications because you won't know that you've made the error. Even if alpha and beta are set to be low, these errors can occur.

What are the ramifications of a correct decision or of a Type I or Type II error? Imagine that I am doing a study where I want to examine the dose-response relationship between a cholesterol-lowering drug and cholesterol level. My expectation is that more of the drug leads to a greater reduction in cholesterol level, that there is a relationship between dose and response. The null hypothesis (H_0: $\rho_{xy} = 0$) is that there is no linear relationship, and the alternative hypothesis (H_1: $\rho_{xy} \neq 0$) is that there is a linear relationship.

Cell A in Table 7.6 represents the correct decision to fail to reject (i.e., to accept) the null hypothesis. If it is true that there is no relationship between drug dose and treatment response and we conclude this, then we won't be prescribing this medicine for people with high cholesterol since it has no impact on cholesterol level. This is a good decision on a number of grounds: instead of giving people a useless treatment we shall, I hope, be directing them to a more effective treatment. And people won't be wasting money or having false expectations for this drug.

Cell D represents another correct decision: rejecting the null hypothesis and concluding that the drug works in reducing cholesterol level when it really does. As a result, we'll have another weapon in our armamentarium of ways to improve people's health. If we prescribe this drug for someone, it should be effective in helping him or her reduce serum cholesterol.

Cells B and C represent Type II and Type I errors respectively, and both errors have serious consequences. One error is not more serious than the other, in my opinion. Cell B, Type II error, means that we would conclude that the treatment is ineffective when it really is effective. What are the consequences of this? Well, we would end up withholding this effective treatment from people with elevated cholesterol levels. If there were no other effective treatments available, or if a person could not tolerate the existing treatments, the ramifications of this could be quite serious. How great a risk do you want to have for making this error? Are you willing to run a 20% risk of making it? 10%? 5%? 1%? .1%?

Type I error, cell C, could lead to just as serious consequences. If Type I error occurred, we would conclude that the treatment was effective, though it wasn't. As a result, we would start prescribing this medication for people with high cholesterol levels. These people would have false expectations for treatment, would be spending money on an ineffective treatment, and most seriously, would be using an ineffective treatment rather than another, effective treatment. How great a risk do you want to have for making this error? Are you willing to run a 20% risk of making it? 10%? 5%? 1%? .1%?

Having spent many pages exploring the hypotheses statisticians use, we are ready to turn to the next Tom-and-Harry step, the decision rules that statisticians use. But, before we do so let me review the material on hypotheses by going over our study of whether there is a relationship between height and foot size. Remember, we are using a Pearson product moment correlation coefficient because we are examining the relationship between two ratio-level variables. Even though we violated one of the assumptions for the Pearson r, that our sample is a random sample, that assumption is a robust one and we can proceed.

Our hypotheses, written in symbolic notation, are the following:

$$H_0: \rho_{xy} = 0$$
$$H_1: \rho_{xy} \neq 0$$

Here is what the hypotheses mean in English:

1. The null hypothesis says that even though there is no linear relationship between height and foot size in the population, when we draw our sample and calculate the correlation for it, the observed correlation will not be exactly zero. The observed correlation, however, should be close enough to zero that the discrepancy from zero can be explained by sampling error.
2. The alternative hypothesis says that in the population there is a linear relationship between foot size and height and that the observed correlation in our sample will reflect this. In other words, the discrepancy

between the observed correlation and the expected population value of zero is too great for sampling error to be a tenable explanation. Rather, the observed correlation is an accurate reflection of the nonzero linear relationship that exists in the population.

Group Practice 7.3

For each of the following scenarios, assume that no assumptions for the Pearson r have been violated. Then, (a) state both the null and alternative hypotheses in symbolic notation and in English, and (b) describe the population to which the results can be generalized. Why worry about the population to which results can be generalized? Remember, we're using Pearson r as an inferential statistic, so we need to think about the population to which we can generalize the results. Researchers often don't provide many details about how their samples were obtained, so you are going to need to use your common sense to answer this question.

1. A psychology researcher believes that physical similarity predicts marital success. That is, she believes that couples with similar levels of physical attractiveness are more likely to have successful relationships. To test this she obtains wedding photos from a large sample of couples and has them rated for the physical attractiveness of the bride and the groom. She constructs an interval-level physical dissimilarity scale that ranges from zero (bride and groom are equally attractive) to 10 (one is much more attractive than other). She then waits 10 years, finds each couple, and ascertains whether they are still married. If a couple is divorced, she finds out how long the marriage lasted. Thus marital longevity, which can range from 0 to 10 years, is her measure of marital success. In her sample she examines the relationship between scores on the physical dissimilarity scale and marital longevity.

2. A pediatric nurse practitioner has a theory that parental anxiety predicts how likely it is that a parent will bring a child in for a nonnecessary visit to the primary care provider. (A nonnecessary visit is one where there turns out to be no medical problem requiring attention.) To eliminate the concern that inexperienced parents are more likely to have nonnecessary visits, he decides to focus on second children. At the child's first visit, he administers an anxiety questionnaire to the parent. Then, over the next 2 years, he tracks the number of nonnecessary visits for each child so that he can calculate the percentage of visits that are nonnecessary.

Step 4: Despise

The fourth step in "Tom and Harry despise crabby infants," my six-step procedure for conducting a null hypothesis significance test, involves the *decision rule* that we will use to decide whether to reject the null hypothesis. Two subdecisions determine the decision rule, decisions about alpha (the significance level) and about whether one is doing a one- or a two-tailed test. This step is also a good time to think about whether a sample size is adequate, whether it gives you enough "power" to have a reasonable chance to be able to reject the null hypothesis if it should be rejected.*

---

*My discussion of sample size and power will wait until the next chapter. But, to foreshadow, power is the probability that one will correctly reject the null hypothesis (which is what we usually want to do) and it is calculated as $1 - \beta$, where β = the probability of making a Type II error.

LOOKING CLOSER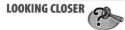

As you should remember, α represents the probability of making a Type I error and is something that researchers decide on, or set, in advance. Your willingness to make a Type I error should be determined by how serious the consequences of that error are. If you are doing a dose-response study where the drug under investigation has damaging side effects, then a Type I error will lead to prescribing an ineffective drug with serious side effects, and you would want to avoid this error. But there are situations where the costs of a Type I error aren't as serious. If we find in our sample a relationship between drinking eight glasses of water a day and decreased risk of getting the flu, and there really is no such relationship in the population, no great harm will be caused by people's increased water consumption.

You may think that we should always want to avoid a Type I error, and that is true. It is always better to avoid errors. However, there is a cost to avoiding Type I error: increasing the likelihood of a Type II error. If we make it less likely that we'll incorrectly reject the null, we make it more likely that we'll erroneously fail to reject it.

When looking at the linear relationship between height and foot size, the ramifications don't appear to be too great if we conclude that there is a relationship between the two when there really isn't. Though I still don't want to make a Type I error, I am not going to be obsessively concerned about making one.

In this instance I will follow statistical tradition and say that I am willing to make a Type I error 5% of the time. That is, I'm willing to live with 19-to-1 odds: I expect that if I were to do this study 20 times I would make a Type I error once and end up concluding that a relationship exists when it does not. If I do the study only once, as I am doing here, there is a chance, a 5% chance, that the current study is the one in which I lose on that 19-to-1 bet.

Statisticians, of course, never use English when they can find some more obscure way of saying something. So, rather than saying that they are willing to make a Type I error 5% of the time, they say either (a) that they have set α at .05 (or $\alpha = .05$), or (b) that $p < .05$, meaning that the probability of a Type I error is less than .05.*

Setting α at .05 is a convention in statistics, and I am not sure how it started, but $\alpha = .05$ is arbitrary. There is no reason other than tradition that an α level of .04, or .06, or .09 can't be used. There are two other α levels commonly used. Researchers who are more concerned about making a Type I error will likely set α at .01, allowing a 1% chance of making a Type I error. Those who are very worried about making a Type I error will set α at .001 in order to have only a .1% chance of making a Type I error. These alpha levels are commonly used, but they are just as arbitrary as the .05 level.

LOOKING CLOSER   *Yes, I agree. They should say $p \le .05$, not $p < .05$. But, the tradition is to say $p < .05$.

After all that we've discussed about the arbitrary nature of the alpha levels and choosing an alpha level based on the consequences of a Type I error, I would like to simplify your introduction to statistics. Thus, for now, simply adopt $p < .05$ as your decision rule. To paraphrase Nancy Reagan, "Just say .05." And when someone, like me, asks why you have set α at .05, say that you have chosen $\alpha = .05$ because you are willing to run the risk of making a Type I error 5% of the time.

After deciding on the alpha level, you need to choose between a one-tailed and a two-tailed test. To understand the difference, let's look at the alternative hypothesis. The alternative hypothesis usually represents how we think the world is really set up and the null hypothesis is the antithesis. Therefore, if we can reject the null hypothesis, we are forced to accept the alternative. To do this, we build a sampling distribution of the test statistic based on the null hypothesis being true.

In our scenario involving the linear relationship between height and foot size, the hypotheses are the following:

$$H_0: \rho_{xy} = 0$$
$$H_1: \rho_{xy} \neq 0$$

The alternative hypothesis claims a relationship between height and foot size, but it doesn't take a stand on the *direction* of the relationship. If the relationship were either a direct one (taller people have longer feet) or if it were an inverse one (shorter people have longer feet), the alternative hypothesis would be true. Statisticians call this a *nondirectional* hypothesis.

Now, just moments ago we decided to set α at .05. So, we need to mark off 5% of the sampling distribution of r as the rare zone. (The *rare zone* is the part of the sampling distribution that will lead to our rejecting the null hypothesis if $r_{observed}$ falls within it. I call the remaining area the *common zone* since it is the area where the observed r should commonly fall if the null hypothesis is true.) Since our hypothesis is nondirectional, we are going to split that 5% into two equal parts and put 2.5% in each end, or *tail*, of the distribution. Thus, a nondirectional hypothesis is a *two-tailed* test.

In Figure 7.12, I take the correlations that I calculated for the 1,000 repeated, random samples of size $N = 6$ from my population where $\rho_{xy} = 0$, and I've marked off the bottom 25 and the top 25 correlations, putting 2.5% of the correlations in each of the tails.

We use a two-tailed test when we have a nondirectional hypothesis, but let's be honest. Do you really think it is likely that there is an inverse relationship between height and foot size? That is, do you think it possible that, in general, short people have longer feet than tall people? I'm pretty sure that if a linear relationship exists between height and foot size, it is a direct one—that tall people have longer feet than short people. In symbolic notation, the alternative hypothesis would be $\rho_{xy} > 0$, since correlations have positive values when there are direct relationships.

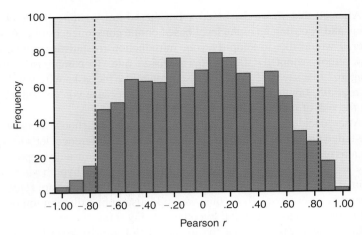

Figure **7.12** Two-tailed distribution of the extreme 5% of 1,000 correlations in a sampling distribution of r_p.

What impact does this have on the null hypothesis? Since the null is mutually exclusive from the alternative, and because the two have to cover all the options, the null would become $\rho_{xy} \leq 0$. Here are the two hypotheses:

$$H_0: \rho_{xy} \leq 0$$
$$H_1: \rho_{xy} > 0$$

Given these *directional* hypotheses, when would I reject the null? Only when the observed correlation falls in the rare zone. However, the rare zone, all 5% of it, is located *only* in the upper end of the sampling distribution, only in *one tail* of it. Thus, I am conducting a one-tailed test. In Figure 7.13, I show the 1,000 correlations in my sampling distribution, with a vertical line indicating the spot that separates the top 50 correlations from the lower 950.

Look carefully at these two figures. Notice that the vertical line at the top of the one-tailed distribution is at a different position than the vertical line at the top of the two-tailed distribution. In the two-tailed version, the top 2.5% of scores are greater than or equal to an *r* of .83, whereas in the one-tailed version the top 5% of scores are greater than or equal to an *r* of .74. And this makes sense: a 5% bite out of a distribution should be bigger than a 2.5% bite.

There are important ramifications to this. It means that if you are doing a one-tailed test and your alternative hypothesis is correct, it is *easier* to reject the null. If our observed correlation between *X* and *Y* is .75, that falls in the rare zone for the one-tailed test but not for

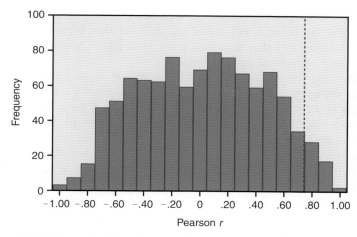

Figure **7.13** One-tailed distribution of the extreme 5% of 1,000 correlations in a sampling distribution of r_p.

the two-tailed test. Thus, there are occasions where we would reject the null hypothesis for a one-tailed test, but wouldn't if we were doing a two-tailed test.

Having a larger rare zone—doing a one-tailed test—sounds like a good thing, no? Shouldn't we always do a one-tailed test? You should use a one-tailed test if you have a reason to believe, *in advance of doing your study*, that there is a specific direction to the relationship. Why might you believe this in advance? Perhaps prior research has indicated a direction to the relationship, or perhaps the theory surrounding your variables suggests a direction.

However, here is what you cannot do: you cannot start out doing a two-tailed test, calculate your correlation, find out that the correlation falls into the rare zone–no man's land between a one-tailed and a two-tailed test, and *then* say, "Oh, I'm going to do a one-tailed test now because I will be able to reject the null." Statisticians view that as cheating.

Why not always do a one-tailed test? Because there is a downside to a one-tailed test. Suppose, given the scenario I've outlined above, we calculate the correlation coefficient and find it to be −.85, indicating a strong inverse relationship between height and foot size. With a one-tailed test, we can only reject the null if our *r* is positive. Thus we'd be forced to fail to reject the null hypothesis and would have no evidence to conclude that there is a linear relationship between the two variables. With a two-tailed test, however, we'd be able to reject the null and conclude that there appears to be an inverse linear relationship between our two variables.

Statisticians, almost without thought, set α at .05 and choose to use a nondirectional, two-tailed test. This isn't always wise, but for now, with you just starting out in statistics, I want you to follow suit. When asked why you are doing a two-tailed test, respond that because you have nondirectional hypotheses, you are using a two-tailed alpha level. (By the bye, this is also called a two-tailed *p* value.)

The next part of Step 4 involves figuring out the critical value of *r*. Now, you might think that we would need to construct a sampling distribution of *r* for repeated, random samples of size *N* from a population where $\rho = 0$. And, conceptually, you are right. Luckily, though, someone has already done the hard work and has figured out the rare zone cutoff points for different α levels, both one- and two-tailed, for different sample sizes. Before we examine such a table, let's take a look at the sampling distributions of r for sample sizes of 6, 25, and 100.

Note, in Figure 7.14, that as *N* increases the sampling distribution becomes more compact and more peaked, that the values of *r* cluster closer to zero. There are two reasons it makes sense that the distribution of *r* gets more compact and more peaked. First, as sample size increases, each sample provides a better estimate of the population value. Thus when $\rho = 0$, larger samples are more likely to yield correlation coefficients closer to zero. In addition, think back to the formula for the standard error of the mean: $\sigma_M = \dfrac{\sigma}{\sqrt{N}}$. As *N* gets larger, the standard error of the mean—the standard deviation of the sampling distribution of the mean—gets smaller. In other words, when the sample size is larger there is less variability in the sampling distribution of the mean. Ditto for the sampling distribution of *r*. As sample size gets larger, the rare zone cutoff point creeps closer to a value of zero, because there is less dispersion from the value of zero for the correlations.

Appendix Table 4 shows the **critical values of *r***, r_{cv}, for Pearson product moment correlation coefficients for different sample sizes, different alpha levels, and one- or two-tailed tests. What is a critical value? It is the point in a sampling distribution that marks off the rare zone, the cutoff point for rejecting the null hypothesis. Our rule is that if the calculated value of $|r|$ is greater than or equal to r_{cv}, it falls in the rare zone and we reject the null hypothesis.

Table 7.7 is a selection from Appendix Table 4. Let's take a few moments to orient ourselves to this table.

First, note that this is called a table of *critical values* for *r* for the Pearson product moment correlation coefficient. Thus, the values in the body of the table are r_{cv}s, the critical values that represent the cutoff point for the rare zones for Pearson *r*s. If the absolute value of *r* that we calculate, $r_{observed}$, is greater than or equal to r_{cv}, then it falls in the rare zone and we will reject the null hypothesis.

Each row in the table represents a different sample size. Again, statisticians never use a common word when they can find something more confusing, so in this instance the first column is labeled *df*, which stands for degrees of freedom. For Pearson *r*s, *df* is calculated as *N* – 2, as the sample size minus two. Because the smallest number of cases on

---

critical value of r

The point in a sampling distribution of *r*s that separates the rare zone from the common zone; abbreviated r_{cv}; if $|r_{observed}| \geq r_{cv}$, reject H_0.

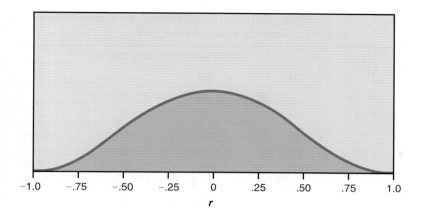

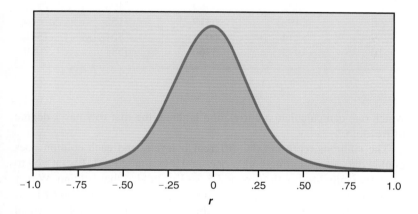

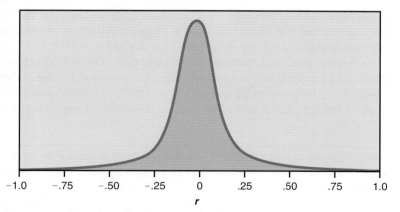

Figure **7.14** Sampling distributions of r_p for *N*s of 6, 25, and 100. (Redrawn from sampling distributions from "Concepts and Applications of Inferential Statistics" by Richard Lowry, http://faculty.vassar.edu/lowry/webtext.html.)

TABLE **7.7**   **Section of Appendix Table 4: Critical Values of *r* for Pearson Product Moment Correlation Coefficients When $\rho_{xy} = 0$**

	LEVEL OF SIGNIFICANCE, ONE-TAILED TEST			
	.05	.025	.01	.005
	LEVEL OF SIGNIFICANCE, TWO-TAILED TEST			
df = N − 2	.10	.05	.02	.01
1	.9877	**.9969**	.9995	.9999
2	.9000	**.9500**	.9800	.9900
3	.8054	**.8783**	.9343	.9587
4	.7293	**.8114**	.8822	.9172
5	.6694	**.7545**	.8329	.8745
6	.6215	**.7067**	.7887	.8343
7	.5822	**.6664**	.7498	.7977
8	.5493	**.6319**	.7155	.7646
9	.5214	**.6021**	.6851	.7348
10	.4973	**.5760**	.6581	.7079

which one can calculate a correlation is three, the first row has 1 degree of freedom.*

The columns represent the different α levels, and each column does double duty, representing both a one- and a two-tailed test. I want you to use a two-tailed test with α set at .05, so I've bolded that column. With 1 degree of freedom and a two-tailed test with $\alpha = .05$, $r_{cv} = .9969$ with α set at .05. This means that r_{xy} falls in the rare zone if it is less than or equal to −.9969 or greater than or equal to +.9969. Since *r* ranges from −1.00 to +1.00, a correlation must be very near perfect for it to be significant if $df = 1$. Note that as *df* increases, as *N* increases, r_{cv} decreases. Thus, by the time one reaches $df = 10$, the rare zone for a two-tailed test has moved to less than or equal to −.5760 and greater than or equal to +.5760.

As I mentioned, each column does double duty. The bolded column represents the critical values for a two-tailed test with $\alpha = .05$, but it also represents r_{cv} for a one-tailed test with $\alpha = .025$. This makes sense since an alpha level of .025 is half of .05, and so the upper (or lower) tail of a

---

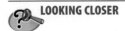 **LOOKING CLOSER**

*Want a way to think of degrees of freedom? Think of *df* as indicating how much of the sample is undetermined. Imagine a sample of three people with a mean weight of 125 pounds. If I don't tell you any more, then you can't determine the weights of any of the people. If I tell you the weight of one person, you still don't know the weights of the other two. But, if I tell you the weights of two people, then the weight of the third person can be calculated. If the first two people each weigh 150 pounds, for a total of 300 pounds, then the third person has to weigh 75 pounds so that the average is 125. Thus, there are two degrees of freedom in this example.

two-tailed test at $\alpha = x$ is equivalent to the critical value for a one-tailed test at $\alpha = x/2$.

Oh yes, and what should we do if the correlation has a negative value? Well, like the normal distribution, the sampling distribution is symmetric and is centered around a value of zero, so the same percentage of the distribution falls in the rare zone *below* a negative correlation as in the rare zone *above* a positive correlation. This means that, as long as we are doing a two-tailed test, we can ignore the sign of the correlation, either by treating $r_{observed}$ as a positive number or by treating r_{cv} as a negative number. If, for example, we have 6 degrees of freedom and calculate $r = -.75$, we will reject the null hypothesis, since $r_{observed}$ $(-.75)$ falls below r_{cv} of $-.7067$.

Let's explore the table for a bit. If $N = 10$, r_{cv} at the .05 level, two-tailed, = _____ .*

If $N = 10$ and I am doing a two-tailed test at the .05 level, is $r_{xy} = .60$ in the rare zone? How about an r of $-.63$? Of .6319? Of $-.67$?†

I trust that it makes sense that as N gets larger (i.e., as df increases), r_{cv} gets smaller—gets closer to zero. Remember, the sampling distributions in Figure 7.14: if $\rho_{xy} = 0$ and we have a large sample, the sample statistic will provide a better estimate of the population value (i.e., sampling error will play less of a role), and we should get an r that is very close to ρ. The largest df I've ever found in a table of r_{cv} is 10,000; when $N = 10,002$ $r_{cv} = .0196$! Yes, that's right. If your N is over 10,000 and you observe a correlation as small as .02 in your sample, you can reject the null hypothesis and conclude that the correlation is statistically different from zero. (This should make you think about the difference between statistical and practical significance, a topic I'm saving for the next chapter.)

It makes sense, I hope, that r_{cv} decreases as N increases. Let's now go across the columns and see what happens to r_{cv} as the α level decreases. Let's focus on two-tailed tests and look at the bottom row ($df = 10$) of the partial table in Table 7.7. Note that as we move from left to right and the α level gets smaller, moving from .10 to .01, that the r_{cv} gets larger, gets further away from zero. Phrased differently, the rare zone gets smaller as α decreases and, as a result, it gets harder to reject the null hypothesis. This should make sense, since the rare zone should be larger when $\alpha = .10$ and there is a 10% chance of making a Type I error, compared to when $\alpha = .01$ and there is only a 1% chance of making a Type I error. When we are less willing to make a Type I error—to reject H_0 by mistake—the rare zone should be smaller so that it is harder to reject the null.

I do need to mention what to do if there is no row with your degrees of freedom in the table of critical values. For example, the table in the appendix goes up one df at a time to 50 degrees of freedom ($r_{cv} = .2732$ for $\alpha = .05$, two-tailed) and then jumps to $df = 55$ ($r_{cv} = .2606$). What

---

*Since $df = N - 2$, the answer is .6319.

† No. No. Yes. Yes.

LOOKING CLOSER

should you do if your $df = 53$? Well, you have four options. The first, and the best, is to go and find a more detailed table.* Failing that, there are three more options. One is that you could interpolate, say that 53 is 60% of the way between 50 and 55 and then add 60% of the difference between the two critical values to the lower critical value. This is not a great idea since, like z scores, critical values are not spread evenly through an interval. Thus there is a chance that you could calculate a critical value that is lower than the real critical value, resulting in rejecting the null erroneously. For the same reason the next option doesn't make sense, that is, using the smaller critical value—the one with the larger degrees of freedom—as the critical value. If you can't find a more detailed table, use the final option: use the more extreme critical value associated with the *smaller* degrees of freedom. Statisticians are a very conservative lot, and they want to make it as unlikely as possible that they mistakenly reject the null hypothesis. By selecting $r_{cv} = .2732$ for $df = 50$ instead of $r_{cv} = .2609$ for $df = 55$, we make it harder to reject the null hypothesis and make the chance of a Type I error less likely.

We've already covered all parts of the decision rule of Step 5, but let me formalize for you how the decision rule works depending on whether $|r_{xy}| \geq r_{cv}$ or $|r_{xy}| < r_{cv}$.

If $|r_{xy}| \geq r_{cv}$, then we shall follow this course:

1. Reject the null hypothesis and be forced to accept the alternative hypothesis.
2. Say that the correlation between X and Y in the sample is statistically different from zero, and conclude that there is probably a nonzero linear relationship between the two variables in the population.
3. Write the results as r $(df) = .xx$, $p < \alpha$ (In place of df you would put the actual degrees of freedom, in place of $.xx$ you would put the actual calculated correlation [not r_{cv}!], and in place of α you would put the actual alpha level that you had decided on. Thus your results might look something looking like: r $(17) = .67$, $p < .05$.)[†]

LOOKING CLOSER

*Far and away the most detailed table I've ever found is by Alan Sockloff and John Edney of Temple University. Their table has critical values of r up to 1,000 by ones and then it quickly skips up to 10,000. Their table, "Some extensions of Student's t and Pearson's r central distribution," was published as Technical Report 72-5 by Temple University's Measurement and Research Center in 1972. I've been encouraging the Measurement and Research Center to post it on their website, so go there and check: http://www.temple.edu/marc/ If it is not there, complain to them about its absence and help in my campaign to get it posted.

[†]This format is called APA format, after the style manual published by the American Psychological Association in which it appears (of which the most recent version, the fifth edition, was published in 2001). You'll be pleased to know that you can ignore my rounding rules when reporting the value of a correlation in APA format since the APA requests that values of test statistics be reported only to two decimal places. Thus, when calculating a Pearson r, you only need to calculate it to four decimal places so you can end up rounding it to two.

4. Worry about the possibility of having made a Type I error.*

What does $p < \alpha$ mean, as shown in point 3 above? Well, let's assume that we have set α at .05, so $p < \alpha$ is written as $p < .05$. This means that the results fall in the rare zone—that a result occurred that should happen less than 5% of the time when the null hypothesis is true. So, when $p < .05$, we reject H_0.

If $|r_{xy}| < r_{cv}$, then we do the following:

1. Say that we have failed to reject the null hypothesis. (Remember, never say that you have proven the null.)
2. Say that the correlation, in the sample, between the two variables is not statistically different from zero. As a result, we don't have sufficient evidence to conclude that there is a nonzero linear relationship between X and Y in the population.
3. Write the results in APA format as $r\,(df) = .\text{xx}, p > \alpha$, or as $r\,(df) = .\text{xx}$, ns where .xx = the observed r and where the ns stands for not significant. (For example, $r\,(23) = .04, p > .05$ or $r(23) = .04, ns$.) This means that the correlation is a common one—that it happens more than 5% of the time when the null hypothesis is correct—so there is no reason to question the null hypothesis.
4. Worry about the possibility that we've made a Type II error.[†]

I've just introduced American Psychological Association (APA) format, the most common way that results of statistical tests are reported. APA format will return for other statistical tests in subsequent chapters, so you might as well start getting used to it. APA format may seem like a code, but it simply requires that you provide four bits of information:

1. What test was done? (In this case, r.)
2. How many cases were there? (In this case, df gives us that value as long as one knows that the degrees of freedom for a Pearson r equals $N - 2$.)
3. What was the *observed value* (NOT the critical value) of the test statistic?
4. Was the null hypothesis rejected? That is, was $p < .05$ (rejected) or was $p > .05$ (not rejected)?

Except for the final part of the fourth step of Tom-and-Harry, worrying about whether our sample size is adequate, we're done with the "*d*espise" stage (perhaps an aptly named one). You'll be happy to hear that I am going to leave worrying about sample size until the next chapter when we learn in detail about β, the probability of Type II error. But, before we move on to actually calculating an r, let's do Step 4 for the height–foot size data set.

The $df = 4$ because $N = 6$. I set α at .05 because I am willing to make a Type I error 5% of the time. I am doing a two-tailed test because I do not

---

*Remember that earlier I had said that we would need to worry only about one of the two possible errors at a time? If we reject the null, we need to worry about Type I error.

[†] And, if we fail to reject the null, we only need to worry about having made a Type II error.

LOOKING CLOSER

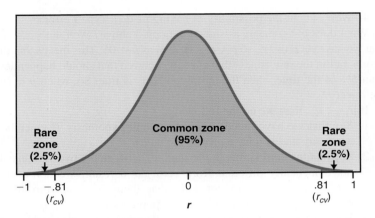

Figure **7.15** Sampling distribution of *r* for *N* = 6, *α* = .05, two-tailed, with common and rare zones indicated.

have a directional hypothesis. Given this, my r_{cv} = .8114. If $|r_{xy}| \geq$ .8114, then I shall report $p <$ .05, reject the null hypothesis, say that the correlation is statistically different from zero, conclude that there is probably a nonzero linear relationship between height and foot size in the population, and worry about having made a Type I error. If $|r_{xy}| <$ .8114, then I shall fail to reject the null hypothesis, report $p >$ .05, say that the correlation is not statistically different from zero, say that there is not sufficient evidence to conclude that there is a linear relationship between height and foot size, and worry about having made a Type II error.

The decision rule is easier to understand if you see it graphically. In Figure 7.15, I am approximating the sampling distribution of *r* by drawing a normal distribution. I've marked the midpoint, where *r* = .00, and the upper and lower limits, where *r* = −1.00 and +1.00. I've also marked −.8114 and .8114, the critical values of *r* for a two-tailed test when *df* = 4 and *α* = .05. The middle part of the distribution is labeled as the *common zone,* and the two tails of the distribution are labeled as *rare zones.* The common zone, the middle part of the sampling distribution, comprises 95% of the area under the curve, which leaves 5% of the area under the curve falling in the two rare zones.

If the null hypothesis is true, if there is no correlation between height and foot size, then the curve in Figure 7.15 is an approximation of the sampling distribution of *r*. That is, if ρ_{xy} = 0 and we draw repeated, random samples of size six from the population, the observed correlation between *X* and *Y* will fall in the common zone 95% of the time and will fall in the rare zone only 5% of the time. The logic of hypothesis testing says that if something happens that could happen, but should happen only rarely if the null hypothesis is true, then we reject the null hypothesis. Thus, if the observed correlation falls in the rare zone we call it a rare event, an event unlikely to happen by chance if the null hypothesis is true,

TABLE **7.8** Implications of and Differences between $|r_{xy}| \geq r_{cv}$ and $|r| < r_{cv}$ with $\alpha = .05$, Two-Tailed

	$|r_{xy}| \geq r_{cv}$	$|r_{xy}| < r_{cv}$
Where the observed r falls	Rare zone	Common zone
Statement about H_0	It is rejected	Failed to reject it
Statement about H_1	Forced to accept it	Failed to support it
Error to be concerned about	Type I	Type II
Probability of that error	.05 (α)	To be determined (β)
Report probability of results occurring if H_0 is true as	$p < .05$	$p > .05$
The correlation is called...	...statistically different from zero (statistically significant)	...not statistically different from zero (not statistically significant)
Conclusion about linear relationship that exists between X and Y in the population	A linear relationship probably exists	Not sufficient evidence that a linear relationship exists*

*Though, technically this is the correct conclusion, most statisticians make statements like, "The results were not statistically significant and so there appears to be no linear relationship between X and Y." But, that is the *interpretation* of the results, a topic for the next chapter.

and we reject the null hypothesis. (The $p < .05$ that we write in APA format when we reject the null hypothesis is a shorthand way of saying, "This result is rare, it happens less than 5% of the time when H_0 is true." The $p > .05$ that we write in APA format when we fail to reject H_0 is shorthand for, "This result is common, it happens 5% of the time or more, when H_0 is true.")

Believe it or not, we are ready to do the calculations. However, to help keep all this decision rule information straight, Table 7.8 highlights the differences between when the observed r falls in the rare and the common zone of the sampling distribution.

Group Practice 7.4

1. Buffy plans to calculate a Pearson r for a study with 24 cases. She is using a two-tailed test with α set at .05. Draw a sampling distribution of r, and use r_{cv} to label the rare and common zones. What is her decision rule? Be sure to mention concerns about Type I and Type II error.

2. Skip plans to calculate a Pearson r for a study with 18 cases. He is using a two-tailed test with α set at .01. Draw a sampling distribution of r, and use r_{cv}

to label the rare and common zones. What is his decision rule? Be sure to mention concerns about Type I and Type II error.

3. Desdemona also plans to calculate a Pearson r. She has 76 subjects and is using a two-tailed test with α set at .05. Draw a sampling distribution of r, and use r_{cv} to label the rare and common zones. What is her decision rule? Be sure to mention concerns about Type I and Type II error.

Step 5: Crabby

After all the lead in-to *calculating* a Pearson product moment correlation coefficient, I'm afraid that the actual calculations are going to be anti-climactic. The formula is short and the calculations aren't too difficult; they just involve a bit of tedium and require attention to detail.

For most statistics there are two types of formulae: definitional formulae and calculating formulae. A definitional formula explains, or defines, what is being calculated. A calculating formula has been algebraically rearranged so that it still leads to the right answer, but is easier to use.

You probably won't be too surprised to learn that I prefer definitional formulae since they give additional insight into what the statistic is doing. So, here is the formula that I want you to master for calculating a Pearson *r*.*

F O R M U L A

Pearson Product Moment Correlation Coefficient (r_p)

Equation 7.1

$$r_p = \frac{\Sigma(z_x z_y)}{N}$$

Where:
r_p = the Pearson product moment correlation coefficient being calculated
z_x = an *X* score converted to a *z* score
z_y = a *Y* score converted to a *z* score
N = the number of cases (i.e., the number of pairs of scores)

This is a definitional formula, so let's pause for a moment and think about what the formula does. We have a group of *N* cases, and for each case we have its values on two variables, *X* and *Y*. We take all the *X* values, find M_x and s_x, and use these to convert each *X* score into a *z* score. We do the same thing, using M_y and s_y, to convert each *Y* score into a *z* score. For each case we take its pair of *z* scores, z_x and z_y, and multiply them together. These resulting numbers are called cross-products. Once we have done this for all the pairs of scores, we add up the *z* score cross-products and then, finally, divide this sum by *N*, the total number of pairs of scores we have, to yield r_p. Thus, a Pearson *r* is, simply, the average of the cross-products of the *z* scores.[†]

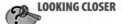 **LOOKING CLOSER**

*Once you leave this class you'll probably never again calculate a correlation by hand. Computers do the calculations faster than you and are much less likely to make a math error. So, humor me and use the definitional formula, not a calculating formula.

[†] See footnote on opposite page.

What does it mean to say that a Pearson r is the average of the z score cross-products? Think of a situation in which there is a strong, direct (i.e., positive), linear relationship between two variables. Imagine, for example, a group of children of varied ages from 1 to 10 years. Each child's height and weight have been measured. In general there is a strong, direct, linear relationship between height and weight in kids: taller kids are heavier, and shorter kids are lighter. Let's pick one kid whose height and weight are both well above average for the sample. When this kid's height and weight are converted to z scores, they'll be positive and fairly large. What happens when we multiply together two positive and large numbers? We get an even larger positive number. What would happen with a kid from this sample who is both short and light? His or her height, when converted to a z score, would be relatively far below the mean, a large, negative number. Ditto for the weight. When we multiply this child's two large, negative z scores together, we get, again, a large, *positive* number. And when we add up all these large positive numbers that are the cross-products of the z scores and take their average, we'll end up with a large and positive value for our Pearson r.

A corollary situation occurs when there is an inverse relationship between two variables, let's say, between days of excessive alcohol consumption and GPA in college students. A student who is well above average in GPA and well below average in terms of alcohol consumption will have a large, positive z score for GPA and a large, negative z score for alcohol consumption. These two large z scores multiplied together will yield a large number, but a negative one. A student with a low GPA and a high alcohol consumption will also yield a large, negative score when his or her two scores are multiplied together. Thus in this situation, the sum of the cross-products of the z scores will be large, negative numbers and the average of these, the Pearson r, will be a large negative number.

What about the situation in which there is no relationship between two variables, say between intelligence and shoe size? In this situation some very intelligent people will have very big feet, some will have average-size feet, and some will have very small feet. When you turn these into cross-products of z scores, the first group will have big positive numbers, the second group numbers near zero, and the third group large, negative numbers. When you add all these numbers together the sum will be near zero, as will be the average of the cross-products. The Pearson product moment correlation coefficient is the average of the cross-products of the z scores, and when the correlation is near zero, so is the sum of the cross-products of the z scores.

(Continued) [†]And now I can tell you why the Pearson r is called, formally, the product moment correlation coefficient. z scores are the first moment about the mean (in the section about skewness and kurtosis in Chapter 6, I talked about moments about the mean), and so r is calculated by finding the products of these moments.

LOOKING CLOSER

TABLE **7.9**   **Data for Calculating Pearson Product Moment Correlation Coefficient between Foot Size (X) and Height (Y)**

	X	Y	z_X	z_Y	$z_X z_Y$
	9.00	64.00	.0000	−.6222	.0000
	9.00	67.00	.0000	.3111	.0000
	10.00	67.00	1.2247	.3111	.3810
	8.00	62.00	−1.2247	−1.2443	1.5239
	10.00	72.00	1.2247	1.8665	2.2859
	8.00	64.00	−1.2247	−.6222	.7620
M:	9.0000	66.0000			$\Sigma = 4.9528$
s:	.8165	3.2146			

So, let's calculate r_p for our height–foot size data set. Table 7.9 displays the original data set, the scores converted to z scores, and the cross-products of the z scores.

As is shown in the table, the sum of the cross-products of the z scores is 4.9528. The mean of this, $\dfrac{4.9528}{6}$, is the Pearson r, .8255, which rounds to .83. Figure 7.16 shows that the observed value of r fell in the rare zone, that it is a rare event when H_0 is true. Following the decision rule, we find that $|.8255| \geq .8114$, that $|r_{observed}| \geq r_{cv}$, so we reject the null hypothesis, say that the linear relationship observed in the sample is statistically different from zero, and conclude that there is probably a nonzero, linear relationship between height and foot size in the population. In APA format, $r(4) = .83, p < .05$. There is a possibility we have we made a Type I error, that we have concluded there is a linear relationship between the two variables in the population when there really isn't.

Having learned how to calculate a Pearson r, it is time to turn attention to the last stage of the six-step hypothesis testing procedure, the interpretation. But, to be honest, I think that this has been enough material for one chapter, so I'm going to end here and give the final step its own chapter.

Group Practice 7.5

For each data set below, calculate the Pearson product moment correlation coefficient. Don't worry about whether any assumptions have been calculated, and don't write out the decision rule; just calculate Pearson r and report the results in APA format. Use a two-tailed test with $\alpha = .05$. For the first data set you have to calculate the mean and standard deviation yourself.

1.	**X**	96.7	103.0	97.3	102.0	98.5	100.5	99.0	99.8
	Y	.4	4.8	2.7	6.5	3.3	2.6	2.5	2.7

2.	**X**	23	21	28	23	33	17	29	*M:*24.8571	*s:* 5.0265
	Y	12	28	13	41	22	34	18	*M:*24.0000	*s:*10.0712

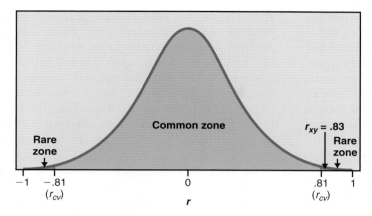

Figure **7.16** Sampling distribution of *r* for height–foot size data set showing r_{cv} and $r_{observed}$ (r_{xy}).

SUMMARY

Broadly speaking, inferential statistics can be divided into two categories, relationship tests and difference tests. Relationship tests reveal whether there is a relationship between two variables, the predictor and the criterion. Difference tests reveal whether two (or more) groups differ in their scores on a dependent variable.

The first step in conducting a null hypothesis significance test is choosing the statistical test to be used. One should base this decision on the type of question being asked (relationship or difference) and the level of measurement of the variables (categorical vs. continuous and whether nominal, ordinal, interval, or ratio). A relationship question can be addressed with one of three correlation coefficients: a Pearson product moment correlation coefficient if both variables are interval or ratio level, a Spearman rank order correlation coefficient for two ordinal-level variables (or if one is ordinal and the other interval or ratio), and a chi-square test of association for two nominal level variables. (If one variable is categorical and the other is not, then a difference test is used to answer a relationship question.)

Once the test has been chosen, evaluate whether the test can be completed. Null hypothesis significance tests should only be used if the assumptions on which they are based have not been violated. There are five assumptions for the Pearson *r*: random sample, interval- or ratio-level variables, normality, linearity,

and homoscedasticity. Some assumptions are robust (they can be violated to some degree and under some conditions), and others are not robust (they can't be violated).

If the assumptions have been met, the next step is to state the null and alternative hypotheses. The null hypothesis for the Pearson product moment correlation coefficient states that there is no linear relationship between the two variables in the population. The alternative says that there is a nonzero linear relationship in the population. Obviously, only one of these can be true. Interestingly, we usually believe that the alternative hypothesis is true. Since it is possible to disprove a negative, we set up the null to try to knock it down and be forced to accept the alternative hypothesis.

In order to decide which hypothesis to believe, we compare the observed correlation between the two variables in our sample to the expected sampling distribution of correlations that should occur if the null hypothesis is true. This sampling distribution is centered around a correlation value of zero, the value from the null hypothesis. This sampling distribution is divided into the common zone—the middle section where sampling error can explain the deviation of the observed correlation from the expected value of zero—and the rare zone, where the observed correlation value is too far away from zero for sampling error to be a likely explanation for the deviation. The common zone of the sampling distribution is separated from the rare zone by the critical value of r. If something happens that could happen, but should happen only rarely if the null hypothesis is true, then we reject the null hypothesis. In other words, if the observed value of the statistic falls in the rare zone, then it is not likely to have come from a population like the one defined by the null hypothesis and so we conclude that H_0 is probably not true.

We determine the size of the rare zone when we set the alpha level. Most commonly, alpha is set at .05 and is two-tailed, meaning that the rare zone comprises the bottom 2.5% and the top 2.5% of the sampling distribution. In this case there is a 5% chance of obtaining, owing to sampling error, a sample that has a statistically significant degree of linear relationship between the variables, even though the sample comes from a population where there is no linear relationship between the variables. Such a situation, where the null hypothesis is erroneously rejected and a relationship between the variables is mistakenly confirmed, is called a Type I

error. The corollary error, called Type II error, occurs when the observed correlation falls in the common zone but should have fallen in the rare zone. When this happens, we fail to reject the null hypothesis when we should have and conclude, erroneously, that there is no evidence that a linear relationship exists between the variables. The probability of this happening is called beta, abbreviated β; the method used to calculate beta is reserved for the next chapter.

As well as the two errors, two correct conclusions can occur. In one correct conclusion, there is no linear relationship between the variables in the population and this is the conclusion that we draw. The other correct conclusion occurs when there is a linear relationship between the two variables in the population and this is the conclusion we reach.

The final part of the chapter involved learning to calculate the value for a Pearson product moment correlation coefficient and report it in APA format. The Pearson r is calculated as the average of the cross-products of the two variables when each variable has been converted to a z score.

Review Exercises

A reminder about Review Exercises and Homework Problems: it is up to you to choose the correct statistical procedure to apply. For right now that is fairly simple: you only know how to do the Pearson product moment correlation coefficient. However, it is possible that the data I give you are not appropriate for a Pearson r. In that case, explain why the Pearson r is inappropriate and identify the appropriate test.

Go through the *first five* steps of Tom-and-Harry for questions 1 to 3. *Save your answers: you'll need them in Chapter 8!* Be sure to think through which variable is X and which is Y, and make sure that you state the hypotheses in English as well as in statistics. Unless otherwise mentioned, use a two-tailed test with α set at .05.

1. An intensive care unit (ICU) nurse in a small, community hospital is interested in seeing if the patients' health statuses when they enter the ICU predicts how long they stay there. So, she administers the APACHE III, an interval-level measure of severity of illness, to all the ICU patients

admitted in a 1-month period and then measures, in days, their ICU stays. The APACHE III is scored based on the information from the first 24 hours in the patient's chart. Scores range from 0 to 299; higher scores indicate greater severity of illness.

Here are the data:

APACHE	# ICU Days
90	1
290	12
100	3
275	14
120	8
255	9
180	7
230	9
215	5

In case you are wondering (and you should be) the skewness and kurtosis for the APACHE are −.291 and −1.631 with standard errors, respectively, of .717 and 1.4000; for the number of ICU days, skewness and kurtosis are −.072 and −.466, with the same standard errors. (SPSS was used to calculate skewness and kurtosis for both variables.)

Be sure to discuss the population to which the results can be generalized.

2. College administrators are always concerned about retention, about keeping students in school so that they can graduate. A college administrator had a theory that the first month of college determined whether a student would return for a second year of college. Specifically, she thought that the more often a student drank alcohol to excess during his or her first month of college, the less likely he or she was to make it to a second year of college. So, she obtained a random sample of first-year students at her college and, at the end of their first month, asked how many days they had drunk alcohol to excess. Scores could range from 0 (0 days of alcohol to excess) to 30 (30 days of alcohol to excess). She then waited a year to see how many of them returned for a second year of college. Scores on this variable are either 0 (did not return for a second year) or 1 (did return for a second year).

Here are the data:

Days of Alcohol	Return to School?
18	0
3	1
12	0
0	1
9	0
1	1
5	1
2	1

Here are descriptive statistics for the data:

M	s	Skewness (SE)	Kurtosis (SE)
Alcohol days			
6.2500	5.8683	1.027 (.752)	.177 (1.481)
Return to school			
.6250	.4841	−.644 (.752)	−2.240 (1.481)

To what population can the results be generalized?

3. An elementary-school gym teacher wonders about the relationship between vision and the eye-hand coordination skills necessary for athletics. He took a sample of children at his school and gave them an interval-level eye exam. The eye exam he used reported vision as a percentage of average. That is, a score of 100 means average vision, scores above 100 mean better than average, and scores below 100 mean worse than average. The highest score a person could obtain was 200; the lowest was 0. He then measured the children's eye-hand athletic coordination by tossing 50 tennis balls to each child from 15 feet away. To reduce variability owing to the toss, he used an automatic ball-tossing machine with the toss velocity set at "easy." The number of balls caught, which could range from 0 to 50, was the measure of eye-hand athletic coordination.

Here are the data:

Vision	# Caught
25	10
170	34
130	10
50	34
150	17
100	61
90	66
75	42
110	45
100	15

Here are descriptive statistics for the data:

M	s	Skewness (SE)	Kurtosis (SE)
Vision			
100.0000	41.5331	−.112 (.687)	−.218 (1.334)
# caught			
33.4000	19.3298	.355 (.687)	−1.148 (1.334)

To what population can the results be generalized?

4. You are having dinner with your parents, two reasonably intelligent people who don't know very much about statistics. Explain to them the difference between Type I and Type II error. Use the example of tossing a coin to determine if it is fair.

5. Give two examples (not ones from the book!) of variables that you think should have a positive correlation, two examples of variables that you think should be negatively correlated, and two things that you think should not be correlated.

6. In Figure 7.12, I indicate the values (−.75 and .83) associated with the extreme 5% of the 1000 Pearson rs for samples of size $N = 6$ I calculated. Do these values differ from the r_{cv} that is found in the table of critical values for Pearson r? Why?

7. A cardiovascular researcher decides that she wants to study people in the United States with low diastolic blood pressure. If she wants to have, for her sample, 50 people with diastolic blood pressures of 55 or lower, how many people must she screen to find her subjects? (In case you want to know, in the United States the mean diastolic blood pressure is 77, and $s = 11$. Let's assume that diastolic blood pressure is normally distributed.)

8. A respiratory therapist wants to examine the effect of exercise on oxygen saturation levels in blood. He obtains a group of healthy college students and has them run on a treadmill for different amounts of time. After each student has run, he measures oxygen saturation levels. In statistical notation and in English, what are his null and alternative hypotheses? To what population can he generalize his results?

9. Xerxes is doing a one-tailed Pearson r with α set at .05; he expects to find a positive correlation. He has 12 cases. What is his decision rule? Be sure to draw a sampling distribution of r, and use r_{cv} to mark off and label the rare and the common zones.

10. A public health researcher has developed a program to encourage the wearing of bicycle helmets. She gets 10 school districts and implements the program at 5 randomly selected schools. She then goes to each of the 10 school districts and measures the percentage of kids who wear helmets while riding bicycles. What test should she do to see if the program has had any impact on helmet wearing?

11. A pharmaceutical company researcher was testing a new sleep aid medication. To test it, he gave different doses of the drug (ranging in 5-mg increments from 0 to 50 mg) to a large group of people with insomnia. Each person took his or her assigned dose only 1 night. That night each person measured how long, in minutes, it took to fall asleep. The researcher wants to see if there is a relationship between the dose of drug taken and the length of time it takes to fall asleep. What statistical test should he use?

Homework Problems

1. Having violated no assumptions, I complete a Pearson product moment correlation coefficient for 19 cases and find $r = -.4555$, with $\alpha = .05$, two-tailed. Which type of error do I need to worry about?
   a. Type I
   b. Type II
   c. Both
   d. Neither
   e. Not enough information to tell
   f. Since the correlation is negative, the polarity of the error is reversed.

2. I violated no assumptions and found $r = -1.38$ for 92 cases. I used $\alpha = .05$, two-tailed. What is the best descriptor of the *linear* relationship between X and Y?
   a. It is an inverse relationship.
   b. It is a linear relationship.
   c. It is not significantly different from zero.
   d. Both (a) and (b)
   e. There was some error in calculating r.

3. If N remains constant, in which situation is it easiest to reject the null hypothesis?
   a. $\alpha = .05$, two-tailed
   b. $\alpha = .01$, two-tailed
   c. $\alpha = .05$, one-tailed
   d. $\alpha = .01$, one-tailed
   e. Not enough information to tell

4. An assumption for which the calculation of the Pearson r is not robust has been violated. The test can still be conducted if which of the following is true?
   a. $N \geq 50$
   b. $N < 50$
   c. The test shouldn't be conducted.

5. $r_{observed}$ falls in the common zone of the sampling distribution when $\alpha = .05$, two-tailed.
   a. This proves the null hypothesis.
   b. This disproves the null hypothesis.
   c. This proves the alternative hypothesis.
   d. This disproves the alternative hypothesis.
   e. None of the above
   Go through the *first five* steps of Tom-and-Harry for the next three questions. *Save your answers to these questions: you'll need them in Chapter 8!* Don't forget to think about which variable is X and which is Y. Unless otherwise mentioned, use $\alpha = .05$, two-tailed.

6. The owner of a hair salon is curious about the relationship between the amount of hair cut and the amount of money earned by the stylists. So, at the end of a day he weighs the amount of hair around the chairs of his eight stylists and tallies the amount of money, excluding tips, that they have earned. Here are the data. Be sure that you discuss the population to which these results can be generalized.

Lbs of Hair	Earnings ($)
1	170
11	185
2	150
8	165
4	125
7	130
5	100
6	110

(Using SPSS I calculated skewness [and SE] and kurtosis [and SE] for pounds of hair as .266 [.752] and −.223 [1.481]; for dollars earned they are .021 [.752] and −1.431 [1.481].)

7. A dentist is interested in the relationship between fluoride consumption and cavities. She takes a random sample of adult patients from her practice and counts how many cavities they have had in their permanent teeth. From each person she also finds the number of years he or she drank fluoridated water as a child; the maximum value is 18 years. Here are the data. Be sure to describe the population to which the results can be generalized.

Yrs Fluoride	# Cavities
0	10
18	0
0	5
18	1
0	8
18	2
2	7
12	3
3	6
11	2
7	6
9	4

Here are descriptive statistics for the data:

M	s	Skewness (SE)	Kurtosis (SE)
Yrs fluoride			
8.1667	6.9502	.264 (.637)	−1.546 (1.232)
# cavities			
4.5000	2.9011	.247 (.637)	−.748 (1.232)

8. A psychologist is interested in the relationship between machismo and anxiety. Specifically, he has a theory that men use machismo as a defense against anxiety, as a way to make themselves appear less scared than they really are. He obtains a sample of men who are about to have their blood drawn and gives each of them an interval-level measure of machismo. Scores on this test can range from 0 to 60, with higher scores indicating a greater level of machismo. He then has the man take a seat in a phlebotomy chair while the phlebotomist draws blood from the person who had been ahead of the man in line. This person is a confederate of the researcher. The phlebotomist pretends to have a lot of trouble finding a vein on this person and this person starts to scream in pain, curse the phlebotomist, and ask how long the phlebotomist has been drawing blood. The phlebotomist mentions that it is her first day on the job. Finished with the confederate, the phlebotomist then turns to the real subject on whom she measures a heart rate (the measure of

anxiety) before drawing blood. The psychologist measures heart rate rather than asking the men to tell how anxious they are, because he believes they cannot fake their heart rate whereas they could misreport their level of anxiety. The psychologist considers higher heart rates to indicate a greater level of anxiety. Here are the data for determining the relationship between machismo and anxiety. Be sure to comment on the population to which the results can be generalized.

Machismo	Heart Rate
5	88
56	95
10	72
43	52
22	98
37	75
24	72
32	57
29	85

M	*s*	Skewness (*SE*)	Kurtosis (*SE*)
Machismo			
28.6667	14.9369	.155 (.717)	−.137 (1.400)
Heart rate			
77.1111	15.0144	−.303 (.717)	−.934 (1.400)

9. Buffy and Skip both draw samples of $N = 45$ from a population where $\sigma = 10.00$. Buffy calculates a 95% confidence interval for her sample, and Skip calculates a 90% confidence interval for his sample. Buffy finds a mean of 56.52 for her sample, and Skip finds a mean of 55.98 for his sample. Whose confidence interval is wider? Why?

10. If we fail to reject the null hypothesis, why is it incorrect to say that we have proved the null?

11. A public health researcher decides to investigate if men or women are more likely to wash their hands after using a public restroom. She sends colleagues into restrooms to observe men and women and to note whether they wash their hands, coded yes or no, after using the restroom. What statistical test should she use to determine if there is a relation between gender (male or female) and hand washing (yes or no)? To what population can she generalize the results?

12. After having completed that study, the public health researcher decides that she needs to have a more detailed measure of hand washing. She constructs a hierarchy of hand washing behavior ranging from no hand washing (scored as 0), to rinsing with water (scored 1), to brief washing with soap (scored 2), to thorough washing with soap (scored 3). What statistical test should she now use to determine if there is a relationship between gender and hand washing?

13. Clothilde measured how open people were to trying new foods on a 9-point interval scale where higher scores indicate a greater willingness to try new foods. Below is an *un*grouped frequency distribution that shows what she found. What score would be associated with someone whose percentile rank score was 24?

Score	Frequency
9	3
8	5
7	7
6	10
5	8
4	7
3	6
2	4
1	2

14. Buffy is told that her systolic blood pressure is very low. In fact, as a percentile rank, her systolic blood pressure is a 7. What percentage of people have a blood pressure that is higher than hers? If systolic blood pressure is normally distributed with a mean of 125 and a standard deviation of 16, what is her blood pressure?

8

Interpreting Pearson Product Moment Correlation Coefficients

Learning Objectives

After completing this chapter, you should be able to do the following:

1. Determine whether the null hypothesis is rejected for a Pearson product moment correlation coefficient.
2. Determine and interpret the direction of a Pearson product moment correlation coefficient.

(Continued)

3 Determine the strength and meaningfulness of a Pearson product moment correlation coefficient by calculating and interpreting (a) a 95% confidence interval, (b) a coefficient of determination, or (c) a binomial effect size display.

4 Differentiate between prediction for cases in general and prediction for a specific case; calculate and interpret Y' and a 95% prediction interval for a specific case.

5 Identify which type of error may have occurred for a Pearson product moment correlation coefficient, and explain the implications of that error.

6 Calculate and interpret power and β for a Pearson product moment correlation coefficient; calculate the sample size needed to have sufficient power for a correlation coefficient.

7 Explain the difference between association (correlation) and causation.

8 Explain the impact of outliers on a correlation coefficient.

9 Write a complete interpretative statement for a Pearson product moment correlation coefficient that addresses statistical significance, direction, strength, predictive ability, limitations, and strengths.

Chapter Roadmap

In this chapter we reach a major destination: interpreting the results of a Pearson product moment correlation coefficient. Interpretation is a human endeavor and thus a subjective one. Just as people differ in how they interpret the outcome of trials (think OJ Simpson or Michael Jackson), people differ in how meaningful they find a correlation coefficient.

Interpretation involves talking about the direction of a correlation coefficient and its strength. Direction refers to whether the relationship between the two variables is direct (higher scores on X are associated with higher scores on Y), inverse (higher scores on X are associated with lower scores on Y), or zero (there is no association between the scores on the two variables). Strength can be measured a number of different ways: (a) the 95% confidence interval, the range within which we are confident that the population value, ρ, falls; (b) the coefficient of determination, how much of the variability in one variable can be predicted by knowing the other; (c) the binomial effect size display, how likely a case is to have an above average score on one variable if it has an above-average score on the other; and (d) a case's estimated score on one variable given its score on the other. This last measure of strength will show the difference between prediction for cases in general as opposed to prediction for a specific case. We'll see that a correlation that appears to be strong in general may appear weak when predicting the value for a specific case.

In this chapter we also discuss how to calculate the probability of a Type II error, which leads to an exploration of power—the probability of correctly rejecting the null hypothesis—and how many cases one needs to have a reasonable chance of achieving this.

t took me one chapter to lead you through the first five steps (what test is chosen, whether assumptions are met, null vs. alternative hypotheses, decision rule, and calculations) of my procedure for null hypothesis significance testing. Now it will take a full chapter to cover the final step, the interpretation of the results.

STEP 6, *INFANTS*

Though people may think that the purpose of statistics is calculation, they're wrong. Calculations are just a prelude to the real reason we do statistics, to *interpret* them. The objective of statistics is answering a question. And it is via the interpretation of the statistic that we calculate that we both answer the original question posed *and* explain the meaning of the answer. For example, is there a relationship between height and foot size? If so, what does the relationship mean?

Interpreting a correlation coefficient is a very human endeavor. Computers can do the calculations and spit out the results, but they can't tell us what the results mean. I liken the interpretation part of hypothesis testing to the role of a jury in a trial. In a trial, the prosecution and the defense present, and rebut, evidence. But it is the jury that decides what the evidence means.

Psychologists differentiate between sensation and perception, and this difference is helpful in understanding the difference between results and interpretation. A sensation is a physical stimulus that is *objective* and can be measured. For example, if you've ever had your hearing tested, then you were exposed to sounds of different frequencies and different intensities. But, whether you heard these stimuli or not is a question of *perception*. It is possible for two people to perceive the same stimulus quite differently, for one to think it loud and the other soft, for one to find it pleasant and the other unpleasant. Thus, perception is *subjective*.

The results of a statistical test, the statement that $r = .30$, is the objective stimulus. How it is perceived or interpreted is subjective. One person may perceive a correlation of .30 as indicating a strong and meaningful relationship between two variables, and another may perceive it as indicating a weak and trivial relationship between the variables. I don't mean to suggest that there is no such thing as an incorrect interpretation, since that is certainly not true. An interpretation can be wrong! One person may view a glass as half empty and the other may view it as half full, but they are in agreement that it contains some liquid.

My objective is that by the end of this chapter you'll be able to explain, *in plain English*, how you interpret the results of a Pearson product moment correlation coefficient, what you think the results *mean*. I want your interpretations to be comprehensible to someone who is reasonably intelligent but who doesn't have a lot of statistical savvy.

There are two parts to the interpretation of a Pearson correlation coefficient: first, a conclusion as to whether the results show a relationship that is statistically different from zero, and then an explanation of what the results mean.

The first part, whether the results are statistically significant, is far and away the easier part, especially as we've already done the work in Steps 4 and 5, when we made our decision rule and put the results in American Psychological Association (APA) format.

However, before I review the decision rule, let me remind you of what a statistically significant result means for a correlation coefficient. A correlation that is *statistically different from zero* means that we have rejected the null hypothesis and that we conclude that there is probably some nonzero relationship between the two variables *in the population*. It tells us nothing about how far away from zero the presumed nonzero relationship is, or in which direction it deviates from zero. We can infer that if we replicate the study, if we draw another sample and calculate a correlation coefficient for the new sample, we would expect the observed correlation coefficient to land in the rare zone again.

Don't forget that there is a difference between statistical significance and practical significance. If the sample size is large enough, even a trivial linear relationship is large enough to be statistically different from zero. That doesn't mean, however, that it is enough of a relationship to be meaningful, to make a difference. For example, as you'll remember from the last chapter, if one has over 10,000 cases, an *r* of .02 is statistically significant. A correlation of .02 reflects a trivial relationship between two variables, an almost zero relationship. Yet with enough cases we would conclude that it is, statistically, indicative of a nonzero relationship.

If the results are *not statistically different from zero*, it means that the observed results from this sample have fallen in the common zone—that we have failed to reject the null hypothesis. Speaking technically, if we fail to reject the null hypothesis we can only conclude that there is insufficient evidence to conclude that the observed correlation is statistically different from zero. In double negative terms, this means there is no reason to disbelieve that there is no relationship between the two variables.

Many researchers find such language cumbersome and the conclusion unsatisfying. Human nature being what it is, they end up making an interpretation that goes beyond the logic allowed by hypothesis testing, just as some perceive a "not guilty" verdict as indicating innocence. Thus, researchers often suggest (or even state explicitly), when they fail to reject the null, that the null hypothesis is supported, that the observed correlation is a zero correlation, and that it is likely that $\rho = 0$. I'll try to be pure in my interpretations, but I am also a pragmatist about the power of human nature. In some instances, when a jury says "not guilty," even I conclude that the defendant is innocent.

REJECTING THE NULL: RESULTS STATISTICALLY DIFFERENT FROM ZERO

Our decision rule had two outcomes, either rejecting or failing to reject the null hypothesis, depending on where the observed correlation fell—in the common or the rare zone—in the sampling distribution. If the absolute value of $r_{observed}$ is greater than or equal to r_{cv}, we conclude that this outcome is an unusual one if H_0 is correct and we report that the probability of this outcome occurring, if H_0 is true, is less than alpha. This is what is called a statistically significant result, which means that we reject the null hypothesis and are forced to accept the alternative hypothesis: we conclude that there is likely a nonzero relationship, in the population, between the two variables. Another way of phrasing this is to say that the linear relationship between X and Y in the sample is statistically different from zero, that the observed correlation is so large that it is unlikely that it occurred as a result of sampling error from a population where $\rho_{xy} = 0$. Hence, it is plausible that $\rho_{xy} \neq 0$. There is, of course, the risk that this conclusion is wrong.

FAILING TO REJECT THE NULL: RESULTS NOT STATISTICALLY DIFFERENT FROM ZERO

The other path for our decision rule occurs when the absolute value of $r_{observed}$ is less than r_{cv}; this means that we have failed to reject the null hypothesis, that we call our results not statistically significant. In this case we conclude that the observed correlation is a common one when the null hypothesis is true, that it is not statistically different from zero, that the fact that it is not exactly zero can be attributed to sampling error. Thus, we say that the probability of observing this outcome, if the null hypothesis is true, is greater than alpha, and we have no reason to reject the null hypothesis that $\rho_{xy} = 0$.

In the height–foot size example we've been working with, our r_{cv} was .8114 and we observed, or calculated, $r_{xy} = .8255$. Thus, we reject the null hypothesis of $\rho_{xy} = 0$ and are forced to accept the alternative hypothesis of $\rho_{xy} \neq 0$. In other words, we conclude that the correlation between X (foot size) and height (Y) in the sample is statistically different from zero and that there is a probably a nonzero, linear relationship, in the population, between these two variables. Following APA format, we write: $r(4) = .83$, $p < .05$. This is shorthand for: "With a sample size of six, we observed a correlation of .83. If the null hypothesis that $\rho_{xy} = 0$ were true, then we would observe a correlation this large very rarely, less than 5% of the time. Because the observed correlation fell in the rare zone, something that should happen only rarely if the null hypothesis is true, we reject the null hypothesis and conclude that the correlation between X and Y in the population is probably different from zero."

Suppose that our calculated correlation had been .4589, not .8255. Then we would have failed to reject the null hypothesis and would have concluded that there is not sufficient evidence to conclude that there is a nonzero linear relationship between X and Y in the population. In APA format we would have written: $r(4) = .46, p > .05$. In English, that means that we observed a correlation of .46 between height and foot size in our sample of size six. We conclude that this correlation is a common one, it occurs more than 5% of the time when $\rho_{xy} = 0$, so there is no reason to question the null hypothesis. Since the correlation is not statistically different from zero, we end up with insufficient evidence to conclude that there is a linear relationship between height and foot size in the population.*

Group Practice 8.1

For all questions, assume $\alpha = .05$, two-tailed, unless it is otherwise indicated.

Answer all of the following for each scenario:

(a) Draw an approximation of the sampling distribution for r on which you place r_{cv}, and use it to label the rare and common zones. Place r_{xy} in the sampling distribution and decide if it falls in the rare or the common zone.

(b) What is H_0? is H_0 rejected, or do we fail to reject it?

(c) Write the results in APA format. Is r_{xy} statistically different from zero?

(d) Is it reasonable to conclude that it is likely that there is, in the population, a linear relationship between X and Y? Speculate about the direction (direct, inverse, or zero) of the relationship.

(e) What type of error could have been made? In English, what does that error mean? What is the probability of that error having been made?

1. $N = 10, r_{xy} = .6100$
2. $N = 24, r_{xy} = -.4534$
3. $N = 39, r_{xy} = -.3160$
4. $N = 177, r_{xy} = .1513$

We now have a handle on whether the correlation is statistically significant, but we haven't really begun to *interpret* the correlation. Also, what we've done so far doesn't pass the intelligent-consumer test. Would an intelligent but not statistically savvy person understand if you said that you just finished conducting a study and failed to reject the null hypothesis? Let us turn to a variety of ways of making sense of a correlation coefficient. There are really two questions to address: (1) the direction of the relationship and (2) its strength. Direction is easy, but strength is hard. When we discuss the strength of a correlation we are talking about how meaningful it is, about its practical significance. On that people can disagree.

In terms of strength, first we'll build confidence intervals for our correlations so that we can get a sense of the range within which we think

---

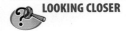

LOOKING CLOSER

*I do want to point out that you will occasionally see the abbreviation "*ns*," which is short for "not significant," used instead of $p > .05$.

ρ, the population value of the correlation, falls. After all, null hypothesis significance testing means using inferential statistics, using a sample statistic to draw some conclusions about a population parameter. Then we'll examine a number of different ways of judging the strength of the linear relationship between two correlated variables. Some methods examine prediction in general, and some examine prediction for specific cases. We'll look at two ways to examine predictive strength in general: the percentage of variance explained and the binomial effect size display. Finally, we'll examine the predictive utility of correlations for a specific case, the degree to which the correlation allows us to estimate a case's value for Y if we know its value on X.

How you interpret a correlation depends on whether it is statistically significant. For example, if we conclude that it is unlikely there is anything but a zero relationship between the two variables, we will not want to estimate a case's score on Y from its score on X. So, first I'll address interpreting correlations that are statistically different from zero. Then I'll turn to interpreting nonsignificant correlations.

INTERPRETING CORRELATIONS THAT ARE STATISTICALLY DIFFERENT FROM ZERO

DIRECTION

When we say that a correlation is statistically significant, when $p < \alpha$, we are concluding that the linear relationship between X and Y in the population is probably different from zero.* And yet, we know more than that. We know whether the correlation coefficient we calculated was positive or negative, whether the probably nonzero linear relationship is direct or inverse. So, rather than just saying that we conclude the correlation is nonzero, we can start our interpretation by making a statement about direction.

In our height–foot size example, the correlation was positive, .83, and so to say that there is a relationship between height and foot size is accurate, but it is inadequate. Better, more informative, is to say something like, "There is a positive (or direct) relationship between height and foot size that is statistically different from zero: in general, college students at Penn State Erie who have longer feet are also taller." †

---

*Don't forget that our decision is probabilistic, that there is an α level chance of being wrong when we say that we reject the null hypothesis.

†Note the use of the term "in general" in my interpretation. "In general" means that I expect that the rule won't be true in all situations. I wouldn't be shocked to meet someone who was taller than me yet had shorter feet. In general, the older the used car, the lower the price. But, I'm pretty sure that if you are selling a 1990 Rolls Royce and I am selling a 2003 Subaru, you'll be getting more for your car than I will. Exceptions to a rule *probe* the rule, they don't disprove it.

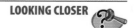 LOOKING CLOSER

If the correlation were negative, as it was when I examined the relationship between the age of used cars and their prices in Chapter 7, we would make a statement like, "There is a statistically significant inverse relationship between the age of a used car and its price. In general the older the car, the lower the price." You can see what an inverse relationship looks like in Figure 7.8 on p. 202.

That's all there is to interpreting direction: pay attention to the sign associated with the correlation, positive or negative, and then explain what it means for the association between X and Y. As values on X go up (or down), what happens to values on Y?

STRENGTH

Having addressed direction, it is now time to turn to examining the strength and the meaningfulness of the correlation, the practical significance. For this to make sense, let me spend a little time showing what correlations of different strength look like.

Figure 8.1 shows scatterplots for eight positive values of r.* Note that as the r values increase from .00 all the way up to 1.00—as the correlation coefficient gets *stronger*—that the points converge until they all fall on a diagonal line.

Let's think about the strength of these scatterplots in a predictive sense: if you know a case's value on X, how well can you predict its value on Y? If it helps, think of the predictor variable as SAT score and the criterion (predicted) variable as college GPA. Might not a college want to choose students for admission at least partly on the basis of how well they think a student will do in college?

If you look at the very last scatterplot in Figure 8.1, Panel H, where r is as strong as possible (1.00), you will note that we can perfectly predict a person's GPA if we know his or her SAT score since all the cases fall on a straight line. And if you look at the very first scatterplot, Panel A, where the correlation of zero is as weak as possible (.00), knowing a student's SAT gives no information about his or her potential GPA. Look at the other scatterplots: where, between Panel A and Panel H, would you draw the line and say that the scatterplots above this point indicate a strong and meaningful relationship between SAT and GPA?

Look at the third scatterplot, Panel C, where $r = .30$. Do you think it would help much in predicting GPA from SAT? Look at how much spread there is in Y for each X value. This does not look as if it would

---

LOOKING CLOSER

*If these were negative correlations they would have the same pattern, but the slope would be down and to the right, not up and to the left.

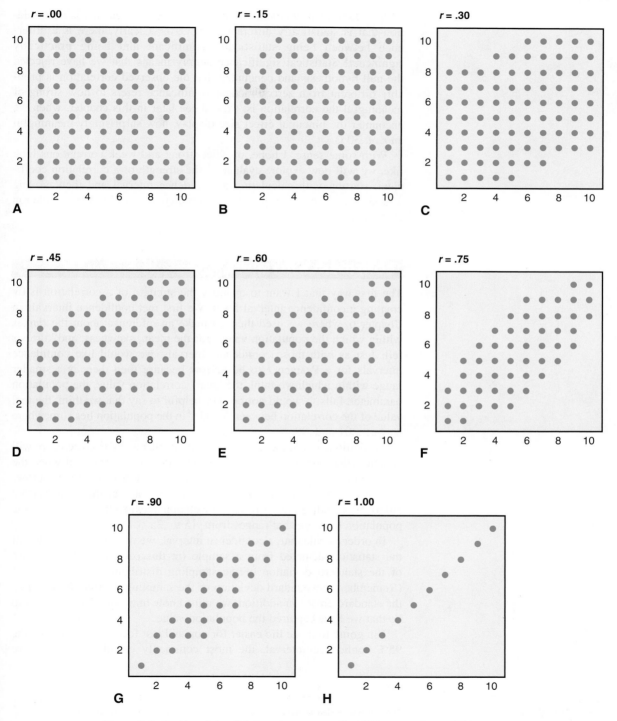

Figure **8.1** Scatterplots of data sets representing different values of Pearson *r*.

be very helpful in predicting a *Y* value for an *X*. Yet, this is a correlation that is statistically different from zero.* Clearly, there is a difference between being statistically significant and being practically significant! Statistical significance simply means that we have rejected the null hypothesis and concluded that the observed correlation is probably different from zero. Practical significance refers to how strong or meaningful the correlation is. (You'll see later in this chapter, when we encounter the binomial effect size display, how surprisingly meaningful an *r* of .30 is.)

With some sense, I hope, of what strong and weak correlations look like, we will now explore evaluating the strength of a correlation coefficient, starting with calculating a confidence interval and then moving to a number of ways to quantify the predictive capacity of a correlation coefficient.

CONFIDENCE INTERVALS

The first way that I want to quantify the strength of a correlation is by creating a confidence interval for it. We first met confidence intervals in Chapter 6, where we used them to make an inference about the ranges within which the population values for the mean, skewness, and kurtosis fell. Just as with those confidence intervals, we would like confidence intervals for a Pearson *r* to be narrow because then there is a smaller range within which we think the "real" correlation value, the population parameter, falls. It would not be very helpful to say that we think the real value of the correlation between *X* and *Y* in the population lies somewhere between .01 and .99.

In addition, as stronger correlations are further away from zero, we will conclude that our correlation is stronger and more meaningful when the lower end of the confidence interval, the end closer to zero, is further away from zero. Thus I'd view a confidence interval that ranges from .40 to .50 as indicating a stronger correlation between the variables in the population than one that ranges from .15 to .25.

In order to calculate a confidence interval, we need to have a value of the statistic calculated from a sample (in this case, *r*) and a measure of the standard deviation of the sampling distribution of the statistic. (Remember, the standard deviation of the sampling distribution is called the standard error.) In addition, we must know how confident we want to be that we have captured the population value.

I'm going to make life easier for you and just focus on calculating the 95% confidence interval, the most commonly calculated one. We've

---

LOOKING CLOSER   *The only two correlations in Figure 8.1 that aren't statistically significant are Panels A and B.

already learned to calculate r, the test statistic, so there's really only one step left, figuring out the standard error of r, which I abbreviate as s_r (pronounced "s sub r").

Unfortunately, the whole process of calculating a confidence interval turns out to be a bit more complex because the sampling distribution of r is not normally distributed. This is especially true as $|r|$ gets further away from zero. Thus we shall need to convert r to a normal distribution, calculate our confidence interval around this converted score, and then convert this new metric back to r.

We'll convert r to **Fisher's z transformation of r,** what is sometimes simply called an **r-to-z transformation.*** (The transformation back will be called a z-to-r transformation.) When discussing an r that has been transformed to a z, I'll use the abbreviation z_r (pronounced "z sub r"), differentiating it from the z score of Chapter 5.

Why do we need this r-to-z transformation? Because, as mentioned previously, the sampling distribution of r is not normally distributed, especially when r is large. And a moment's thought should convince you that this is so. Imagine a population in which $\rho = .90$. If we draw repeated, random samples from this population and calculate r each time, the rs should center around .90. But, wouldn't they be limited in terms of how much higher they could go? It would be impossible to draw a sample and find an r that is larger than 1.00. However, we could find correlations that are much smaller than .90 as a result of sampling error and, as a result, the sampling distribution will tail off to the left—it will be negatively skewed. The r-to-z transformation is a logarithmic transformation of rs into z_rs, a transformation that changes the shape of the sampling distribution to normal.

There is a formula for doing the transformation, but the convention is to provide an r-to-z table, such as Table 5 in the Appendix. A small piece of Table 5 is given in Table 8.1.

The rows in this table represent the first two decimal places of a correlation, and the columns represent the third decimal place. Our observed correlation in the height–foot size data set was .8255, which rounds to .826. Looking at the intersection of the row (.82) with the column (.006), we find that z_r is 1.175. To put this in words, an r of .826 is transformed to a z_r of 1.175. If the r had been negative ($-.826$), then the z_r would have been negative (-1.175).

Now that our r has been transformed so that it is normally distributed, we build the 95% confidence interval around it by subtracting and adding 1.96 s_r.

Fisher's z transformation of r

An r value transformed into a normally distributed z score.

---

*Why is this called Fisher's transformation? Because it was developed by Ronald Fisher, a famous statistician.

LOOKING CLOSER

TABLE **8.1**   **Part of Appendix Table 5: Fisher's transformation of *r* to *z*ᵣ**

	.000	.001	.002	.003	.004	.005	.006
.80	1.099	1.101	1.104	1.107	1.110	1.113	1.116
.81	1.127	1.130	1.133	1.136	1.139	1.142	1.145
.82	1.157	1.160	1.163	1.166	1.169	1.172	1.175
.83	1.188	1.191	1.195	1.198	1.201	1.204	1.208
.84	1.221	1.225	1.228	1.231	1.235	1.238	1.242
.85	1.256	1.260	1.263	1.267	1.271	1.274	1.278

F O R M U L A

Standard Error of the Sampling Distribution of *r* (s_r)

Equation 8.1

$$s_r = \frac{1}{\sqrt{N-3}}$$

Where:

s_r = standard error of the sampling distribution of *r* that is being calculated

N = the number of pairs of cases used in the calculation of the correlation coefficient

This formula says that the standard error for the sampling distribution of *r* is calculated as the numerator of 1 divided by the denominator of the square root of the number of cases minus 3. For the height–foot size data set, N was 6. Thus

$$s_r = \frac{1}{\sqrt{6-3}} = .5774$$

As you can see by the equation, the standard error of the sampling distribution has an inverse relationship with N: when N is small, s_r is large; and when N is large, s_r is small.

Equation 8.2 shows the formula for calculating the 95% confidence interval for z_r. Let me be clear: this formula calculates the 95% confidence interval for an *r* that has been transformed to a *z*. Thus, once we have done the calculations, we will need to transform the z_r back to an *r* value.

F O R M U L A

95% Confidence Interval for z_r

$$95\% \, CI_{z_r} = z_r \pm 1.96 s_r$$

Equation 8.2

Where:

$95\% \, CI_{z_r}$ = the 95% confidence interval for z_r that is being calculated

z_r = the r-to-z transformation of the correlation coefficient (via Appendix Table 5)

s_r = the standard error of the sampling distribution of r (via Equation 8.1)

NOTE: If you wish to calculate the 90% confidence interval, substitute 1.65 for the 1.96 in the equation. If you want to calculate the 99% confidence interval, substitute 2.58.

This formula says that the 95% confidence interval for z_r ranges from z_r minus 1.96 standard errors of the sampling distribution of r to z_r plus 1.96 standard errors of the sampling distribution of r. For the height–foot size data set, the $95\% \, CI_{z_r} = 1.175 \pm 1.96(.5774) = 1.175 \pm 1.1317$. When we do the subtraction and addition, we find that the 95% confidence interval for z_r ranges from a low of .0433 to a high of 2.3067.

Remember, though: this is the confidence interval in terms of z_r units, not in terms of r units. So, we need to convert this back to r. Just as we used a table (Appendix Table 4) to convert from r to z_r, we will use a table (Appendix Table 6) to convert from z_r to r. I have a portion of this table in Table 8.2.

In this table the rows represent the first decimal place of the z_r, and the columns represent the second decimal place. The low end of the 95% confidence interval (CI) that we calculated was .0433, and this rounds, with two decimal places, to .04. The intersection of the highlighted row

TABLE **8.2**   **Part of Appendix Table 6: Transformation of z_r to r**

	.00	.01	.02	.03	.04	.05	.06
.00	.000	.010	.020	.030	.040	.050	.060
.10	.100	.110	.119	.129	.139	.149	.159
.20	.197	.207	.217	.226	.235	.245	.254
.30	.291	.300	.310	.319	.327	.336	.345
.40	.380	.388	.397	.405	.414	.422	.430
.50	.462	.470	.478	.485	.493	.501	.508

(.00) and column (.04) yields a transformation from a z_r of .04 to an r of .040. If you look at the rest of the table in the Appendix, you'll find that the upper limit of our confidence interval converts from a z_r of 2.3067, which rounds to 2.31, to an r of .980. Thus, the 95% confidence interval for the correlation ranges, in r units, from .04 to .98.

What does this confidence interval mean? Well, remember that we started down this path as a way of examining how strong or meaningful a correlation coefficient was. So, let's see what this confidence interval tells us about the strength of the relationship between height and foot size.

We already know that the relationship is statistically significant and positive, meaning that we have concluded that the population parameter, ρ, is likely greater than zero. Consistent with this, the 95% confidence interval does not capture zero and is above zero. The 95% confidence interval tells us the range within which we think it tenable that ρ falls. The real relationship between height and foot size may be as great as .98, almost a perfect linear relationship, or it might be as low as .04, verging on a zero relationship. With a range that large, I'm not very confident that the relationship is a strong or meaningful one. As I said earlier, we like our confidence intervals to be narrow, not wide. And here, with a range from .04 to .98, it is about as wide as it can be for a correlation that is statistically different from zero.

The problem is that our N is so low. When one has a small sample from a population, sampling error is more likely to yield a sample that is not representative of the population. If our sample had been larger, say 26, then the standard error of the sampling distribution of the r would have been smaller, .21 instead of .58, yielding a narrower confidence interval, from .64 to .92. If this were the situation, I would be more comfortable in concluding that the relationship between height and foot size was a meaningful one since my projected low value for ρ was .64.

However, our N is 6, not 26. So, how do I interpret our actual results? By saying something like, "The linear relationship observed between height and foot size (r (4) = .83, $p < .05$) is statistically different from zero, suggesting that there is a positive (or direct) relationship between height and foot size among college students at Penn State Erie. It appears, in general, that college students at Penn State Erie who have longer feet are also taller. Because the sample size is so small ($N = 6$), the 95% confidence interval within which the correlation between height and foot size in the Penn State Erie population is predicted to fall is quite large, ranging from .04 to .98. Thus, based on this sample, the real relationship between height and foot size in the population, though statistically different from zero, may be very strong or quite weak. I recommend replicating this study with a larger sample size to get a better estimate of the real strength of the linear relationship. In addition, the original sample was not a random sample from the population of college students, making it difficult to generalize the results to college students in general, I recommend trying to obtain a more representative sample to increase generalizability."

Please note that the interpretation provides a platform for you to comment on the weaknesses (or strengths) of the study and to make suggestions for improving it. In this instance, I've commented both on the small sample size and the generalizability problem that I noted back in Chapter 5 when I was analyzing the assumptions for the Pearson r. By the time you get to the interpretation, you probably know the data (and their limitations) better than anyone else, so don't be shy about sharing your insights.

If the sample size for the correlation between height and foot size had been 26 instead of 6, I would have said, "The results of this study showed a direct linear relationship between foot size and height that was statistically different from zero (r (24) = .83, p < .05.) This suggests that, in general, college students at Penn State Erie who have longer feet are also taller. The 95% confidence interval within which the correlation between foot size and height likely falls in the population ranges from .64 to .92. Thus, the correlation between foot size and height seems to be strong and meaningful. However, as the sample on which these results are based was not a random sample from the population of college students, the degree to which these results can be applied to college students in general is unknown."

Remember, to consider a correlation strong the confidence interval should be narrow and relatively far from zero. Table 8.3 outlines some interpretative options for six types of confidence intervals. You'll note that I recommend replication when the confidence interval is wide. Replication, drawing a new sample and redoing the study, is a wonderful thing. If one replicates and finds the same results, that greatly increases one's faith in the original results. And, if the results of the replication turn out dramatically different—well, that's OK too. One then needs to figure out why the results are different: whether the effect is not very robust, or what the conditions are in which the effect is observed.

TABLE **8.3**   **Guidelines for Interpreting Confidence Intervals (*CIs*) for Pearson Correlations**

	CI captures zero	*CI* is near zero	*CI* is far from zero
***CI* is narrow**	Plausible that ρ is zero (e.g., *CI* ranges from −.05 to .05)	Plausible that ρ is near zero and weak, likely not a meaningful relationship (e.g., *CI* ranges from .05 to .15)	Plausible that ρ is strong and meaningful (e.g., *CI* ranges from .70 to .90)
***CI* is wide**	Provides little useful information about ρ so replication is advisable (e.g., *CI* ranges from −.55 to .55)	ρ could be weak or moderate; replication advisable (e.g., *CI* ranges from .05 to .55)	ρ likely moderate to strong, may be meaningful; replication advisable (e.g., *CI* ranges from .35 to .85)

Group Practice 8.2

1. Create a 95% confidence interval for the following: $r = .4519$, $N = 25$. Based on the confidence interval, should we reject the null hypothesis? Write the results in APA format.

2. If $r = .1634$ and $N = 29$, what is the 95% confidence interval? Based on the confidence interval, should we reject the null hypothesis? Write the results in APA format.

3. I have a sample of 77 people who had strokes, came to the hospital emergency room (ER), and received treatment. At the time of admission, I calculate how many hours elapsed from the onset

of stroke symptoms to ER admission and initiation of treatment. At the time of discharge, I administer a test that measures the degree of stroke-induced impairment. (Higher numbers on this interval-level measure indicate greater impairment.) I correlate the number of hours from symptom onset to ER admission with the degree of stroke-induced impairment and find $r = .6385$. Write a paragraph of interpretation for this correlation. (See my interpretation of the height–foot size correlation for an example of an interpretation. Be sure to comment on any strengths or weaknesses of the study.)

STRENGTH OF ASSOCIATION

So far we've examined the strength of correlations by seeing how wide and how far from zero the confidence interval is. Now, let's think about the strength of the correlation in a different way by examining how well, for cases *in general*, we can predict *Y* if we know *X*—how strong the *association* is between the two variables. There are two such approaches that we'll explore: the percentage of variance predicted approach and the binomial effect size display approach. Interestingly, they appear to give different answers as to how predictively useful a correlation is. The answers are actually the same, but one, the binomial effect size display, gives its results in a more intuitively understandable metric. Since that one makes more sense, of course I'm going to start with the percentage of variance predicted, the less intuitive one.

PERCENTAGE OF VARIANCE PREDICTED

coefficient of determination

The amount of the variability in one variable that is predicted by another variable.

The percentage of variance predicted, called the **coefficient of determination,** tells how much of the variability in *Y* can be explained by *X*.* (And since correlations are ambidextrous, the coefficient of determination also tells how much of the variability in X can be predicted by *Y*.)

A concrete example should make this easier to understand. The students at your college do not all have exactly the same GPA; that is, there is variability in GPA. In Figure 8.2, an amorphous blob (Panel A) represents the variability that exists in GPA. The area inside that blob encompasses all of the variability, 100% of it, that exists in GPA.

Now, let's think of some factors that are associated with GPA. Intelligence is one, since smarter people usually have higher GPAs, but intelligence is not the only determinant of GPA. Other factors include the

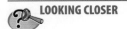

LOOKING CLOSER

*The coefficient of determination is also called "percentage of variance explained" or "percentage of variance accounted for."

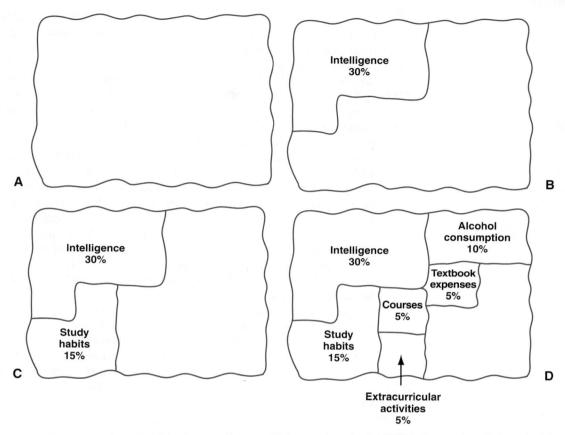

Figure **8.2** Hypothetical example demonstrating sources of variability in GPA.

difficulty of the courses taken, study habits, number of extracurricular activities, alcohol consumption, and ability to afford textbooks. Of course there are more factors and if we knew all of them we could account for all the variability that exists in GPA, but here I have only listed six factors.

Let's (arbitrarily) say that intelligence predicts/explains/accounts for 30% of the variability in GPA, as indicated in Panel B of Figure 8.2. Study habits accounts for another 15% of GPA (again, arbitrarily determined), as shown in Panel C. Finally, Panel D illustrates the other four factors, totaling 65% of the variability being explained, and 35% left unaccounted for, or unpredicted.*

---

*In real life, things aren't quite this neat. Intelligence may account for 30% of the variability in GPA, and study habits may account for 15%, but the two factors together would account for less than 45%. Why? Because they overlap, they are not independent! In general, smart people have better study habits. Thus, taken together, study habits and intelligence may account for only 40% of the variability in IQ. (And don't forget that I am just making these numbers up.)

LOOKING CLOSER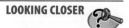

If I did a study in which I correlated measures of intelligence and GPA for a representative sample of college students, then I should find that intelligence predicts about 30% of the variability in GPA scores. I could flip this around and say that although intelligence predicts 30% of the variability in GPA, 70% of the variability in GPA is left unpredicted.

The difficulty with the coefficient of determination lies in how to interpret it. Is 30% of the variability in one variable predicted by another variable a lot? When you put it in the context of 70% remaining unexplained, it certainly doesn't sound like very much.

In actuality, predicting 30% of the variability in a variable is a heck of a lot of variability accounted for. Cohen, a respected statistician, talked about variables having small, medium, or large effects in a 1988 book. He offered these "effect sizes" as rough guides, not as hard and fast rules, so don't make too much of them. When he talked about correlations *in the social and behavioral sciences*, he said that a variable that predicts ≈1% of the variance has a small effect, one that predicts ≈10% of the variance has a medium effect, and one that predicts ≈25% has a large effect. In that context, if intelligence really did explain 30% of the variability in GPA, it would be a very large effect.*

You are probably wondering how to figure out the coefficient of determination, the percentage of variance in one variable that is predicted by the other in a Pearson product moment correlation coefficient. I've been putting it off because it is remarkably easy: you simply square the *r*. Yes, r^2, pronounced "*r* squared," tells the amount of variability in one variable (either *X* or *Y*) that is predicted by the other (either *Y* or *X*) for a Pearson *r*. Not that this needs a formula, but here it is:

F O R M U L A

Coefficient of Determination (r^2)

Equation 8.3 $r^2 = (r)^2$

Where:
r^2 = the coefficient of determination (percentage of variance predicted) that is being calculated
r = Pearson *r*

Let's work backwards from Cohen's rough guidelines for strength of an effect to figure out the level of correlation coefficient associated with small, medium, and large effects. If we know the percentage of variance

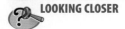
LOOKING CLOSER

*I need to stress that Cohen's examples of small, medium, and large effects of 1%, 10%, and 25% refer to research in the social and behavioral sciences and that things can be different in other disciplines like engineering or medicine.

that is predicted, we can take the square root of that value to find the correlation ($r = \sqrt{r^2}$). Thus, a correlation that predicts 1% of the variance (a small effect) is an r of about .10. A correlation that predicts 10% of the variance (a medium amount) works out to an r of about .30. Finally, a large-effect correlation, predicting about 25% of the variance, is an r of about .50. Thus, according to Cohen, in the social and behavioral sciences, a small r is $\approx$ .10, a medium r is $\approx$ .30, and a large r is $\approx$ .50. Cohen meant for these numbers to be rough guides, not cast in stone, but they have become the embodiment of the definition of small, medium, and large effect sizes and people treat them with reverence. Because these numbers are useful, here they are highlighted in Table 8.4.

Now that we know how to calculate the coefficient of determination and have some rough guidelines for interpreting them, let's move on to our second way of calculating strength of association, the binomial effect size display.

TABLE **8.4** **Cohen's guide to small, medium, and large effect sizes in the social and behavioral sciences**

Effect size	r	r^2
Small	$\approx$.10	$\approx$.01
Medium	$\approx$.30	$\approx$.10
Large	$\approx$.50	$\approx$.25

BINOMIAL EFFECT SIZE DISPLAY

The binomial effect size display, or BESD for short, is a way of translating a correlation to show how much of an effect one variable (the predictor variable or the independent variable) would have on the other (the criterion variable or the dependent variable) if both variables were binomial variables (Rosenthal and Rubin, 1982).* What does it mean for a variable to be a binomial variable? It simply means that the variable has only two categories, for example child vs. adult, healthy vs. sick, inpatient vs. outpatient. It is possible to take a continuous variable and to turn it into a binomial variable by splitting it in two. Using foot size for example, we could take our measure of foot length in inches and classify people whose foot length is below the mean as having smaller feet and those whose foot length is greater than or equal to the mean as having larger feet. In a binomial effect size display, each variable is treated as a binomial (or dichotomous) variable in order to examine how one variable affects the other. Thinking of height and foot size, for example, the question the BESD addresses may be, "How likely are people who are tall to have big feet?" And, again, I have to point out that since correlations are ambidextrous, the question the BESD addresses could also be, "How likely is it that someone who has big feet is tall?" It all depends on what you want to predict.

Let's imagine that we are interested in studying the effects of parental happiness on weight gain in premature infants. For this study we have a sample of 200 premature infants. While they are in the hospital we administer a test of parental happiness to these infants' parents. The parental happiness test measures how happy and excited the parents are

---

*Rosenthal, R., & Rubin, D. B. (1982). A simple, general-purpose display of magnitude of effect. *Journal of Educational Psychology*, 74, 166-169.

LOOKING CLOSER

	Lower weight gain	Higher weight gain	
Parents less happy with new baby	A	B	100
Parents more happy with new baby	C	D	100
	100	100	200

NOTE: I've put the predictor variable (the IV) as the row variable and the criterion variable (the DV) as the column variable.

Figure **8.3** Two-by-two matrix for parental happiness/infant weight gain data with marginal frequencies only.

by the arrival of their new baby. Higher scores indicate more excitement and happiness and lower scores indicate less excitement and happiness. (Please note: lower scores don't mean that the parents are unhappy or not excited, only that they are *less* happy or *less* excited.) During the time that the infants are in the hospital we keep track of their weight gain in grams. Obviously, higher numbers indicate a greater weight gain and, just as obviously, it is important for premature infants to gain weight.

After we have collected all our data we classify the parents as "more happy" or "less happy" on the basis of some reasonable decision rule. I'm going to do something called a **median split**, in which we split the sample at the 50th percentile. As a result, half the parents (100) are classified as being more happy with having a new baby, and half (100) are classified as being less happy with having a new baby.

We also do a median split on weight gain. Thus, half the infants (100) are classified as having a higher weight gain, and half (100) are classified as having a lower weight gain. Figure 8.3 shows a two-by-two **matrix** (that's the word statisticians use for this sort of table) that has parental happiness as the row variable and infant weight gain as the column variable. Note that whereas I have the *marginal* frequencies indicated in the table for both rows (e.g., there are 100 parents who are happier with their new baby) and columns (e.g., there are 100 infants with a higher weight gain), I have not indicated the frequencies for any of the cells.

Now, let's imagine that parental happiness has no relationship to in-hospital weight gain. A baby with a happier parent is as likely to have a higher weight gain as a lower weight gain and ditto for a baby with a less happy parent. To put that in the language of this chapter, the correlation between parental happiness and weight gain is zero. What does that

median split

Dividing a sample at the 50th percentile of a variable.

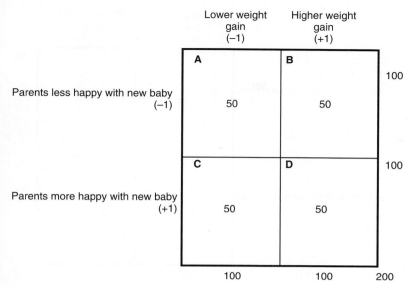

Figure **8.4** Two-by-two matrix showing no relationship (*r* = .00) between two variables.

mean for the frequencies that go in the cells in our two-by-two matrix? How should the 100 infants of happy parents be distributed between "high–weight gainers" and "low–weight gainers?" Since there's no relationship between the two variables, since parental happiness has no impact on how much weight is gained in hospital, the 100 infants should be evenly split (50/50) between the two cells. And ditto for the infants of the unhappy parents. This outcome is shown in Figure 8.4.

I've made one other change to this figure: I've added numerical values to the variables. Thus, high parental happiness is classified as a +1, low parental happiness as −1, high weight gain as +1, and low weight gain as −1. Thus an infant whose parents were relatively happy and excited with its arrival and that had a relatively high weight gain would be classified as +1, +1. I could similarly classify all the other 199 infants.

I know that I've told you that Pearson product moment correlation coefficients should only be calculated for interval-level variables, and the variables that we have here are ordinal at best. But, if we went ahead and calculated the correlation for these pairs of scores for the 200 infants anyway, we'd end up with an *r* of zero.*

Now, let's imagine that there were a perfect relationship between parental happiness and weight gain. That is, all the premature infants

---

*To be exact, this is a special kind of a correlation coefficient, a phi (the Greek letter φ) coefficient, that is meant to be used with two dichotomous variables. Phi is pronounced "fie," as in "fee, fie, foe, fum."

LOOKING CLOSER

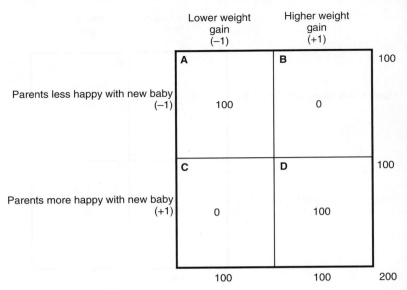

Figure **8.5** Two-by-two matrix showing a perfect, direct relationship between two variables.

whose parents were more excited at their arrival, and none of the premature infants whose parents were less excited at their arrival, had above-average weight gains. The results of this would look like Figure 8.5 and would yield $r = 1.00$ if we calculated the correlation for the pairs of scores.

The binomial effect size display takes a correlation and transforms it into this two-by-two matrix format, showing what the values in the cells would be if the marginal frequencies for each row and for each column were 100. As a result, we can calculate the percentage of cases for each level of the predictor variable that are at each level of the criterion variable.

Let's imagine that we really did the study involving parental happiness and weight gain in infants and found that $r = .30$. We know, thanks to Cohen's terminology, that this is a moderate correlation and we know, via the coefficient of determination, that 9% of the variability in hospital weight gain is explained by parental happiness and excitement. That doesn't sound like much variability being explained, does it? Here's where the BESD comes in.

Let's convert that .30 correlation into a binomial effect size display. To do so, we start with the two-by-two matrix shown in Figure 8.4, the one with no relationship between the two variables, and we adjust the values of 50 in the cells up and down so that they reflect $r = .30$. Let me explain it first, and then I'll put it as a formula. We take the correlation and multiply it by 100 ($.30 \times 100 = 30$). We then take this value and

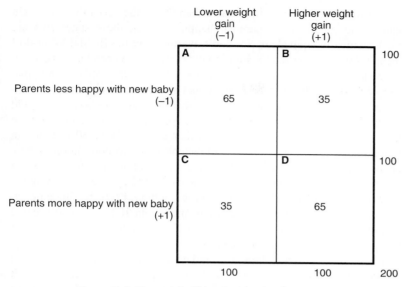

Figure **8.6** Binomial effect size display for *r* = .30.

divide it by two (30 ÷ 2 = 15). Next, we add this value to the 50 in cell A, subtract it from the 50 in cell B, subtract it from the 50 in cell C, and add it to the 50 in cell D. Thus, we'll end up with a two-by-two matrix that looks like Figure 8.6.

We now have a correlation redisplayed as a binomial effect size display, something that is easier to interpret than the coefficient of determination.* The BESD can be interpreted as showing that if parents are more excited about having a new baby there is a 65% chance that their premature infant will have an above-average weight gain. How do I get to that 65%? By looking at the row with 100 parents who have above-the-median levels of happiness about their new baby. Look at Cell D: 65 of them have infants with above-average weight gain, and 65 of 100 = 65%. Similarly, we conclude that premature infants born to parents who have below-average amounts of happiness about their arrival have a 65% chance of their infant having a below-average weight gain.

I do have one warning about the binomial effect size display. It is an easier metric to grasp than the coefficient of determination, and it gives a different, and apparently stronger, view of the world than does *r*². Doesn't a 65% chance of having a baby that gains more weight if the parents are

---

*If you calculated a correlation where there were 65 cases with values of −1 and −1, 35 with values of +1 and −1, 35 with +1 and −1, and 65 with +1 and +1, you would end up with *r* = .30. If you don't trust me, try it.

LOOKING CLOSER

more excited sound more impressive than 9% of the variability in weight gain being predicted by parental happiness? Yet, these statements are mathematically equivalent. So, don't overinterpret the BESD! What do I mean? Suppose you read a study that examined the correlation between shoe size and intelligence and concluded, "There is a 50% chance that people who have larger-than-average feet also have above-average intelligence." That sounds impressive. After reading that statement you would probably surreptitiously start comparing your feet to those of others in hopes of finding that yours were larger than average. But a 50% chance in a binomial effect size display is equivalent to a zero correlation, a 50% chance represents a coin flip. Fifty percent is baseline in a binomial effect size display; it is not like saying that one has a 50% chance of winning the lottery. If I had a 50% chance of winning a lottery, I'd be buying a ticket. If I had a 50% chance of being more intelligent if I had longer feet, I wouldn't buy any foot stretchers since I'd also have a 50% chance of being less intelligent if I had longer feet.

I hope that you know how to calculate and interpret the BESD, but it always helps to have a formula, and so I've put one in Equation 8.4. It helps to think of the binomial variables as having values of plus one or minus one. The pluses and minuses can represent high and low values or good (e.g., alive) vs. bad (e.g., dead) outcomes. I habitually make the predictor variable (the independent variable) the row variable and the criterion variable (the dependent variable) the column variable, but this is a matter of preference.

F O R M U L A

Binomial Effect Size Display (BESD)

	$Y = -1$	$Y = +1$	
Equation 8.4	**A**	**B**	100
$X = -1$	$50 + \dfrac{100(r)}{2}$	$50 - \dfrac{100(r)}{2}$	
	C	**D**	100
$X = +1$	$50 - \dfrac{100(r)}{2}$	$50 + \dfrac{100(r)}{2}$	
	100	100	200

Where:
r = the observed correlation between X and Y

With two ways to measure strength of association, percentage of variance predicted and the BESD, let's see how to use them with our height–foot size data set. The last time I interpreted the correlation (in our discussion on calculating confidence intervals) I concluded that the confidence interval was so large that it was unclear whether the relationship between height and foot size was very strong or quite weak. How would I change this interpretation in light of either the coefficient of determination or the binomial effect size display? In this case, I wouldn't change anything at all because the value of the correlation is possibly as low as .04 (in which case .16% of the variability in height is predicted by foot size), or it is possibly as high as .98 (in which case 96% of the variability in height is predicted by foot size). Similarly, with the BESD there may be a 52% chance that a person with an above-average foot size will be above-average in height, or there may be a 99% chance that a person with an above-average foot size will be above-average in height. These ranges are so great that I don't have much confidence in knowing how strong the association is between the two variables.

How would the interpretation have changed if N had been larger? Earlier, when I magically increased the sample size to 26, I concluded that the correlation between height and foot size was direct, strong, and meaningful. What would I add to this from our investigation of strength of association? Well, it depends on who my audience is. If my audience were statisticians, I would be more likely to use the coefficient of determination since this is a metric with which they are familiar. I would say something like, "The correlation between foot size and height seems to be a strong and meaningful one in which one variable predicts about 68% of the variability in the other." Statisticians would recognize 68% as indicating a very strong relationship. If my audience were a more general one, I would use the BESD and say something like, "The correlation between height and foot size seems to be a strong and meaningful one. If the correlation in the population were on the low end of the confidence interval, .64, then a college student who is above average in foot size would have about an 82% chance of also being above average in terms of height compared with the 18% chance of being above average in height for a college student who is below average in foot size." *

Note that I did not include both the coefficient of determination and the BESD in my interpretation. It is not wrong to include both, but I find the "kitchen sink" approach leans toward overkill, and I prefer to be more focused. I agree with Mies van der Rohe: less is more.

*Note that I chose to use the low end of the confidence interval (.64) to calculate the binomial effect size display and not the observed correlation of .83. It would not be wrong to calculate the BESD using .83, but I tend to be conservative and would rather err on the side of underestimating the strength of a relationship.

LOOKING CLOSER

Group Practice 8.3

NOTE 1: We've focused on interpreting correlation coefficients that are statistically significant, but I'm sure you can handle a *brief* statement if an *r* is not statistically significant. If *r* is not significant, I calculate the confidence interval (see Table 8.3 for interpretative guidelines), but I don't calculate either the coefficient of determination or the binomial effect size display. (Can you figure out why not?)

NOTE 2: Decide how to focus your interpretation and how to make sense of conflicting information. What do you do when one measure of strength says that the correlation is strong and the other says that it is weak? You can always suggest obtaining more information, that is, replicating the study to gain more confidence in the results. Also, note that some measures of strength (e.g., confidence intervals) are influenced by sample size, and others (e.g., BESD) are not. When sample sizes are small, you should be concerned about the robustness of results.

NOTE 3: Be conservative and creative in your interpretations. (No, the two are not mutually exclusive.) After calculating a confidence interval you have three options for a correlation to interpret: $r_{observed}$, the low end of the confidence interval, or the high end of the confidence interval. Which one you interpret is up to you, but here are my guidelines.

If the confidence interval is narrow, then I would go with $r_{observed}$. However, if the confidence interval is wide, I tend to be conservative and go with r_{low}, the end of the interval that is closer to zero.

1. In examining the relationship between amount of exercise (higher numbers = more exercise) and amount of weight lost (higher numbers = more weight lost), a nurse found that $r = .4238$ for the 45 participants he had in his study. (No assumptions for the Pearson *r* had been violated.) Using a two-tailed test with α set at .05, report the results in APA format, and calculate the 95% confidence interval, the coefficient of determination, and the BESD. Then write an interpretative paragraph.

2. A nutritionist recruited 11 participants who wanted to lose weight and who were willing to be hospitalized so that she could monitor their actual caloric consumption. She measured caloric consumption (higher numbers = more calories consumed) and weight loss (higher numbers = more weight lost) during 7 days of hospitalization and, with no assumptions violated, found $r = -.5578$. Using a two-tailed test with α set at .05, report the results in APA format, and calculate the 95% confidence interval, the coefficient of determination, and the BESD. Then write an interpretative paragraph.

USING CORRELATIONS FOR SPECIFIC PREDICTIONS

When the *r* is statistically different from zero, we can use the correlation coefficient to estimate, or predict, a *Y* value for a specific *X* value. When we do so, the estimated *Y* is called *Y'*, pronounced "Y prime."

Why would we want to do so? As one example, this would allow us to predict a future variable (e.g., college GPA), from something measured in the present (e.g., SAT score). This approach, technically called linear regression, has almost certainly been used on you. In deciding whom to accept, most colleges rely on linear regression. They take high school GPA and/or SAT scores and use them to predict college GPA. If they predict that you will perform well at their college, they are likely to admit you. If they predict that you won't do well at their college, …

The accuracy of our estimates, the *Y'*s, depends on the strength of the correlation: the stronger the correlation, the more accurate the estimates.

Think back to the scatterplots of different correlations, which are reprised in slightly altered form in Figure 8.7. In Panel A, where $r = .00$, the points in the scatterplot are arrayed as a rectangle where each X value is associated with the whole range of possibilities for Y values. Thus, for any value of X the associated Y value can range anywhere from 1 to 10. Given this, if a case has an X value of 1, what is our best predictor of its Y value?

It turns out that the best predicted value of Y, Y', is the mean of all the Y values, in this case 5.5. Why is this the best predicted value? Well, it depends on how one defines "best." In this instance, I am defining best as the value that minimizes the difference from the actual Y to the predicted Y'. If a case has an actual Y value of 6 there is a .5 difference between Y and Y'. Since the smallest possible value of Y is 1, and the largest possible value of Y is 10, the largest possible discrepancy between a Y and a Y' is 4.5. If we use any other value for the predicted value—say, 6.0 instead of 5.5—then the possible discrepancy will be greater. (The distance from 1 to 6 is 5, which is half a unit larger than the distance from 1 to 5.5.)

If we connect all the dots of our *predicted values* in Panel A, we get a *straight* line (it's called *linear* regression) going horizontally through the scatterplot. You can see this **regression line** in Panel A of Figure 8.7.

How is this regression line used? Well, for any X value, we can draw a line vertically up from the X value to where it intersects with the regression line, then horizontally over to where it intersects with the ordinate (the Y axis). The Y value at the Y axis is Y' for X. In panel A of Figure 8.7, no matter what X value we have the Y' value will always be 5.50. Thus, if $X = 2$, we predict that $Y' = 5.50$; if $X = 7.37$, we predict $Y' = 5.50$, and so on.

Contrast what happens when $r = .00$ with what happens for the other extreme value of a correlation, a perfect correlation of 1.00. A perfect correlation means that if we know a case's standing on X then we can perfectly predict its standing on Y. A scatterplot of a perfect correlation has all the points falling on a diagonal line, as shown in panel H of Figure 8.7. Note that the regression line travels straight through all of the data points.

The X values in these scatterplots range from 1 to 10, as do the Y values. In panel H, if a case has an X score of 1, we predict its Y' to be 1, and if a case has an X of 8 we predict its Y' to be 8. We are not limited to predicting Y's only for existing values of X: we can predict a Y' for any value of X. If, for example, $X = 5.3$, Y' will be 5.3.*

Note that the angle of the regression line increases from horizontal to a 45-degree-diagonal as the correlation increases from $r = .00$ to $r = 1.00$. (The angles would also change from horizontal to diagonal, as r increased in strength from .00 to -1.00, but would move in the other direction.)

regression line

The "best-fitting" straight line that allows one to predict a case's score on the criterion from its score on the predictor.

---

*It is just because there is a perfect synchrony between my X values and my Y values that the Y' for a given X is the same as the X. Usually this is not the case.

LOOKING CLOSER

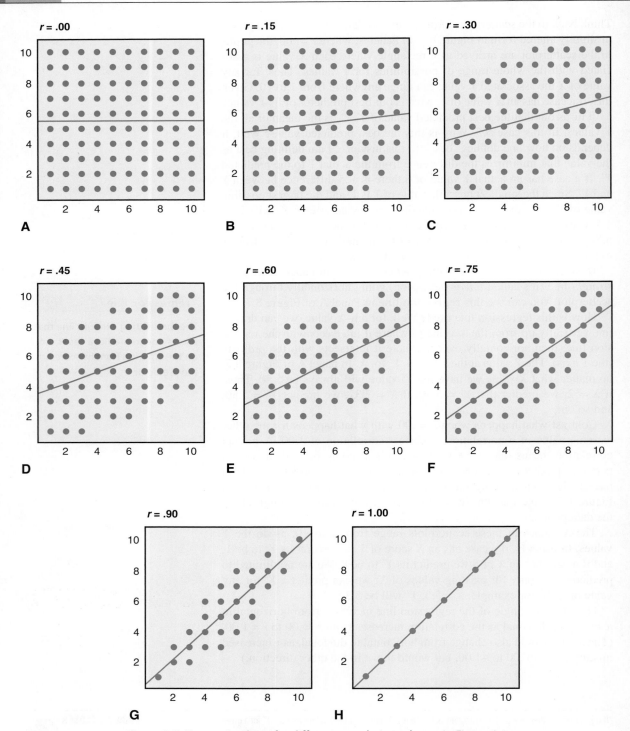

Figure **8.7** Regression lines for different correlations shown in Figure 8.1.

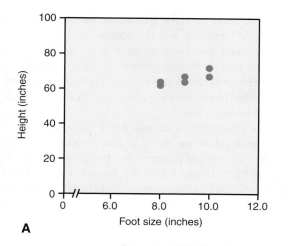

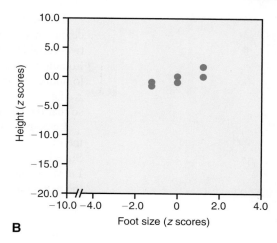

A   B

Figure **8.8** Height–foot size scatterplots for raw scores and z scores.

No matter what the angle of the regression line may be, it is used in the manner outlined above: draw a vertical line up from X and then draw a horizontal line over to the Y axis to find Y'. However, drawing lines is not a terribly accurate approach. So, of course, there is a formula for Y'. Most of the formulae that are given for this are a bit tedious because they work with the raw scores of X and Y. But, if one is willing to work with z scores, with z_x instead of X and $z_{Y'}$ instead of Y', the formula is simplicity itself. We'll transform a raw X score into z_x, find $z_{Y'}$ for that, and then transform $z_{Y'}$ back into a raw score, into Y'. As we go through this process, I'll explain why this prediction procedure is called linear *regression*.

But, before I show you the formula (Equation 8.5), I want to remind you that transforming a set of scores to z scores does not change the shape of the set of scores. Figure 8.8 displays scatterplots for the height–foot size data set, both as raw scores (A) and as z scores (B). Note that the two scatterplots look exactly the same, although the values on the abscissa and the ordinate are different.

FORMULA

Predicted Y Score As a z Score ($z_{Y'}$)

$z_{Y'} = r(z_X)$

Equation 8.5

Where:
$z_{Y'}$ = the predicted Y score (Y') as a z score
r = the Pearson r between X and Y
z_x = the X score converted to a z score

To use this equation we need to know the mean (M) and standard deviation (s) for each of the variables and the correlation between the two variables. Then, we convert the raw score of X to a z score, z_x (via Equation 5.1), and multiply that by the correlation (r). That's all there is to finding Y' as a z score. However, we'll almost certainly want to convert $z_{Y'}$ (i.e., the Y' in z score format) back to raw score units, via Equation 5.2, so that the answer is more interpretable.

Let's imagine, using our height–foot size data, that I find a footprint in the mud outside my campus window one morning and, suspecting a Penn State Erie student, wonder how tall the person was who left the footprint. I measure the footprint and find it to be 11.75″ long. From Table 7.8, I find the mean (and standard deviation) for foot size is 9.0000 (.8165), and for height it is 66.0000 (3.2146). I have already calculated the correlation between height and foot size as .8255.

First I transform the raw score (11.75) into a z score:

$$\frac{11.75 - 9.0000}{.8165} = 3.3680$$

Then, I multiply that z_x (3.3680) by r (.8255) to find $z_{Y'} = 2.7803$. Since that number represents the person's height as a z score, I want to convert it back to raw score units, back into inches. Using Equation 5.2, I calculate the raw score for this as $(2.7803 \times 3.2146) + 66.0000 = 74.9376$. Thus, I estimate that this person's height, his or her Y', is 74.94″—that he or she is almost 75 inches tall.

This is a "point" estimate since it gives the value as a single point. The other option is an "interval" estimate, an estimate that gives the value as a range within which the population value likely falls. Confidence intervals are interval estimates and have the advantage of giving a range within which the estimate falls, making us aware of the inaccuracy, the error, inherent in any single point estimate. When an interval is predicted for a specific case—not for the value of a parameter—it is called a **prediction interval,** not a confidence interval.

To calculate a prediction interval for the estimated Y score, we need to know something called the standard error of the estimate ($s_{Y-Y'}$, pronounced "s sub Y minus Y prime"), which is the standard deviation of the sampling distribution of the Y's. In other words, if you draw repeated, random samples from the population and each time calculate the correlation between X and Y and use that to estimate Y' for X, you will have a sampling distribution of Y's. This sampling distribution would have a standard deviation, $s_{Y-Y'}$. To use the standard error of the estimate for calculating a prediction interval, we must adjust it a bit. The adjustments involve making it larger so that it estimates a population value and, yet again, making it larger to account for sample size and for how far away the X score is from the mean. We'll call this new standard error

prediction interval

The interval within which it is predicted that a score is likely to fall for a specific case.

of the estimate the "corrected standard error of the estimate" and abbreviate it as $\hat{s}_{Y-Y'}$.*

The formula for calculating the standard error of the estimate, in raw score units, is shown in Equation 8.6, and the formula for using this to calculate a 95% prediction interval for Y' is shown in Equation 8.7.† It looks, and it is, a bit tedious.

F O R M U L A

Corrected Standard Error of the Estimate ($\hat{s}_{Y-Y'}$) for Y'

Equation 8.6

$$\hat{s}_{Y-Y'} = s_Y \sqrt{(1 - r^2)} \; \sqrt{\frac{N}{N-2}} \; \sqrt{1 + \frac{1 + z_X^2}{N}}$$

Where:

$\hat{s}_{Y-Y'}$ = corrected standard error of estimate being calculated

s_Y = the standard deviation of Y

r = correlation between X and Y

N = the number of cases used to calculate the correlation coefficient

z_x = the X score for which Y' is being calculated, expressed as a z score

---

F O R M U L A

95% Prediction Interval for Y'

Equation 8.7

$$95\% \; PI = Y' \pm t(s_{Y-Y'})$$

Where:

$95\% \; PI$ = the 95% prediction interval being calculated

Y' = the predicted value of Y for a given X, calculated via Equation 8.5 and turned back into a raw score via Equation 5.2

t = t value with $df = N - 2$ from Appendix Table 3 ($\alpha = .05$, two-tailed)

$\hat{s}_{Y-Y'}$ = the corrected standard error of the estimate via Equation 8.6

Let's use these equations. Equation 8.6 says that to calculate the corrected standard error of the estimate we multiply the standard deviation of Y by the square root of the difference, $1 - r^2$. This product is then

---

*Just as with the correction to the estimated population variance, $\hat{s}^2$, the correction for the standard error of the estimate will be smaller when N is larger. In addition, it is smaller when X is closer to the mean.

†This formula is based on equations in Cohen and Cohen, 1983.

LOOKING CLOSER

multiplied by the square root of the quotient of N divided by $N - 2$. Finally, this product is multiplied by the square root of the sum of one plus the quotient of the sum of one plus the squared z score divided by N. Whew. Using the height–foot size data set where $x = 11.75$ and $z_x = 3.3680$, we calculate

$$S_{Y-Y'} = 3.2146 \sqrt{(1 - .8255^2)} \sqrt{\frac{6}{6-2}} \sqrt{1 + \frac{1 + 3.3680^2}{6}}$$

$$= 3.2146 \times .5644 \times 1.2247 \times 1.7485$$

$$= 3.8852$$

Thus the corrected standard error of the estimate is 3.89.

Using Equation 8.7 to calculate the 95% prediction interval for the predicted Y score, we take Y' (74.9376) and subtract from it and add to it t corrected standard errors of the estimate. Appendix Table 3 tells us that the t value with 4 degrees of freedom is 2.7764. Following this equation, we calculate the 95% prediction interval:

$$95\% \ PI = 74.9376 \pm (2.7764 \times 3.8852)$$

$$= 74.9376 \pm 10.7869$$

When reporting a prediction interval we go from low to high, so we report the 95% prediction interval for Y' as ranging from 64.15″ to 85.72″. The height of the person who left the footprint is fairly certain to fall in this ≈22-inch range. It doesn't eliminate very many subjects, does it, to know that the person who left the footprint outside my window is likely be anywhere from a bit taller than 5′4″ to almost 7′2″?

In this situation, given the width of the confidence interval for r, it makes some sense that our prediction interval is wide as well. With small sample sizes our statistical estimates are not robust, and we cannot have much confidence in the results. If we actually did a study with only six subjects, we would be foolish. If N had been 26 the prediction interval would have been smaller, about 9 to 10 inches wide, from 5′10″ to 6′8″; if N had been dramatically larger, say 260, the prediction interval would shrink to ≈7″ wide, ranging from 5′11″ to 6′7″. That's still wide, though we would be fairly certain that the person is close to or above 6′ tall.

Unfortunately, prediction intervals remain wide even when a lot of stars line up in our favor. Imagine that there is a very strong correlation, say, a correlation of .90, between IQ and the quantitative section of the SAT. We know, thanks to the binomial effect size display, that a person who has an above-average level of intelligence has a 95% chance of getting an above-average score on the SAT. But what does this mean for a specific person—say, for Skip, who has an IQ of 115? Skip's IQ score was one standard deviation above the mean, and his predicted SAT score is 590, or nine tenths of a standard deviation above the mean. However, since a point estimate provides more precision than we really have, let's find the 95% prediction interval for Skip's score, and let's assume that the .90 correlation is based on an N of 1,000,000. Even under these favorable

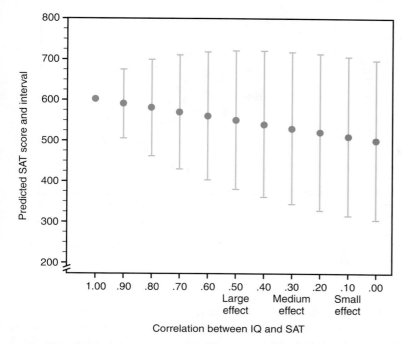

Figure **8.9** Impact of size of correlation on width of prediction interval for an IQ score of 115. NOTE: Small, medium, and large effect sizes as defined by Cohen (1988).

conditions—a very strong correlation, a predictor score that is close to the mean, and a very large *N*—the 95% prediction interval is large, ranging from a low of 505 to a high of 675. I doubt that Skip would find it useful to be told that he will probably score somewhere in this 170-point range on the SAT.

This points up the difference between making a prediction "in general" and "in specific." In general, Skip should do well on the SAT, he has a 95% chance of scoring above average according to the binomial effect size display. But in specific, where will he score? Well, that one is a lot tougher to nail down with confidence unless *r* = 1.00.

Figure 8.9 shows the impact of the size of the correlation on the width of the prediction interval for the IQ and SAT example I was using above. Note how quickly the prediction interval increases in width as *r* moves away from a perfect correlation. As *r* gets smaller, we are less certain of the range in which a predicted score will fall. When *r* = 1.00, prediction is perfect, but as soon as we step away from that, the interval becomes wide. In fact, if *r* were .99, the prediction interval would be 55 SAT points wide. Look how wide the prediction interval for *r* = .50, what Cohen (1988) considers a large effect! Our ability to have certainty in predicting criterion scores for specific cases is limited.

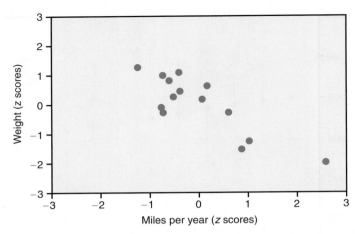

Figure **8.10** Scatterplot showing relationship between amount I exercise and amount I weigh.

This figure also shows why linear regression is called linear *regression*. Note that as *r* gets smaller, our predicted SAT score, *Y'*, gets closer and closer to the mean. As *r* gets closer to zero the predicted value of *Y* *regresses* more and more toward 500, the mean SAT value. This makes sense, for if *r* = .00, then knowing *X* tells us nothing about *Y*, and our best guess for *Y'*, in that situation, is the mean. As we know less and less, our prediction should fall back closer and closer—regress—to the mean.

It follows from this that if a correlation coefficient is not statistically different from zero, there is no reason to worry about calculating *Y'*. The reasoning for this is fairly straightforward. If the correlation coefficient is not statistically significant, then we fail to reject the null hypothesis and have no evidence that *r* is anything but zero. If *r* is zero, then our best estimate of *Y'* is simply the mean of *Y*, no matter what *X* value we are given.

My final thought on the topic of using a statistically significant correlation to predict *Y* from *X* is that one always needs to stop and think about one's results. Just because you can calculate a *Y'* doesn't mean that it is right. Remember, interpretation involves a human factor. Here's a real life example to drive that point home.

My favorite physical exercise is riding a bicycle. You may find this hard to believe about me, but I am compulsive enough to keep track of how many miles I ride every year. I also, like most Americans, keep an eye on my weight. Once, with a little spare time on my hands, I decided to look at the relation between how much I exercised per year and how much I weighed at the end of the year. You can see the relationship in the scatterplot in Figure 8.10.*

LOOKING CLOSER

*Please note: I am a little bit shy and don't want to overwhelm you with the physical prowess evident in my yearly mileage or tell you how much I really do weigh. So I have transformed both into *z* scores.

The relationship is statistically significant (r (9) = −.86, $p < .05$) and appears quite strong. This is a great example of an inverse relationship: the more I ride my bicycle in a given year, the less I weigh at the end of that year. It seems reasonable, then, that I could use this to plan a weight-loss program. That is, I could pick the weight that I want to be, and then calculate how many miles I need to ride in a given year to reach my desired weight. I could also turn things around and estimate how much I would weigh if I rode a certain number of miles in a given year.

And it is here that we run into trouble. Just because you can calculate it, doesn't make it so. It turns out that if I bike 21,000 miles in a year, I should reach a weight of −15 pounds. Don't forget that the final step of Tom-and-Harry, the interpretation phase, is a human one. That is, a machine can calculate that biking 21,000 miles leads to a weight of −15 pounds, but it takes a human being to realize the absurdity of such a prediction. Yes, I could certainly bike 21,000 miles (though I would have to give up my day job and move to a better climate), and if I did so I would be in very good, and very lean, shape. Still, I guarantee you that I wouldn't weigh negative 15 pounds.

I can't leave this biking example without making one last point. And, I promise that this is the last point for this section: never forget the four most important words in statistics, "Correlation is not causation." Just because two variables are correlated does not mean that one causes the other. There are always three possibilities that must be considered: that X causes Y, that Y causes X, or that something else causes both X and Y.*

In thinking about what causes what for a correlation, the human factor in interpretation is important. I suppose it is possible that weight causes miles ridden, that the more I weigh, the harder it is for me to pedal my massive carcass up and down hills and so my riding decreases. More plausible, however, is that exercise has an impact on weight—that the more I ride, the less I weigh.

I would like to propose a third option, that something else causes both X and Y. And the something else that I would like to propose is age. If you look at Figure 8.11 you'll see a graph showing that as the years go by (and I get older), the number of miles I ride has tended to decrease. There's also a bar chart showing that as the years go by, my weight has tended to increase. Though I would like to believe that simply increasing my exercise will cause me to shed my excess weight, I don't think it is that simple. I think that my increasing age is having an impact both on my increasing weight and my decreasing miles.[†]

---

*Actually, there is a fourth option: that we have made a Type I error and concluded that there is a relationship where none exists. That is, X doesn't cause Y, Y doesn't cause X, and something else doesn't cause both X and Y, rather the apparent relationship is spurious.

[†]I don't mean to propose that exercise has no impact on weight; it certainly does. There is a type of correlation, called a partial correlation, that allows one to remove the effect of a third variable when examining the relationship between the original two variables. When I remove the effects of age from the correlation between miles ridden and weight, the correlation drops down from −.86 to −.66. The −.66 is still a significant correlation, but the change indicates that age does play a role.

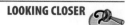

LOOKING CLOSER

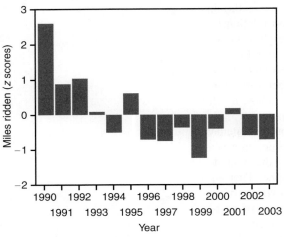

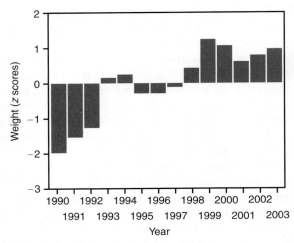

Figure **8.11** Exploring the impact of increasing age on my exercise and my weight.

Y' is typically used to make predictions for a single case or for a set of cases, but there are situations when it may be used as part of an interpretative statement for a correlation. If, for example, one were looking at the relationship between SAT and college GPA, it might be of interest to report the predicted GPA for a modal student. You'll have a chance to do so in this set of group practice problems.

Group Practice 8.4

1. In a group of 57 cases, $r_p = .4387$. If $M_X = 29.3512$, $s_X = 8.3419$, $M_Y = 423.1385$, and $s_Y = 57.5282$. Given $X = 19.76$, fill in the blanks:

   a. $z_X =$ _____

   b. $z_{Y'} =$ _____

   c. $Y' =$ _____

   d. $\hat{s}_{Y-Y'} =$ _____

   e. 95% prediction interval for Y' ranges from _____ to _____ .

2. A researcher is interested in the impact of parental reading on children's vocabulary. To a sample of 235 sixth-grade students, he administers a vocab- ulary test that is scored on the interval level. (The mean score on this exam is 10.00 with a standard deviation of 3.00.) The researcher also finds out how many hours the parents spend reading books each week. The mean for this is 5.00 with a standard deviation of 1.50. After checking assumptions and finding that normality, linearity, and homoscedasticity are OK, the researcher calculates $r = .58$. Interpret this correlation. In your discussion, be sure to talk about the predicted vocabulary score for someone whose parents read 3.5 hours per week compared to someone whose parents read 6.5 hours per week.

INTERPRETING CORRELATIONS THAT DO NOT STATISTICALLY DIFFER FROM ZERO

If the correlation is not statistically significant, if it is not statistically different from zero, then our interpretative job is actually more chal- lenging. Remember, if the correlation is not statistically significant then we have failed to reject the null hypothesis, but we have not proven the null hypothesis. Failing to prove a defendant guilty is not the same as proving the defendant innocent.

In Chapter 7 we covered the fact that failing to reject the null doesn't prove the null, but understanding this is even more important now that we are venturing into the world of interpretation. So, let's look at this again. Suppose we want to know whether seawater contains gold. We randomly select 50 spots from all the oceans of the world and from each one remove a gallon of seawater. We bring the gallons back to the laboratory and, using a very sensitive and well-calibrated scale, measure how much gold each gallon contains. We use a difference test to decide between the null hypothesis that seawater contains no gold and our alternative hypothesis that seawater contains some gold. Completing our measurements, we find that each gallon contains, on average, .0000000093 ounces of gold and that this amount of deviation from the null-hypothesized value of zero is small enough that we *fail* to reject the null hypothesis. Here's my question: Having failed to reject the null hypothesis, is it reasonable to conclude that the null hypothesis—that seawater contains no gold—is true?

No, that would not be a reasonable conclusion. Clearly, seawater contains *some* gold, though a very, very small amount in each gallon. So, via the logic of null hypothesis significance testing, what conclusion can we draw? The official conclusion is that our results are not statistically different from zero, that's all. We can't say that the value is zero, and we can't say that it isn't: we can only say that (a) it is not statistically different from zero, and (b) we may be mistaken.

But, in the human endeavor of interpretation, in how we perceive these results, we may draw a different conclusion. I might conclude that the amount of gold in a gallon of seawater is functionally zero, and I would probably decide that my wife wouldn't be very excited if, when our fiftieth wedding anniversary rolled around, I gave her a gallon of seawater to celebrate the event. That is, I might *interpret* the results as indicating that seawater contains no gold.

But, on a larger scale, that interpretation is wrong. Quite wrong. A gallon of seawater contains almost no gold, but there are approximately 360 quintillion gallons of seawater in the world. And that means that there are about 200 billion pounds of gold in the ocean. Do you still want to conclude that seawater contains no gold? Or do you want to figure out how to mine seawater?*

Interpreting results that are not statistically different from zero is more challenging than interpreting results that are statistically different from zero because, technically, all we know is that the results are not statistically different from zero. The verdict of "not guilty" has been returned, and now we have to decide if we interpret that as "innocent."

---

*By the bye, seawater really does contain that small amount of gold per gallon. Thus, dissolved in all the oceans of the world there really floats 200 billion pounds of gold.

LOOKING CLOSER

Sometimes, as a pragmatic decision, we interpret results that are not statistically different from zero as indicating that it is likely that there is no association, no correlation, between X and Y in the population. Imagine a pharmaceutical researcher trying to find new ways to lower cholesterol level. The researcher believes she has a promising drug and has done a number of studies with it, each in the population of interest. Each study has shown no statistically significant relationship between use of the drug and decreased cholesterol level. Further, imagine that the researcher has limited resources of time and money to spend on her research. (OK, limited resources is hard to imagine with a pharmaceutical company, but stick with me.) At some point, shouldn't she stop investigating this drug and turn her attention to another, to one that will, she hopes, show more promise?*

With regard to writing interpretative statements for correlations that are not statistically different from zero, I see little reason to calculate a coefficient of determination, or to calculate a binomial effect size display, or to predict Y'. Why? Because if we conclude that there is not sufficient evidence of a nonzero linear relationship between X and Y in the population, then there is no reason to believe that knowing X tells us anything about Y—so there is no need to find out how much of the variability in Y is accounted for by X. Ditto for the binomial effect size display: if there is insufficient evidence to conclude that X is related to Y, cases that are above average on X will be just as likely to have a score above average on Y as below average on Y. And, finally, if there is no relationship between X and Y, knowing a case's X score gives us no useful information about its Y score, and our prediction of Y' will always be the mean.[†]

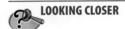 **LOOKING CLOSER**

*Though, let me continue with my gold metaphor to explain why it is dangerous to conclude that $\rho = 0$. Imagine that I have a gold mine in the ground and that over time the vein of gold gets thinner and thinner. Might I not reach a point where the cost of mining the gold gets greater than the worth of the gold I retrieve? And, at this point I'll make the pragmatic decision to stop mining the gold. That doesn't mean that there is no gold there, it just means that it costs too much to retrieve it. But, over time, might not things change? Might a new and cheaper mining technology come along, or might the price of gold increase? And, under those conditions, might it not make financial sense, again, for me to start mining? So, even though our researcher's cholesterol drug hasn't shown promise so far, do you want to conclude that it will never, under any conditions, be helpful?

At the same time, pragmatically, it is not showing any utility now. So, it is reasonable to conclude that it is ineffective under the current conditions and she should turn her attention to other avenues.

[†]Many statisticians—your instructor perhaps is one—advocate calculating and reporting effect sizes even when one fails to reject the null hypothesis. Their reasoning is that failing to do so increases the possibility of discounting the importance of a large but not-statistically-significant effect. This is called a Type II error, and it occurs when the null hypothesis actually is false but one fails to reject it. Type II error certainly is a problem when it occurs, and it is an error to be avoided. But, as I advocate calculating the probability of this error occurring—and am about to teach you how to do it—and as I advocate calculating confidence intervals for not-statistically-significant correlations in order to have some sense of how strong the effect might be, I think that you will adequately be on the alert for Type II errors.

So, what do I advocate in terms of interpretation when a correlation is not significant? Well, first we should calculate the confidence interval for the correlation. Obviously, this confidence interval will capture zero because we have failed to reject the null hypothesis. But, the width, location, and lopsidedness of the confidence interval will give us useful information. Consider the following confidence intervals that capture zero, either from −.07 to .17 ($r = .05$, $N = 250$) or from −.47 to .55 ($r = .05$, $N = 15$). If the confidence interval is relatively narrow and centered around zero, as in the first scenario, then we could be reasonably comfortable concluding that it is unlikely that there is a linear relationship between the two variables. Being mindful of the possibility of a Type II error (after all, the confidence interval ranges up to .17) we would be more comfortable giving up on the search for a relationship if the results had been replicated a few times. We would start to entertain the possibility of making an interpretative statement about the lack of a linear relationship between the two variables.

This is in contrast to the second scenario, where the confidence interval is wide with possible population correlations on either side (−.47 and .55) that are quite strong. We would want similar statistically nonsignificant results from multiple replications before feeling comfortable making an interpretative statement about the lack of a relationship between the variables.

There's a third scenario, one in which the confidence interval is lopsided: it captures zero, but most of it is on one side. An example would be a correlation of .15 with 147 cases, resulting in a confidence interval ranging from −.01 to .30. The official conclusion in such a situation remains that there is not sufficient evidence that the population value of the correlation is anything but zero, but I am quite concerned about Type II error. Though ρ may fall anywhere in the interval from −.01 to .30, the odds are greater that ρ is positive. Yes, there is not sufficient evidence that ρ is anything but zero, but we came close to rejecting the null hypothesis and finding a statistically different from zero direct relationship. I want to replicate, and I suspect, especially if we increase our sample size, that we'll end up rejecting the null hypothesis on replication.

When we fail to reject the null hypothesis, we worry about making a Type II error, about concluding that there is no linear relationship when there really is one. Being concerned about Type II error will lead us (a) to calculate β, the probability of this error, (b) to explore something called the power of a statistical test, and (c) to explore the adequacy of sample sizes for a correlation coefficient. Thus, we'll finally be able to address the missing piece of the Tom-and-Harry Step 4 (the decision rule), whether the sample size is adequate.

As always, it is better to have a concrete example. So, let's imagine a random sample of 15 people from the population of adult men in the United States. For each person, we calculate body mass index and measure total cholesterol level. For those who don't know, body mass index, or BMI, is a measure of body fat based on a person's height and weight: higher BMI scores indicate that a person is more overweight.

TABLE **8.5**   **Cholesterol and BMI Data for 15 Adult Males***

BMI	Cholesterol
17	220
18	190
19	230
20	240
21	190
23	260
25	240
27	210
29	200
31	260
32	280
33	256
34	230
35	240
29	250

*Note: According to the National Heart, Lung, and Blood Institute, a BMI ≤ 18.5 indicates a person is underweight, BMIs from 18.5 to 24.9 are in the normal range, overweight is from 25 to 29.9, and greater than 30 indicates obesity. Cholesterol levels ≥ 240 are considered high, from 200 to 239 is borderline, and below 200 is considered OK.

Total cholesterol level is a measure of the total amount of cholesterol (LDL and HDL) carried in the blood. Higher numbers indicate greater amounts of cholesterol. The data are shown in Table 8.5.

As prelude to the interpretation of the correlation coefficient for these data, let's march through the first five steps of Tom and Harry for these data.

Test

The statistical test that we will use is a Pearson product moment correlation coefficient since we're examining the relationship between two ratio-level variables.

Assumptions

There are five assumptions for the Pearson r: (a) random sample, (b) interval or ratio level variables, (c) normality, (d) linearity, and (e) homoscedasticity. Our sample is a random sample of men from the population of adult men in the United States, and both of the variables are ratio-level, so we have not violated either of the first two assumptions. The 95% confidence intervals for skewness and kurtosis for both variables capture a value of zero, indicating a reasonable possibility that both variables are normally distributed in the population. The scatterplot, shown below in Figure 8.12, neither suggests that there is a nonlinear relationship between the two variables nor does it show marked heteroscedasticity, suggesting that neither of the last two assumptions was violated. Thus, with no assumptions violated, we proceed with the test.

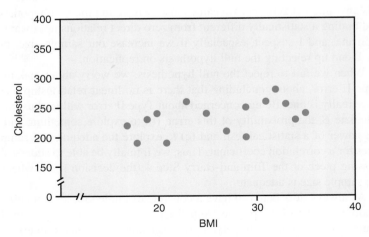

Figure **8.12** Scatterplot for body mass index and cholesterol level.

Hypotheses

The null hypothesis (H_0) is $\rho_{xy} = 0$ and the alternative hypothesis (H_1) is $\rho_{xy} \neq 0$. The null hypothesis states that there is no linear relationship between the two variables in the population. Even so, when we take a sample from the population and calculate the value of the correlation for that sample, the observed correlation will not be exactly zero. However, it should be close enough to zero that the deviation from zero is explained by sampling error. The alternative hypothesis states that in the population, there is a linear relationship between the two variables, and that the observed correlation in the sample will reflect this. That is, the observed correlation in the sample will be far enough away from zero that the deviation from zero is too great to be explained by sampling error from a hypothesized parameter of zero.

Decision rule

Our hypothesis is nondirectional, so we will do a two-tailed test. Because we are willing to make a Type I error (reject the null when it is correct) 5% of the time, we set α at .05. Thus r_{cv} is .5140. If the absolute value of the observed value of r is $\geq$ .5140, then we shall reject the null hypothesis, report $p < .05$, and conclude that there is probably a nonzero linear relationship between BMI and cholesterol level in the population. If the absolute value of the observed r is $<$ .5140, then we shall fail to reject the null hypothesis, report $p < .05$, and conclude that there is not sufficient evidence to reject the hypothesis that there is anything but a zero relationship between BMI and cholesterol level in the population.

Calculation

$r(13) = .48$, $p > .05$.*

And now we are ready for the interpretation!

Interpretation: Worrying about Type II error

The first part is easy as we've already planned it out in Step 4, the decision rule. Thus, I would make a statement like, "I have failed to reject the null hypothesis and thus conclude that the relationship between body mass index and total cholesterol level is not statistically different from zero. Based on this sample, a man's weight relative to his height (his BMI) appears to be unrelated to his cholesterol level."

---

*Remember, $p > .05$ means that results like this are likely, that they should occur 5% of the time or more, if the null hypothesis is true.

LOOKING CLOSER

I bet that that statement doesn't feel right to you. We all know, don't we, that weight is related to cholesterol level? Thus we are confronted with two options. Either the received wisdom that weight and cholesterol level are related is wrong, that is, $\rho_{xy} = 0$ is true and my interpretation is right or, for some reason, we have made an error in failing to reject the null hypothesis.

This error, which is the opposite of what we are concerned about when we reject the null hypothesis (Type I error), is Type II error. What if, in the population, there really is a relationship between BMI and cholesterol, but our results have failed to show this? There are two reasons why this could occur. First, we may have obtained a nonrepresentative sample. That is, as a result of the luck of the draw of random sampling (remember those M&M's!) we may have obtained a sample that doesn't look like the population. That is, in the whole population there is a relationship between the two variables, but in our sample there wasn't.

The other option is that the level of correlation we observed is true. Meaning, in this case, that ρ really is somewhere in the region of .48, but we didn't have enough cases for it to be found to be statistically different from zero.

How could this be so? Take a look at the table of critical values of r (Table 4) in the Appendix and look down the bolded column. Note that as N (i.e., df) increases, r_{cv} decreases. If the N had been 17, not 15, our results would have been statistically significant.* That is, if N had been larger, we would have been able to reject the null hypothesis!

In either event, whether we have a bad sample or not enough cases, we may have made a Type II error. How concerned should we be about making a Type II error?

Unlike Type I error, where we set the likelihood of making a Type I error (α) before we do any calculations, the likelihood of making a Type II error (β) is not commonly set in advance. Researchers tend to worry about the probability of having made a Type II error after the statistical test is over. I think that this is unfortunate, and I want you to help reverse this trend by showing concern for Type II error before you begin your statistical test. As we shall see, the easiest way to keep β low is to keep N high.

I've mentioned before that statisticians always seem to be confusing the situation by giving things odd names. Well, here's another thing they do. Rather than talk about β, the likelihood of making a Type II error (incorrectly failing to reject the null), they talk about **power,** the likelihood of rejecting the null hypothesis when it is in fact wrong. Power,

power

The probability of correctly rejecting the null hypothesis.

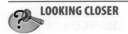 **LOOKING CLOSER**

*Remember, null hypothesis significance testing is like pregnancy, not horseshoes. Close doesn't count. We made the agreement that if the $|r|$ was ≥ the critical value of r, we would reject the null. We can't weasel out now and say that our results were "approaching" statistical significance so we have almost rejected the null. If you live by the sword, you have to be willing to die by the sword.

defined as $1 - \beta$, is the likelihood of correctly rejecting the null hypothesis. So, if $\beta = .20$, power $= .80$. That is, if there is a 20% chance of mistakenly failing to reject the null hypothesis, then there is an 80% chance of correctly rejecting it. Remember: we set up a statistical test in hopes of rejecting the null, so we want statistical power to be as high as possible.

Though the decision about α level is arbitrary, the accepted convention is to set it at .05. The decision about β is just as arbitrary, and it is just as codified: the convention is to set β at .20, making power .80.

I'll be honest: this mystifies me. Why is it acceptable to make a Type I error only 5% of the time and a Type II error 20% of the time? As I've said before, both of these errors have serious ramifications. In the present BMI-cholesterol scenario, a Type I error would involve telling people to lose weight in order to lower cholesterol levels, when doing so would have no impact on cholesterol level. This might keep them from seeking a more effective treatment for their elevated cholesterol levels, and this is not a good outcome. Even a worse outcome, however, occurs with a Type II error. If a Type II error occurred, then we would not tell people to lose weight, even though losing weight would help lower their cholesterol levels. As a result, people might die. Why we are 4 times more willing to make this error than having people lose weight for no reason is a mystery to me.

Well, not a total mystery. As we are about to see, power is tied to sample size. And, if we held β to the same standard as α (i.e., set both at .05), then the sample sizes necessary to carry out research might be so large as to be impractical. I encourage you to consider setting β at .05, not .20.

Because researchers often don't set power in advance, they commonly want to know the statistical power of the test that was just conducted. Given the sample size that we have (in this case 15) and assuming that ρ really equals the observed correlation (in this case .48), how likely is it that we have made a Type II error?* Phrased another way, what is the probability, if the null hypothesis is false, that we will correctly reject it if $N = 15$ and $\rho = .48$? That is a question of statistical power.

Power depends on three things. One is the α level, and this makes a certain sense. If α were set at .25, then it would be much easier to reject the null hypothesis since the rare zone in the sampling distribution would be larger than it is when α is set at .05. When α is larger, since it is easier to reject the null, statistical power is greater. (Remember, power equals the probability of correctly rejecting the null hypothesis.)

Another thing that determines power is the sample size. Larger Ns mean more power! The simplest way to see this is to look at the table of

---

*Why are we willing to assume that $\rho = .48$? Because that is the only information we have! Sure the value may be inaccurate, but do you have anything better to use?

LOOKING CLOSER

critical values of r in the Appendix Table 4. Look down the bolded column and note again that as N increases, r_{cv} decreases. Isn't it easier to reject the null if $r_{cv} = .27$ ($df = 50$) than if $r_{cv} = .38$ ($df = 25$)?

Finally, statistical power depends on the effect size, on how big the correlation is. Look at the eight scatterplots in Figure 8.1 or 8.7. Imagine taking a sample of size 10 from the scatterplot of panel D ($r = .45$) and from panel G ($r = .90$). Which sample of 10 is more likely to allow us to reject the null hypothesis of $\rho = 0$? It would be more likely for the sample from $r = .90$ than from $r = .45$, because we are more likely to get a sample that falls close to the regression line, that has a linear relationship. And since power is the probability of rejecting the null hypothesis, then power is greater for the larger correlation.

Calculating power is a pain, because it depends on these three factors and the formula is complex. No one I know calculates power directly; all rely on tables that do most of the heavy lifting. Typically there are multiple power tables, one for each α level (both one-tailed and two-tailed), in which the rows and columns represent different levels of N and r. Table 7 in the Appendix is a simple one-scenario power table; it shows power for different sample sizes and different rs when, *and only when*, $\alpha = .05$, two-tailed. But, since a two-tailed alpha level of .05 is the most commonly used option, this is not much of a limitation.

Look at the section of Appendix Table 7 shown in Table 8.6. The rows represent different Ns, and the columns represent different r values. Each column represents either the observed r or what you hypothesize as the value in the population, ρ. Note that the values increase by .05 increments. Because statisticians are always conservative and like to underestimate things, we will take a "The Price Is Right" approach: if your exact r or ρ is not available, pick the value that is closest without going over. In the example that we've been working with, $r = .48$, so we'll focus on the column for $r = .45$.

What do we do with N? For sample sizes from 5 to 30, I've tabled each N value, and then I start skipping, first every other, then by 10s, then by 50s, and so on. Use "The Price is Right" approach for N as well: if the exact value isn't there, use the next lower value.

TABLE **8.6**   **Part of Appendix Table 7: Power of Pearson *rs*, $\alpha = .05$, Two-Tailed**

	Observed or Hypothesized *r* Value									
N	.05	.10	.15	.20	.25	.30	.35	.40	.45	.50
5	.02	.03	.04	.04	.05	.06	.07	.08	.10	.11
6	.03	.03	.04	.05	.06	.07	.09	.11	.13	.15
7	.03	.03	.04	.06	.07	.08	.10	.13	.16	.19
8	.03	.04	.05	.06	.08	.10	.12	.15	.19	.23
9	.04	.04	.05	.07	.09	.11	.14	.17	.21	.26

So, how does the table work, and what do the values at the intersection of the rows and columns mean? Let's imagine that we have a sample of size 9, and an observed correlation of .283 in our sample. At the intersection of the highlighted row of $N = 9$ and column of $r = .25$, we find the value of .09. This value, .09, is the power of a correlation with nine cases, where the null hypothesis is false, and where the real ρ is .25: if $\rho = .25$ and you draw a sample of nine cases from the population, then you have only a 9% chance of rejecting the null hypothesis with a two-tailed α set at .05. In such a situation there is less than a 10% chance of correctly rejecting the null hypothesis, and these are not good odds. Phrased differently, β (the probability of making a Type II error) is 91%: there's over a 90% chance that we will make a Type II error if we draw a sample of size nine from the population where $\rho = .25$. Thus, we have likely made an error in failing to reject the null hypothesis. Would it be reasonable to conclude that there is no relationship between X and Y on the basis of our observed correlation of .283? No! Our statistical test was *underpowered,* it didn't have enough cases for us to have a fighting chance to reject the null hypothesis.*

Go down any column in the table and you will note that as N increases, so does the power: given any ρ, when you have a larger N you are more likely to be able to conclude that the relationship between X and Y is statistically different from zero. Similarly, if you go across a row, you will note that power increases as r increases: given any N, it is easier to find a nonzero relationship between X and Y when the relationship between X and Y is stronger. Both of these make sense since we know that power depends on sample size and effect size.

If you turn to the complete table in the Appendix, you'll be able to find that the power for our BMI-cholesterol correlation is .38. That means that *if* the real relationship between BMI and cholesterol were equivalent to $\rho = .45$ *and* if we are doing a two-tailed test with α set at .05 *and* if we have 15 subjects, *then* we have only a 38% chance of correctly rejecting the null hypothesis. Phrased differently, we have a 62% chance of making a Type II error. Thus when our N is only 15, it is very likely that we would end up concluding that BMI has no impact on cholesterol level when it really does if there is a real relationship between the two variables at the .45 level.

With this information we are ready to update our interpretative statement. Before I said that there appeared to be no relationship between

---

*Here's another way to think about what it means to be underpowered. Imagine that there is a nonzero relationship between X and Y in the population, that $\rho = .25$, and that we have drawn a random sample of size nine from that population. How large a correlation must we find to be able to reject the null hypothesis and conclude that there is a nonzero relationship? If $N = 9$, $df = 7$, and $r_{cv} = .67$. Yes, that's right, we'd need to observe a correlation greater than or equal to .67 to conclude that a nonzero relationship exists when $N = 9$ and $\rho = .25$. The odds of drawing a sample of nine cases from a population where $\rho = .25$ and finding $r_{observed} = .67$ are low. We'd need to be quite lucky to end up rejecting H_0.

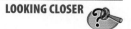

LOOKING CLOSER

BMI and cholesterol level. Now I would say, "Though I have failed to reject the null hypothesis and am forced to conclude that there is no evidence in this sample that a man's body mass index has an impact on his cholesterol level, I do not have faith that these results are true. Given the small sample size, my statistical test was underpowered and has over a 60% chance of leading to the wrong conclusion. I recommend redoing this study with a larger sample size before drawing any conclusions about the relationship between BMI and cholesterol."

It is imperative to calculate power when one fails to reject H_0, but it also makes sense to calculate power when one does reject H_0. Let's imagine that our N had been larger—say, 21—for the BMI-cholesterol study and that we had still found $r = .48$. This would have been significant (r (19) = .48, $p < .05$). Calculating the power, we find that it was .53. Thus we had only a 53% chance of rejecting the null hypothesis, and we did so. Did we just get lucky and correctly reject the null, or did we have a nonrepresentative sample? Calculating power raises that question and should lead to the suggestion that before we conclude that these results are true, we should replicate the study with an adequate N.

This returns us to the question of how we decide what is an adequate value for N. This question was raised in Step 4 of our six-step hypothesis-testing procedure but was left unaddressed, awaiting our arrival at the interpretation phase.

Appendix Table 7 can be used in reverse to figure out sample sizes. Let's take the .48 correlation that I found for my 15 BMI-cholesterol subjects and use it in Appendix Table 7. Taking my conservative "closest-without-going-over" approach, I'm going to use the column with a correlation coefficient of .45. Then, I'm going to proceed down that column until I reach the first row that has power at or above .80. If you look at the complete table in the Appendix, you'll find that the N associated with this is 38. Thus we need at least 38 cases to have a sample size that supports an 80% chance of rejecting the null hypothesis that $\rho = 0$ when ρ really is .45, with $\alpha = .05$ and a two-tailed test.

Appendix Table 8 provides a direct approach to finding the adequate sample size. It gives the values of N needed for different levels of correlations *and* for different levels of power. A section of Appendix Table 8 is shown below in Table 8.7.

The rows in this table represent different levels of ρ; the columns represent different degrees of power. The intersection of a row and column represents the sample size necessary to have the specified degree of statistical power to reject the null hypothesis when the alternative hypothesis (the ρ in the row) is true. Look at the intersection of $\rho = .475$, highlighted, with power = .80: we can see that if $\rho = .475$ and we wish to have a power of .80—to have an 80% chance of being able to reject the null hypothesis—then we need to have at least 34 cases in our sample. (Note that this is not the same value that we found above when we were using Appendix Table 7 backwards; I have made Appendix Table 8 a bit more detailed in terms of the options for the level of the correlation.)

TABLE **8.7** **Part of Appendix Table 8: Values of *N* Necessary to Detect Different Levels of *r* for Different Levels of Power When $\alpha = .05$, Two-Tailed**

	POWER					
r or *p*	.75	.80	.85	.90	.95	.99
.400	43	48	54	63	77	107
.425	38	42	48	55	67	94
.450	34	38	43	49	60	83
.475	30	34	38	44	53	73
.500	27	30	34	39	47	65

Remember the earlier example where $N = 9$ and we hypothesized that $\rho = .25$, and we found that power was less than .10? In the footnote on page 281, I mentioned that with nine cases, the critical value of r is .67, meaning that we would need to find a correlation that large or larger to reject the null hypothesis. Obviously, the odds of drawing a sample in which $r_{observed} \geq .67$ from a population in which $\rho = .25$ are quite low. That's why such a study would be underpowered. If we wanted to have power of .80 where $\rho = .25$, an appropriate N would be 125. Given an N of 125, $r_{cv} \approx .18$. This means that in order to reject the null hypothesis and conclude that there is probably a nonzero correlation in the population, we need to find $r_{observed} \geq .18$. The odds of drawing a sample of 125 cases from a population where $\rho = .25$ and finding $r_{observed}$ of .18 or greater are fairly high. In fact, the chances are 8 out of 10.

The advantage of using Appendix Table 8 over Table 7 backwards is that it allows us to see the sample size required for different levels of power. For our BMI data, if we desire that β, like α, be set at .05 (i.e., that power = .95), then we will need to have at least 53 cases in our sample. Increasing the power from .80 to .95 means increasing the sample size by over half, from 34 to 53.

And, this is why many research studies are underpowered: it takes a lot of cases to have sufficient power, especially if the expected effect is small. Further, studies are underpowered because researchers don't want to think in advance about how large the expected effect is, and when they do think about it they often, optimistically, predict it to be stronger than it really is.

Appendix Table 8 can—and should!—be used in advance of completing a study in order to decide how many cases are needed. This can help a researcher decide whether it is feasible to proceed with a study. Suppose we believe, based on previous research or on theoretical grounds, that the correlation between our two variables is .25. We then need to decide how willing we are to make a Type II error. Say we decide the consequences of a Type II error are just as serious as the consequences of a Type I error and set both at .05. Consulting Appendix Table 8 we learn that we need at least 204 cases to achieve the desired level of power. If it is unlikely that we can obtain 204 cases for our study, we will need to rethink our study before proceeding.

Back in Group Practice 8.3, there was a question involving a nutritionist who did a study on caloric consumption and weight loss and found that $r(9) = -.5578$, $p > .05$. That is, though the correlation was negative (the more calories consumed, the fewer pounds lost), it was not statistically significant. Now that we know about power and sample size, I want to rethink this problem with you. First of all, with $N = 11$, the researcher engaged in an underpowered study, with a power of only about .41. That means that if there really were a relationship between caloric consumption and weight loss (and I think we all agree that there probably is), the researcher had only a 41% chance of finding it with 11 subjects. How many subjects should the researcher have had? Well, one option is to say 25, which is the suggested N for $r = .55$ (remember, we use the absolute value of the correlation in power calculations) and $\beta = .20$. However, we want to make sure that we have enough subjects to find the relationship if it exists and if the relationship is weaker than we thought it was. Thus, it makes sense to base our decision on the lower bound, $-.49$, of the confidence interval that ranged from $-.49$ to $-.95$. Using the "Price-is-Right" value of .475, the calculated minimum N is 34, not 25. Thus, to be safe, and have a fighting chance of rejecting H_0, the researcher should redo the study with at least 34 participants. Being even more conservative, and setting β at .05, yields a sample size of 53. With apologies to the Bauhaus school of architecture, more is more.

Group Practice 8.5

1. Buffy is planning a correlational study. Though she will set her null hypothesis as $\rho_{xy} = 0$, she actually believes that $\rho_{xy} = .38$. (This belief is based on her prior research.) She will do a two-tailed test with α set at .05. How many cases should she have if she wants to have a 20% chance of making a Type II error? A 5% chance?

2. Skip decides to do a research project for his senior-year project. He is interested in the impact of television violence on the behavior of children. He obtains a sample of 19 children in a kindergarten class and finds the number of hours of commercial television each one watches per week. He also has the kindergarten teacher rate, on an interval-level scale where higher numbers indicate greater aggressiveness, how aggressive each child is. He checks the assumptions for a Pearson r and, finding that he has violated none, he calculates r_p as .4330. Using a two-tailed test with α set at .05, interpret his results.

Believe it or not, we are about done with our exploration of the interpretation step of our first null hypothesis significance test. The only thing left to stress is how to begin and how to end your interpretation. It is a good idea to start an interpretation by stating, briefly, what the study was about. This way the interpretation can stand on its own.

Also, by the time you have done all the work for an interpretation, you should have a pretty good sense of the strengths and weaknesses of the research conducted. These insights should not go to waste, so end the

TABLE **8.8** **Interpreting a Pearson Product Moment Correlation Coefficient**

I. State the purpose of the study and the results in APA format.
II. If fail to reject H_0
   A. Report found linear relationship in sample not statistically different from zero
   B. Conclude not sufficient evidence to conclude that linear relationship in population is nonzero
   C. Calculate confidence interval. [Some statisticians recommend calculating and reporting effect sizes (e.g., r^2 and BESD) even when the null hypothesis is not rejected.]
   D. Calculate power and sample size
   E. Discuss possibility of Type II error
   F. Mention strengths, limitations, and/or suggestions
III. If reject H_0
   A. Report found linear relationship in sample statistically different from zero
   B. Conclude linear relationship in population is likely nonzero
   C. Report direction of relationship
   D. Calculate confidence interval
   E. Calculate r^2 and/or BESD
   F. Calculate Y' (and, where appropriate, a prediction interval)
   G. Calculate power and sample size
   I. Discuss possibility of Type I error
   J. Mention strengths, limitations, and/or suggestions

interpretation by discussing the strengths and limitations of the research. Please note that I have been doing this throughout the chapter for the foot size–height data set, that I have noted that my sample came from only one college, that the results cannot be generalized to all college students, and I suggest that the study be redone with a more representative sample. So, use the interpretation section to make suggestions for improving the study. Similarly, you can use the discussion section to spread some praise around. If there was a particular strength of the study—for example, the sample was randomly drawn from the population—mention that as well.

To help guide you in interpreting Pearson correlations, Table 8.8 lists all the interpretative options I have discussed for Pearson correlations. Notice that I am not stating that you must use all of these interpretative options for a Pearson r—they are simply the options from which you can select when you interpret a correlation coefficient.

Why are there so many options? Well, why do I have so many screwdrivers? I just took a walk through my house and found that I have more than a dozen screwdrivers. If all screwdrivers drive screws, just as all measures of effect size measure the size of an effect, then why do I need so many? Well, some are for Phillips-head screws, and some are for flat-head screws; some are for big screws, and some are for small screws. Thus it makes sense to pick the right screwdriver for the job. But, if it is a flat-head screw of a certain size, there are several screwdrivers I could pick. What do I do? I pick the one that is most convenient, or if all are equally convenient, I pick my favorite.* The same is true for statisticians: they develop habitual ways of interpreting results, tried and true methods with which they are comfortable. I taught you a lot of different ways that you can interpret Pearson product moment correlation coefficients so that you will be familiar with them and, for the present, I want you to be able to calculate all of them. But, in the future, I expect that you will select the one that is most appropriate for the task at hand.

To end this chapter, let me do two final interpretations. The first is a complete, final, interpretative statement for the observed correlation (r (4) = .83, $p < .05$) between foot size and height. Note that although I have, throughout this chapter, calculated all the interpretative options for the data, I don't use them all in my interpretation.

"I completed a study in which I examined the relationship between height and foot size for six college students randomly selected from Penn State Erie. The linear relationship observed between height and foot size observed in the sample was statistically different from zero (r (4) = .83, $p < .05$), suggesting that there is a positive (or direct) relationship between height and foot size among college students at Penn State Erie. It appears, in general, that college students at Penn State Erie who have longer feet are also taller. Because the sample size was so small ($N = 6$), the 95% confidence interval within which the correlation between height and foot size in the Penn State Erie population is predicted to fall is quite large, ranging from .04 to .98. Thus, the real relationship between height and foot size in the population may be very strong or quite weak. I recommend replicating this study with a larger sample size to attain adequate power and to get a better estimate of the strength of the linear relationship. Though a sample size of 13 would be adequate if the actual correlation between height and foot size were of the size observed in the current study, I recommend using a larger sample to provide a better estimate of the population value of the correlation. In addition, the original sample was not a random sample from the population of college students, making it difficult to generalize the results to college students in general. I recommend trying to obtain a more representative sample to increase generalizability."[†]

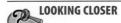

LOOKING CLOSER

*And yes, I do have a favorite screwdriver.

[†]Note that I don't give an exact value for a recommended sample size. I say that $N = 13$ would be adequate, but I recommend using a "larger" sample. If I based sample size on the low end of the confidence interval ($\rho = .04$), I'd recommend having 12,560 cases and this seems absurdly high. So, I'm going to rely on the common sense of the next researcher: 13 cases are enough in terms of power but not adequate for a representative sample.

The other interpretation is for a new example. Imagine that I have gone to New York City and obtained a random sample of married couples who were about to have their first child. To each couple I administered a measure of marital harmony, an interval-level measure scored so that higher scores indicate greater marital harmony. Eighteen years later I administered a measure of psychological health to the 475 children I was able to track down. (There had been 537 couples in the original study.) The measure of psychological health was also an interval-level measure and was scored so that higher scores indicated greater mental health. I found $r = .4482$ with a 95% confidence interval that ranged from .3373 to .5173. With α, two tailed, set at .05, here is my interpretation:

"I completed a study in which I examined the impact of parental marital harmony at the time of the birth of a child on the child's psychological health 18 years later. I found a direct linear relationship between parental marital harmony and the psychological well-being of that child that was statistically different from zero (r (473) = .45, $p < .05$). This relationship indicates that the children of couples with more marital harmony at the time of the birth are more likely to have greater degrees of psychological health when they are young adults.

"The relationship appears to be meaningful and at least moderately strong. Since I had a random sample of couples from New York City who were about to have their first child, I can generalize to this population. I am 95% certain that the level of the relationship in this population between marital harmony and the child's psychological health 18 years later falls in the range from .34 to .52. If the relationship is at the low end of this range (.34), this translates into a child who is born to parents above average in terms of marital harmony having a 67% chance of turning out above average in terms of psychological health. This is in contrast to the 33% chance that a child born to parents below average in terms of marital harmony would have to turn out above average in psychological health. Thus, as the actual correlation in the population is likely .34 or higher, having maritally harmonious parents at birth seems to more than double a child's likelihood of being psychologically healthy as he or she enters adulthood.

"There is, of course, a chance that this conclusion is in error and that there really is no relationship between parental marital harmony and a child's psychological outcome. Though the relatively large sample size in the present study makes this less tenable, it still is advisable to replicate the findings before making any policy decisions based on these results.

"There are a few strengths and limitations of the present study worth noting. A strength is that the sample size was large and the study had adequate power for rejecting the null hypothesis. Four limitations are worth noting. First, the results are based on a sample from New York City, so they may only apply to people from large, diverse urban settings in the northeastern United States. Secondly, they are based on the outcomes of first children, and so the results may not apply to later-born children. Third, the only couples included in this study were married

couples, and so the results cannot be generalized to single parents or unmarried couples. The fourth limitation is the most serious: since this was a correlational study, we cannot draw cause-and-effect conclusions. It does seem reasonable to believe that couples with greater relationship harmony will produce children who are psychologically healthier. However, this study does not prove that one causes the other. It is a viable possibility that some other variable, for example socioeconomic status, causes both. Perhaps having more financial resources yields both more harmonious relationships and happier children."

OUTLIER ADDENDUM TO CHAPTER 8

This section is an addendum, something that I want to mention but that I am not sure where to place. Logically, it should have gone in the previous chapter where I talked about making scatterplots, but you didn't have enough knowledge about correlations to understand it then. You do now; so, here it is.

What I am talking about is outliers, data points that fall far away from the rest of the data set and that have an unusually large influence on a correlation. When you make a scatterplot I want you to keep an eye out for them, and here is why. Figure 8.13, *A* shows a scatterplot for a small data set that has no outliers. There is no relationship between *X* and *Y*; $r = 0$, as indicated by the rectangular shape of the data and the horizontal position of the regression line. No matter the *X*, our predicted *Y*, *Y*′, is always the same, M_Y. However, note what happens when I add an outlier, the data point in the upper right hand corner of Figure 8.13, *B*. That single data point changes the correlation from $r = 0$ to $r = .71$ and redraws the regression line.

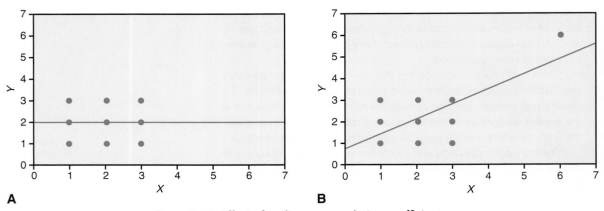

A　　　　　　　　　　　　　　　　　　**B**

Figure **8.13** Effect of outliers on correlation coefficients.

Outliers are a problem because they change the value of a correlation, either increasing it or decreasing it. How do you decide whether a data point is an outlier and what do you do about it? Deciding whether a data point is an outlier is a subjective affair. An outlier is a data point with an abnormally high or low value. And yet, what *I* think is far enough away from normal to be an outlier may not be what *you* think is far enough away from normal. The simplest test for an outlier is to eyeball the scatterplot—and at this point that is all that I am suggesting that you do.*

Once you have identified an outlier, you must decide what to do with it. First, check whether it is a data entry error. If so, correct it. If it is not a data entry error, it probably is a rare but possible event. After all, even in the middle of summer there is occasionally a very cold day.

However, that rare event can seriously distort a correlation and thus the interpretation. If you were looking at the correlation between temperature and heat stroke and, in your random sample of summer days had one day in which the high temperature was 20° F, might that not affect your results by making the linear relationship between temperature and heat stroke look different than it is?

So, what to do? One option is to delete outliers from analysis. But, that is not satisfactory, since the definition of outliers is subjective and you leave yourself open to questions as to whether you simply deleted data points because they failed to help make your case. Additionally, those data points do really exist, so you also leave yourself open to questions as to whether you are representing reality in your analysis.

Another option is to scale your data down to the ordinal level and use what are called nonparametric statistics.[†] A correlation like Spearman's *r*, because it is based on ranks and not on actual values of the data, is less affected by outliers.

A third option, and one that I like as much as using a nonparametric statistic, is to do the analysis both ways and report both ways. That is, do the analysis with the outlier in place, report that one is concerned about the effect of the outlier, and then redo the analysis without the outlier. As the outlier represents a real data point, this serves to give an idea of the range within which the real correlation probably falls.

---

*If you want to do more, here's what SPSS® does. Calculate the interquartile range *(IQR)* and then add 1.5 *IQR*s to the top of the *IQR* range and subtract 1.5 *IQR*s from the bottom of the *IQR* range. Any value that is more than 1.5 *IQR*s beyond the *IQR* is an outlier.

[†] I haven't given them this title yet, but statistics like Spearman's *r* or the chi-square are called nonparametrics because to use them one doesn't need to make assumptions about the skewness and kurtosis, the parameters, of the data.

LOOKING CLOSER

SUMMARY

Interpreting the results of a statistical test means explaining, in clear English, what the results mean. This is a subjective enterprise: just as people can disagree over whether a glass is half full or half empty, different people may interpret the same correlation differently. This does not mean that all interpretations are correct (after all, there is water in the glass), only that different people can perceive, or interpret, the same result differently.

Interpretation involves commenting on the direction (direct, inverse, or zero) and strength of the observed linear relationship. The strength of a correlation can be examined in general—that is, for all cases; or in specific—that is, for individual cases. Overall strength can be assessed by examining the 95% confidence interval, which tells the range within which we predict ρ is likely to fall, the coefficient of determination, which tells how much of the variability in one variable can be predicted by knowing the other, or the binomial effect size display, which tells how likely a case is to be above average on one variable if it is above average on the other. The specific strength of a correlation is examined by predicting a case's score on one variable from its known score on the other variable; the inaccuracy of this is shown by calculating the 95% prediction interval, the range within which we are reasonably confident that a case's actual score on the criterion variable will fall.

How results are interpreted depends in part on whether the results showed a correlation statistically different from zero. If the relationship were statistically different from zero, then all of the above applies. If the results were not statistically different from zero, then since there is no reason to conclude that there is a relationship between the two variables in the population, we are not interested in predicting one variable—either in general or in specific—from the other. However, since we would now be concerned with having made a Type II error, we would be concerned with calculating β, the probability of this. In addition, interpreting results when we fail to

reject the null hypothesis is more challenging since all that we can conclude is that the results are not statistically different from zero. Finding someone not guilty is not the same as finding him or her innocent.

Power, which is equal to one minus β, is the probability of correctly rejecting the null hypothesis. The commonly accepted minimum for power is .80, which means that there is a 20% chance of making a Type II error. I advocate setting power at .95, which puts the chance of a Type II error at the same level as the commonly set level of Type I error.

Power depends on sample size, alpha, and effect size, so calculating power leads to thinking about what sample size is necessary to be able correctly to reject the null hypothesis. Thus, in this chapter we learned how to find the sample size necessary to have a reasonable chance of meeting our goal of rejecting the null hypothesis. We also learned that it is wise to think about this in advance to make sure that the study is not underpowered.

Outliers are data points that fall far away from the rest of the data and change the value of a correlation coefficient, either inflating it or deflating it, sometimes dramatically. Scatterplots should always be inspected for outliers. If outliers exist, I suggest calculating the correlation coefficient twice, once with all the data and once with the outliers excluded.

Two other interpretative concerns were highlighted in this chapter: the difference between prediction *in general* vs. prediction *in specific*, and the fact that correlation is not causation. Correlation coefficients calculate the degree of relationship, in general, between two variables. Thus a correlation coefficient might be strong enough to say that, in general, people with higher SAT scores obtain higher GPAs. Still, many of us know someone who doesn't do well on standardized tests but who does well in school, or someone who does well on standardized tests but who is a slacker with regard to schoolwork. Thus the overall relationship between SAT and GPA is not correct for these people. When correlations are used to predict the performance of an individual case, even when the correlation is strong and meaningful in general, the range within which the prediction for the individual case falls is often so large as to be of little use. Correlations are meant to capture an overall relationship; when we use them to predict the score for an individual case we need to accept their limitations.

The four most important words in statistics are "Correlation is not causation." The existence of an association, a correlation, between X and Y does not mean that X causes Y. That certainly is one possibility, but it is also possible that Y causes X or that some other variable causes both X and Y. A correlation coefficient merely reports the degree of association between two variables; it is mum on the topic of causality. That is where you come in as the interpreter, either to address cause and effect or to caution the reader from drawing a cause-and-effect conclusion.

Review Exercises

1. You have completed a study in which you took a random sample ($N = 2512$) of college-bound high-school seniors from the United States and found out their combined SAT scores (i.e., the verbal score plus the quantitative score). You then waited until the end of their first year of college, wherever they went, and obtained their GPAs. No assumptions were violated. You correlated the two variables and found that $r = .3714$. Interpret this correlation.

2. Complete the final step of Tom-and-Harry, interpretation, for Chapter 7 Review Exercise 1. If someone is admitted to the intensive care unit (ICU) with an APACHE III score of 231, about a half standard deviation above the mean in terms of severity of illness, what is your prediction for how long he or she will stay in the ICU? Don't forget to calculate the 95% prediction interval for this. (By the bye, $N = 9$, $M_X = 195.000$, $s_X = 71.9182$, $M_Y = 7.5556$, $s_Y = 3.8905$, and $r_{xy} = .8419$.)

3. Complete the final step of Tom-and-Harry, interpretation, for Chapter 7 Review Exercise 3. If a child's vision score is 75, how many balls do you predict that he or she will catch? Don't forget the prediction interval. (By the bye, $N = 10$, $r_{xy} = -.0224$, $M_X = 100.0000$, $s_X = 41.5331$, $M_Y = 33.4000$, and $s_Y = 19.3298$.)

4. I am doing a study in which I believe that ρ really does equal .45. I will do a two-tailed test with α set at .05 and β set at .20. How many subjects do I need? If I set β at .05, what impact will that have on the number of subjects I need? If I change α to .01, how many subjects will I need?

5. Desdemona weighed herself on a scale measuring to the nearest half-pound before she started on a diet, and she weighed 135.5 pounds. Two weeks later she weighed 131.0. What is the most weight she could have lost? The least?

6. A school nurse is interested in finding the best way to put bandages on skinned elbows. Whenever a child comes into her office with a skinned elbow she flips a coin. If the coin turns up heads, she has the child bend his or her arm while she applies the bandage. If the coin turns up tails, she has the child keep his or her arm straight while she applies the bandage. The next day she checks whether the bandage is still in place. What is her dependent variable? Her independent variable?

7. Suppose postoperative quality of life (QOL) is normally distributed and scaled on a score that has a mean of 100 and a standard deviation of 25. Further, imagine that surgeons consider a bad outcome anyone who ends with a QOL score of 70 or below. What percentage of the time should a surgeon obtain a bad outcome?

Homework Problems

1. The difference between a correlation being meaningful in general but not in specific is the same as the difference between which of the following?
   a. Y' and the 95% prediction interval
   b. Setting α at .05 and β at .20
   c. The coefficient of determination and the binomial effect size display
   d. The binomial effect size display and the 95% prediction interval
   e. None of the above

2. A researcher has calculated a 95% confidence interval for a correlation as ranging from .03 to .30. Which of the following should the researcher do?
   a. Reject the null hypothesis
   b. Fail to reject the null hypothesis
   c. Worry about having made a Type II error
   d. Say that the correlation is so weak as to be meaningless

3. I am testing the null hypothesis that $\rho = 0$. What happens as the actual value of the correlation in the population increases from zero?
   a. Power increases.
   b. The N needed to have an 80% chance of rejecting the null hypothesis for a correlation coefficient decreases.
   c. β decreases.
   d. All of the above
   e. None of the above

4. If $r^2 = .36$, what is the probability of a person who has an above average score on X also having an above average score on Y?
   a. 18%
   b. 30%
   c. 50%
   d. 68%
   e. 80%

5. If $r(198) = .10$, $p > .05$, then what would we conclude about the direction of the observed linear relationship between X and Y?
   a. It is probably direct.
   b. It is probably inverse.
   c. There is no evidence it is not zero.
   d. It is probably sloped.

6. You have completed a study on a random sample of 638 adults in the United States who had had the flu. For each person you obtained an interval-level measure of his or her general level of physical health (higher scores meant they were healthier) and found the number of days he or she had been ill with the flu. No assumptions were violated, and you calculated $r = -.4612$. Interpret this correlation.

7. Complete the final step of Tom and Harry, interpretation, for Chapter 7 Homework Problem 7. If a person took fluoride treatment for 9 years, half of his or her childhood, how many cavities do you predict that he or she will have? Don't forget the prediction interval. (By the bye, $N = 12$, $r_{xy} = -.9051$, $M_X = 8.1667$, $s_x = 6.9502$, $M_Y = 4.5000$, and $s_Y = 2.9011$.)

8. Complete the final step of Tom and Harry, interpretation, for Chapter 7 Homework Problem 8. If Skip's machismo score is 35, what do you predict as his heart rate in this stressful situation? (By the bye, $N = 9$, $r_{xy} = -.1143$, $M_X = 28.6667$, $s_x = 14.9369$, $M_Y = 77.1111$, and $s_Y = 15.0144$.)

9. A sociologist wants to investigate the impact of unemployment on suicide rates. He obtains data from 25 cities about their unemployment rates in one year and their suicide rates the following year. He then correlates these two variables. Label these variables as independent and dependent variables or as predictor and criterion variables. Which is correct?

10. Given the following data, calculate the Pearson product moment correlation coefficient. Don't worry about whether any assumptions have been violated, just find r.

X	Y
7	5
5	8
3	6
8	3
11	10

9

Two-Sample Difference Tests

The Independent-Samples *t* Test

Learning Objectives

After completing this chapter, you should be able to do the following:

1 Differentiate difference tests from relationship tests and independent samples from dependent samples; select the appropriate difference test to answer a research question.
2 Evaluate the assumptions, explain the hypotheses, and state the decision rule for an independent-samples *t* test; know what to do if the assumptions for the independent-samples *t* test are not met.
3 Explain the effect of alpha, the number of tails, and sample size on the critical value of *t*.
4 Calculate the standard error of the difference, the pooled variance, and $t_{observed}$.
5 Determine if the observed value of *t* falls in the rare zone or the common zone of the sampling distribution, and tell the direction of the difference between population means.
6 Interpret the strength and practical significance of an independent-samples *t* test using (a) a 95% confidence interval for the difference between population means, (b) the standardized difference between means, (c) the percentage of variance in the dependent variable predicted by the independent variable, (d) *r*, or (e) a binomial effect size.
7 Determine the power of an independent-samples *t* test and the sample size necessary to have an independent-samples *t* test with sufficient power.

In this chapter we move on to our second statistical test, the independent-samples *t* test. The independent-samples *t* test is a two-sample difference test, one of the most frequently used tests in statistics. Two-sample difference tests compare, for example, an experimental group to a control group to see if they differ on some outcome variable.

There are just a few new concepts in this chapter. I spend some time discussing the different difference tests and how they vary in terms of the number of samples, the type of samples (independent vs. dependent), and the number of independent, or grouping, variables. The dependent-independent samples distinction is new; dependent samples occur when the selection of cases for one sample influences or determines the cases selected for the other sample. Another new concept arises in the interpretation phase when we learn a new measure of effect size, *d*, that tells how far apart two means are in standard deviation units.

Otherwise, this chapter covers old ground from a new perspective. Note that in the interpretation phase we will be concerned with (a) whether the difference between two sample means is statistically different from zero, (b) the direction of the difference, (c) the size, or meaningfulness of the difference, and (d) the type of error that could have been made.

Though this chapter focuses on two-sample difference tests, I will introduce you to multiple-sample and one-sample tests as well. I'll cover multiple-sample tests in detail in the next two chapters. I'll mention one-sample tests in this chapter, but I won't cover the calculations for them.

In the last two chapters we covered the Pearson product moment correlation coefficient, a relationship test, as our first null hypothesis statistical test. Now it is time to turn to a different type of null hypothesis test: difference tests.

Imagine data from a sample of students where I have their scores on the first two exams in a class. One question I could ask of these data concerns *patterns*, such as, "Is the pattern of scores on the first test similar to the pattern of scores on the second?" That is, if a student performed relatively well on the first test, is he or she likely to perform relatively well on the second?

Another type of question I could ask concerns *level*. For example, were the scores on the two tests at the same level, or was one test harder than the other? This question could be answered by seeing if the average grades on the two tests were comparable.

The pattern question and the level question are two different questions, and it is possible to imagine many combinations of answers. Perhaps the pattern of scores is similar, but one test was harder than the other. Or, maybe the two tests were equally difficult, but a student's score on one test wasn't predictive of his or her score on the other.

Tests that examine patterns are relationship tests—correlations—and tests that examine level are difference tests. There are times that we'll want to ask both types of questions about the same set of data, and there will be times that only one type of question is appropriate. In this chapter we'll examine difference tests: tests that compare samples to see if they differ in their level of the dependent variable.

You can think of relationship tests as examining the degree of relationship between two variables, X and Y, in *one* sample of cases. The difference tests that we'll start with, two-sample difference tests, have *two* samples of cases, not one as in a relationship test. These samples differ on some grouping variable* and are compared to see if they differ in the amount of the dependent variable that each group contains. For example, a sample of boys and a sample of girls can be compared to see which can run faster. In this case the grouping variable is gender (boys vs. girls), and the dependent variable is running speed.

TWO-SAMPLE DIFFERENCE TESTS

Two-sample difference tests are some of the most commonly used statistical tests. When you think of an experiment, you probably think of two groups, an experimental group and a control group. The experimental group is given the experimental treatment and the control group is not. The outcome variable, the dependent variable, is then measured, and the question to be answered is whether the two groups differ on the outcome variable.

How common is this scenario? Every Tuesday *The New York Times* publishes a special section called "Science Times" that, cleverly, is all about science. The topics covered on a day when I was writing this section (September 7, 2004) are examples of data that should be analyzed using two-sample difference tests:

- Diabetics who get their exercise by walking *down*hill (sample 1) had a bigger improvement in glucose tolerance (the dependent variable) than did diabetics who got their exercise by walking *up*hill (sample 2).
- Some burrowing owls spread cow and horse dung around their nesting holes (sample 1), and some don't (sample 2). Those that decorate with dung catch and eat up to 10 times more beetles (the dependent variable) than do those that don't decorate with dung.

---

*The grouping variable represents the basis on which the groups differ. Often the grouping variable is an independent variable, but not always. Remember, an independent variable is one that the experimenter controls or manipulates. Thus gender, when comparing a group of boys to a group of girls, is a grouping variable, not an independent variable.

LOOKING CLOSER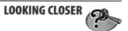

- Does taking a drink of alcohol before bed help one sleep? Sample 1 consisted of people taking a drink before bed and sample 2 of people who didn't take a drink; the dependent variable was sleep quality. (In case you want to know, alcohol doesn't improve sleep quality.)
- People who complete cardiac rehabilitation programs after a heart attack (sample 1) are 5 times less likely to die (the dependent variable) than those who do not take part in cardiac rehabilitation (sample 2).
- Parents of pediatric patients who are given "prescriptions" for medical information Internet sites (sample 1) use the Internet significantly more (the dependent variable) than do parents who aren't given the "prescriptions" (sample 2).

Just as with correlation coefficients, we are not really interested in the specific samples being studied—we want to make inferences about the larger populations from which the samples are drawn. That is, with the diabetes example above, we don't really care that in this specific group of 45 diabetics, those who exercised by walking downhill showed better glucose tolerance than did those who walked uphill. We care about whether these results apply to the larger population of diabetics.

With correlations, we call the result statistically different from zero, or statistically significant, if we conclude that the result observed in the sample is unlikely to occur if the null hypothesis is true. And, we infer from this that there is a linear relationship between the two variables in the population. We'll use similar logic with two-sample difference tests where we address the question, "How big must the difference be between *two samples* before we decide that it reflects a real difference between the *two populations*—that it is not simply due to sampling error?"

This question can be asked of interval- and ratio-level data, of ordinal data, or of nominal data, and it can be asked if the samples are independent or dependent. There are different tests to be used in each of these six situations. You already know how to differentiate interval and ratio from ordinal and ordinal from nominal. But the independent/dependent samples distinction is a new one, so let me explain it to you.

INDEPENDENT VS. DEPENDENT SAMPLES

independent samples

Samples where the selection of cases for one sample has no influence on the selection of cases for the other sample(s).

"**Independent samples**" refers to samples in which the cases in one sample are independent of the cases in the other sample. They are called *independent* because the way in which cases are selected for one sample has no impact on how the cases are selected for the other sample; the cases in one sample exert no influence on the selection of, *are independent of*, the cases in the other sample.

As an example, suppose that we want to compare the intelligence of men to the intelligence of women. We could draw a random sample of men from the population of men and draw a random sample of women from the population of women. Since the men selected for the male sample have no impact on who is in the sample of women, these two samples are independent.

Here's another way that we could obtain the two samples, a way that would lead to **dependent samples:** we obtain a random sample of men from the population of men and then ask each man to bring a woman with him to the testing session. These samples are not independent since who is in one sample, the women, *depends* on who is in the other sample. The composition of one sample influences the composition of the other, so the samples are dependent.

Samples can often be gathered either way. Sometimes it makes more sense to answer the question being asked by using independent samples, and sometimes dependent samples make more sense. In the example above, comparing intelligence of men to women, it makes more sense to have independent samples since that better addresses the question being asked.

But, here's an example where dependent samples seem more appropriate. Suppose that we want to compare the prices at two grocery stores. If we use *independent* samples, then we get a list of all the items at store A and randomly select items from that list to make up the sample for store A. We also get a list of all the items for sale at store B and randomly select items from that list to get the sample for store B. Since each store contains thousands of items, I can almost guarantee that the two samples will have very little overlap. Thus, for example, at one store we might have steak in our sample and at the other we might have bananas.

My guess is that this doesn't seem very fair to you, that it doesn't seem right. What seems intuitively right is to have the same items in our shopping carts at both stores, to have the items in the shopping cart at the second store *depend* on what was in the cart at the first store. Thus, we might draw a random sample of items from one store and then select the same items for our sample at the other store.*

Dependent samples are also called "paired" or "correlated" samples. They are called paired samples because they involve pairs of items, such as husbands and wives, or siblings. And they are called correlated samples because the samples are *related* to each other, again like husbands and wives or siblings. In addition, there are two specific types of dependent samples, matched samples and pre-post samples.

---

*Let me defend independent samples for my grocery store example. If our Ns were large enough and if we used random sampling, we should end up with samples that were representative of each store. Thus if one store carried more expensive items than the other store (e.g., steak, macadamia nuts, imported beer), we would confirm exactly that point: the items at this store are more expensive. The question being answered by an independent-samples test, then, is a little different from the question being answered by a dependent-samples test. A dependent-samples test for the grocery store example answers the question whether, *for the same items*, the two stores differ in price. The independent-samples test answers the question whether one store has higher-priced items than the other. Whether you choose to use independent or dependent samples depends, in good part, on the question you are asking. (Though as we'll see, dependent-samples tests have the advantage of having more power, of making it more likely that one will be able to reject the null hypothesis).

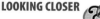 **LOOKING CLOSER**

matched samples

Samples that are equalized on a third variable.

pre-post sample

A group of cases that is followed over time. Also called a longitudinal sample.

Matching, which yields **matched samples,** involves trying to equalize two samples on a third, or *confounding,* variable. A confounding variable is another variable, other than the independent variable, that the researcher thinks might influence the results. For example, in 2004 researchers reported that long-term use of methamphetamine (speed) caused destruction of brain tissue (Thompson et al.*). The researchers used magnetic resonance imaging (MRI) to examine the brains of a group of methamphetamine addicts who had been using the drug for at least 10 years and compared their brains to the brains of control cases who had never used the drug. However, since it was possible that as people get older some brain tissue dies, the researchers *matched* the control group to the experimental group in terms of age. Thus, when they found a difference between the two groups, they could discount the possibility that it was due to an age difference between the two groups.

Pre-post, or **longitudinal, samples** are another type of dependent, or correlated, sample. In a longitudinal or pre-post design, one group of cases is followed over time. For example, the degree of headache pain people feel might be measured before they take aspirin and again an hour later. Since a case can't be in the post group unless it was in the pre group, this is another example of dependent samples. Often the pretest is called Time 1, abbreviated T1, and the post-test is called Time 2 (T2).

Just as it is important to know the level of measurement of the dependent variable to select the right statistical test, you must know whether you are working with independent or dependent samples. The simplest way to think about these two types of samples is to think of the criterion of random sampling. If each sample is a random sample from its respective population, then the samples are independent. If each is not a random sample, then examine how the two samples are gathered to see if there is any connection between them or any way the selection of one sample influences the selection of the other. If there is, the samples are dependent; if not, consider the samples independent.

Another way to differentiate independent from dependent samples is to think about sample sizes. Think of the *independent samples* grocery store example earlier. Isn't it possible that one sample would have 17 items in it and the other would have 21, that is, that the two sample sizes would be different? But wait: we can't have different sample sizes for dependent (paired) samples! So, if the two sample sizes are different, or could be different, we have independent samples. If the two sample sizes are the same, we could have either independent or dependent samples.

Since there are three levels of measurement for the dependent variable and two types of samples, there are six two-sample difference tests (listed in Table 9.1) that you will need to know about. Though in this chapter we shall only learn to calculate one, the independent-samples *t* test, you must know about the other five to answer the "what test when" question.

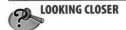 **LOOKING CLOSER**

*Thompson, et al. (2004). Structural abnormalities in the brains of human subjects who use methamphetamine. *The Journal of Neuroscience,* 24(6), 6028-6036.

TABLE **9.1** **Two-Sample Difference Tests**

	LEVEL OF MEASUREMENT OF DEPENDENT VARIABLE		
	Interval/ratio	Ordinal	Nominal
Independent Samples	Independent-samples *t* test	Mann Whitney *U* test	Chi-square difference test
Dependent Samples	Dependent-samples *t* test	Binomial sign test	McNemar test

If a researcher has interval- or ratio-level data *and* independent samples *and* the relevant assumptions have been met, then the appropriate two-sample test is the independent-samples *t* test. This test is sometimes called the Student's *t* test because the man who developed it, William Sealy Gossett, published under the pseudonym "Student."* There is also a version of the *t* test, the dependent-samples *t* test (also known as the paired-samples *t* test or the correlated-samples *t* test) that can be used when one has interval- or ratio-level data and dependent samples.†

For ordinal data and independent samples, the test to choose is the Mann Whitney *U*. For ordinal data and dependent samples, use the binomial sign test. For nominal-level data and independent samples, the chi-square difference test is the correct choice. For nominal-level data and dependent samples, use the McNemar test. Though I expect you to know when to use all of these, we won't learn how to calculate the Mann Whitney *U*, the binomial test, or the McNemar test.

MULTIPLE-SAMPLE AND ONE-SAMPLE DIFFERENCE TESTS

Two samples, as used in the context of two-sample significant difference tests, refers to how many samples or groups the researcher is comparing.‡ I would like to introduce you now to two other types of difference tests: multiple-sample and one-sample difference tests.

---

*Why did he publish under a pseudonym? According to Salsburg (2001), he worked for the Guinness Brewing Company (yes, that Guinness!), and they had forbidden their employees from publishing anything for fear of giving away any of their beer-making secrets. So, to protect his job he published under a pseudonym. (Salsburg, D. [2001]. *The lady tasting tea: how statistics revolutionized science in the twentieth century.* New York: W. H. Freeman and Company.)

†I'll explain, when we get to Chapter 11, why I prefer a test called repeated measures analysis of variance over the dependent-samples *t* test. For now, for the sake of simplicity and symmetry, I'm sticking with the dependent-samples *t* test.

‡Sometimes this is hard to figure out on account of the way language is used. Thus a researcher might talk about obtaining one sample from a population, a sample that she divides into three groups. Does she have one sample or three? Assuming that she's comparing group A to group B to group C, she has three samples.

LOOKING CLOSER

Sometimes the question that we want to answer is more complex than simply comparing an experimental group to a control group; sometimes we need more samples. For example, we may want to compare different pain relievers (e.g., aspirin, acetaminophen, ibuprofen, and placebo) to see which is more effective. Suppose we do this by taking a group of people with pain and randomly assigning each one to receive a different drug. Because we have four samples, one for each drug, this is considered a **multiple-sample difference test.** To be more specific, this is called a **one-way** or a **one-factor test** where the word "way" or "factor" refers to the number of independent variables. In this example there is one independent variable (type of drug) with four **levels,** or categories (aspirin, acetaminophen, ibuprofen, and placebo).

It is also possible to have multiple ways or multiple factors, to have multiple independent variables. For example, we might have samples of men and samples of women who are randomly assigned to receive the four different drugs. Thus we have two independent variables, drug and gender, where the first independent variable (drug) has four levels and the second (the grouping variable, gender) has two levels. This type of study is called a **factorial design** to indicate that there is more than one factor, or a two-way design to indicate that there are two independent variables. It is also called a *4 × 2* (pronounced "four by two") design to indicate that there are four levels of one independent variable and two levels of the other independent variable. Since it doesn't matter which independent variable is first or which is second, this study could also be called a *2 × 4* design.

Factorial designs can get even more complex. We might be interested in the effects of these drugs on different types of pain in the two genders. That is, we might be interested in their effectiveness on headache pain, back pain, and dental surgery pain. Thus, our factorial design would now be a three-way design, a *4 × 3 × 2* design (i.e., four levels of drug, three levels of pain, and two levels of gender). Though the number of factors is unlimited (we could add pain tolerance, prior experience with analgesics, age, etc.), there are practical reasons for limiting them. First, the sample size gets large. If we stayed with our *4 × 3 × 2* design, we would have 24 cells to fill. (A **cell** is what we call each intersection of the factors.) Thus, one cell—or sample—is men with headache pain receiving aspirin, another is men with back pain receiving aspirin, and so on. If each cell has five cases, we would need to have 120 participants in all. If we added pain tolerance (high, medium, and low) as another factor, we would triple the number of participants needed. That's a lot of subjects.

Another reason to limit the number of factors is that as the number of factors increases, interpretation of the results gets more difficult. When there is more than one factor, statisticians calculate the interaction effect, which is how two or more factors influence each other. With the *4 × 2* (drugs and gender) study, there is one interaction effect (drugs by gender), and it examines whether the drugs work differently for the different genders. If we move to a *4 × 3 × 2* study (drugs, type of pain, and gender), we now have four interaction effects to worry about: drugs by pain,

---

multiple-sample difference test

A difference test involving more than two samples.

---

one-factor test

A difference test with only one grouping or independent variable. Also called a one-way test.

---

levels

Categories of a grouping or independent variable.

---

factorial design

A study design having more than one grouping or independent variable.

---

cell

Each level in a one-way design or the intersection of two or more grouping or independent variables; each cell is equivalent to a sample.

drugs by gender, pain by gender, and drugs by pain by gender. In the terminology that statisticians use, those are two-way interactions (drugs by pain, drugs by gender, and pain by gender) and a three-way interaction (drugs by pain by gender). Two-way interactions are relatively easy to interpret, and three-way interactions are interpretable. But once one gets to four-way interactions (e.g., type of drug by type of pain by level of pain tolerance by gender)—well, many statisticians just throw up their hands and ignore them.

I have two more things to say about multiple-sample significant difference tests and then we'll let them lie fallow for a few chapters. First, one can have either independent or dependent samples with multiple-sample significance tests. When the samples are dependent, the multiple-sample significant difference tests are called **repeated measures tests.** For example, each person could receive, in a random order, each of the four drugs. In addition, we could measure the effect of each of the four drugs on pain at three points in time (at time of ingestion, 1 hour later, and 2 hours later). This would be a two-way design with two repeated measures (drugs and time) with four levels of one independent variable (drug) and three levels of the other (time).

And finally, it is possible to mix independent and dependent samples. For example, rather than giving each participant each drug, we could randomly assign each participant to receive only one drug and then measure the effect of that drug at the three points in time. This is still a *4 × 3* design, but only one of the factors is a repeated measure.

Having learned about multiple-sample difference tests, let's turn to **one-sample difference tests.** One-sample difference tests are, as you might guess, used when the researcher has only one sample of cases, or one group. To what is the sample being compared to find out if there is a significant difference? To the population.

Why would you want to do this? Well, most commonly one-sample tests are used to see whether a sample is representative of or comes from a population. For example, suppose that I obtain a sample of adults from the United States and find out how likely they are to get vaccinated for the flu next year. In your role as the National Vaccination Czar, before you make any decision about how much flu vaccine to produce for next year based on my sample results, you should be reasonably certain that the sample is a good one—that is, that it is representative of the population of the United States. If I tell you that my sample is not statistically different from the American population in terms of age, race, gender, marital status, and so on, wouldn't that support the notion that the sample may also be similar to the U.S. population in terms of flu vaccine behavior? Thus, I could use one-sample tests to compare the information from my sample to the information from the U.S. census data to see if there are any statistically significant differences.

There are three one-sample difference tests displayed in Table 9.2. If you have nominal data (e.g., race or marital status), then the appropriate test to choose, if assumptions are not violated, is the chi-square

repeated measures test

A difference test for dependent samples.

one-sample difference test

A difference test in which a sample is compared to a population.

TABLE **9.2**   **One-Sample Significant Difference Tests**

Level of Measurement of Dependent Variable	Test Choice
Interval/ratio	One sample t test
Ordinal	Kolmogorov-Smirnov goodness-of-fit test
Nominal	Chi-square goodness-of-fit

goodness-of-fit test, often abbreviated as χ^2 *GOF*. If you have ordinal-level data, rank data, and assumptions are not violated, choose the Kolmogorov-Smirnov goodness-of-fit test. If you have interval- or ratio-level data, such as age or income, and if assumptions are not violated, choose the one-sample t test. Again, though I expect you to know when to use these, we won't be learning how to calculate them. There has to be some reason to take another statistics course.

Group Practice 9.1

1. For each scenario, (i) list the grouping variables; (ii) count the number of levels; (iii) count the samples being compared; (iv) write the research question using either the word "relationship" or "difference"; and (v) decide what statistical test should be used to answer the question. When answering the "what test when" part of the question, be as specific as possible. You have 15 tests to choose from: three relationship tests, six two-sample difference tests, three one-sample difference tests, and three multiple-sample difference tests (one-way, factorial, and repeated measures). Plus, I may throw you a curve and present a scenario for which we don't have a test.

    (HINT: To find the number of samples involved, draw the design as a matrix. The number of cells in the matrix is the number of samples/groups.)

    a. A psychologist compares gender (boys vs. girls) *and* handedness (right-handed vs. left-handed) to see which group has the fastest reaction time.

    b. A cardiologist compares resting heart rates of people who live in multistory apartment buildings with elevators, multistory apartment buildings without elevators, ranch-style houses, and multistory houses.

    c. An industrial/organizational psychologist compares an interval-level job satisfaction rating given by respiratory therapists to the known average country-wide rating of job satisfaction for workers in general.

    d. An economist has a sample of 100 factories in which he is examining the relationship between average age of the work force at the factory and the factory's absentee rate.

2. For each scenario, (i) identify the samples as independent or dependent, and (ii) decide what statistical test should be used to answer the question. (See question 1 for guidelines in answering the "what test when" part of the question.)

    a. A swimming coach compares the times of male and female swimmers in the 400-meter individual medley at the summer Olympics.

    b. A researcher for an automobile company compares reaction times in a driving simulator between people who are regular drinkers of alcohol and people who never drink alcohol. (All are sober at the time of testing.)

    c. A school principal gets a sample of families with two, and *only* two children, and compares high school grade point average (GPA) for the first child to that for the second child.

Group Practice 9.1—cont'd

d. A political scientist gets representative samples of college students from two types of colleges: large, state universities and small, liberal arts colleges. For each student she measures his or her degree of political conservatism on an interval-level scale at the start of college, then waits 4 years and measures his or her degree of conservatism again. She wants to know whether political conservatism changes over time and whether this change is different in large, public universities vs. small, liberal arts colleges.

e. A drug company is developing a drug that its researchers think will slow the development of Alzheimer's disease. They take a group of people in early stages of Alzheimer's, administer an interval-level test of cognitive functioning, give them the drug for 6 months, and then readminister the test of cognitive functioning.

3. Read each scenario and (i) label it as a relationship or a difference question, (ii) determine the level of measurement of the dependent variable, and (iii) decide what the appropriate statistical test is to answer the question. (See question 1 for guidelines on deciding "what test when.")

a. A criminologist is interested in the effects of poverty on criminal behavior. He obtains a group of men whose childhoods have been spent in poverty and a group whose childhoods have not been spent in poverty. From each man he learns whether he has an adult criminal record (measured as yes or no). What statistical test should he use to see whether there is a relationship between childhood poverty and adult criminal behavior?

b. What statistical test should he use to determine whether the two groups (poverty vs. no poverty) differ in terms of adult criminal behavior?

c. A college administrator returns from a conference at which she learned that on an average day in an average class at an average college in the United States, only 78% of the enrolled students are present in class. She is curious whether attendance at her college differs, so she takes a random sample of classes at her college and records attendance on a randomly selected day. What statistical test should she choose to answer her question?

d. A theology professor obtains a sample of students who are opposed to the death penalty and a sample of those who are in favor of the death penalty. He is curious whether these two groups differ in terms of their religiosity. He administers a religiosity scale to them, a scale that ranks people into five categories: very positive about religion (2), positive about religion (1), neutral about religion (0), negative about religion (–1), and very negative about religion (–2). What statistical test should he use to see if the two groups differ in their feelings about religion?

e. The theology professor is also curious about the effect of a parent's level of religiosity on a child's level of religiosity. Using the same measure of religiosity, he collects information about the religiosity of the same-gender parent for each student. What statistical test should he use to see whether there is a difference between a parent's and a child's degree of religiosity?

THE INDEPENDENT-SAMPLES *t* TEST

It is time to learn the details of our first difference test, the independent-samples *t* test. The independent-samples *t* test is used to compare two groups or samples—say, boys and girls—to see if they differ on some interval- or ratio-level dependent variable, such as intelligence quotient (IQ). That is, we have one grouping variable (in this case, gender) with two levels (in this case, boys and girls) and one interval- or ratio-level dependent variable (in this case, IQ).

I'll summarize the independent-samples t test first and then go back and cover the six steps of "*Tom and Harry despise crabby infants*" (though I've already covered *Tom*—what test should be chosen—in the previous paragraph).

Let's start with the assumption that boys and girls are equally intelligent, that the population mean of IQ for boys is equal to the population mean of IQ for girls (i.e., $\mu_{boys} = \mu_{girls}$). Imagine drawing a large and random sample of boys from the population of boys. *Thanks to sampling error* it is unlikely that M_{boys} would exactly equal μ_{boys}. They should be close to each other, but I'd be surprised to find them equal down to the last decimal place. Similarly, if I drew a random and large sample of girls from the population of girls, I'd be surprised to find M_{girls} exactly equal to μ_{girls}. Again, I would expect this discrepancy because of the role that sampling error plays.

There's nothing malicious going on: this is just the way that sampling error works. Thanks to sampling error, we don't expect that a sample mean will be an exact reflection of a population mean.*

So here we are in a situation where $\mu_{boys} = \mu_{girls}$, but where, almost certainly, $M_{boys} \neq \mu_{boys}$ and $M_{girls} \neq \mu_{girls}$.

Think about that for a moment. What are the ramifications of that for the concordance between the mean IQ for my sample of boys (M_{boys}) and the mean IQ for my sample of girls (M_{girls})?

It means that it is unlikely that the means of the two samples will be exactly equivalent. Even if $\mu_{boys} = \mu_{girls}$, I can almost guarantee, thanks to sampling error, that $M_{boys} \neq M_{girls}$. Even if two population means are equal, when we draw samples from each population and compare the sample means, we shall almost certainly find that there is a difference between the two sample means.

As evidence of this, I constructed a large ($N = 10,000$) data set and drew repeated random samples of size 50. For each sample I calculated M. When I had two sample means I subtracted one from the other to calculate a difference score, and then I started over. I did this 500 times, ending with 500 values of $M_1 - M_2$. Since each was a sample from the same population, the two sample means should be similar. Yet, only 1.60% of the time did $M_1 = M_2$! This demonstrates that even when the samples come from the same population, it is an unusual event when two sample means are exactly the same.

We are in the world of inferential statistics now, in the world where we don't know, we can't know, population values. (As it is impossible to measure the IQ of every boy and every girl in the world, we can never know the actual value of μ_{boys} or μ_{girls}.) Though we don't know the population values, we want to make *inferences* about them, which is why *inferential* statistics are called inferential.

LOOKING CLOSER

*As we saw with the M&M's, random error—sampling error—will occasionally yield a sample that is quite unlike the population.

So, imagine this as our situation. We draw one sample of boys from the population of boys and one sample of girls from the population of girls. For each sample we calculate a mean IQ score, and we find that the two sample means are different from each other. What should we conclude about the relative intelligence of boys and girls in general?

We have two choices:

1. The two population means really are equal. The difference we found between the two sample means was caused by sampling error.
   –*or*–
2. The two population means really are not equal. The difference we found in the sample means reflects that difference, that reality.

If we draw a large and random sample of boys and a large and random sample of girls and find that the two sample means aren't that different, that they are something like 100.12 and 100.13, then we would likely conclude that this is not enough of a difference to reflect a real difference, that this difference is due to sampling error. We would conclude that option 1 is the correct conclusion.

But suppose that our two large and random samples yield means of 75 and 125. In this instance wouldn't we opt for conclusion 2, that the two population means are different? I certainly would lean in that direction.

Given large, random samples and either a large or small difference, the conclusion seems obvious. But what about when the difference is somewhere in the middle? Or when the samples aren't large? What about when there is a lot of variability in the samples? How then do we decide between the two options?

Difference tests reveal the size of a sample difference necessary to be considered representative of a real difference between two populations. A result is statistically significant if we conclude that the observed deviation from the null-hypothesized value is larger than expected due to sampling error. The probability of the observed difference resulting from chance—from sampling error—is less than 5% if the null hypothesis is true, so we conclude that the difference found between the two samples probably represents a real difference between the two populations. As we infer from this that it is a "real' difference between the two populations, for two-sample difference tests we conclude that if we replicate the study, we should again find a difference between the two samples as large (or larger) than we found before.

We're now ready to work through some data. Imagine that we want to study the effect of fear on behavior. We develop a maze and train mice to run from one end to the other, from the start box to the goal box, where they find a piece of cheese. After we train the mice to run the maze, we randomly select 10 mice from the population of trained mice and then randomly assign these 10 to two groups, a control and an experimental group. For the control group, we simply time how many seconds it takes each mouse to run the maze. For the 5 mice in the experimental group, we also time how long it takes to run the maze, but they run the maze while a cat is watching. (Don't worry, though visible to the mouse running the maze, the cat can't get its paws on the mouse.) Here are the data, in seconds, for the two groups.*

Control (no cat)	5.47	5.48	5.12	5.67	4.89	($M = 5.3260$)
Experimental (cat)	4.43	4.27	4.78	4.12	4.99	($M = 4.5180$)

The two groups run the maze in different times (5.33 sec vs. 4.52 sec), and although you might be tempted to conclude that this difference means that a fear stimulus causes mice to run the maze more quickly, we need to determine if the difference reflects a real difference. We need a statistical test.

Let's go through the six steps of the mnemonic "Tom and Harry despise crabby infants" for completing a null hypothesis significance test. As a reminder, here are the six steps:

1. **Test** : What statistical *T*est is being chosen and why?
2. **Assumptions** : What are the *A*ssumptions for the test? Can the test be completed?
3. **Hypotheses** : What is the null *H*ypothesis? What is the alternative hypothesis?
4. **Decision rule** : What is the *D*ecision rule? Is the sample size adequate?
5. **Calculation** : *C*alculate the test statistic.
6. **Interpretation** : *I*nterpret the results.

Test

What test are we doing and why? Well, we are comparing one sample (cat present) to another sample (no cat) to see whether there is a *difference* in maze-running time that is due to the presence of a fear stimulus. We have two samples, so we are doing a two-sample difference test.

Examination of Table 9.1 shows that there are six different two-sample tests. Which one we choose depends on whether we have independent or dependent samples and on the level of measurement of our dependent variable.

Sample sizes are equal, $n = 5$ for each sample, so that gives us no information as to whether the samples are independent or dependent.[†] We must figure out what types of samples we have without such an obvious clue.

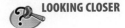 **LOOKING CLOSER**

*We have a real independent variable here since we randomly assigned mice to groups and controlled whether they received the manipulation. It is OK to refer to this as a grouping variable, which is a broader term.

[†]According to APA format, an uppercase letter (*N*) refers to the total number in a sample and a lowercase letter (*n*) refers to the number of cases in a subsample. Thus, in the present scenario $N = 10$, but for each group $n = 5$.

The basic question for determining types of samples is whether the selection of cases in one group influences the selection of cases for the other group. If the two groups are independent of each other, as they are here thanks to the fact that we randomly assigned the mice into the control and experimental groups, then they are independent samples.

In addition, we must decide the level of measurement of the dependent variable. The dependent variable is the time it takes to run the maze, and that is being measured in seconds. Thus, this is a ratio-level measure.

With two independent samples and a ratio-level measure, the appropriate test is an independent-samples *t* test.

Assumptions

The second step in my six-step procedure for hypothesis testing involves listing the assumptions for the chosen test, seeing if any were violated, and then deciding whether to proceed with the test. Remember, some assumptions are robust (i.e., they can be violated) and some are not, but even a robust assumption can be stretched beyond the breaking point.

There are five assumptions for the independent-samples *t* test, two of which—the first two—are not robust. These are the assumptions:
1. Independent samples (not robust to violations)
2. Interval- or ratio-level data (not robust to violations)
3. Random samples (robust to violation, but implications for interpretation if violated)
4. Normality (robust to violation if *n*s are large and about equal)
5. Homogeneity of variance (robust to violation if *n*s are large and about equal)

The first two assumptions, that the two samples are independent and that the dependent variable is being measured at the interval or ratio level, are not robust assumptions. They must be met in order to choose the independent-samples *t* test from the available options of two-sample difference tests. If the samples are not independent, or if the dependent variable is measured at the nominal or ordinal level, you should not calculate an independent-samples *t* test but rather you should fall back to one of the other tests in Table 9.1.

If any or all of the other three assumptions is violated then you *may* be able to complete an independent-samples *t* test. It depends.

The third assumption, what I abbreviate as "random samples," says that each of the two samples is a random sample from its respective population. This assumption is commonly violated, and the *t* test can still be meaningfully calculated. However, if this assumption is violated it means that there are limitations to the interpretation that can be made of the test results.

This assumption exists because the critical value of *t* to which the observed value of *t* will be compared is based on random samples being used to generate the sampling distribution. Thus it makes sense, in a comparing-apples-to-apples-and-not-to-oranges kind of way, that the observed value of t should be calculated from random samples since it is being compared to a sampling distribution built from random samples.

Ideally, if comparing a sample of boys to a sample of girls to determine whether they differ in terms of some dependent variable, we should have a random sample of boys from the population of boys and a random sample of girls from the population of girls. In actual fact, this ideal situation almost never exists. Rather, we might have samples of boys and girls from some elementary school, samples whose parents agreed to let them participate in a research project. Though these are not random samples from the populations of boys and girls, we still want to know if there is a statistically significant difference between the samples. However, we would want to be careful in claiming that the results obtained in these specific circumstances apply to the broader populations of boys and girls. In this sense, lack of random samples limits interpretation.

The fourth assumption, "normality," holds that the dependent variable is normally distributed in the population. Continuing with the comparison of boys to girls in terms of some dependent variable, say size of vocabulary, this means that vocabulary size is normally distributed in the population of boys and that it is normally distributed in the population of girls. This assumption is relatively robust to violations (i.e., one can go ahead and compute the t value) as long as the sample size is relatively large (i.e., $N \geq 50$) and the two samples are about equal in size.* That this assumption is robust if total sample size is relatively large is due to the central limit theorem, which asserts that a sampling distribution should be normally distributed as long as the sample size is large.

In addition to N having to be large for this assumption to be robust, the two sample sizes should be "relatively" equal in size. What does "relatively" mean? One rule of thumb says that if the larger sample is more than 1.5 times the size of the smaller sample, then the sample sizes are unequal (Welkowitz, Ewen, and Cohen, 2002).[†] Thus, if one sample has a size of 10 and the other is 14, they are relatively equal since $10 \times 1.5 = 15$ and 14, the size of the other sample, is less than 15. If the two samples had sizes of 10 and 16, however, they would be considered unequal.

In any event, we need to assess normality for each of the samples. To do this we use the techniques learned at the end of Chapter 6 for creating confidence intervals for skewness and kurtosis. Remember, if a variable is normally distributed, skewness and kurtosis should equal zero. If we construct a 95% confidence for both skewness and kurtosis for each of our samples, and if all four confidence intervals (that's two for each sample)

LOOKING CLOSER

*Remember, N refers to the total sample and n refers to a subsample.

[†] Welkowitz, J., Ewen, R.B., & Cohen, J. (2002). *Introductory statistics for the behavioral sciences* (5th ed.). New York: John Wiley & Sons, Inc.

capture the value of zero, then it is reasonable to conclude that the *population* values of skewness and kurtosis may be zero.

There is a pragmatic warning that I want to raise here. Whenever sample sizes are small, as they are with the mouse-maze data and many other data sets used as examples in this book, one needs to be leery of drawing conclusions about population values. When sample sizes are small, the value of a statistic can vary greatly from sample to sample and you should be careful about generalizing from the sample to the population.

The fifth assumption, what I abbreviate as "homogeneity of variance," means that the variances of the two populations are equal. In English, this means that the two populations have equal spread or variability. Using the example of comparing boys to girls in terms of size of vocabulary, this assumption means that the degree of variability in boys' vocabularies is as great as the degree of variability in girls' vocabularies, that $\sigma^2_{boys} = \sigma^2_{girls}$.

This assumption, like the previous one, is robust if N is relatively large (≥ 50), and the two sample sizes, n_1 and n_2, are relatively equal. There is also a rule of thumb, given that sample sizes are relatively equal, for deciding whether the degrees of variability in the two samples are similar enough to proceed: as long as the larger standard deviation is not twice as large as the smaller standard deviation, homogeneity of variance is probably not violated (Bartz, 1999).* Given that we are interested in drawing conclusions about the population variances, it makes sense to use $\hat{s}$, not s, for our standard deviation measures for this rule of thumb.

Let's now examine the five assumptions for the mouse-maze data. We can address the first two assumptions (independent samples and interval- or ratio-level data) quickly, since we already determined that we had random samples and a ratio-level measure when we selected the independent-samples *t* test. Remember, the 10 mice that we randomly selected from the population of trained mice were randomly assigned to the experimental and control groups, so the selection of cases for one group did not influence the selection for the other. In simpler terms, the two groups are independent.

Furthermore, our dependent variable is time measured in seconds, a ratio-level variable. So, neither of the two non-robust assumptions for the independent-samples *t* test has been violated.

The third assumption says that our samples are random samples from the population, and this one will take a little more thought. We randomly sampled the mice from the population of mice trained to run the maze. However this is clearly not a random sample from the world's population of mice, and so the generality of our findings will be limited.

The mice trained to run the maze were a specific breed from an animal supply agency.† Clearly, these mice are different from free-range mice that inhabit houses and fields. Free-range mice very likely have had

---

*Bartz, A. E. (1999). *Basic statistical concepts* (4th ed.). Upper Saddle River, NJ: Prentice-Hall, Inc.

†By the bye, I didn't really do this study.

LOOKING CLOSER

prior experience with cats, something our laboratory mice did not. The laboratory mice ate more regularly than do free-range mice and were almost certainly in better health. They probably differed from free-range mice in a number of other ways as well. Do any of these things have an impact on the results of the study? They very well may, and so when we interpret the results we'll need to bear this in mind.

The fourth assumption is normality, and it is robust if N is large and the two sample sizes are relatively equal. Well, although the two sample sizes are equal, N is not large, and so we have to be concerned about having violated normality. Thus we need to calculate 95% confidence intervals for skewness and kurtosis for each sample and also consider modality.

Using Equation 6.4 (a and b) to calculate skewness and kurtosis and Equation 6.5 (a and b) to calculate their standard errors, the 95% confidence intervals for, respectively, skewness and kurtosis for the control condition are from −2.55 to 1.75 and from −5.60 to 2.99. Because both intervals capture the value of zero, there is no reason to question whether the dependent variable may be normally distributed in the population. Similarly, with 95% confidence intervals for the experimental group ranging from −1.88 to 2.41 for skewness and from −5.75 to 2.84 for kurtosis, it is reasonable to conclude that the dependent variable is normally distributed in this population as well. Thus, the fourth assumption does not appear to have been violated. (With only five cases per group, it does not make much sense to evaluate modality.)

The fifth assumption, homogeneity of variance, says that the population variances for the two groups are equivalent. This assumption is robust as long as N is large and if the two samples are about equal in size. As N is not large here, we need to examine the degree of variability found in our sample for an apparent difference between the two populations. Using the rule that the homogeneity of variance assumption is not violated if the standard deviation ($\hat{s}$) of one sample is not twice the standard deviation of the other, I calculated the corrected standard deviation of the control group as .3144 and of the experimental group as .3602, and found the ratio of the larger divided by the smaller:

$$\frac{.3602}{.3144} = 1.1457$$

Since 1.15 is less than 2.00, this assumption does not appear to be violated.

Thus, only one of the five assumptions, the one requiring that our samples be random samples from their respective populations, has been violated, and this is a robust assumption. It seems reasonable to go ahead and conduct the t test even though this assumption has been violated. However, when it comes time for interpretation we shall have to bear this limitation in mind.

Group Practice 9.2

For each scenario that follows, (a) list the assumptions for the appropriate statistical test and decide whether to proceed with the test; (b) whether or not you decide to proceed with the test, describe the population to which the results of the study can be generalized.

1. A psychologist wants to examine the effects of scary movies on dreams. He obtains a sample of 72 people who say that they dream regularly and randomly divides them into two groups. To one group he shows a scary movie before bedtime, and to the other group he shows a nonscary movie. Each person then goes to sleep and tells him, in the morning, whether he or she can recall a dream from the night. If a person cannot recall a dream, he or she gets a score of zero. If a person recalls a dream and it is not scary, he or she gets a score of one; a scary dream gets a score of two. The mean score for the control group (the nonscary movie group) is 1.13 with a standard deviation (s) of .37. For the experimental group, the scary movie group, the mean is 1.47 with a standard deviation (s) of .53. Skewness for the two groups is .51 and .43, respectively; kurtosis, respectively, is –.03 and .14.

2. An anesthesiologist is interested in whether preoperative anxiety level is influenced by marital status. For the next 100 surgeries in which she is involved, she uses an interval-level scale to measure preoperative anxiety level in the patients and notes whether the patients are married. Fifty-nine patients are married. Their M on the anxiety scale is 17.34, with $\hat{s} = 8.86$, skewness = .43, and kurtosis = –.37. For the nonmarried patients, $M = 24.67$, $\hat{s} = 11.43$, skewness = .65, and kurtosis = –1.17.

3. A nutritionist wonders whether children's levels of courtesy have any impact on the amount of candy they collect for Halloween. She has a third-grade teacher rate the politeness of all 24 students in his class on an interval-level scale where higher scores indicate more politeness. The mean politeness level is 43.47 with $\hat{s} = 15.93$; skewness is –.47 and kurtosis is .56. The kids all go trick-or-treating and count the number of pieces of candy that they obtain. The nutritionist is interested in how many pieces of candy each child obtains, so a large piece of candy is considered equivalent to a small piece. For the candy measure, $M = 75.49$, $\hat{s} = 29.11$, skewness = .88, and kurtosis = 1.73.

Hypotheses

The next step in hypothesis testing involves specifying both the null and alternative hypotheses, if possible both in symbolic notation and in English. For a *t* test, as it was for the Pearson *r*, the null hypothesis is set up so that we can reject it and be forced to accept the mutually exclusive alternative hypothesis.

Research studies are almost always done because the experimenter believes that the independent variable, the grouping variable, makes a difference.* The study we are using for our example, the effect of a fear stimulus on behavior, is being done because I think that the presence of a

---

*There is a group of statistical tests, called tests of equivalence, that can be used when one wants to show that there is not a statistically significant difference between two groups (Cribbie, R.A., Gruman, J.A., & Arpin-Cribbie, C.A. (2004). Recommendations for applying tests of equivalence. *Journal of Clinical Psychology*, 60(1), 1-10.)

LOOKING CLOSER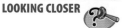

cat will have an impact on mouse behavior. If I didn't think that having a cat watch mice while they run a maze would have an impact on the mice's behavior, then either I wouldn't be doing the study or I would be doing the study with what I thought was a more effective fear stimulus, such as the sound of hissing cats.

This is the null hypothesis for two-sample significant difference tests: The means for the two *populations* are the same, and any difference found between the two *sample* means can be accounted for by sampling error. Statisticians express this as $\mu_1 = \mu_2$ where μ_1 represents the population mean for one group and μ_2 represents the population mean for the other group.

The null and the alternative hypotheses must be all-inclusive and mutually exclusive. Thus if the null hypothesis says that the two population means are equal, the alternative hypothesis is that the two population means are not equal. Expressed in symbolic notation, the alternative hypothesis reads $\mu_1 \neq \mu_2$. Expressed in English, the alternative hypothesis says that the observed difference between the two samples is too large to be due to sampling error for samples drawn from one population—that a difference this large occurs because the samples were drawn from populations with different means.*

So, for the study investigating the effect of a fear stimulus on mouse behavior, this is how we write the hypotheses in symbolic notation:

$$H_0: \mu_1 = \mu_2$$
$$H_1: \mu_1 \neq \mu_2$$

I would explain them, in English, as follows. The null hypothesis, H_0, says the mean maze-running time for the population of mice that run a maze while a cat is present is the same as the mean maze-running time for the population of mice that run a maze without a cat present. Though the two population means—the μs—are the same, I don't expect to find that the sample means will be exactly the same. That is, I expect to find that M_1 is not exactly equal to M_2, though the difference between the two sample means should be small enough that it can be explained by sampling error.

The alternative hypothesis says that the difference between the two sample means is so large that sampling error is unlikely to account for it; it is probably not due to a deviation from a sampling distribution of difference scores that would come from samples drawn from the same population. Thus, the two samples come from populations with different means.

Group Practice 9.3

For question 2 from Group Practice 9.2, regardless of whether the assumptions are violated, express the hypotheses in symbolic notation and in English.

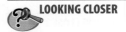 **LOOKING CLOSER**

Just as I did with correlations, I am going to focus on nondirectional hypotheses. It is possible to have directional hypotheses, for example, those who exercise will lose more weight than those who don't exercise. (The nondirectional version of this would say that there is a difference in weight loss between those who exercise and those who don't, but it wouldn't make a prediction about which group would end up weighing less.) The null hypothesis for the directional prediction would be $\mu_{Exercise} \leq \mu_{NoExercise}$, and the alternative hypothesis would be $\mu_{Exercise} > \mu_{NoExercise}$.

Decision Rule

The fourth step of null hypothesis significance testing involves finding the critical value of the test statistic, determining the decision rule (when do you reject H_0?), and making sure that the sample size is adequate.

The critical value of the *t* statistic, t_{cv}, separates the area of the sampling distribution of *t* that is the rare zone, the area where observed values of *t* are unlikely to fall if the null hypothesis is true, from the common zone. The logic here is the same as that used for the Pearson *r*: if something happens that *could* happen, but *should* happen only rarely if the null hypothesis is true, then we reject the null hypothesis. Since this is only the second time that we've confronted this logic, and since it is the logic that undergirds all null hypothesis significance testing, let me explain it in detail again.

Earlier I mentioned constructing a population of 10,000 cases and repeatedly drawing random samples of size 50 from this population. Each time I drew a sample, I calculated its mean; after every two samples, I subtracted the second sample mean (M_2) from the first (M_1), creating a difference score. I did this for 500 pairs of sample means. Since each sample came from the same population, we would expect the sample means to be very similar. However, we would also expect that random error—sampling error—would make it unlikely that any two pairs of means would be exactly the same. In fact, as I reported earlier, only 1.60% of the time were the two sample means exactly equal.

We could think of the 500 difference scores as comprising a sampling distribution of difference scores. Figure 9.1 shows this distribution.

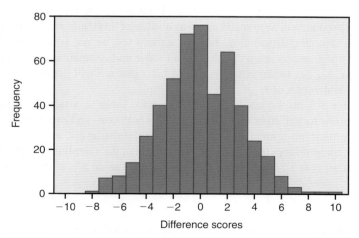

Figure **9.1** Sampling distribution of 500 difference scores for 500 pairs of samples randomly drawn from the same population.

Note that this sampling distribution centers around a value of zero and tails off to each side. Just as the central limit theorem predicts, it looks somewhat normally distributed. In addition, note that we do get some difference scores that are fairly far from the expected value of zero, with a range of difference scores from −7.95 to 9.60. Even when sample sizes are relatively large (50 in this instance) and the samples are drawn from the same population, we do occasionally get two samples that differ by a large amount, an amount large enough that it should cause us to pause and think it a real possibility that the samples came from two different populations.

We are going to use the same decision rule that we used with the Pearson r. That is, we will compare our observed result to the sampling distribution that would be expected to occur if the null hypothesis were true. If the observed result is one that would occur commonly under H_0— if it falls into the common zone of the sampling distribution—then there is no reason to question the null hypothesis. But, if the observed result falls into the rare zone of the sampling distribution—into the extreme 5% of the sampling distribution—then we shall say that though it is possible that this result could occur when H_0 is true, it is unusual enough that we doubt that H_0 is true. In this case, we shall reject H_0 and be forced to accept H_1.*

The actual sampling distribution to which we shall compare our calculated t value is the sampling distribution of the t, but we haven't yet learned how to calculate a t value. So, for the moment, I have demarcated the top and bottom 2.5% of the sampling distribution for the 500 difference scores in Figure 9.2. This means, just as I did with the Pearson r, that I am using a two-tailed test of significance.

Based on this sampling distribution, if I drew two samples from populations that I expected to be like the population from which this sampling distribution comes, and I found a difference of, say, 8.00 between the two sample means, then I would not believe that the two population means were really equal as a value of 8.00 falls in the rare zone of the sampling distribution. For our actual t test we are going to do this same thing, except we will calculate a t value and compare our calculated t value, $t_{observed}$, to the critical value of t, t_{cv}, that we will get from a table of critical values of t.

Table 9.3 displays a section of Appendix Table 9, a table of critical values of t for different alpha levels and for both one- and two-tailed tests. I hope that you remember that the different alpha levels, abbreviated α, represent how large (or small) the rare zone is in the sampling distribution. If you set α at .05, that means that you have set aside 5% of the sampling

---

LOOKING CLOSER

*I hope it is clear that this 5% I am talking about is the alpha level and that you could set α at whatever level you wanted. For the sake of simplicity, I am going to use the most often used alpha of .05.

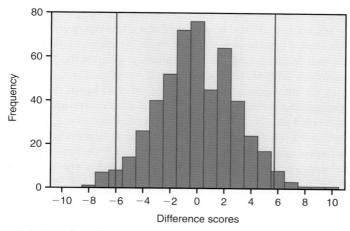

Figure **9.2** Sampling distribution of 500 difference scores with the extreme 5% of scores indicated.

distribution as the rare zone and that you are willing to make a Type I error—mistakenly reject H_0—5% of the time. If that seems like too great a risk of making a Type I error, you can choose a smaller α level, say .01, where you run the risk of making a Type I error only 1% of the time. Note that as α gets smaller, the rare zone gets smaller and t_{cv} gets larger, making it harder to reject the null hypothesis.

The one-tailed vs. two-tailed distinction is based on whether your hypotheses are directional. The hypotheses for the mouse-maze data (H_0: $\mu_1 = \mu_2$ and H_1: $\mu_1 \neq \mu_2$) are nondirectional, that is, they make no prediction about whether the presence of the fear stimulus causes the mice to run the maze more quickly or more slowly.

TABLE **9.3** **Section of Appendix Table 9, Critical Values of *t***

	ONE-TAILED TEST			
	.05	.025	.01	.005
	TWO-TAILED TEST			
df	.10	.05	.02	.01
6	1.9432	**2.4469**	3.1427	3.7074
7	1.8946	**2.3646**	2.9980	3.4995
8	1.8595	**2.3060**	2.8965	3.3554
9	1.8331	**2.2622**	2.8214	3.2498
10	1.8125	**2.2281**	2.7638	3.1693
infinity	1.6449	**1.9600**	2.3263	2.5758

Just as with the Pearson r, I want you, as a beginning student of statistics, to opt for $\alpha = .05$ and a two-tailed test when doing an independent-samples t test. I have bolded that column in the table of critical values.*

Note that in this table of critical values, just as for the Pearson r, the first column is labeled "df" for degrees of freedom. The t_{cv} for a t test is found at the intersection of the appropriate row, based on df, and the appropriate column based on the α level and whether you are doing a one- or a two-tailed test. Note that, just as with the Pearson r, t_{cv} gets smaller as df increases. This means that the rare zone is larger when the sample size is larger, making it easier to reject the null hypothesis with a larger sample size. The degrees of freedom for an independent-samples t test, shown in Equation 9.1, are calculated by subtracting two from N.

F O R M U L A

Degrees of Freedom (df) for an Independent-Samples t Test

Equation 9.1 $df = N - 2$

Where:
df = degrees of freedom being calculated
N = total number of subjects in the two samples

Thus, if one sample has nine cases and the other sample has seven, the total N—what is sometimes called the grand N—is 16 and degrees of freedom is 14. Some people prefer to think of degrees of freedom for an independent-samples t as the sum of each sample n minus one, that is, as $(n_1 - 1) + (n_2 - 1)$, which in this case is $(9 - 1) + (7 - 1)$, or $8 + 6$, or 14. Whichever way works for you is acceptable.

If each sample has five cases, as is the case for our mouse-maze example, then the grand N is 10 and the degrees of freedom equals 8. Looking at Table 9.3 we see that the critical value of t with 8 degrees of freedom (highlighted) and at the two-tailed level with α set at .05 (bolded) is 2.3060. Figure 9.3 shows the sampling distribution of t, marked by common and rare zones for $\alpha = .05$, two-tailed, with $df = 8$. Our decision rule is the same as it was for the Pearson r: If the *observed value* of the test statistic is greater than or equal to the *critical value* of the test statistic, we shall reject the null hypothesis.† To phrase it another way, if $|t_{observed}|$ is $\geq t_{cv}$, we conclude that $t_{observed}$ falls in the rare zone of the sampling distribution, that it is unlikely to have occurred as a result of

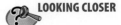

LOOKING CLOSER

*Just as with the Pearson r, for a given α level it is harder to reject the null hypothesis with a two-tailed test than with a one-tailed test.

†Calculated values of t can be positive or negative and so our decision rule, just as it did for the Pearson r, uses the absolute value of t.

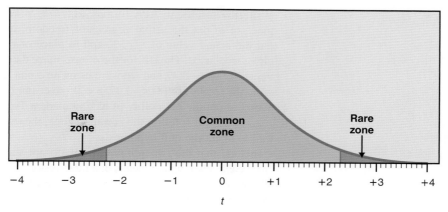

Figure **9.3** Sampling distribution of *t* for *df* = 8, separated into rare and common zones for α = .05, two-tailed. (Sampling distribution of *t* from Lowry R: *Concepts and applications of inferential statistics,* available on the Internet at http://faculty.vassar.edu/lowry/webtext.htm.)

sampling error if H_0 were true. The logic of hypothesis testing is that if something happens that could happen, but should happen only rarely if the null hypothesis is true, then we reject the null hypothesis. If $|t_{observed}| \geq t_{cv}$, we end up concluding that the probability of this rare result occurring if the null hypothesis is true is less than α, is low. Thus we reject the null hypothesis and report that $p < \alpha$. When we reject the null hypothesis and are forced to accept the alternative hypothesis, we conclude that the difference between the two groups is statistically different from zero, a result that is *probably* due to $\mu_1 \neq \mu_2$ being true. Of course, we will need to keep in mind the possibility that we have made a Type I error.

If $|t_{observed}|$ is $< t_{cv}$, then the observed difference between M_1 and M_2 is small enough that it falls in the common zone of the sampling distribution of the difference scores, and we conclude that it can be explained by sampling error when $\mu_1 = \mu_2$. Thus, we say that the difference is not statistically different from zero and we fail to reject the null hypothesis.* The type of error we need to worry about in this situation is Type II.

To summarize the decision rule:

I. If $|t_{observed}| \geq t_{cv}$, if $t_{observed}$ falls in the rare zone, then we would
   1. Reject the null hypothesis and be forced to accept the alternative hypothesis;
   2. Conclude that the two *sample* means statistically differ from each other and that this probably means that the two *population* means differ from each other;

---

*When they fail to reject H_0, many researchers believe in their hearts, or even say out loud, that the two population means are the same. This is an erroneous conclusion. Why? Because we don't prove the null, we can only provide evidence against it. The strongest statement one should make when one fails to reject the null hypothesis is that the evidence was not sufficient to support rejecting the null hypothesis.

LOOKING CLOSER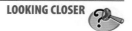

3. Write the results, in APA format, as: $t\ (df) = $ x.xx, $p < \alpha$.* In place of df put the actual degrees of freedom, in place of x.xx put the actual value of $t_{observed}$, and in place of α put the actual alpha level used. Thus, if for the mouse-maze data the calculated value of t was -3.47 and we were using an alpha level of .05, we write the results as $t\ (8) = -3.47$, $p < .05$ since our t_{cv} was 2.31; and

4. Worry about the possibility of having made a Type I error.

II. If $|t_{observed}| < t_{cv}$, if it fell in the common zone, then we would

1. Fail to reject the null hypothesis;

2. Conclude that the two *sample* means do not statistically differ from each other, which means that there is not sufficient evidence to conclude that the two *population* means differ from each other;

3. Write the results, in APA format as: $t\ (df) = $ x.xx, $p > \alpha$. In place of df put the actual degrees of freedom, in place of x.xx put the actual value of $t_{observed}$, and in place of α put the actual alpha level that you had chosen. Thus, if for the mouse-maze data the calculated value of t was 1.23 and I was using an alpha level of .05, I write the results as $t\ (8) = 1.23$, $p > .05$;[†] and,

4. Worry about the possibility of having made a Type II error.

There is one more part to Step 4, deciding if one's sample size is adequate. I want to put that aside until after Step 6, when I have explained another way to calculate effect sizes. So, to end this section, let me summarize in Table 9.4 the differences between when $t_{observed}$ falls in the rare zone or the common zone.

TABLE **9.4**   **Implications of and Differences between $|t_{observed}| \geq t_{cv}$ and $|t_{observed}| < t_{cv}$ with $\alpha = .05$, Two-Tailed**

	$|t_{observed}| \geq t_{cv}$	$|t_{observed}| < t_{cv}$
Where the observed t falls	Rare zone	Common zone
Statement about H_0	It is rejected	Failed to reject it
Statement about H_1	Forced to accept it	Failed to support it
Error to be concerned about	Type I	Type II
Probability of that error	.05 (α)	To be determined (β)
Report probability of results occurring if H_0 is true as	$p < .05$	$p > .05$
Results are called	Statistically significant	Not statistically significant
Conclusion about sample means	Statistically different	Not statistically different
Conclusion about population means	Probably different	Not sufficient evidence that are different

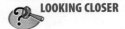

LOOKING CLOSER

*What does $p < \alpha$ mean? That $t_{observed}$ fell in the rare zone, that the probability of these results having occurred by chance, due to sampling error, if the null hypothesis were true is very low. These results would occur less than 5% of the time if the null hypothesis were true.

[†] See footnote on opposite page.

Calculations

The next step in hypothesis testing, Step 5, involves actually calculating the test statistic. Before showing the formula that we will use, I want to discuss the logic of what we are calculating.

For the mouse-maze data we know that $M_{Experimental} = 4.52$ seconds and $M_{Control} = 5.33$ seconds. We want to know if this .81 second difference is statistically significant, if it is sufficiently large to be suggestive of a population difference. We know that if the null hypothesis, $\mu_1 = \mu_2$, is true, then the difference between the two *M*s should be zero, though because of sampling error we don't expect it to be exactly zero. We also know that if the null hypothesis is true and our samples are large enough, the mean of the sampling distribution of the difference scores of $M_1 - M_2$ should be zero and the sampling distribution of the difference scores should be normally distributed.

Hold those thoughts for a moment while I remind you about *z* scores and the normal distribution. z scores are calculated by the formula $\frac{X - M}{s}$ and represent how far from the mean (*M*) a score (*X*) is in standard deviation (*s*) units. In a normal distribution, 95% of the cases will fall within 1.96 standard deviations of the mean, as shown in Figure 9.4.

So, why this excursion to *z* scores? Because I want to make the point that a *t*, which we are about to calculate, is a lot like a *z*. We know that the observed difference between our two means is .81 seconds away from what should be the mean of the sampling distribution (.00) if the null hypothesis is true. The question that we want to answer, since we are using a two-tailed test with α set at .05, is this: does this observed difference score of .81 fall within 1.96 standard deviations of the sampling distribution from the mean of the sampling distribution? Does it fall in

---

(Continued) [†]What does $p > .05$ mean? That $t_{observed}$ fell in the common zone, that there is a reasonably large probability, more than a 5% chance, that these results would occur by chance if the null hypothesis were true.

LOOKING CLOSER

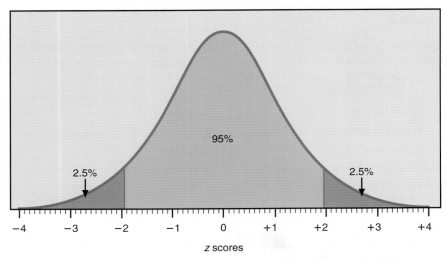

Figure **9.4** Percent of the area under the normal curve that falls within 1.96 standard deviations of the mean.

the rare zone of the sampling distribution or in the common area? If it falls in the rare zone we'll draw one conclusion, and if it falls in the common zone a different conclusion. All we need to answer this question is the standard deviation of the sampling distribution, because then we can calculate a kind of z score, called a t score, that tells us how far from the mean, in standard score units, our observed difference score falls. Got it?

Equation 9.2a is the "official" formula for calculating an independent-samples t test.

F O R M U L A

Independent-Samples *t* Test

Equation 9.2a

$$t = \frac{(M_1 - M_2) - \mu_{M_1-M_2}}{\hat{s}_{M_1-M_2}}$$

Where:

t = independent-samples t value being calculated

M_1 = mean of first sample

M_2 = mean of second sample

$\mu_{M_1-M_2}$ = mean of the sampling distribution of difference scores

$\hat{s}_{M_1-M_2}$ = standard error of the difference (the standard deviation of the sampling distribution of difference scores)

Note the similarity between this formula and the formula for a *z* score. In the numerator, we have an observed score, the difference between our two sample means. From the observed score we subtract a mean, the mean of the sampling distribution of the difference scores. The new difference score is then divided by a standard deviation, the standard deviation of the sampling distribution of the difference (called the standard error of the difference) to yield the independent-samples *t* value.

If the null hypothesis is true, and null hypothesis significance testing depends on our assuming that the null hypothesis is true, the mean of the sampling distribution of the difference is zero. Thus, assuming H_0 is true, the second part of the numerator becomes zero and we can simplify the equation for the independent-samples *t* test to Equation 9.2b.

F O R M U L A

Simpler Independent-Samples *t* Test

Equation 9.2b

$$t = \frac{M_1 - M_2}{\hat{s}_{M_1 - M_2}}$$

Where:

t = independent-samples *t* value being calculated

M_1 = mean of first sample

M_2 = mean of second sample

$\hat{s}_{M_1 - M_2}$ = standard error of the difference (the standard deviation of the sampling distribution of difference scores)

This formula says to calculate a *t* value by finding the difference between the two sample means and dividing this difference by the standard error of the difference.

All that remains is calculating the standard error of the difference, which is easier than Equation 9.3 looks. All we need to know are the number of cases (*n*) for each sample and the estimated population variance ($\hat{s}^2$) for each sample.

F O R M U L A

Standard Error of the Difference for an Independent-Samples *t* Test

Equation 9.3

$$\hat{s}_{M_1 - M_2} = \sqrt{\left[\frac{(n_1 - 1)\hat{s}_1^2 + (n_2 - 1)\hat{s}_2^2}{n_1 + n_2 - 2} \right]\left[\frac{n_1 + n_2}{n_1 n_2} \right]}$$

Continued

Standard Error of the Difference for an Independent-Samples *t* Test—cont'd

Equation 9.3	Where:

$\hat{s}_{M_1-M_2} =$ standard error of the difference (the standard deviation of the sampling distribution of difference scores) being calculated

$n_1 =$ the number of cases in the first sample

$\hat{s}_1^2 =$ the estimated population variance for the first sample

$n_2 =$ the number of cases in the second sample

$\hat{s}_2^2 =$ the estimated population variance for the second sample

This formula looks forbidding, but it is primarily tedious. Here, in English, is what it does:

1. Subtract 1 from the *n* for the first sample and multiply this by the estimated population variance for the first sample.
2. Do the same thing using the *n* and the estimated population variance for the second sample.
3. Add the values of step 1 and step 2.
4. Find the grand *N* (i.e., add the *n*s for the two samples together) and subtract two from this. (NOTE: this value is the same as the degrees of freedom for an independent-samples *t* test.)
5. Divide step 3 by step 4.
6. Divide the grand *N* by the *n* for the first sample multiplied by the *n* for the second sample.
7. Multiply step 5 by step 6.
8. Find the square root of step 7.

Let's calculate $\hat{s}_{M_1-M_2}$ for the mouse-maze data and then use that to calculate a *t* value. We know that each sample has an *n* of 5, and earlier I calculated $\hat{s}$ for each sample as .3144 and .3602 for control and experimental groups respectively. Squaring these estimated populations' standard deviations gives an $\hat{s}^2$ for the control group of .0988, and for the experimental group of .1298. Plugging these into Equation 9.3:

$$\hat{s}_{M_1-M_2} = \sqrt{\left[\frac{(5-1).0988 + (5-1).1298}{5+5-2} \right]\left[\frac{5+5}{5\times5} \right]}$$

$$= \sqrt{\left[.1142 \right]\left[.4000 \right]}$$

$$= .2137$$

We have everything needed to calculate our first *t* value—but first, a practical matter. Under the square root sign in the formula for calculating $\hat{s}_{M_1-M_2}$, there are two sections in brackets. The first bracketed part,

$\dfrac{(n_1 - 1)\hat{s}_1{}^2 + (n_2 - 1)\hat{s}_2{}^2}{n_1 + n_2 - 2}$, has a name, the pooled estimate of the population variance or $\hat{s}^2{}_{pooled}$. We will need this when we interpret the *t* test, so it is a good idea to make a note of the value. For our mice-maze data, $\hat{s}^2{}_{pooled} = .1142$.

And now let's calculate *t*! The mean of the control group is 5.3260, the mean of the experimental group is 4.5180, and the standard error of the difference is .2137. Plugging these values into Equation 9.2 yields this:

$$t = \frac{5.3260 - 4.5180}{.2137} = 3.7810 = 3.78$$

I have a couple of small but important points to make before I put this answer in APA format and follow through on Step 4, the decision rule. First, it doesn't matter which sample mean is subtracted from the other. In this instance I subtracted the experimental mean from the control mean, but I could just as easily have subtracted the control mean from the experimental mean. If I had done so, my *t* value would have been −3.78 instead of 3.78. In either event the absolute value of the *t* is the same, and it is the absolute value that we compare to the table of critical values of *t*. Because it doesn't matter, I usually make my life easier by avoiding negative numbers and subtract the smaller mean from the larger.

Second, note that I only carried four decimal places through my calculations. APA format says that results should be reported to two decimal places, so I am carrying two more than I'll need. Though I report the *t* value as 3.78, when I use it to calculate other values (e.g., as we'll do in Equation 9.7), I'll revert to the more exact value of 3.7810.

Let's now put the answer in APA format.* Since the critical value of *t* with eight degrees of freedom and a two-tailed α set at .05 was 2.31, and the absolute value of the observed value of *t* (3.78) was greater than or equal to this, it falls in the rare zone of the sampling distribution that exists if the null hypothesis is correct (see Figure 9.5). This is an observed value that falls in the rare zone, that has a less than α probability of occurring—which means that we reject the null hypothesis. We write this as: *t* (8) = 3.78, *p* < .05. (Note that it is the *observed* value of *t* that is placed in APA format, *not* t_{cv}!)[†]

---

*Remember, APA format has you give four pieces of information: (1) what test was conducted, (2) *N*, (3) test statistic results, and (4) statistical significance level.

[†]If $t_{observed}$ had been less than t_{cv}—say it had been 2.30—then we would have written the results in APA format as *t* (8) = 2.30, *p* > .05 or *t* (8) = 2.30, *ns* (where *ns* stands for "not significant"). The *p* > .05 means that these results are common ones—they occur more than 5% of the time if H_0 is true—and so there is no reason to reject the null hypothesis. Thus, we end up concluding that there is no statistically significant difference between the two populations. Note that we are not saying that the two population means are the same, just that there is no reason to conclude that they aren't.

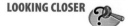
LOOKING CLOSER

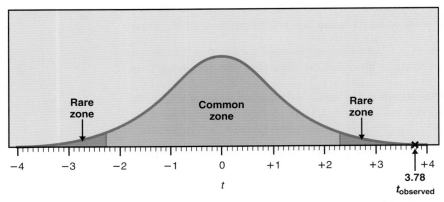

Figure **9.5** Observed value of *t* for mouse-maze data in relation to t_{cv} in sampling distribution of *t*. (Sampling distribution of *t* from Lowry R: *Concepts and applications of inferential statistics,* available on the Internet at http://faculty.vassar.edu/lowry/webtext.htm.)

Since I am rejecting the null hypothesis, I find that there is a statistically significant difference between the two sample means. I conclude that the two population means are probably, but not certainly, different. There is a lot more that I can conclude, but I am going to save that for the final step, Step 6, interpretation.

Group Practice 9.5

For the following scenario, assume that no assumptions have been violated and calculate *t*. Using $\alpha =$ .05, two tailed, write the results in APA format. Save your answer; you'll need it later.

1. A nurse educator at a large university wants to help student nurses feel more comfortable administering injections. She thinks that using visualization techniques, having students go through the process of administering injections in their minds, will be helpful. She takes 12 student nurses from her school and randomly assigns them to two groups. The control group receives standard training in administering injections. The experimental group receives standard training plus the visualization technique. The student nurses then practice on real patients, and each records the number of injections it takes for him or her to feel comfortable in administering injections. The number of injections until comfort is reached is the dependent variable. The nurse educator finds that the control group takes 6, 5, 12, 5, 7, and 9 injections to feel comfortable ($M = 7.3333$, $\hat{s} = 2.7325$); the experimental group needs 6, 3, 2, 5, 3, and 5 ($M = 4.0000$, $\hat{s} = 1.5492$).

Interpretation

The final step involves interpreting the results, saying in English what the results mean. If you told your parents, "Mom, Dad, I just completed a *t* test and rejected the null hypothesis!" would they have any idea what you had found? Statistics are used to answer questions, and though

$p < .05$ may be meaningful to a statistician it is not meaningful to the vast majority of people. Plus, as we saw with correlations, saying that the relationship is statistically different from zero is only the beginning. Interpretation involves thinking about the question you set out to answer, thinking about your data in the context of the calculated statistics, and drawing a conclusion. Interpretation is not for the faint of heart: when you interpret, you take a stand.

Interpreting a *t* test means addressing several questions. First, is the observed difference statistically different from zero? Then, if the difference is statistically significant, what are the direction and size of the difference? Finally, what is the power of the test?

Presence of a Difference

The question that we have set out to answer is whether, for mice, the presence of a fear stimulus has an impact on maze-running behavior. We found that the control group mice ran the maze in 5.33 seconds and the experimental group mice in 4.52 seconds. We calculated that $t(8) = 3.78$, $p < .05$. Since the result fell in the rare zone, meaning it happens less than 5% of the time when H_0 is true, we rejected the null hypothesis. So let's start our interpretation by saying, "I reject the null hypothesis that the running time of the experimental population (mice running the maze when a fear stimulus *is* present) is equivalent to the running time of the control population (mice running the maze when a fear stimulus *is not* present). The difference in time between the two sample means is likely too great to have been due to sampling error; it probably reflects a real difference between the two populations." (If we had failed to reject H_0, I would have said something along the lines of: "I fail to reject the null hypothesis that the mean time it takes to run a maze is equal for mice whether or not a fear stimulus is present. The observed difference between the mean times for the experimental group (fear stimulus present) and the control group (no fear stimulus present) is small enough that it can be accounted for by sampling error. There is not sufficient evidence to suggest that maze running time is affected by the presence of this fear stimulus in mice.

Direction of the Difference

My interpretation, so far, is not very informative. Just as with correlations, the next step, *when the difference is statistically significant*, is to talk about the direction of the difference.* We know that there is a statistically

---

*Notice that I avoid calling the difference *significant*; I always call it *statistically significant*. Calling it *significant* makes it sound meaningful; calling it *statistically significant* leaves open the possibility that the difference could be practically meaningless.

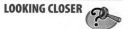

LOOKING CLOSER

significant difference; now let's examine the sample means and tell the direction of the difference. Examination of the sample means (5.33 for the control group and 4.52 for the experimental) allows me to say something like this: "The difference between the two groups is statistically significant. The presence of a cat fear–stimulus caused mice to run the maze faster, reducing the mean time from 5.33 to 4.52 seconds." Now, not only have you told your reader that there is a difference, but you have told them the direction of the difference.

If there had not been a statistically significant difference between the experimental and control groups, then I would have said something like this: "The difference between the two sample means is not statistically significant. There is no evidence from the present study that the presence of a cat has any impact, positive or negative, on maze-running times for mice."

Size of the Difference I: Confidence Intervals

Knowing that a direction exists and the size of the difference, we'll now want to how big—or meaningful—the difference is. Generically, this is called an effect size, as in, "How much of an effect did the independent variable have?" We'll see four different ways of calculating effect sizes for *t* values: (1) confidence intervals, (2) the effect size *d*, (3) the percentage of variance predicted, and (4) correlation coefficients.

The first way to examine the size of the difference is to compute a confidence interval for the difference between the two population means. When results are statistically significant, the confidence interval should not capture zero, indicating that the absolute value of the difference between the two population means is almost certainly more than zero.* However, the confidence interval tells us more. It tells the size that we can reasonably expect for the "real" difference that probably exists between the two population means. Just as with confidence intervals for correlations, we will be concerned both with how tight or narrow the confidence interval is and with how far away from zero it falls. We're going to use confidence intervals to judge how meaningful the difference between the two populations is—if it exists.

Calculating a confidence interval, Equation 9.4, is not difficult since we've already done most of the hard work: We found the critical value of *t* in Step 4 and calculated the standard error of the difference using Equation 9.3.

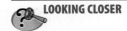

LOOKING CLOSER

*Just as with correlation coefficients, I will advocate calculating confidence intervals for results that are not statistically significant. We know in advance that these confidence intervals will capture zero, but we'll want to know how far from zero they reach and how lopsided they are.

95% Confidence Interval for the Difference between Two Population Means for an Independent-Samples *t* Test

$$95\% \; CI_{\mu_1 - \mu_2} = (M_1 - M_2) \pm t_{cv} \, (\hat{s}_{M_1 - M_2})$$

Equation 9.4

Where:

$95\% \; CI_{\mu_1 - \mu_2}$ = the 95% confidence interval for the difference between two population means being calculated

M_1 = the sample mean for group one

M_2 = the sample mean for group two

t_{cv} = the critical value of *t*, two-tailed, $\alpha = .05$*

$\hat{s}_{M_1 - M_2}$ = the standard error of the difference, calculated via Equation 9.3

To calculate a confidence interval, take the difference between the two sample means and add to and subtract from this difference the product of the critical value of *t* (two-tailed, $\alpha = .05$) times the standard error of the difference.

For our mouse-maze data set, we would calculate the 95% confidence interval for the difference between two population means as (5.3260 − 4.5180) ± 2.3060(.2137) = .8080 ± .4928 and report it as ranging from .32 to 1.30.

$$95\% \; CI = (5.3260 - 4.5180) \pm 2.3060(.2137)$$
$$= .8080 \pm .4928$$

I would interpret this as meaning that the mean difference between the *populations* of control mice and experimental mice may be as little .32 seconds or as much as 1.30 seconds. In other words, the presence of a fear stimulus may cause the experimental population of mice to run this maze as little as almost a third of a second faster to 1.3 seconds faster than the control population. Given the short amount of time it takes a mouse to run the maze (≈ 5 seconds), a difference of a third of a second (about a 6% improvement) seems like a lot, leading me to conclude that not only is the difference *statistically* significant but it is *practically* significant as well. Fear stimuli lead mice to run the maze faster! Thus my interpretative statement would read, "I calculated the 95% confidence interval for the difference between the population means and found that in their

---

*If you want to calculate a different confidence interval, say 99% or 90%, use t_{cv} for the appropriate two-tailed α level, say .01 or .10.

LOOKING CLOSER

Group Practice 9.6

Calculate the 95% confidence interval for the question in Group Practice 9.5 and write an interpretative statement using the confidence intervals. Don't forget to comment on the direction of the difference.

respective populations the increase in speed for mice running the maze with a fear stimulus present is most likely to range from .32 to 1.30 seconds. Given that the overall average time to run the maze was around 5 seconds, I think that the presence of a fear stimulus substantially increases the speed with which mice run the maze."

Size of the Difference II: Effect Size *d*

In making sense of the confidence interval I just eyeballed it in relation to the time it took to run the maze and concluded that the fear stimulus had a meaningful effect. It is also possible to calculate something called an effect size in order more objectively to quantify the effect of the independent variable on the dependent variable. When discussing the interpretation of correlations in Chapter 8, I introduced the concept of effect sizes in relation to the percentage of variance predicted (accounted for), and we went on to learn how to calculate a binomial *effect size* display. Now we will learn to calculate another effect size, one that is abbreviated as *d* or, in Greek, δ. Why *d*? Because the uppercase version of the Greek letter δ, Δ, is used in science to indicate change, and the effect size tells how much *change* there is in the dependent variable from the mean of one group—call it the control group—to the mean of the other—the experimental group. The effect size is useful because, like a *z* score, it converts the change score into a common metric: *d* is the distance between the means of the two samples in terms of a standard deviation unit. Unfortunately, the standard deviation used varies a bit from statistician to statistician. Some recommend using the standard deviation of the control group as the denominator, arguing that this gives the distance between the experimental group and the control group in control group units. And this is a perfectly reasonable option. I prefer, however, to use a different denominator, $\hat{s}_{pooled}$, pronounced "s hat pooled." $\hat{s}_{pooled}$ is an estimate of the population standard deviation based on both groups, on both groups being *pooled* together. It has a couple of advantages over using the standard deviation of the control group. First, it is not always clear which group is the control group, and which is the experimental group. For example, if I am comparing boys to girls to see which are taller, should the boys be the control group or should the girls? Depending on which group I use, *d* will vary. The second reason is that $\hat{s}_{pooled}$ will be larger than at least one of the individual standard deviations on which it is based. This occurs because there will be more variability in two groups combined than there is in one group by itself. Thus, using $\hat{s}_{pooled}$ will often result in a smaller, a more conservative, estimate of *d*.

Calculating $\hat{s}_{pooled}$ isn't too hard if you saved the value you calculated for the first bracket under the square root sign in Equation 9.3. The value in the bracket was the pooled estimated population variance, $\hat{s}^2_{pooled}$, and all you need to do is take the square root of that to find $\hat{s}_{pooled}$. However, if you didn't save that value and if you would like a formal equation for $\hat{s}_{pooled}$, here it is:

F O R M U L A

$\hat{s}_{pooled}$, The Pooled Estimate of the Population Standard Deviation

Equation 9.5

$$\hat{s}_{pooled} = \sqrt{\frac{(n_1 - 1)\hat{s}_1^2 + (n_2 - 1)\hat{s}_2^2}{n_1 + n_2 - 2}}$$

Where:

$\hat{s}_{pooled}$ = the pooled estimate of the population standard deviation being calculated

n_1 = the sample size for the first group

$\hat{s}_1^2$ = the estimated population variance for the first group

n_2 = the sample size for the second group

$\hat{s}_2^2$ = the estimated population variance for the second group

This formula says: (1) Take the estimated population variance for each sample, multiply it by the number of the cases in the sample, and add them up. (2) Divide this sum by the degrees of freedom for the *t* test. (3) Take the square root of this quotient.

Using this formula, here is how we calculate $\hat{s}_{pooled}$ for the mouse-maze data set:

$$\hat{s}_{pooled} = \sqrt{\frac{(5 - 1).0988 + (5 - 1).1298}{5 + 5 - 2}} = \sqrt{.1143} = .3381$$

Knowing how to calculate $\hat{s}_{pooled}$, we can now learn the formula for calculating an effect size for an independent-samples *t* test, Equation 9.6.

F O R M U L A

Effect Size (*d*) for an Independent-Samples *t* Test

Equation 9.6

$$d = \frac{M_E - M_C}{\hat{s}_{pooled}}$$

Where:

d = the effect size being calculated

M_E = the mean of the experimental group sample

M_C = the mean of the control group sample

$\hat{s}_{pooled}$ = the pooled estimated population standard deviation

This formula says that d is calculated by finding the difference between the two means and dividing it by the pooled estimate of the population standard deviation. For the mouse-maze data set we calculate d this way:

$$d = \frac{4.5180 - 5.3260}{.3381} = -2.3898 = -2.39$$

This tells us that the mean of the experimental group is 2.39 standard deviations *lower* than the mean of the control group. Though you may not recognize it as such yet, this is a whopping effect size.

One way to interpret d is via Cohen's (1988) small, medium, and large effect sizes.* A small effect size ($r = .10$) is equivalent to $d \approx .20$, a medium effect size ($r = .30$) is equivalent to $d \approx .60$, and a large effect size ($r = .50$) is equivalent to $d \approx 1.20$.

Another way to make sense of an effect size is to put it in terms of a variable with which you are familiar and for which you have an intuitive sense or context. As a psychologist, I use IQ, which has a mean of 100 and a standard deviation of 15. If you're in the health sciences, you might want to consider blood pressure. In the United States, the average systolic blood pressure is 124 mm Hg with a standard deviation of 16. (Diastolic blood pressure has a mean of 77 mm Hg and a standard deviation of 11.) Thus, an effect size of 2.39 means a change of ≈ 36 IQ points, a systolic blood pressure change of ≈ 38 mm Hg, or a diastolic blood pressure change of ≈ 26 mm Hg. That's a lot of effect.

Another way to make sense of an effect size is to treat it as a z score and use it to envision how two normal distributions would overlap. Imagine that the distribution of maze-running times for the experimental mice (the dotted line) is shifted 2.39 standard deviations below the mean of the distribution of maze-running times for the control mice (the continuous line), as shown in Figure 9.6. The darkly shaded section of the distribution represents the control mice times that are faster than the average time for the experimental mice. Consulting a table of area under the curve for the normal distribution tells us that only .84% of the mice in the control group are faster than the "average" mouse in the experimental group. Phrased differently, the average mouse in the experimental group is faster than over 99% of the mice in the control group.[†] The fear stimulus seems to speed up mice quite a lot. My interpretative statement for the

*Cohen, J. (1988). *Statistical power analysis for the behavioral sciences.* Hillsdale, NJ: Lawrence Erlbaum Associates.

[†]Be aware that if two distributions overlap perfectly, the average case in the experimental group has performed better than 50% of the cases in the control group. A statement like "the average case in the experimental group performed better than 55% of the cases in the control group" sounds like the experimental group did dramatically better than the control group. But this is not really the case since it is only an increase of 5%. I hope that you remember that the same interpretative limitation held for the binomial effect size display.

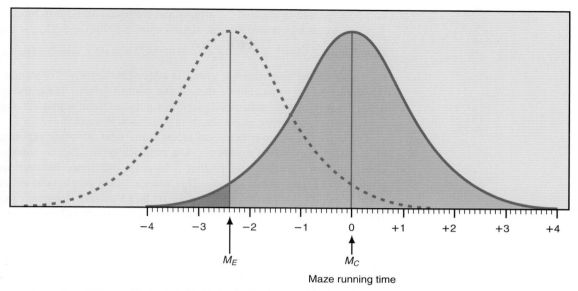

Figure **9.6** Graphic display of effect size (*d*) for effect of fear stimulus on maze-running time for mice.

effect size would read, "I calculated an effect size and found it to be very large, −2.39. This means that the mean of the experimental group was 2.39 standard deviations below the mean of the control group. Assuming that both populations are normally distributed, the "average" mouse, running the maze when a fear stimulus is present, runs the maze faster than 99% of the mice do when there is no fear stimulus present. The presence of a fear stimulus substantially decreases the time it takes mice to run a maze."

It is possible to calculate a confidence interval for *d,* and I show how to do so in the context of Group Practice 9.7.

Many statisticians feel that reporting effect sizes has an advantage over reporting statistical significance. The truth about the statistical significance of *t* is that it is heavily dependent on the size of the samples. Think about IQ and how meaningful a change of one IQ point is. If your IQ were average, such as 100, do you think it would make much difference in your life if someone waved a magic wand over your head and increased your IQ score by one point, to 101? I don't think this difference would have any impact on any aspect of your life. In other words, if we had a group of people who we randomly divided into control and experimental groups, and we did something to the experimental group that increased their IQ by one point, neither you nor I would consider that change to be of any practical significance. But, since the standard error of the difference is heavily influenced by sample size, if *N* is large enough, a *t* value will be statistically significant even if the difference is small. For example, if we had 5000 people in each of the groups and we found an IQ difference of 1 point, we would find statistical significance: $t(9998) = 3.33$, $p < .05$. Calculating d yields $d = \dfrac{101 - 100}{15} = 0.0667 = 0.07$,* which says that the mean of the experimental group is only very slightly, .07 standard deviations to be exact, above that of the control group. Thus, though saying that results are statistically significant makes them sound like they are important, reporting effect size brings us back to earth.

For a similar reason, there are statisticians who advocate reporting effect sizes even when results are *not* statistically significant. Imagine doing another IQ study and finding a 15-point difference between the control and experimental groups. This sounds like a meaningful difference. Wouldn't you like to improve your IQ by 15 points? However, since the sample size is small, only seven per group, we would fail to reject the null hypothesis, finding $t(12) = 1.73$, $p > .05$. Some statisticians advocate reporting the effect size anyway, which in this case is 1.00, to decrease the risk of making a Type II error. Their thinking is that when d is large and results are not statistically significant, a researcher should be alerted to the possibility that the independent variable really does make a difference.

I hate to be old-fashioned, but I disagree. The point of hypothesis testing is to help us decide whether a difference between samples is large enough to reflect a difference between populations. If there is a difference between populations then we would expect, fairly consistently, to find a difference between samples. In that sense a statistically significant difference represents a reliable difference. If the observed difference is not large enough to be considered to represent a real difference, then there's little reason to believe that such a difference will be observed again. In other words, results that are not statistically significant mean that when the study is repeated, we may find, instead of an effect size of 1, an effect size of −1, or 0, or any other value. That is, the effect size is not consistent. This shows once again that you can't have practical significance without statistical significance, and so I don't advocate calculating d if the t value is not statistically significant.

I think that my practice of reporting the confidence interval and power or sample size (which I am about to teach you for independent-samples t tests) is adequate to alert you to the likelihood of a Type II error. At the same time, I recognize that it is becoming standard practice to report effect sizes whether or not there is statistical significance and I won't stand in your, or your instructor's, way if you choose to do so.

Size of the Difference III: Percentage of Variance Predicted

Another way that an independent-samples t can be interpreted is by calculating the percentage of variance in the dependent variable that

Group Practice 9.7

Calculate and interpret the effect size for the question in Group Practice 9.5. Be sure to make a graph for the questions, as shown in Figure 9.6.

To learn how to calculate a confidence interval for d, be sure to read the answer to this Group Practice problem.

LOOKING CLOSER

Here I'm using the population value of the standard deviation for IQ scores to calculate d.

is predicted by the grouping variable.* We saw this concept back in Chapter 8 when we learned to calculate the coefficient of determination, r^2. r^2 tells, for a correlation, how much of the variability in X is predicted by Y and vice versa. As we saw in Chapter 8, the greater the percentage of variability predicted, the stronger the correlation.

The same holds true for an independent-samples *t* test, although (just to confuse things) what is called r^2 or the coefficient of determination for a correlation is called omega squared, abbreviated ω^2, for the *t* test.[†] Not only do they differ in name, but they differ in a substantive way as well: r^2 tells the percentage of variance in one variable predicted by the other *for the sample*, but ω^2 estimates the percentage of variance in the dependent variable that is predicted by the grouping variable *in the population* (Kirk, 1995).[‡] Let me give you the formula for ω^2 and then we'll see how to interpret it for a *t* test.

FORMULA

ω^2, The Estimated Proportion of Variance in the Dependent Variable in the Population That Is Predicted by the Grouping Variable, for an Independent-Samples *t* Test[§]

$$\omega^2 = \frac{t^2 - 1}{t^2 + df + 1}$$

Equation 9.7

Where:

ω^2 = an estimate of the population proportion of variance in the dependent variable that is predicted by the grouping variable

t = the observed independent-samples *t* test value (from Equation 9.2b)

df = the degrees of freedom for the independent-samples *t* test

---

To calculate ω^2, one takes $t_{observed}$, squares it, and subtracts one from the squared value. This difference is then divided by the sum of the squared *t* value plus the degrees of freedom plus one. With our mouse-maze data, we calculate the percentage of variance in running time (the dependent

---

*Researchers also speak of the percentage of variance predicted as telling the percentage of variance *explained* in one variable by the other, or as the percentage of variance in the dependent variable that is *accounted for* by the independent variable.

[†] ω is the lowercase version of the Greek letter "omega" and, though it is not the last Greek letter we are going to learn, it *is* the last letter in the Greek alphabet. Thus, where we might say that we have covered a topic from a to z, Greeks would say that they had covered a topic from alpha to omega.

[‡] Kirk, R. E. (1995). *Experimental design: procedures for the behavioral sciences,* (3rd ed.). Pacific Grove, CA: Brooks/Cole Publishing Company.

[§] This formula is only for an independent-samples *t* test. You'll have to wait until Chapter 11 to learn what to do with a dependent-samples *t* test.

 LOOKING CLOSER

variable) that is predicted by the presence/absence of a fear stimulus (the independent variable) as follows:

$$\frac{3.7810^2 - 1}{3.7810^2 + 8 + 1} = .5707 = .57$$

Note that though I am carrying all my decimal places in the calculations, the convention is to report ω^2 only to two decimal places. ω^2 is usually reported as the *percentage* of variance predicted, so I'm transforming the proportion (.57) to a percentage (57%).

What does this 57% mean? An inspection of the maze-running times tells us that not all mice run the maze in exactly the same time: there is variability in maze-running time. What explains this variability? Well, there probably are individual differences among mice (some are faster, some are smarter, some are lazier, some have had better nutrition, some find the temperature in the room oppressive) that explain a lot of the variability. But in this experiment there is another factor—the independent variable—that differs from one group of mice (the control group) to the other (the experimental group). And this independent variable, the presence/absence of a fear stimulus, predicts (or explains) a very large percentage, 57% to be exact, of the variability in maze-running time. With 57% explained by the independent variable, only 43% is left to be explained either by individual mouse differences or some other systematic variable.* This 57% is a very large effect for an independent variable, and so my interpretative statement would be something like this: "The presence or absence of the fear stimulus explains a very large amount of the variability, 57% to be exact, in the speed with which mice run the maze. Having a fear stimulus present has a substantial impact on making mice run a maze more quickly."

Size of the Difference IV: From *t* to *r* and the Binomial Effect Size Display

We just calculated ω^2 for a *t* test, which is similar to r^2 for a Pearson *r* since both calculate the percentage of variance predicted in one variable by the other. I want you to see the connection between these two, ω^2 and r^2, and hope that makes you wonder whether we can take the square root of ω^2 and turn a *t* into an *r*. The short answer is yes, we can. Why would we want to do this? Because back in Chapter 8 we learned a number of techniques for interpreting correlations, and we could then apply them to interpreting a *t* test.

Above we calculated ω^2 for our mouse-maze data set as .5707. The square root of this is .7554 or, rounded to two decimal places, .76. Thus

---

Group Practice 9.8

Calculate and interpret ω^2 for the question in Group Practice 9.5.

To learn how to calculate a 95% confidence interval for ω^2, be sure to read the answer to this group practice problem.

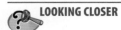 **LOOKING CLOSER**

There's another factor that could account for part of the 43% of unexplained variability: random error. There may be some error in measurement, in how accurately we timed the maze-running times, that accounts for variability in mouse running times. As well, there may be random, mouse to mouse, fluctuations in temperature or other environmental factors that influence maze-running times.

we can *estimate* the correlation between the presence or absence of a fear stimulus and the time it takes to run the maze as .76. But, remember that ω^2 is a *population* estimate, so the r that we have just calculated is an estimate of the correlation between the independent and dependent variables in the population. I'm going to call it $\hat{r}$, that's "r hat," to keep the difference clear.* Here's the equation for it:

FORMULA

$\hat{r}$ For an Independent-Samples *t* Test

$$\hat{r} = \sqrt{\omega^2}$$

Equation 9.8a

Where:

$\hat{r}$ = an estimate of ρ for the relationship between the independent and dependent variable

ω^2 = the estimate of the percentage of variance in the population in the dependent variable that is predicted by the grouping variable for an independent-samples *t* test (from Equation 9.7)

Of course, there's another way to turn a *t* test into a correlation coefficient that is not as simple as taking the square root of ω^2. Technically, this type of correlation coefficient is called a point-biserial correlation, abbreviated r_{pb}, pronounced "r sub pb." Earlier I said that correlations should only be calculated for two interval/ratio variables, and our grouping variable here, whether a fear stimulus is present or not, is a nominal variable. Well, when one variable is dichotomous (that is, there are only two options: fear stimulus present vs. fear stimulus not present) and the other variable is continuous, we can use a special form of the Pearson r, r_{pb}, assuming that the dichotomous variable is scored as having values of zero and one. r_{pb} calculates the *sample* value for the correlation between the grouping and dependent variables. Thus, if we calculated r^2 from r_{pb}, we would expect it to be different from ω^2, and larger than ω^2.[†]

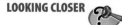

LOOKING CLOSER

*Thus, there are three types of Pearson correlation coefficients (r, $\hat{r}$, and ρ) just as there are three types of standard deviations (s, $\hat{s}$, and σ).

[†]Why larger? Because ω^2 is an estimate of the population value, and r^2 is a sample value. Statisticians make the assumption that there may be chance factors that inflate the value of a statistic for any given sample and so they "shrink" the value when they estimate a population value from a sample value. (Yes, I know that this is not the case for s vs. $\hat{s}$, but that's a different story.)

And, how much larger? Well, that depends both on N and t. As N gets larger, the estimate of the population value shrinks less. And as t gets larger the estimate shrinks less also.

F O R M U L A

Point Biserial Correlation Coefficient from an Independent-Samples *t* Test

Equation 9.8b

$$r_{pb} = \sqrt{\frac{t^2}{t^2 + df}}$$

Where:

r_{pb} = the point biserial correlation coefficient being calculated

t = the independent-samples *t* test value

df = the degrees of freedom for the independent-samples *t* test

This formula says to square the *t* value, and then divide the squared *t* value by itself plus the degrees of freedom. Finally, one takes the square root of this quotient. For the mouse-maze data, this is what we calculate:

$$\sqrt{\frac{3.7810^2}{3.7810^2 + 8}} = .8007 = .80$$

Note that if I went on to calculate r^2 from r_{pb} I would find it to equal .64. As I predicted, this is larger than our ω^2 value of .57.

I'm going to use and interpret r_{pb}, not $\hat{r}$. So why did I introduce and explain $\hat{r}$? Because I thought it would help you see the connection between r and t via the connection between r^2 and ω^2.

Before we go on, note that squaring the *t* value obscures information about direction. So, after we find r_{pb} we must go back and look at the sample means to draw conclusions about direction. With that proviso, let's forge ahead with our $r = .80$ from the mouse-maze data.*

Again, why have we turned *t* into *r*? So that we can take advantage of some of the interpretation techniques we learned for the Pearson *r*. For the Pearson *r* we learned to calculate a confidence interval, which we've already done for the *t*, and we learned to calculate r^2, which we've already done for the *t*. Now let's apply the binomial effect size display and power analysis to the *t* test.

The binomial effect size display, or *BESD*, which we covered in Equation 8.4, takes a correlation and converts it into a statement about the likelihood of the cases in the two groups having high or low scores on the dependent variable. In this case we will examine the likelihood that a case in the control group (no fear stimulus present) runs the maze quickly or slowly vs. the likelihood that a case in the experimental group

LOOKING CLOSER   *Most researchers simply abbreviate the point biserial correlation coefficient as *r*, not r_{pb}.

(fear stimulus present) runs the maze quickly or slowly. Remember that when we turn a *t* into an *r* we always get a positive *r*, so we will need to think about direction. In this case we know, from the mean of 5.33 seconds for the control group and 4.52 seconds for the experimental group, that the experimental group cases run the maze faster. Thus, when we do the *BESD* calculations for *r* = .80, we end up with this:

	Run maze slowly	**Run maze quickly**	
Control Group	A $50 + \dfrac{100(.80)}{2} = 90$	B $50 - \dfrac{100(.80)}{2} = 10$	100
Experimental Group	C $50 - \dfrac{100(.80)}{2} = 10$	D $50 + \dfrac{100(.80)}{2} = 90$	100
	100	100	200

Thus we conclude that mice in the control group have a 10% chance of running the maze quickly, whereas mice in the experimental group have a 90% chance of running the maze quickly. As an interpretative statement I would say, "I converted the *t* value into an estimate of *r* and found it to be .80. When I converted this into a binomial effect size display, I found that mice running the maze when a fear stimulus was present (mice in the experimental group) had a 90% chance of running the maze quickly, whereas mice in the control group had only a 10% chance of running the maze quickly. Mice in the experimental group were about 9 times more likely than mice in the control group to run the maze quickly. This shows that fear stimulus has a substantial impact on mouse–maze-running behavior, that it significantly speeds up maze-running times."

Group Practice 9.9

For the question in Group Practice 9.5, calculate *r* and the binomial effect size display. Interpret the binomial effect size display.

To learn to calculate a 95% confidence interval for r and BESD, be sure to read the answer to this group practice problem.

Power

Our final aspect of interpretation considers power and sample size. Power, as I hope you remember from interpreting correlations, is related to *β*, the likelihood of making a Type II error. Power tells how likely it is that one has made the correct choice of rejecting the null hypothesis. For independent-samples *t* tests, power tells the likelihood, given a certain *N* and a certain effect size, of finding a statistically significant difference between two samples *when the two population means actually are different*.

Having converted our *t* score into r_{pb}, it is easy to calculate power by using Appendix Table 7. We know that *r* = .80 for the mouse-maze data set, and our *N* was 10. Looking at the intersection of the column for *r* = .80 and the row for *N* = 10, we find that power = .82. In percentage terms, this means that we have an 82% chance of correctly rejecting the null hypothesis if the population value of the correlation (ρ) is .80 with a sample of size 10. Commonly, statisticians like power to be set at .80 or higher (i.e., an 80% chance or higher), and this value meets that criterion. We had sufficient power to have at least an 80% chance of rejecting the null hypothesis. Looking at Appendix Table 8, we can see that a total sample size of ten was what was required to have an 80% chance of finding a significant difference between two groups with α set a .05, two-tailed. If we wanted more power, power set at .95, we, should have had a total of 15 cases, or seven to eight cases per group.

There's another way to calculate sample size for an independent-samples t test, a quick calculation from vanBelle's book (2002) of statistical rules of thumb.* All one needs to know is d, the effect size calculated in Equation 9.6. However, as I want to use this equation to calculate sample size *in advance* of doing a t test, I am going to use a simpler version of d, the mean of the experimental group minus the mean of the control group, divided by the standard deviation of the control group.[†]

F O R M U L A

"Rule of Thumb" Estimate of Sample Size per Group for Independent-Samples t Test with α Set at .05 and Power Set at .80

Equation 9.9

$$n = \frac{16}{\left(\dfrac{M_E - M_C}{\hat{s}_C}\right)^2}$$

Where:
n = sample size for each group in an independent-samples t test
M_E = the mean of the experimental group
M_C = the mean of the control group
$\hat{s}_C$ = the corrected standard deviation of the control group
NOTE: Since this formula is calculating sample size, an integer value, round the answer for *N up* to an integer value.

This formula says that we take the constant 16 and divide it by the square of one group mean minus the other divided by the estimated population standard deviation of the control group.[‡] Applying this formula to the mice-maze data set we calculate the following:

LOOKING CLOSER

*VanBelle, G. (2002). *Statistical rules of thumb*. New York: John Wiley & Sons.

[†]If you want to be conservative and would rather err on the side of having a larger sample size, use the larger of the standard deviations for the control and experimental groups, not the control group standard deviation.

[‡]Want a shorthand way of thinking of this? Think of it as $\dfrac{16}{d^2}$.

$$n = \frac{16}{\left(\dfrac{4.5180 - 5.3260}{.3144} \right)^2} = \frac{16}{-2.5700^2} = 2.4224 = 3$$

Thus we conclude that we need about three cases per group, a grand total of six cases, to have an 80% chance of rejecting the null hypothesis when the effect size is $|-2.57|$. Note that the total N calculated here, six, is less than the value of 10 calculated via Appendix Table 8. Do we need three cases per group or five? For two reasons I'm going to select the larger number, five per cell. First, it is not calculated via a "rule of thumb" formula. In addition, I want to be conservative and select a value that means I will have a larger sample size. However, I also want you to have this "rule of thumb" formula in your bag of statistical tricks since it provides a quick way to estimate sample size for an independent-samples t test.

In my interpretative statement about power and sample size for the mouse-maze data I would say something along these lines: "My study had adequate power for me to be able to reject the null hypothesis and conclude that the presence of a fear stimulus had a significant effect on maze-running speed for mice. Though the sample size was adequate, I recommend redoing the study with a larger sample size to increase confidence in the results."

Ideally, you should think about whether your sample size is adequate before completing the t test. If you think back to Step 4, the decision rule, I broached the topic of sample size there. Thus, before you go on to calculate a t test you should determine whether you have enough subjects to have a powerful enough test, to have a reasonable chance of being able to reject the null hypothesis. This is where VanBelle's rule-of-thumb formula comes in.*

Imagine conducting a study to test a new antihypertensive medication. We expect that the traditional blood pressure medication will reduce the systolic blood pressure to 130, whereas the new medication will reduce the systolic blood pressure to 124. We know, from previous research, that the standard deviation for systolic blood pressure is around 16. Thus, we calculate d as being .3750. Using Equation 9.9 we find that we need 114 people in each of the two groups in order to have a reasonable chance, an 80% chance, of being able to find that the new medicine is better than the old medication in reducing blood pressure. This large sample size may cause us to rethink the feasibility of doing the study. Conducting a study with enough cases is better than doing the study with too few cases in each group and making a Type II error, concluding that the new medication is no better than the old when in reality it is.

Back to our mouse-maze study: There's only one more bit of interpretation required before putting it all together. Talking about power—about

---

*VanBelle, G. (2002). *Statistical rules of thumb*. New York: John Wiley & Sons.

LOOKING CLOSER

Group Practice 9.10

For the question in Group Practice 9.5 calculate α, β, power, and the sample size necessary to have an 80% chance of rejecting the null hypothesis when $\alpha = .05$, two tailed. Write an interpretative statement that addresses the possibility that the results of the t test are in error.

Type II error—should remind you that we need to address the likelihood of error in our results. Might the results be the consequence of an unusual sample from the population? Since we rejected the null hypothesis, we need to be worried about Type I error—the possibility that we have rejected the null hypothesis by mistake. So, here's how the next interpretative statement to add would read: "Since I rejected the null hypothesis, I need to be worried about Type I error—that I have rejected the null hypothesis in error. I set the probability of this error at .05, meaning that there is a 5% chance that this error has actually occurred. To increase confidence that I did not reject the null hypothesis in error, I recommend replicating the study with a larger sample size. Though five mice per group is all that is needed to have the standard level of statistical power, I suggest using a larger sample size to have more confidence that the results are reflective of the larger population."*

Had we failed to reject the null hypothesis I would have worried about the possibility that we made a Type II error and I would have calculated β, the possibility of a Type II error, as $1.00 - \text{power}$.

Putting the Interpretation All Together

There have been many parts to the interpretation of an independent-samples t test that we have calculated and thought about, more than we can possibly use. So, let me list all the interpretative aspects that we generated and then pick and choose from them for a meaningful, coherent, and not-too-long interpretation. The options for interpretation are listed in Table 9.5. Remember, these are all tools—many of them screwdrivers—that we have in our toolbox. Which screwdriver you use depends in part on what type of screw you are confronting—small or large, Phillips or slotted—but also on what screwdriver is handy and/or if you have a favorite.

There is one item in Table 9.5 that I have not yet discussed: strengths, limitations, and suggestions. Having completed the data analysis, having been intimately involved in a study, you are in a good position to know the strengths and weaknesses of the study. Thus, the final part of an interpretation should be an acknowledgment of the strengths and weaknesses of a study and suggestions for future research. In the present study, the small sample size is a major weakness. We found statistically significant results with only five mice per group, but five is not a very large number. I'd feel more comfortable that the results are reflective of the larger population if either the sample size had been larger or if the study was replicated. In addition, I feel compelled to make some mention of the limits of generalizing from this study. This study tells me that having a cat watch laboratory mice when they run a maze leads to the mice running

---

LOOKING CLOSER   *Type I means that our conclusion is wrong, not that our results are wrong.

TABLE **9.5** **Interpreting an Independent-Samples *t* Test**

I. Report, briefly, objective of study and results

II. If fail to reject H_0:
   A. Report no statistical difference between sample means (difference between sample means is not statistically significant)
   B. Conclude not sufficient evidence to conclude is a mean difference between the two populations
   C. Calculate confidence interval, power, and sample size. (Many statisticians recommend calculating and reporting effect sizes [e.g., d] even when the null hypothesis is not rejected.)
   D. Discuss possibility of Type II error
   E. Strengths/limitations/suggestions

III. If reject H_0:
   A. Report difference between sample means is statistically different from zero (is a statistically significant difference between sample means)
   B. Conclude there is likely a difference between the two population means
   C. Report direction of difference
   D. Report size of difference
      1. Confidence interval
      2. Effect size
         a. d
         b. area under the normal curve
      3. ω^2
      4. r_{pb}
         a. *BESD*
   E. Calculate power and sample size
   F. Discuss possibility of Type I error
   G. Strengths/limitations/suggestions

the maze more quickly. Can we generalize that the effect would hold for wild mice, with more experience with cats? Can we conclude that all fear stimuli speed up all behaviors for all species? I don't think so, and so we need to mention these limitations. Oh yes, one more thing: don't forget to start out your interpretation with a brief recapitulation of what was done and what was found. Doing so puts the interpretation in context and allows it to stand on its own.

Be aware that different parts of the interpretative calculations may appear to be in conflict: they may lead to different conclusions. One part may, for example, suggest that the effect is not strong, and another may suggest that the effect is meaningful. The reason often comes down to sample size, so let me explain why I am going to end up, for the mouse-maze data, suggesting that the study be replicated with a larger sample size.

Larger samples provide more robust estimates of population values since they are more likely to be representative of the population. Say that we are taking a sample from your college to determine the mean height of its students. I presume that you agree that a sample of 60 is preferable to a sample of six in terms of representing the population of college students. At some point, diminishing returns set in, and the added benefits may not be worth the added cost of increasing the sample from 60 to 200. As we saw in Chapter 6, it is possible to calculate the sample size needed for a confidence interval of a given width. Pollsters routinely draw accurate conclusions about 300 million Americans with samples of 2500.

Other things being equal, larger samples provide better estimates of population values. Sample size also has a ripple effect on t tests and other statistics. If everything else is held constant and only the sample size is increased, a larger sample size will yield a smaller standard error of the difference, the denominator in the independent-samples t test. A smaller $\hat{s}_{M_1 - M_2}$ will result in a larger t value, which means that one is more likely to reject the null hypothesis. In addition, a larger sample size will yield a narrower confidence interval, a bigger d, a larger ω^2, a larger r, and more power. Clearly, getting more cases buys one a lot.

This all said, here's my interpretative statement for our mouse/maze data set. Remember, interpretation is a human endeavor. It is where the researcher makes sense of the results, where he or she explains what is important about the results. As a human endeavor it is personal: what I think should be highlighted about the results may not be what you think should be highlighted, so my interpretative statement will almost certainly differ from yours.* Finally, note that I'm not afraid to play with numbers—to calculate percentages for example, to put results in context. That said, here 'tis:

> *"We conducted a study in which we examined the effect of a fear stimulus, the presence of a cat, on the behavior of mice. We took mice that had been trained to run a maze and randomly assigned them to two groups. For the control group we did nothing but time how long it took them to run the maze; the experimental group ran the maze while being observed by a cat. The control group mice ran the maze in a mean of 5.33 sec ($\hat{s} = .31$) and the experimental mice ran it in 4.52 sec ($\hat{s} = .36$). The difference between the two groups was statistically significant ($t(8) = 3.78$, $p < .05$), suggesting that the presence of a cat caused mice to run the maze faster.*
>
> *"The 95% confidence interval for the difference between the two population means suggests that when the fear stimulus of a cat is present, mice run the maze from .32 to 1.30 seconds faster than when there is no fear stimulus. This is a large effect since it indicates that a fear stimulus causes mice to run from 6% to 24% faster. In my view, even*

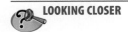 **LOOKING CLOSER**

*I don't mean to suggest that an interpretative statement is entirely subjective, that there is no right or wrong about it. There is right and wrong in interpretation! Still, interpretations differ in their emphases.

'only' a 6% increase in speed is a substantial increase. As another way to view the strength of this effect, I converted the t value into a binomial effect size display, which showed that about 90% of the mice in the experimental group (the group that sees the fear stimulus) run the maze quickly, compared to only about 10% of the mice in the control group running the maze quickly.*

"There is, of course, a chance that the conclusion that a fear stimulus has a significant effect on mouse behavior is in error. In the current experiment, the chance of this conclusion being in error is 5%. To increase certainty in the results of the current study, I recommend replicating the study with a larger sample size.

"Finally, I want to caution against overgeneralizing these results. These results indicate that the presence of a cat, a presumed fear stimulus, makes laboratory mice run a maze faster. Whether the effect holds for wild mice or for mice that have had prior experience with cats is unknown. Similarly, whether other fear stimuli have a similar effect on other behaviors in mice or whether fear stimuli have a similar effect on other species must be determined."

> ### Group Practice 9.11
>
> Based upon your answers to Group Practices 9.5 through 9.10, write a final interpretative statement for the question in Group Practice 9.5. The goal of interpretation is to tell the story of what the results mean. Be thorough, but remember, less is more!

PRACTICING INDEPENDENT-SAMPLES *t* TESTS

For practice, let's work through two more independent-samples *t* tests. The first involves a problem that anyone who has ever baked a cake has encountered, getting the cake out of the pan in one piece. Imagine that a chef has developed a new cooking spray that he thinks lets cakes slide more easily out of pans. He tells one of his clients about this and the client, a scientist, helps the chef test the effectiveness of the new spray. They decide to compare the new spray to the traditional technique of buttering the pan. They prepare the batter for a cake and flip a coin to decide whether they will spray the pan (experimental group) or butter the pan (control group). After they have prepared the pan and put the batter in, they give the cake to someone else to bake. This person then bakes the cake until it is done, removes the cake from the oven, lets it cool for a specified period, and removes the cake from the pan. (They have someone else do this, someone who does not know whether butter or spray was used, so that this person can't influence the outcome of the study. The chef, who hopes to make a lot of money if his spray works, might—consciously or unconsciously—bias the results.) After the cake has been

---

*Note that I chose to interpret the binomial effect size display, not the effect size. The effect size, *d*, led to the conclusion that the average mouse running the maze with a fear stimulus present ran it faster than 99% of the mice in the no-fear condition. This seems like a very large effect, larger than I really believe was at play, especially with such a small sample size. So, I decided to be conservative and interpret the smaller effect size observed with the binomial effect size display.

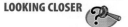 **LOOKING CLOSER**

TABLE **9.6**   **Grams of Cake Left in the Pan: Experimental Spray vs. Butter**

	Control (Butter)	Experimental (Spray)
	1.84	.83
	1.93	1.79
	1.56	2.36
	1.98	2.33
	2.23	1.33
	3.14	1.34
	.98	.77
	1.73	1.67
	3.19	2.53
	2.92	1.62
	1.37	2.35
	3.43	1.15
		1.13
n	12	13
M	2.1917	1.6308
$\hat{s}$	.7951	.6064
Skewness (SE)	.2604 (.7071)	.1529 (.6794)
Kurtosis (SE)	−1.1951 (1.4142)	−1.3071 (1.3587)

removed from the pan, this third person scrapes out any pieces of cake that have been left in the pan and weighs them to determine how much cake stuck to the pan. More weight indicates more cake stuck to the pan. They do this for a baker's dozen of each type, a total of 26 cakes. Unfortunately, their helper tripped and dropped one of the cakes, so they ended up with 12 control cakes and 13 experimental cakes. Here, in Table 9.6, are their data.

It certainly looks like the new spray is working better than the butter since there is about a half gram less cake left in the pan when the new spray is being used, 2.19 grams vs. 1.63 grams. Still, is this difference large enough to be a statistically significant difference? Or, is it just due to sampling error, and the next time we did the study we might find a very different outcome? Let's march through the six steps of Tom and Harry and find out.

Test

The first question is what test we are doing and why. We will use an independent-samples t test because we have two samples (spray vs. butter), the samples are independent (remember that flipped coin that determined whether spray or butter was used), and we have a ratio-level variable, grams of cake left in the pan.

Assumptions

There are five assumptions for the independent-samples *t* test: independent samples, interval- or ratio level-data, random samples, normality, and homogeneity of variance. We've determined that we have independent samples and ratio-level data so the first two assumptions, which are not robust, were not violated. The third assumption, that we have random samples from the respective populations of buttered and sprayed cakes, was violated since we don't have a sample from the population of all cakes being baked. However, violating this assumption is not problematic, so we can proceed.

The fourth assumption, that the data—in the population—are normally distributed can be violated if *N* is large. In this case, however, *N* is small, less than 50, so we need to worry about the assumption.* With such small sample sizes, I am not going to worry about multimodality. The calculated 95% confidence intervals for skewness and kurtosis for each variable reveal that each confidence interval captures zero, so I'm comfortable assuming that each population is normally distributed.†

The final assumption can be assessed by looking at the two standard deviations (.63 and .37) and noting that one is not twice the other. Thus, the only assumption that was violated, random samples from the population, is a robust assumption, and we are good to go with the *t* test.

Hypotheses

The null hypothesis says that the means of the two populations are the same, and the alternative says that the two means are different. This is written, in symbolic notation, as follows:

$$H_0: \mu_E = \mu_C$$
$$H_1: \mu_E \pm \mu_C$$

In English, the null hypothesis says that the means of the two populations are the same. Though the two population means are the same, we don't expect to find that the two sample means are exactly equivalent to each other. However, the two sample means should be close enough to each other that any observed difference can be explained by sampling error for two samples drawn from one population.

---

*And even if *N* were large we would need to calculate the confidence intervals for skewness and kurtosis. Why? Because assumptions are robust to a point. If the violation of normality were extreme, it might push our robust assumption to the breaking point. So, to know whether the assumption is violated to this extreme point, we must calculate the confidence intervals. Sorry.

†The *95% CI* for skewness for the control group is −1.13 to 1.65; for kurtosis it is −3.97 to 1.58. The two CIs, respectively, for the experimental group are −1.18 to 1.48 and −3.97 to 1.36.

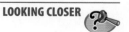 **LOOKING CLOSER**

The alternative hypothesis says that the two population means are different. Thus, when we obtain the two sample means they should be far enough apart that they reflect this real difference between the two populations.

Decision Rule

The next step involves the decision rule. I'm opting for the default options, a two-tailed test with alpha set at .05. (Why am I setting α at .05? Because I am willing to make a Type I error 5% of the time.) With $N = 25$ and $df = 23$, $t_{cv} = 2.0687$. Thus, the decision rule is that if $|t_{observed}| \geq 2.0687$, it is a rare occurrence if H_0 is true, we will reject the null hypothesis, report $p < .05$, and conclude that there is probably a significant difference between the two population means. If $|t_{observed}| < 2.0687$, then we conclude that this is a common outcome when H_0 is true, and we'll fail to reject the null hypothesis. As a result, we would report $p > .05$ and conclude that there is insufficient evidence to conclude that there is a difference between the two population means.

The last part of the decision rule step involves deciding if our sample size is adequate. The easiest way to do this is to use vanBelle's formula (Equation 9.9) to estimate sample size. Using that formula, we see that if the difference between the two population means is really .56 grams, that we would need about 21 cakes per group to have at least an 80% chance of rejecting the null hypothesis. Thus, the current study with only 12 to 13 cakes per group is underpowered. Therefore, I recommend that before the data are analyzed the chef should bake more cakes so that he will have a fighting chance of rejecting the null hypothesis if the null hypothesis should be rejected.

Calculations

Since the chef will not take my advice but wants to conclude the study without collecting any more data, we proceed. We calculate $t(23) = 1.99$, $p > .05$.* As shown in Figure 9.7, this is a commonly observed result when the null hypothesis is true, so we have failed to reject the null hypothesis and have concluded that there is no statistically significant difference between the use of butter or the experimental spray in terms of how much cake sticks to a pan.

Interpretation

There's less math to do when the t value is not significant, but one still needs to explain, in English, what one found: "I analyzed the data from a study that compared two methods of greasing pans for baking cakes to

---

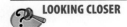 **LOOKING CLOSER**   *If you want to do the calculations, which I heartily recommend, you should find that $\hat{s}_{M_1-M_2} = .2814$.

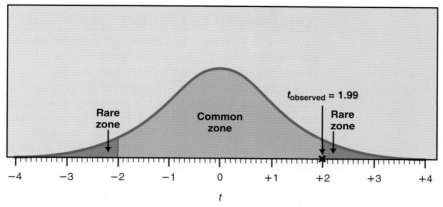

Figure **9.7** Graphic display of $t_{observed} = 1.99$ in relation to $t_{cv} = \pm 2.07$ for the cake-baking experiment. (Sampling distribution of *t* from Lowry R: *Concepts and applications of inferential statistics,* available on the Internet at http://faculty.vassar.edu/lowry/webtext.htm.)

see whether the new method (an experimental spray) differed from the traditional method (buttering the pan) in terms of how easily the baked cake could be removed from a pan. I found that there was not a statistically significant difference between the experimental spray or butter in terms of how much cake remained stuck to a pan (2.19 grams for butter vs. 1.63 grams for spray; $t(23) = 1.99$, $p > .05$). That is, the experimental spray did not work significantly better than butter in reducing baking adhesion. However, the present study was underpowered and should not be taken as the last word on the effectiveness of the new cooking spray. Given the size of the observed difference between the two sample means the present study had only about a 40% chance of rejecting the null hypothesis. Most statisticians recommend having at least an 80% chance of being able to reject the null hypothesis, and in order to have this level of power one would need to have about 21 cakes in each group. Thus I recommend doing this study again, but with 21 cakes in each condition, before concluding anything about the effectiveness of the new cooking spray.* In addition, I want to note that the results of the present study can only be generalized to a specific type of batter used in a specific type of pan in a specific oven. To the effect that these factors, or others such as altitude or humidity, affect cake adhesion they must be controlled and/or studied."

---

*Note that I did not address the issue of error, Type II error, by name. Type II error involves the possibility that a person has mistakenly accepted the null hypothesis. My interpretation addresses this issue, though it doesn't label it as such.

LOOKING CLOSER

ONE MORE BIT OF PRACTICE...

So far we've seen one *t* test that turned out to be statistically significant and one that didn't. There's one more possible outcome when we're planning to use a *t* test, and let's see what that is.

Imagine that an exercise physiologist has developed a new technique that she thinks will be effective in increasing muscle mass. To test it out she obtains 30 women interested in increasing their muscle mass, and randomly assigns them either to receive the new treatment (experimental group) or to be in the control group. After the 4 weeks of treatment she measures how much weight each person can lift. The results are listed in Table 9.7.

It certainly looks like the experimental treatment made a difference since the experimental group lifted almost 30 more pounds per person, on average, than the control group. However, to be sure we need to do a statistical test.

The appropriate test is an independent-samples *t* test since we are comparing the means (we have interval- or ratio-level data) for two groups, groups that are independent of each other. The assumptions for the independent-samples *t* are independent samples, interval- or ratio-level data, random samples, normality, and homogeneity of variance, and

TABLE **9.7**   **Pounds of Weight Lifted: Experimental Group vs. Control Group**

	Control	Experimental
	67	68
	85	195
	70	70
	68	145
	70	70
	98	133
	56	72
	39	126
	99	66
	67	115
	78	74
	97	103
	65	81
	50	90
	48	75
n	15	15
M	70.4667	98.8667
ŝ	18.3765	37.3743
Skewness (*SE*)	.1420 (.6325)	1.2503 (.6325)
Kurtosis (*SE*)	−.8279 (1.2649)	.7930 (1.2649)

it is here that we run into trouble. We already know that we haven't violated the first two assumptions, but we have violated each of the remaining three. The third assumption, random samples, is robust; our violation of this only means that we are limited in the conclusions we can draw from our study. The next two assumptions, normality and homogeneity of variance, are robust if (1) N is large, which it isn't here, and (2) the sample sizes are relatively equal, which they are here. With regard to normality, the 95% confidence interval for skewness for the experimental group does not capture a value of zero. Thus, it is not reasonable to conclude that the amount of weight lifted is normally distributed in the population of women receiving this experimental treatment. If our N were large I might be tempted to proceed, but with only 15 cases per sample I am going to decide not to proceed with the t test.

My decision not to proceed with the t test is made easier by the fact that the fifth assumption, homogeneity of variance, appears to be violated as well. My rule of thumb is to say that as long as one standard deviation is not twice the other we don't worry about violating this assumption. Well, in this instance one $\hat{s}$ is more than twice the other, so we worry about violating the assumption. Again, if the sample size is large the assumption is robust, but N is not large in this instance.

So, what do we do? Statisticians hate to quit and go home; they always try to think of a fallback option. The appropriate thing to do, if one has violated the assumptions for the independent t, is to scale one's variable back to the ordinal level and attempt the Mann Whitney U. If the assumptions for the Mann Whitney U are not met, then scale the variable back to the nominal level and use a chi-square difference test. If the assumptions for the chi-square aren't met—well, then we'll have to scratch our heads and try to figure a way to salvage something. But, for right now, I haven't taught the Mann Whitney U, so we can just recommend it without evaluating its adequacy and then pack up our tents and go home.

SUMMARY

Difference tests are used to compare group averages to see whether groups differ in terms of how much of the dependent variable they possess. There are difference tests that compare a group to a population (one-sample tests), difference tests that compare two groups (two-sample difference tests), and difference tests that compare more than two groups (multiple-sample difference tests). Which difference test one uses in a specific situation depends on four things: (a) how many groups are being compared, (b) at what level the dependent variable is being measured (i.e., nominal, ordinal, interval, or ratio), (c) whether the samples are independent or dependent, and (d) whether the specific assumptions for the chosen test have been met. The independent vs. dependent samples distinction involves whether the selection of cases for one sample determines or influences the selection of cases for the other sample. If there is no connection between the two samples then they are independent, but if they are paired, matched, or yoked in some way they are dependent.

The independent-samples t test is used to compare two independent samples to see if there is a statistically significant difference between the means, a difference that is likely reflective of a difference between the means of the two populations from which the samples came. The logic of null hypothesis testing is the same for the independent-samples t test as for the Pearson r: We have a theory about the two populations—that they are really the same population—and we call this theory the null hypothesis. We then generate a sampling distribution of t values based on the null hypothesis and compare the observed t value for the two samples to the sampling distribution. If the observed value of t is a common outcome—if it falls in the common zone of the sampling distribution—then there is no reason to disbelieve the null hypothesis. However, if the observed value of t is an unusual event, if it falls in the rare zone of the sampling distribution, then we have reason to question the null hypothesis.

As with the Pearson r, we almost always have the objective of showing that the null hypothesis should be rejected. And, as with the Pearson r, we are never sure of our results. If we reject the null hypothesis we have α chance of having made an incorrect decision, and if we fail to reject the null hypothesis we have β chance of having made an incorrect decision.

Once the t value has been calculated and it has been decided whether the null hypothesis is rejected or not, the human endeavor of interpretation begins. Techniques that can be applied include (a) reporting the direction of the difference, (b) calculating the 95% confidence interval for the size of the difference between the two population means, (c) calculating a measure of effect size (ω^2 or d), (d) turning the t value into a correlation and calculating the binomial effect size display, (e) discussing the possibility of Type I or Type II error, (f) making sure that the sample size was adequate, and (g) discussing the strengths and limitations of the study.

It is important to have an adequate sample size, perhaps even larger than what power calculations suggest is minimally necessary. Other things being equal, larger sample sizes provide better estimates of population values and have a ripple effect: not only do they make t values larger, they also change widths of confidence intervals, and increase ω^2 and d. Of course, at some point diminishing returns set in and the cost of having more cases outweighs the benefits they bring. But, other things being equal, larger sample sizes are desirable.

Review Exercises

1. A political scientist obtains a random sample of 37 U.S. senators and gives each an intelligence test. She concludes that the mean IQ of these senators indicates they are smarter than 91% of the United States' population. What can we conclude about the mean IQ of the entire population of U.S. senators? (Remember, for IQ tests we accept that $\sigma = 15$.)

2. What happens to t_{cv} as we move from a one-tailed to a two-tailed test? Does a one-tailed test make it harder or easier to reject the null hypothesis?

3. To adopt a child in the United States, potential adoptive parents must be screened by a social service agency. In essence, they have to get a "license" to have a child. This is in contrast to nonadoptive parents, who can have children without any agency's approval. A family practice nurse wants to investigate whether, as a result of this, adoptive parents were mentally healthier than nonadoptive parents. He obtains convenience samples of 25 adoptive mothers and 25 nonadoptive mothers, all of whom are first time parents with a child younger than 2 years. To each mother he administers an interval-level mental health inventory on which higher scores indicate better mental health. (The mental health inventory was developed so that in the general population $\mu = 50$ and $\sigma = 10$.) Here are his results:

M	$\hat{s}$	Skewness (SE)	Kurtosis (SE)
Nonadoptive			
51.3200	8.6381	.0610 (.4899)	−.3490 (.9798)
Adoptive			
61.4400	10.8888	−.5870 (.4899)	−.6856 (.9798)

Go through all six steps of the hypothesis testing procedure for this scenario.

4. For each scenario that follows, select the appropriate statistical test:

a. A nurse midwife is interested in seeing whether amount of pain experienced during delivery, as measured on an interval-level scale, differs between women who have taken Lamaze classes and women who have not. In addition, she examines whether it makes a difference whether the woman's partner is or is not in the delivery room with her. What test should she do to see if these variables influence amount of pain during delivery?

b. A demographer working for the U.S. Census Bureau investigates whether people who are self-employed are more or less likely to live in urban or rural areas. What test should he do to see if place is related to employment status?

c. A neurologist who specializes in working with people with spinal cord injuries wants to know whether the degree of physical impairment following a spinal cord injury is associated with the degree of depression experienced. What statistical test should she use to investigate this? (By the bye, both variables are measured on interval level scales.)

d. A sports psychologist classifies marathoners, based on their body mass index, heart rate, and lung capacity, as (a) above average in terms of fitness, or (b) below average in terms of fitness. He then records their order of finish in a marathon to see whether fitness level has an impact on how well they do. What test should he use to analyze these data?

e. A survey researcher wants to predict a gubernatorial election in a state where 47%

of the registered voters are Democrats, 43% are Republicans, and 10% are independents or other. She obtains a sample of 2300 voters and finds out their party affiliations, as well as the gubernatorial candidate for whom they plan to vote. What test should she do to determine if the sample is representative of the population in terms of political affiliation?

f. Some people have white coat hypertension. That is, they are anxious when visiting a medical office and, as a result, their blood pressure increases when a person with a white lab coat and a stethoscope walks into the room to take a blood pressure. A family practitioner is concerned that this is more common than suspected, so he makes it a practice to take two blood pressures, one when first walking into the room and a second, unexpected, one after about 15 minutes have passed. He is primarily concerned with diastolic blood pressure (that's the lower number for all you nonmedical types). What test should he do to see if there is a change in blood pressure over this 15 minute time period?

g. A dietitian measures how much food her subjects eat for breakfast and lunch, measures how much energy each person expends during the day, and finds each person's body mass index. She then has each person rate his or her hunger at 6 P.M. (The subjects rate this on an interval-level scale.) The nutritionist wants to see if the three independent variables (consumption, expenditure, and BMI) *combined* can predict hunger level. What is the appropriate statistical test?

Homework Problems

1. If N is larger for an independent-samples t test and everything else remains constant, that means
   a. One is more likely to be able to reject H_0.
   b. One is less likely to be able to reject H_0.
   c. That there is no impact on the likelihood of rejecting H_0 as N does not affect M.

2. If I complete an independent-samples t test and find that the probability of the results occurring if the null hypothesis is true is less than α, then
   a. $\mu_1 = \mu_2$
   b. $\mu_1 \neq \mu_2$
   c. There probably is a difference between the two population means.

d. There probably is not a difference between the two population means.

e. There is not sufficient evidence to draw any conclusion.

3. Which statement cannot be true for an independent-samples t test?

a. I reject the null hypothesis and find $d = 1.50$.

b. I fail to reject the null hypothesis and find $d = 1.50$.

c. I reject the null hypothesis and find $d = .10$.

d. I fail to reject the null hypothesis and find $d = .10$.

e. None of those statements can be true.

f. Any of those statements can be true.

4. If power is greater than .80, what is the result?

a. The null hypothesis will be rejected.

b. The null hypothesis will not be rejected.

c. Power does not determine whether the null hypothesis will be rejected.

5. If N is constant, for which will it be easiest to reject the null hypothesis if the difference is in the expected direction?

a. $\alpha = .05$, one-tailed

b. $\alpha = .05$, two-tailed

c. $\alpha = .01$, two-tailed

d. $\alpha = .01$, two-tailed

e. N does not affect the critical value of t.

6. Assuming that no assumptions have been violated, complete and interpret an independent-samples t test for the following scenario using the six-step hypothesis testing procedure. A gerontologist, concerned about osteoporosis, wants to investigate whether people who have been more active earlier in life have lower risk of osteoporosis. He gains access to a representative, national database that has bone mineral density (BMD) scores on 3782 women above age 60. (The BMD test, an interval level test, has scores that range from 20 to 80. Scores above 40 are not considered problematic. Scores from 25 to 39.9 are indicative of low bone mass; scores below 25 indicate osteoporosis.) Using one-sample significant difference tests, he shows that the sample of 3782 does not significantly differ from the population of women above 60

in the United States on the basis of age, race, marital status, cigarette use, or socioeconomic status. He finds that 1583 of these women were on athletic teams in high school. He compares the BMD scores of the student athletes ($M = 43.98$, $\hat{s} = 12.47$) to the BMD scores of the nonathletes ($M = 35.83$, $\hat{s} = 11.83$).

7. For the following scenarios, tell what statistical test should be done. Be as specific as possible:

a. A cardiologist compares cholesterol levels between people with differing amounts of fish consumption (0 times per week, once a week, or more than once a week), differing body mass indices (underweight, normal, overweight, or obese), and differing levels of stress (low, normal, or high), and men vs. women.

b. A nurse educator compares ordinal-level scores on a licensing exam between RNs who completed 2-year nursing programs vs. 4-year nursing programs.

c. An educational researcher randomly assigns high-school students who regularly use instant messaging to practice a task either on a computer that was or was not connected to instant-messaging software. Later, she measures how well the students in the two groups have learned to do the task using an ordinal-level measure of learning.

d. A religion professor wants to study a sample of college students at his university. Concerned that his sample is not representative of the larger population in terms of its degree of religiosity, he finds data from a large and representative sample of college students that provides information about the percentages of college students who fall into five categories of religiosity: very positive about religion, positive about religion, neutral about religion, negative about religion, and very negative about religion. What statistical test should he do to see if his sample is similar to the larger population?

e. A social scientist obtains a large and representative sample of middle-aged men and has each report how many months were spent in poverty before age 18. She also has each report how many criminal activities have been engaged in since age 18. What test should she do to determine the extent to which childhood poverty is associated with adult criminal behavior?

8. A nutritionist is concerned about the effects of lack of exercise on junk food consumption. He takes 32 teenage boys from a neighborhood high school and randomly assigns them to two evenly sized groups. One group, the exercise group, is given sports equipment and plays games such as football and basketball for an hour. The other group, the no-exercise group, is given access to sedate pastimes such as television, computer games, and books for an hour. After the hour is up, each group is given free access to junk food (potato chips, soda, etc.), and the nutritionist records how many calories each boy consumes. For the exercise group $M = 1196$ and $\hat{s} = 383$; for the no-exercise group $M = 1453$ and $\hat{s} = 458$. Assuming that no assumptions were violated, analyze and interpret these data using the six-step hypothesis testing procedure.

9. Is it OK to proceed with a statistical test for these data? An education researcher wants to see whether using red ink to mark papers has any effect on the self-esteem of children. She obtains a sample of 36 third-graders and randomly assigns them to two equal-sized groups. She has each group take a spelling test that consists of sixth-grade level words so that they will get many words wrong. She grades each spelling test and passes them back. For the control group she uses red ink to grade the tests, for the experimental group she uses green. She then administers an interval-level measure of self-esteem to see if the two groups differ. Higher scores on the self-esteem scale, which is constructed so that it has a mean of 50 and a standard deviation of 10, mean higher, more positive, levels of self-esteem. For the control group $M = 49.87$ and $\hat{s} = 11.45$; for the experimental group $M = 51.33$ and $\hat{s} = 12.99$. Skewness values for the two groups are, respectively, -1.45 and -1.37; kurtosis measures for the two groups are -1.23 and 1.41.

10

Multiple-Sample Difference Tests I

One-Way Analysis of Variance

Learning Objectives

After completing this chapter, you should be able to do the following:

1 Describe how completing multiple null hypothesis statistical tests increases the overall alpha level whereas using a multiple-sample difference test keeps the overall alpha level low.

2 Decide which multiple-sample difference test to use depending on the type of samples and level of measurement of the dependent variable.

3 Explain how variability in individual scores is due to individual differences, error, and treatment effect, and explain how analysis of variance (ANOVA) calculates an F ratio, the ratio of between-group variability to within-group variability.

4 Evaluate the assumptions, explain the hypotheses, generate a decision rule, and estimate the required sample size for a one-way ANOVA.

5 Calculate an F ratio for a one-way ANOVA and complete an ANOVA summary table.

6 Interpret a one-way ANOVA, including measures of effect size, post-hoc tests, confidence intervals, and power.

Two-sample difference tests compare two samples, but researchers often want to examine differences among three or more samples. For example, investigators might want to compare the effectiveness of three different ways of teaching math, or four different treatments for a disease. To deal with these situations, statisticians have developed multiple-sample difference tests, the focus of this chapter. Multiple-sample tests have the advantage of keeping the overall alpha level where initially set, usually at .05; whereas if one uses multiple two-sample tests to compare the samples pair by pair, the overall probability of having committed a Type I error rises. The trade-off, though, is that a multiple-sample difference test only tells that there is a difference between at least one of the pairs of samples; you then must perform an additional test, called a post-hoc test, to find out which pair(s) of samples differ.

In this chapter we learn a specific multiple-sample difference test, the one-way analysis of variance used to compare the means of three or more independent samples. Analysis of variance provides a new way of thinking about the variability in individual scores: partitioning the variability into the subcomponents of (a) variability between groups (variability due to the independent variable) and (b) variability within groups (variability due to individual differences and random error). It is the ratio between these two, what is called an *F* ratio, that is used to determine if the independent variable has a statistically significant effect on group means.

In this chapter, pay special attention to the concept of partitioning the variability. You'll also see how concepts from previous chapters, such as confidence intervals and omega squared, play a role in interpreting the results of ANOVA.

In the last chapter we learned how to compare *two* sample means to decide if it was reasonable to conclude that there was a central tendency difference between the populations from which the samples came. This type of test—an independent-samples *t* test, or more generally a two-sample difference test—is one of the most used tests in statistics because it shows if there is a difference between a control group and an experimental group, a common experimental situation. Often, however, researchers ask more complex questions, questions that involve three, four, or even more groups. Answering this sort of question involves a more complex statistical test than a two-sample difference test.

The easiest way to think about this is with a concrete example. Imagine that I want to know which medication—aspirin, ibuprofen, or acetaminophen—does a better job of getting rid of headaches. I get 100 people with headaches and randomly assign them to five groups. Three of the groups are experimental groups, receiving a standard dose of aspirin, ibuprofen, or acetaminophen, and two are control groups, receiving either a placebo or no pill. When I give each person the pill, I also give him or her a stopwatch to time how long it takes for the headache to go away. Thus, my independent variable is "medication," and it has five levels; my dependent variable is time, in minutes, until the headache goes away.

The reason that a *t* test is not an appropriate choice in this situation is that we would need to perform 10 different *t* tests to answer all the questions posed by our five groups. That is, we would need one *t* test to find out if aspirin differed from ibuprofen, another to see if aspirin differed from acetaminophen, a third to see if aspirin differed from placebo, a fourth to see if aspirin differed from no treatment, a fifth to see if ibuprofen differed from acetaminophen, and so on. Doing 10 *t* tests is tedious, but it can be done. The real problem is that doing 10 *t* tests generates what statisticians call a "runaway alpha" problem. Each individual *t* test has a certain level, α, of having a Type I error, of incorrectly rejecting the null hypothesis. As we commonly set α at .05, this means that for each *t* test there is a 5% chance of concluding that there is a difference between the two conditions when there really isn't. We're willing to accept a 5% chance of making an error for any individual test, but what happens when we are doing 10 tests, each with a 5% chance of an error? This scenario is a bit like having something untoward happen while driving. If there is only a 1% chance of having the front, driver's side tire blow out while you are driving, you might not worry about it. Similarly, if there were a 1% chance of the front, passenger's tire blowing out that might not concern you much either. Ditto for the other two tires and ditto for the 1% chance of hitting a deer and ditto for the 1% chance of the other car running a red light and hitting you. No one of those by itself is very likely. But what about the chance of tire 1 *or* tire 2 *or* tire 3 *or* tire 4 blowing out *or* of hitting a deer *or* of someone running a red light? What about the chance of *any one* of these untoward events occurring? The chance of *any one* of them occurring is greater than the chance of *just one* occurring.

Turning back to the possibility that *t* test 1 *or* *t* test 2 *or* *t* test 3 and so forth for our 10 *t* tests might, erroneously, cause us to reject the null hypothesis: we now have a 40% chance of making a Type I error.* That is, we've gone from having 1 chance out of 20 of making an error to 1 chance out of 2.5 that one of our results will be wrong. I don't like those odds since they are just a little bit better than flipping a coin: heads, no Type I error occurred; tails, a Type I error occurred.

There are a couple of ways around this problem. One is to reduce the alpha levels for the individual tests so that the **experiment-wise** alpha level is .05. In this instance, that means that we set α for each individual test at $\approx$ .005, not .05. That's fine, but we have now made it dramatically

---

experiment-wise alpha level or overall alpha level

The alpha level for an experiment or a series of statistical tests based on the aggregation of the probability of Type I error for all of the individual statistical tests conducted.

---

*Though the simplest way to think of calculating the chance of a Type I error is to multiply the number of tests (10 in this case) by the α level (.05 in this case), that isn't what is done. The overall α level, what is called the experiment-wise alpha level, is calculated by $1 - (1 - \alpha)^k$ where $k =$ the number of tests being done. In this case, with ten tests, the probability equals 40%.

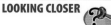
LOOKING CLOSER

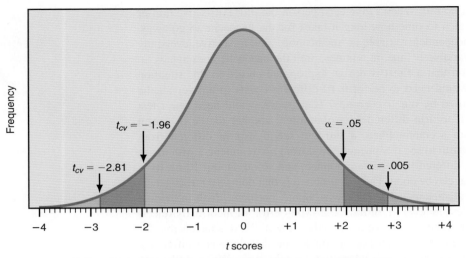

Figure **10.1** Critical values of *t*, two-tailed, for $\alpha = .05$ vs. .005.

harder to reject each individual null hypothesis, as shown in Figure 10.1. In Figure 10.1 the lines separating the rare zone from the common zone are drawn for a two-tailed *t* test with a very large sample size when $\alpha = .05$ vs. when $\alpha = .005$. Note that the shaded area represents the 4.5% of outcomes where the null hypothesis would be rejected with $\alpha = .05$ but not with $\alpha = .005$.

The other option, which is the focus of this chapter, is to do a single test that makes all of our comparisons *and* that maintains our experiment-wise α level at the original level without reducing the α level for an individual comparison. It sounds like it is all done with mirrors—but believe me, it works.

The type of multiple-sample difference test that we shall explore in this chapter is called **analysis of variance,** or **ANOVA** for short.* ANOVAs are used when comparing means, so they are appropriate for interval- or ratio-level data. We will explore, in this chapter, a specific type of ANOVA, a one-way ANOVA for independent samples.† Technically, the ANOVA we shall be working with is called a completely randomized one-way ANOVA, but I'm just going to call it a one-way ANOVA.

analysis of variance (ANOVA)

A multiple-sample difference test used to compare means of three or more samples.

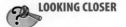
LOOKING CLOSER

*ANOVA is pronounced as a word with a short first and last a, not as individual letters. Oh yes, stress the syllable "no" when you say ANOVA.

†Remember—from previous chapters—what it means to say that something is one-way and that the groups are independent? The number of "ways" is statistics-speak for the number of independent variables. In my example here, there is one independent variable, drug type, though there are five levels of it. (A level is a condition.) Independent samples means that the cases in one sample are independent of, not connected to or influenced by, the cases in the other samples. Since I have randomly assigned people with headaches to receive nothing, placebo, aspirin, acetaminophen, or ibuprofen, the groups are independent.

An analysis of variance yields a test statistic called an F ratio, and an F ratio is a general test. A significant F ratio is a bit like standing outside a football stadium and hearing the crowd roar. You know that something significant happened, but you are not entirely sure what. The F ratio simply tells us that something statistically significant has happened inside the stadium, that the difference between at least two groups is statistically different from zero. We would then need to go into the stadium and do some snooping around to find out which team scored, which two means are statistically different. This snooping around is called, in statistics, doing a post-hoc test. Why post-hoc? Because post-hoc is Latin for "after this," and this is what you do after a significant F ratio.

I like to call ANOVA a Ragu® test in honor of the spaghetti sauce. Years ago there was an ad for Ragu spaghetti sauce in which a potential consumer asked, one by one, if the sauce *really* contained certain spices and ingredients (e.g., oregano or parsley). After each query a matter-of-fact voice-over would intone, "It's in there." If the ANOVA is significant, the F ratio simply indicates that there is a significant difference "in there." We then have to go in there and complete a post-hoc test to decide what pairs of means actually differ. The F ratio tells us only that there is at least one significant difference. And, since the post-hoc test is designed to keep our overall alpha level down, we get to do a lot of tests and not increase our risk of making a Type I error. Talk about having your cake and eating it too.

As you might have guessed, there are a variety of different ANOVAs and a variety of other multiple-sample difference tests. Which one you use depends on (a) the level of measurement of your dependent variable (NOIR), (b) whether the samples are independent or dependent, and (c) the number of independent variables. In this chapter we will focus on situations with only one independent variable, called a grouping variable, as seen in the "What Test When" table, Table 10-1. In the next chapter I'll address tests with more than one independent variable, factorial ANOVAs. Also I'll use that concept to explain how to do a repeated measures ANOVA, how to do a difference test for dependent samples.*

WHY ANALYSIS OF VARIANCE IS CALLED ANALYSIS OF VARIANCE

To understand how analysis of variance works (and why it is called analysis of variance), let's imagine treating some disorder with three different doses of a drug: low, medium, and high. We obtain a random sample from the population of people with the disorder and then randomly assign them to the three treatment conditions. Each person takes his or her assigned dose, and we measure, in days, how long it takes for the

---

*Just to give you a heads up… I never addressed the question of how to calculate a dependent- or paired-samples *t* test in Chapter 9. In the next chapter, when I teach how to do repeated measures ANOVA I'll explain why that is a better test to use than a dependent-samples *t*.

LOOKING CLOSER

TABLE **10.1**   **What Test When: Multiple-Sample Significant Difference Tests with One Grouping Variable**

	Interval/ratio dependent variable	Ordinal dependent variable	Nominal dependent variable
Independent Samples	One-way ANOVA	Kruskal-Wallis one-way ANOVA by ranks	Chi-square difference test
Dependent Samples	Repeated measures ANOVA	Friedman two-way ANOVA by ranks	Cochran's Q test

symptoms of the disorder to go away. We are asking whether different doses lead to different results, whether some doses are more or less effective than others.

In Figure 10.2 I have two options, two extremely different options, of how the results might look. Each panel of Figure 10.2 shows three frequency polygons for the three doses or conditions. In Panel A, the three groups are separated—there is no overlap in time-to-cure for the different doses. Clearly there is a difference in how quickly the three medications take effect. Panel B shows what the results look like if there is little difference in the effectiveness of the three doses: there is a lot of overlap among the three groups, and the three means are very close to each other.

Let's think about *one* of the individual-dose frequency polygons in Panel A: Everyone in the group received exactly the same dose of the medication, but not everybody's disorder went away in exactly the same amount of time. Speaking as a statistician, there's variability *within* the group. What causes this **within-group variability**? The simplest answer is **individual differences,** that individuals differ in how they respond to a stimulus. If a loud sound suddenly went off in your classroom, some students would startle at the sound and others would barely notice it. Why? Because of individual differences! Some people hear better than others, some have nervous systems that are more reactive, some people got more sleep last night, some are more focused on the material that is

within-group variability

The variability within a sample of cases that all receive the same treatment; variability due to individual differences and random error.

individual differences

Naturally occurring differences among cases; a source of within-group variability.

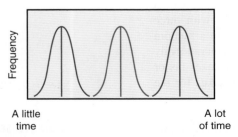
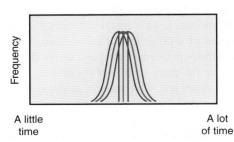

Figure **10.2** Two examples of hypothetical outcomes for a multiple-sample significant difference test.

being covered in class, and so on. There are a whole host of factors that might affect an individual case's response to such a stimulus.

One other factor may play a role in within-group variability: random error. Random error refers to all kinds of uncontrolled error, such as measurement error (e.g., mistiming when the disorder went away), sampling error, and random environmental fluctuations.

We've already learned (in Chapter 4) how to calculate variability within a group when we calculated the variance by finding the mean of the squared deviation scores.* Because it is important to remember how variance is calculated, here's a reprise of the formula for calculating a sample variance:

$$s^2 = \frac{\Sigma(X - M)^2}{N}$$

When we apply this formula to calculate the within-group variance for a single dose level, a single group, we now know that the s^2 we calculate represents the variability within the group, variability that is due to individual differences and random error. We call this, as you have already gathered, the within-group variance.

Let's switch our focus from the variability within each group and think of another way to measure variability: **between-group variability.** That is, we could treat each group as a case and use the group means as our data points. Notice that our focus has shifted here from treating *individual cases* to treating *groups of cases.* Clearly, our sample size has just gotten smaller! (The number of groups, which is now our sample size, is abbreviated as k.)

Having shifted our focus, we could find the mean of the group means (called the grand mean [M_{Grand}] or overall mean),[†] calculate deviation scores from this (the deviation of each group M from M_{Grand}), and find the mean squared deviation. This would be $\frac{\Sigma(M_{Group} - M_{Grand})^2}{k}$. (I hope that you recognize this as the variance formula just reprised a minute ago.) This variance is called the between-group variance.

The sources of variability for between-group variance are (a) random error, (b) individual differences, and (c) treatment effect. Let me explain random error and individual differences first. Why are random error and individual differences a factor in between-group variability as well as for within-group variability? Imagine that each group received exactly the same dose. Even if each group received exactly the same treatment, we

between-group variability

Variability among samples, where each sample is treated as a case; variability due to the effect of treatment as well as individual differences and random error.

---

*There are other ways to calculate variability within a group (range, interquartile range, and standard deviation), but analysis of variance makes use of the variance.

[†]If the groups have different sizes, we'll need to take this into account when calculating the grand mean. But, in my current example our groups all have equal sample sizes, making calculation of a grand mean simply the average of the group means.

LOOKING CLOSER

wouldn't expect each group to end up with *exactly* the same mean. Why? Because random error should give us groups that differ at least slightly from each other and each group will be comprised of individuals with at least slightly different response systems. Thus, even if each group received exactly the same treatment, they would not have exactly the same outcome. This scenario is shown in Panel B of Figure 10.2.

To think about how the treatment affects between-group variability, turn your attention back to Panel A of Figure 10.2. In this scenario the treatment has had an impact: the people who received the low dose of the drug did not do as well as the people who received the medium dose of the drug. Also, the people who received the medium dose did not do as well as the people who received the high dose. So, why do the three group means differ? Partly because of random error and individual differences, but mostly because of the effect of the treatment—because different doses lead to different outcomes.

When we calculate between-group variance for Panel A vs. for Panel B, we should get different outcomes. In Panel A, where the groups have distinctly different means, we have a lot of between-group variability. In Panel B, where the group means are close to each other, we have little between-group variability. Yet in both panels the degree of within group-variability is the same. Hmmm…

In one situation, Panel A, there's more between-group variability than there is in the other situation, Panel B. Yet both situations have the same degree of within-group variability. Can we compare, or analyze, those two variances, between-group and within-group, for the two scenarios to determine if the differences between the group means are statistically significant differences?

Believe it or not, we have just developed one-way analysis of variance as a way to see if groups differ. In one-way analysis of variance we partition the variability in scores into two components: within-group variability and between-group variability. Within-group variability is built of individual differences and random error, while between-group variability is built of those two *plus* treatment effect. We then examine the ratio of the two—it's called an *F* ratio—by dividing between-group variability by within-group variability:

$$\frac{\textit{Between-Group Variability}}{\textit{Within-Group Variability}}$$

If treatment has little or no effect, then between-group variability is due almost entirely to individual differences and random error, the same factors that determine within-group variability. In that case, the ratio of between-group variability to within-group variability, the *F* ratio, will end up close to 1.0. But, when treatment has an effect, when the group means differ, between-group variability is greater than within-group variability, and the *F* ratio is greater than 1.0. It is in this sense that ANOVA is an *analysis* of *variance*: the variance between groups is compared to the variance within groups. With this conceptual overview, let's turn to the mechanics of ANOVA.

TABLE **10.2** **Data from Centripetal Coin Funnel**

	Pennies	Nickels	Dimes	Quarters
Seconds	7.9, 8.7, 8.4	10.0, 10.4, 9.4	7.0, 6.5, 6.4, 7.4	9.4, 9.5, 10.0
M $(\hat{s})$	8.333 (.404)	9.933 (.503)	6.825 (.465)	9.633 (.321)

TOM, HARRY, AND THE ONE-WAY ANOVA

Let's do an analysis of variance. Have you ever been at a zoo or some other public place where they collect spare change for a worthy cause by having a large funnel-shaped device with a hole at the bottom? You place a coin in a slot, let it go, and the coin rolls on its edge into the top of the funnel. Gravity pushes the coin against the wall of the funnel and pulls it down while centripetal force propels the coin around and around in tighter and tighter circles, until, finally, gravity wins and the coin falls into the hole at the bottom. There is something hypnotic about watching coins swirl down, and children love to deposit coin after coin after coin. I was curious whether different denomination coins (pennies vs. nickels vs. dimes vs. quarters) took different amounts of time to swirl through such a funnel.

One of my sons has a bank that is a small version of this coin funnel, and one afternoon I grabbed a stopwatch, a bunch of coins, and collected some data. In Table 10.2 are the raw data along with the means and standard deviations. (By the bye, these are real data from real coins.)

Figure 10.3 is a bar graph showing the results. Looking at the graph, do you think that different coin denominations take different amounts of time to swirl through the funnel?

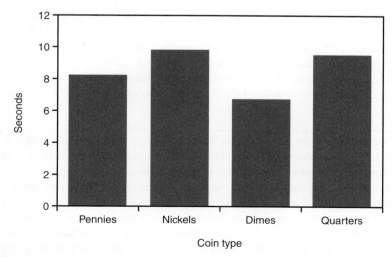

Figure **10.3** Bar graph showing mean time it takes to swirl through the coin funnel for different coin types.

It certainly looks as if "treatment" may have an effect, that different coins take different amounts of time to swirl through the funnel. (Even when nothing was *treated*, as is the case here, statisticians still call the effect of the grouping variable, here coin denomination, the treatment effect.) The question is whether there was more of a difference *between* groups than *within* groups, and simply examining means doesn't answer that question. For the moment all that we can say is that it looks like denomination may affect run-time since the means are different, ranging from 6.8 sec (dimes) to 9.9 sec (nickels). It is not until we complete a statistical test that we determine if it is statistically likely that a treatment effect exists.*

So, let's enter the world of Tom and Harry, where our first step is to determine what statistical test to do.

Test

We are asking here whether there is a *difference* between outcomes for the groups, so we will perform a difference test. Further, we have more than two groups, so we will employ a multiple-sample difference test. Table 10.1 tells us that we must decide both level of measurement for the dependent variable and whether the samples are independent or dependent. The number of seconds a coin takes to swirl through the funnel is a ratio-level variable since the numbers tell a difference, the direction of the difference, and the size of the difference, and the scale has a real zero point. The groups, what are often called cells, are independent because the coins selected for one group did not determine which coins were selected for another group. Given this, the appropriate multiple-sample difference test is the one-way ANOVA.

Assumptions

The assumptions for the one-way ANOVA are the same as the assumptions for the independent-samples *t* test. In fact, the one-way ANOVA is just an extension of the independent-samples *t* test.[†]

These are the assumptions for the one-way ANOVA:
1. Independent samples (not robust to violations)
2. Interval- or ratio-level data (not robust to violations)

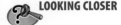

LOOKING CLOSER

*And remember, even then we are not certain. Thanks to the logic of hypothesis testing, our decisions are probabilistic—our decision is probably right. If we reject the null hypothesis there is a chance that we made a Type I error; and if we fail to reject the null, there's a chance that we made a Type II error.

[†]As we'll see and take advantage of in the next chapter, when you have two samples and a dependent variable that is interval- or ratio-level, you can just as readily calculate a *t* value as an *F* ratio. In such a situation, $t = \sqrt{F}$. This also means that the *t* test also examines the ratio of between-group variability to within-group variability—it just does the math differently. There's one more implication to mention: technically, the definition of a multiple-samples difference test should say it is used with two or more samples, not three.

3. Random samples (robust to violations, but implications for interpretation if violated)
4. Normality (robust to violations if ns are large and roughly equal)
5. Homogeneity of variance (robust to violations if ns are large and roughly equal)

The one-way ANOVA is not robust to violations of the first two assumptions, which means that if they are violated we should not proceed with the analysis of variance. To state that as a positive: a one-way ANOVA should only be done with independent samples and interval- or ratio-level data.

The third assumption is almost always violated, and it will still be OK to go ahead and complete the ANOVA. This assumption exists because of how we obtain the sampling distribution of the F ratio to which we shall be comparing our observed F ratio: by taking repeated *random* samples from a population, calculating an F ratio for these samples, and then building the sampling distribution out of these F ratios. The comparison of an observed F ratio to the sampling distribution of F ratios makes sense if one is comparing apples to apples—an F ratio from a random sample of the population to F ratios from random samples of the population.

In actual fact, it is very rare that we have random samples. Thinking back to my headache example, is it realistic to expect that my sample of headache sufferers who were assigned either to no treatment, placebo, aspirin, ibuprofen, or acetaminophen was a random sample from the population of all the people in the world with headaches? Obviously not. Nonetheless, the question of which headache medicine works better is a good one and deserves an answer. So, statisticians forge ahead and are willing to make an apple-to-oranges comparison. We are careful, however, to point out the limits of generalizability when we interpret the results.

The last two assumptions are "robust if" assumptions: if they are violated we can still go ahead and complete the ANOVA, as long as certain conditions are met and as long as the violations aren't too great. The first of these is the normality assumption, that the dependent variable is normally distributed in the population. ANOVA is robust to violations of this assumption as long as N (note: that is N, not n) is large enough and the ns are about equal. The rule of thumb that I use (Diekhoff, 1996) is that as long as $n \geq 15$ it should be OK to do the ANOVA.* Regarding ns being about equal, we will use the rule of thumb that we used for the t test and say that as long as one n is not 1.5 times the size of another, we're good to go.

How do we test this assumption—how do we decide if the variable is normally distributed in the population? We'll use the same approach as for the independent samples t test, that is, we'll use logic (should the variable

---

*Diekhoff, G. M. (1996). *Basic statistics for the social and behavioral sciences.* Upper Saddle River, NJ: Prentice Hall.

LOOKING CLOSER

be normally distributed?) and/or confidence intervals for skewness and kurtosis. If the sample size is large enough, we'll also examine modality.

The second of the "robust if" assumptions is the homogeneity of variance assumption, that the variability of the dependent variability in each of the treatment groups is about equal. We're going to use the rule of thumb that we used for independent-samples t tests: one $\hat{s}$ shouldn't be more than twice as large as another $\hat{s}$. If one is twice as large as another, then this assumption has been violated. But, if N is large and ns are about equal, the assumption can be violated as long as the violation isn't too great. In other words, if ns are large and equal and if one $\hat{s}$ is 2.00 and the other is 5.00, go ahead and calculate the ANOVA. But, if one $\hat{s}$ were 2.00 and the other were 10.00, I'd be leery of calculating the ANOVA even if ns were large and equal. If that were the situation, I'd be looking to scale the dependent variable back to the ordinal level and use a fallback test.

Let's see if the coin data meet the assumptions for a one-way ANOVA. I already know that my data meet the first two assumptions (independent groups and interval- or ratio-level variable) since I satisfied myself on those counts when I selected the one-way ANOVA. I obtained the coins to be tested from the stray coins on my dresser, and thus the coins are not random samples from the population of U.S. coinage. In other words, I violated the third assumption, the assumption of random samples from the population. I'm comfortable believing that there is nothing unusual about the sample of change that sits on my dresser. So, even though this is not a random sample of U.S. coinage, it is probably a *reasonably* representative sample of U.S. coinage.* So, we will go ahead with the ANOVA and not be too concerned, when it comes time to interpretation, with limitations to generalizability.

The last two assumptions, normality and homogeneity of variance, are robust if ns are equal and large. The ns are roughly equal (none is more than 1.5 times the size of the other), but they are small, with $N = 13$. If there are violations of normality or homogeneity of variance, we will not be able to trade on the robustness of the ANOVA.

We could calculate skewness and kurtosis for each of the groups and then calculate the 95% confidence intervals for these. But when the sample size is small, as it is here, estimates aren't very robust.† So, we will use logic instead of math. There is one factor that seems likely to influence how long it takes a coin to swirl through the funnel: size. Size

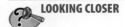
LOOKING CLOSER

---

*Nonetheless, it is a small sample. If I were doing this study for anything other than illustrative purposes, I'd have a larger sample size.

†I mentioned back in Chapter 6 that it is not a good idea to calculate confidence intervals if there are fewer than 12 cases. Statistical Package for the Social Sciences (SPSS), by the bye, won't even calculate kurtosis if $N < 4$.

of coin may be measured by weight or diameter. Still, no matter how it is measured, I think that coins within any denomination vary on it. There are certainly minute variations present in coins as they leave the mint, and the variations grow as the coins circulate. It seems reasonable to me that it is random factors that determine this variability and, as we've seen before, random factors generate normal distributions. So, let's assume normality even without calculating confidence intervals for skewness and kurtosis.

The final assumption to assess is homogeneity of variance. Table 10.2 displays the standard deviations for the four cells; they range from a low of .321 to a high of .503. Since the largest is not more than twice the size of the smallest, there is no reason to question homogeneity of variance.

To recap: only one assumption—that each sample is a random sample from its respective population—is violated, and calculation of ANOVA is robust to violations of this assumption. We'll need to be a bit careful when we interpret the results because I don't have random samples, but other than that we're good to go.

Hypotheses

The next step involves stating the hypotheses. As the one-way ANOVA is an extension of the independent-samples t test, the hypotheses will be very similar, though with one wrinkle. For the t test the hypotheses were $H_0: \mu_1 = \mu_2$ and $H_1: \mu_1 \neq \mu_2$. The null hypothesis for the one-way ANOVA is a direct extension, and we will simply keep adding μs until all the samples being tested have been accounted for. For the coin-funnel data we are analyzing, the null hypothesis is as follows:

$$H_0: \mu_{pennies} = \mu_{nickels} = \mu_{dimes} = \mu_{quarters}$$

In English this means that there is no treatment effect—that all samples come from the same population and thus will generate sample means that are close enough to each other that the differences can be explained by sampling error.

The alternative hypothesis is a little harder to write in symbolic notation. The alternative hypothesis is *not* $\mu_1 \neq \mu_2 \neq \mu_3 \neq \ldots \neq \mu_k$. (Statisticians use the letter k to indicate the number of groups.) That is, the alternative hypothesis doesn't say that *every* population mean is unequal to *every other* population mean. Rather, it says that at least one population mean is different from at least one other population mean. Here's how I'll write this:

$$H_1: \text{Not all } \mu s \text{ are equal}$$

In English: at least two of the groups come from different populations, and the sample means for the groups that come from different populations will be far enough from each other that sampling error is an unlikely explanation for their differences. Rather, the observed differences reflect a real difference between those two populations.

Decision Rule

This step involves (a) finding the critical value of the test statistic, (b) stating the decision rule, and (c) deciding if the sample size is adequate. The last part of this, seeing if the sample size is adequate, is a question of power—of the probability of rejecting the null hypothesis when the null hypothesis should be rejected. Though ultimately I would like you to be able to do so at this stage, I am going to leave off explaining how to calculate power (and sample size) until the interpretation phase of the one-way ANOVA. With that lurking in the background, let's go on to the critical value of F and the decision rule.

The logic of hypothesis testing for the ANOVA is the same as it was for the r and the t. That is, we will calculate a test statistic, in this case the F *ratio,* abbreviated F, and will compare that to a sampling distribution of F.* If our observed F falls in the rare zone of the sampling distribution—if it is one that is unlikely to have occurred by chance when H_0 is true—then we'll reject the null hypothesis. For the F ratio, as for the Pearson r and the independent t, we'll reject the null hypothesis when the F ratio found in our sample, $F_{observed}$, is greater than or equal to the critical value of F, F_{cv}.[†] Similarly, if $F_{observed} < F_{cv}$—if the observed value of F falls in the common zone of the sampling distribution of F—then it is a result that has a high probability of having occurred by chance when the null hypothesis is true, and there is no reason to question the null hypothesis.

The chosen size of the rare zone, the α level, is a decision about how often one is willing to make a Type I error.[‡] As with statistical tests we've already learned, the most common practice is to set α at .05, to be willing to make a Type I error 5% of the time. Table 10 in the Appendix lists critical values of F at the .05 level only. If you are more concerned than this about the possibility of Type I error, you'll need to consult a different table of critical values of F.

The good news about ANOVA is that you don't need to worry about whether you are doing a one-tailed or a two-tailed test. The F distribution

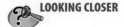
LOOKING CLOSER

*How is the sampling distribution of F created? By taking a single population and drawing k random samples of size n from it. Because the samples are all coming from the same population, the only reason they should differ is sampling error. The F is then calculated for the k samples, and this (drawing k samples of size n and calculating the F ratio) is done again and again and again. The frequency distribution of the F ratios is the sampling distribution of F. In other words, the sampling distribution of F shows what we would expect to find for k samples of size n if the null hypothesis were true.

[†] Because F is always $\geq$ zero, we don't need to talk about the absolute value of the test statistic.

[‡] Here's a quick refresher on the two different types of error. Type I error means that one has incorrectly rejected the null hypothesis. (A fair coin will occasionally turn up heads 5 times in a row.) Type II error occurs when one has incorrectly failed to reject the null. (The coin really is unfair but we conclude that it is fair.) The probability of Type I error occurring is α, and the probability of Type II error occurring is β.

is one-tailed, and the one tail of the F distribution captures the possibility that a pair of means differs in either a positive or a negative direction. Because of the way it is calculated, as the ratio of the variability between groups divided by the variability within groups, an F ratio can never be negative, so we don't need use the absolute value of the test statistic in our decision rule. In a little bit, in Figure 10.4, I'll show an example of the F distribution, and you can see that it is one-tailed and positively skewed.

F has a whole variety of sampling distributions, just as r and t do. And, as is true for r and t, the sampling distributions (and the critical values) of F are determined by degrees of freedom. For r and t, degrees of freedom were determined purely by N; for ANOVA, degrees of freedom depend both on N and k. (Remember, k = the number of groups being compared.) We talk about the degrees of freedom for the numerator of the F ratio and the degrees of freedom for the denominator of the F ratio. I'll abbreviate these, generically, as $df_{numerator}$ and $df_{denominator}$. However, because $df_{numerator}$ for the one-way ANOVA are the degrees of freedom associated with between-groups variability and $df_{denominator}$ are the degrees of freedom associated with within-groups variability, I'll refer to them as $df_{between}$ and df_{within}.*

There is one more degree of freedom term to remember: degrees of freedom total, abbreviated df_{total}. As I've mentioned, analysis of variance partitions the variability that exists in individual scores into the variability that is due to within-group factors (individual differences and random error) and the variability that is due to between-group factors (treatment, individual differences, and random error). Thus the *total* variability is divided into those two factors, and each factor is associated with a certain number of degrees of freedom. Similarly, the total number of degrees of freedom is divided, or partitioned, into two, and so $df_{total} = df_{between} + df_{within}$. Equation 10.1 shows how to calculate the various degrees of freedom for a one-way ANOVA.

F O R M U L A E

Degrees of Freedom Between, Within, and Total for One-Way ANOVA

$df_{between} = k - 1$ **Equation 10.1**

$df_{within} = N - k$

$df_{total} = N - 1$

Continued

---

*Just to make things even more complicated, be aware that the denominator in an F ratio is often called the "error term," and the degrees of freedom associated with this are often called degrees of freedom error, or df_{error}.

 LOOKING CLOSER

FORMULAE

Degrees of Freedom Between, Within, and Total for One-Way ANOVA—cont'd

Equation 10.1

Where:

$df_{between}$ = between-groups degrees of freedom; degrees of freedom for the numerator term for a one-way ANOVA

k = number of samples or groups

df_{within} = within-group degrees of freedom; degrees of freedom for the denominator term for a one-way ANOVA

N = total number of cases for a one-way ANOVA

df_{total} = degrees of freedom total for a one-way ANOVA

NOTE: $df_{total} = df_{between} + df_{within}$

These equations say that $df_{between}$ equals the number of samples minus one, df_{within} equals the total number of cases minus the number of samples, and df_{total} equals the total number of cases minus one. For my coin-funnel data, where I have a total of 13 cases in four groups, the numerator degrees of freedom would be 3 (via 4 − 1), the denominator degrees of freedom would be 9 (via 13 − 4), and degrees of freedom total is 12 (via either 13 − 1 or 9 + 3). For an F ratio, the tradition is to report only degrees of freedom for the numerator and denominator terms and to report them first for the numerator and then the denominator. In this case, the F ratio has 3 and 9 degrees of freedom.*

Because we now know the degrees of freedom for the F ratio we will calculate, we can find the F_{cv} that we'll compare to $F_{observed}$. The table of critical values of F is Appendix Table 10, and I have put a section of it in Table 10.3. The critical values of F are listed at the intersection of a column (the degrees of freedom for the numerator of the F ratio) and a row (the degrees of freedom for the denominator of the F ratio).†

For our coin example, where the degrees of freedom are 3 and 9, F_{cv} = 3.8625. Figure 10.4 shows the sampling distribution of F, on which I have marked off this critical value as well as the rare and common zones. Note that the F ratio does not have values below zero, and that it is one-tailed and positively skewed.

The decision rule for the one-way analysis of variance is the same as for r and t: if the observed value of the test statistic is greater than or equal to the critical value of the test statistic, we reject the null hypothesis; if the observed value of F is less than F_{cv}, we fail to reject H_0.

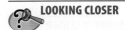

LOOKING CLOSER

*Do you have trouble keeping the numerator, the top number, straight from the denominator, the bottom number? Here's a mnemonic that I've found helpful to keep them in order: Notre Dame.

†Why do I use the labels "numerator" and "denominator" in this table, rather than "between" and "within"? Because that makes this table more generic. In the next chapter we'll learn about factorial and repeated measures ANOVAs, and these use different words for the numerator and denominator terms.

TABLE **10.3** **Critical Values of *F*, a Section of Appendix Table 10**

	1	2	3	4	5
1	161.448	199.500	215.707	224.583	230.162
2	18.5128	19.0000	19.1643	19.2468	19.2964
3	10.1280	9.5521	9.2766	9.1172	9.0135
4	7.7086	6.9443	6.5914	6.3882	6.2561
5	6.6079	5.7861	5.4095	5.1922	5.0503
6	5.9874	5.1433	4.7571	4.5337	4.3874
7	5.5914	4.7374	4.3468	4.1203	3.9715
8	5.3177	4.4590	4.0662	3.8379	3.6875
9	5.1174	4.2565	3.8625	3.6331	3.4817
10	4.9646	4.1028	3.7083	3.4780	3.3258

Columns = Numerator degrees of freedom
Rows = Denominator degrees of freedom

By now you should be familiar with all that follows from this, and I have the details of the decision options listed in Table 10.4. If $F_{observed}$ falls in the rare zone, we'll (a) reject the null hypothesis, (b) report that at least two of the samples have means that are statistically different, (c) conclude that it is likely that at least two of the populations have different means, and (d) worry about having made a Type I error. If $F_{observed}$ falls in the common zone, we'll (a) fail to reject the null hypothesis, (b) report that none of the sample means differs statistically from any other, (c) conclude that there is insufficient evidence to conclude that any two population means differ, and (d) worry about having made a Type II error.

APA format for analysis of variance involves, as always, reporting what statistic was calculated, the value of the statistic, the number of

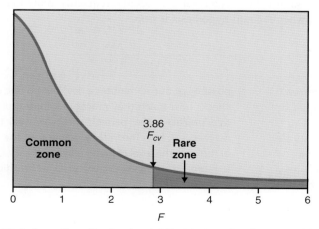

Figure **10.4** Sampling distribution of *F* with 3 and 9 degrees of freedom. (Adapted from Lowry, R. [2006]. *Concepts and applications of inferential statistics* [online]. Available: http://faculty.vassar.edu/lowry/webtext.html)

TABLE 10.4   Conclusion Options for One-Way ANOVA with α Set at .05

	$F_{observed} \geq F_{cv}$	$F_{observed} < F_{cv}$
Where the observed *F* falls	Rare zone	Common zone
Statement about H_0	It is rejected	Failed to reject it
Statement about H_1	Forced to accept it	Failed to support it
Error to be concerned about	Type I	Type II
Probability of that error	.05 (α)	To be determined (β)
Report probability of results occurring if H_0 is true since	$p < .05$	$p > .05$
Results are called	Statistically significant	Not statistically significant
Conclusion about sample means	At least two are statistically different	No statistical difference between any two
Conclusion about population means	At least two are probably different	Not sufficient evidence that any are different

subjects, and whether the results were common or rare under the null hypothesis. If our observed value of *F* had been greater than F_{cv}, say if *F* were 4.13, then APA format would look like this: $F(3, 9) = 4.13, p < .05$. This says that the observed value of *F* with 3 and 9 degrees of freedom was 4.13, and there is less than a 5% chance of this occurring when the null hypothesis is true. It also says, because we know how degrees of freedom are calculated, that there were 13 cases.* If the observed value of *F* had fallen in the common zone—if it were, say, 3.18—then here's how the results would appear in APA format: $F(3, 9) = 3.18, p > .05$. This statement says that this is a result that occurs frequently, more than 5% of the time, when the null hypothesis is true.

For the first six questions, (a) write out the research question and (b) tell what statistical test should be used to answer it.

1. For their first year of piano lessons, students are randomly assigned to different types of practice. One group is forced to practice for 30 minutes a day. Another group is told to practice "as much as possible, about 30 minutes a day," but no one ever checks how much they practice. A third group is told "practice makes perfect," and every week their teachers ask how much they practice. At the end of the year, the level of piano playing of each child is rated on an interval-level scale where higher scores represent greater ability.

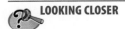   **LOOKING CLOSER**   *We know this because $N = df_{between} + df_{within} + 1$.

Group Practice 10.1—cont'd

2. Groups of college students from three different academic programs (engineering, business, and humanities) are asked at the start of their college careers whether they consider themselves Democrats or Republicans. Four years later, they are asked to rate their party affiliation again.

3. A group of people who have been driving for a number of years have their driving ability tested in a driving simulator. The driving simulator yields a score that tells the percent of time that the driver is on task/attentive. In a random order, each driver drives under three different conditions: (1) no distractions, (2) radio on, and (3) radio on and incoming cell phone calls.

4. Some dorm bathrooms are single-gender (male-only or female-only) and some are multigender. The janitorial crew rates each of the three types of bathrooms as "messy" or "not messy."

5. Some colleges have no general education requirements (i.e., there are no courses that are required of all students), some have general education requirements that require an introductory psychology course, and some have general education that requires other courses but not introductory psychology. The year level (first year, sophomore, junior, or senior) of introductory psychology students was measured at these three types of colleges.

6. Male students and female students are asked to rate the safety of their campuses. The scale used has categories of not at all, slightly, moderately, considerably, and extremely.

7. A researcher was interested in investigating the effect of initial treatment on outcome after a stroke. Some hospitals have specially trained "stroke teams" in their emergency rooms (ER) and the researcher was interested in the extent to which treatment by such a team had an impact on poststroke quality of life. The researcher measured quality of life on a ratio-level scale that ranged from 100 (no loss in quality of life, or 100% of prestroke quality of life is maintained) to zero (complete loss of all quality of life). The researcher found stroke patients from two comparable hospitals in her city, one with a stroke team and one without. It turned out that the patients she followed were initially treated under three different conditions: (1) by the specially trained stroke team in the ER, (2) in the ER that had the specially trained stroke teams, but the patient was not treated by the stroke team, and (3) in an ER without a specially trained stroke team. Here are the data she collected (as well as M and $\hat{s}$):

Group 1: 74, 86, 77 (79.0000, 6.2450)
Group 2: 76, 72, 65 (71.0000, 5.5678)
Group 3: 58, 70, 52 (60.0000, 9.1652)

The researcher plans to analyze her data using a one-way ANOVA. Determine whether she can proceed, state the hypotheses, and state the decision rule. (Be sure to draw a sampling distribution of F.)

Calculations

If you liked calculating variance back in Chapter 4, then you'll love the calculations for ANOVA. We will calculate three different variances: one for the total variability, one for between-group variability, and one for within-group variability. But, of course, statisticians don't call them variances, they call them **mean squares.** Go figure.

To start out, we will calculate the numerator term for a variance. The basic formula for a variance is $s^2 = \dfrac{\Sigma(X - M)^2}{N}$, and the numerator term consists of adding up squared deviation scores. Thus the numerator term is a sum of squares, abbreviated SS. The first step in a one-way ANOVA is

mean square

Estimate of a population variance used in analysis of variance.

to calculate sums of squares for total variability (SS_{total}), for between-group variability ($SS_{between}$), and for within-group variability (SS_{within}).

Sums of Squares for One-Way ANOVA

Equation 10.2

$$SS_{total} = \Sigma(X - M_{Grand})^2$$

$$SS_{between} = \Sigma\left(n_{Group}(M_{Group} - M_{Grand})^2\right)$$

$$SS_{within} = \Sigma(X_{Group1} - M_{Group1})^2 + \Sigma(X_{Group2} - M_{Group2})^2 + \dots + \Sigma(X_{Groupk} - M_{Groupk})^2$$

Where:

SS_{total} = sum of squares total

$SS_{between}$ = sum of squares between groups

SS_{within} = sum of squares within groups

X = the score for a case

M_{Grand} = the grand mean

n_{Group} = the sample size for a group

M_{Group} = the mean for a group

X_{Group1} = the score for a case in the first group

M_{Group1} = the mean for the first group

X_{Group2} = the score for a case in the second group

M_{Group2} = the mean for the second group

$\dots$ = ditto for all the intervening groups

X_{Groupk} = the score for a case in the last group

M_{Groupk} = the mean for the last group

I'll explain each of these in turn and we'll do the calculations for our coin data. Then I'll introduce something called an ANOVA summary table, which will bring order to our calculations and make calculating the rest of the one-way ANOVA a snap.

The formula for sum of squares total says that we subtract the grand mean from each individual score, square these deviation scores, and add them all up. To save you (and me) from flipping back and forth to our coin data, let me reprise and update Table 10.2. In Table 10.5 I've updated the data by including the sample size for each group, increasing the number of decimal places for the means to four (using APA format means we'll end up at two), and including the grand mean.

Table 10.5 provides us with everything we need to calculate SS_{total}. Again, all we do is subtract the grand mean from each score, square the deviation scores, and add them all up. For the coin data this becomes

TABLE **10.5** **Updated Data Set from the Coin Funnel**

	Pennies	Nickels	Dimes	Quarters
Seconds	7.9, 8.7, 8.4	10.0, 10.4, 9.4	7.0, 6.5, 6.4, 7.4	9.4, 9.5, 10.0
N; M	3; 8.3333	3; 9.9333	4; 6.8250	3; 9.6333

Grand mean: 8.5385

the following: $(7.9 - 8.5385)^2 + (8.7 - 8.5385)^2 + (8.4 - 8.5385)^2 + (10.0 - 8.5385)^2 + (10.4 - 8.5385)^2 + (9.4 - 8.5385)^2 + (7.0 - 8.5385)^2 + (6.5 - 8.5385)^2 + (6.4 - 8.5385)^2 + (7.4 - 8.5385)^2 + (9.4 - 8.5385)^2 + (9.5 - 8.5385)^2 + (10.0 - 8.5385)^2 = .4077 + .0261 + .0192 + 2.1360 + 3.4652 + .7422 + 2.3670 + 4.1555 + 4.5732 + 1.2962 + .7422 + .9245 + 2.1360 = 22.9910$. I grant that this is a lot of work, but it is primarily a matter of tedium and bookkeeping. The next one, $SS_{between}$, is easier.

Sum of squares between is calculated by adding up the squared deviations of the grand mean from each group mean. And, to compensate for the fact that the group means are built of individual cases, before we add up the squared deviation scores we multiply each by the number of cases that are in the group. For the coin data, $SS_{between}$ looks like this: $3(8.3333 - 8.5385)^2 + 3(9.9333 - 8.5385)^2 + 4(6.8250 - 8.5385)^2 + 3(9.6333 - 8.5385)^2 = (3 \times .0421) + (3 \times 1.9455) + (4 \times 2.9361) + (3 \times 1.1986) = .1263 + 5.8365 + 11.7444 + 3.5958 = 21.3030$.

The final sum of squares, sum of squares within, is tedious again. It is similar to SS_{total}, but instead of subtracting the grand mean from each case, each case has its respective group mean subtracted from it. Thus, SS_{within} is the sum of the squared deviation scores of each case from its group mean. For the coin data this is how it looks: $(7.9 - 8.3333)^2 + (8.7 - 8.3333)^2 + (8.4 - 8.3333)^2 + (10.0 - 9.9333)^2 + (10.4 - 9.9333)^2 + (9.4 - 9.9333)^2 + (7.0 - 6.8250)^2 + (6.5 - 6.8250)^2 + (6.4 - 6.8250)^2 + (7.4 - 6.8250)^2 + (9.4 - 9.6333)^2 + (9.5 - 9.6333)^2 + (10.0 - 9.6333)^2 = .1877 + .1345 + .0044 + .0044 + .2178 + .2844 + .0306 + .1056 + .1806 + .3306 + .0544 + .0178 + .1345 = 1.6873$.

Now that we've calculated all three sums of squares, I can tell you that we did more work than we needed to. We only needed to calculate two of the sums of squares, since the total variability is partitioned into between-group and within-group variability, i.e., $SS_{total} = SS_{between} + SS_{within}$. That's almost true in this case since $SS_{between} = 21.3030$ and $SS_{within} = 1.6873$. Those two added together equal 22.9903, which is just rounding error away from our calculated value of 22.9910.*

---

*Rounding error crept into all of our calculations. If one carried all decimal places in all calculations, as I advise, $SS_{total} = 22.9908$, $SS_{between} = 21.3033$, and $SS_{within} = 1.6875$.

LOOKING CLOSER

TABLE **10.6**   **Blank One-Way Analysis of Variance Summary Table**

ANOVA summary table for...				
Source	SS	df	MS	F
Between				
Within				
Total				

If you calculate any two sums of squares, you can figure out the third, and this puts you in a Dirty Harry moment: Do you feel lucky today?* Are you comfortable with your math, and are you willing to calculate just two sums of squares? Or, would you feel more comfortable calculating all three as a check on your work? Me, I like to calculate all three.

With all three degrees of freedom and sums of squares calculated, it is time to introduce the ANOVA summary table. An ANOVA summary table, a blank one of which is shown in Table 10.6, is a way to organize the information in an analysis of variance so that it leads you to calculate the correct *F* ratio and makes what was done clear to a reader of your results.

The first thing to note about an ANOVA summary table is that it has a title. In Table 10.6 the title ends with ellipses, but the title is used to explain what data are being analyzed. Next, note that there are five columns, the first of which, "Source," already has the rows labeled. "Source" represents the sources of the variability in the data, and there are two sources of variability, between-group and within-group, that sum together to yield total variability. These are abbreviated as "between," "within," and "total," and each will be followed *across* the rest of the table. It is important that the rows be in this order: first "between," then "within," and finally "total."

The next column is labeled "SS" and this stands for sum of squares. As you might guess, each row's sum of squares is placed in its respective column. In the third column, which is labeled "*df*" for degrees of freedom, each source of variability's degrees of freedom is placed. We've already calculated sum of squares and degrees of freedom, so we could fill in the table to this point.

The fourth column is labeled "MS," which stands for **mean square** and which represents the variance that we will analyze. As a refresher, here's the formula for a sample variance, $s^2 = \dfrac{\Sigma(X - M)^2}{N}$, and here's the formula for the estimated population variance: $\hat{s}^2 = \dfrac{\Sigma(X - M)^2}{N - 1}$. Note that each column has a sum of squares for the numerator term and a denominator term that is based on *N*. The SS column represents the numerator term for a variance, and the *df* column represents the denominator term. Because the degrees of freedom is a corrected term—it doesn't represent the exact number of cases that go into calculating the sum of squares—the *MS* term is more like a corrected variance than a sample variance.

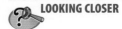 **LOOKING CLOSER**

*Why is this a Dirty Harry moment? In the movie of that name, Clint Eastwood plays a cop who has a shootout with a criminal and then apprehends him. Clint points his gun at the criminal and asks whether the criminal thinks Clint has shot only five bullets or has emptied his gun of all six. If all six are gone, the criminal can run away. But, if the criminal guesses wrong and runs away, then Clint will shoot him with the remaining bullet. So, Clint asks him if he's feeling lucky today.

The fifth and final column is labeled "F" for the F ratio that is being calculated. The F ratio is the ratio $\dfrac{MS_{between}}{MS_{within}}$, and now I hope it is even clearer why I've been referring to $MS_{between}$ as the numerator term and MS_{within} as the denominator term. (In addition, as I've footnoted earlier, the denominator term is sometimes called the "error" term. So, for one-way ANOVA, MS_{within} is the error term.)

One complication to ANOVA summary tables is that they are not filled out completely; some cells are left blank. So, Equation 10.3 includes an ANOVA summary table that shows which cells are filled and how.*

F O R M U L A E

Degrees of Freedom, Mean Squares, and F Ratio for Completing a One-Way ANOVA Summary Table

Source	SS	df	MS	F	**Equation 10.3**
Between	Equation 10.2	$k - 1$	$\dfrac{SS_{between}}{df_{between}}$	$\dfrac{MS_{between}}{MS_{within}}$	
Within	Equation 10.2	$N - k$	$\dfrac{SS_{within}}{df_{within}}$		
Total	Equation 10.2	$N - 1$			

Where:
SS = sum of squares
df = degrees of freedom
MS = mean square
F = F ratio
Equation 10.2 = this value is calculated via Equation 10.2
k = number of groups
$SS_{between}$ = between-groups sum of squares
$df_{between}$ = between-group degrees of freedom
$MS_{between}$ = between-group mean square
MS_{within} = within-group mean square
SS_{within} = within-group sum of squares
df_{within} = within-group degrees of freedom

I have one more point to make regarding the ANOVA summary table, and then I'll fill in the coin data. The final point involves decimal places. It is APA format to report results only to two decimal places, and so our *final* ANOVA summary table will follow that format. However, until I get to that point, I'll carry two more than I'll need. Later, when we use some

---

*I have no idea why statisticians don't calculate MS_{total}, but they don't. So, don't!

LOOKING CLOSER

TABLE **10.7**   **Partially Completed ANOVA Summary Table for Data Regarding Number of Seconds It Takes Coins to Swirl through a Coin Funnel**

Source	SS	df	MS	F
Between	21.3033	3		
Within	1.6875	9		
Total	22.9908	12		

NOTE: See the footnote on p. 375. These are the values calculated when carrying all decimal places.

TABLE **10.8**   **ANOVA Summary Table for Data Regarding Number of Seconds It Takes Coins to Swirl through a Coin Funnel**

Source	SS	df	MS	F
Between	21.30	3	7.10	37.87*
Within	1.69	9	.19	
Total	22.99	12		

NOTE: * = $p < .05$*

of the values in the summary table to calculate other values, we'll resurrect more decimal places.

So, with that proviso, let's go ahead and finish the summary table! As a first step, Table 10.7 contains the information we've calculated so far: the sums of squares and the degrees of freedom with all the decimal places.

I hope that you see how easy it is to complete the rest of the ANOVA summary table. To get the mean square for between and within, we divide the two sums of squares by their respective degrees of freedoms. Then we divide mean square between by the mean square right below it, mean square within, to yield the *F* ratio. When all that work is done, we end up with Table 10.8, where I've followed APA format regarding decimal places.

At this point, we are done with the initial calculations. As the observed *F* value of 37.87 is greater than the critical value of 3.8625, we will reject the null hypothesis and report the results, in APA format, as: $F(3, 9) = 37.87$, $p < .05$.

What do these results mean? Well, that's interpretation, the next step in Tom and Harry.

INTERPRETING ONE-WAY ANOVA

The *F* ratio calculated for an analysis of variance is sometimes referred to as an omnibus test or an **omnibus *F*.** When omnibus is used as an

omnibus *F*

The overall *F* ratio calculated for an analysis of variance; it does not tell which specific pairs of means, if any, statistically differ.

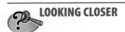

LOOKING CLOSER

*Many ANOVA summary tables use asterisks to indicate if the *F* ratio is statistically significant. A single asterisk (*) commonly indicates $p < .05$, two asterisks (**) indicate $p < 0.01$, and three asterisks indicate $p < .001$. But, there should always be a note on the table that tells what the asterisks mean. I have seen tables where a single asterisk indicates $p < .10$.

adjective like that, it means "providing for many things at once." Thus, analysis of variance is a nonspecific test: When we reject the null hypothesis for a one-way ANOVA, all we can conclude is that at least two of the means of the k groups statistically differ from each other. We don't know which two or if there are more than two. I liken it to hearing a cheer go up from inside a stadium and knowing that something significant happened. But, we don't know how significant or for which team.

In interpreting ANOVA, there are two different techniques that are used: general and specific. The general technique, finding the percentage of variance predicted in the dependent variable by the grouping variable, will summarize the significance of whatever happened. Thus, though we'll find out how many points were scored inside the stadium, we won't know which team scored the points. For that, we'll need to use a more specific approach, to buy a ticket and actually go into the stadium. So, let's start with the general approach and then move on to the specific approach of post-hoc tests.

PERCENTAGE OF VARIANCE PREDICTED

The percentage of variance predicted, what is sometimes called strength of association, is a measure of how much of the variability in the dependent variable can be predicted (or explained or accounted for) by the independent variable. We've already seen this when we calculated r^2 for r and ω^2 (omega squared) for t. Luckily, we won't have to learn a new abbreviation, since ω^2 can also be used for ANOVA.* Let's see the formula (Equation 10.4), calculate it for the coin data, and think about what it means.

F O R M U L A

Omega Squared (ω^2), Percentage of Variance Predicted in the Dependent Variable by the Grouping Variable, for One-Way ANOVA

$$\omega^2 = \frac{SS_{between} - (k-1)\, MS_{within}}{SS_{total} + MS_{within}}$$

Equation 10.4

Where:

ω^2 = omega squared; the percentage of variance predicted

$SS_{between}$ = between-group sum of squares

k = number of groups

MS_{within} = within-group mean square

SS_{total} = sum of squares, total

---

*There are other statistics that are used to calculate percentage of variance predicted for ANOVA. One popular one is η^2. η is the Greek letter "eta," pronounced as in "I *et a* carrot yesterday."

LOOKING CLOSER

The formula says to take $SS_{between}$ and subtract from it the product of MS_{within} multiplied by the difference of the number of groups minus one to find the numerator. The numerator value is then divided by the sum of SS_{total} plus MS_{within}. With the $SS_{between}$ in the numerator and the SS_{total} in the denominator, you can think of this formula as giving the percentage of total variability that is accounted for by the between-group factor. The other factors in the numerator and the denominator—the subtraction from the numerator and the addition to the denominator—are correction factors that shrink the percentage of variance predicted so that it is a population estimate, not just an accounting for a sample.

To do the actual calculations, we must resurrect some decimal places from the information in the ANOVA summary table so that we can follow my rounding rules. Thus, for the coin-funnel data the calculations are as follows:

$$\omega^2 = \frac{21.3033 - (4-1).1875}{22.9908 + .1875} = \frac{20.7408}{23.1783} = .8948$$

This result, almost 90% of the variability being predicted, is a phenomenal amount.* Yes, but what does it mean? First, remember that coins vary in how long it takes them to traverse the coin funnel. One factor that determines time is individual variability, factors that vary from coin to coin within a denomination. Not all dimes are equally round or equally thick, or weigh exactly the same, or have the same pattern of dings and dents from use. In addition, as coins—for example a group of dimes—traverse the coin funnel one after another, there are slightly different patterns of dust and debris on the funnel, slightly different swirls of air, even slight variations in the ambient temperature. These are random error factors. All of these individual difference and error factors have some impact on how long it takes a coin to swirl through the funnel.

There's another factor that can influence run-time, the between-group factor, and that—the grouping variable—is what was tested by the ANOVA. Pennies, nickels, dimes, and quarters differ from each other on a number of dimensions (weight, circumference, thickness, type of metal, milling of the edge) and one, some, or all of these could influence the speed with which a coinlike disk traverses the funnel. The percentage of variance predicted, ω^2, tells how much of the variability in run-times is accounted for by these between-group factors. In this case we can see that almost all the variability, 89.48% of it to be exact, is explained by—is predicted by—the between-group factor, the grouping variable of coin type. Only 10.52% is left unexplained, to be predicted by individual difference and error factors.

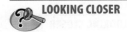

LOOKING CLOSER

*Cohen's rule of thumb, mentioned back in Chapter 8, was this: *for the social and behavioral sciences, predicting 1% of the variance is a small effect size, 10% a medium effect size, and 25% a large effect size.* Here, in a physical science example, we're explaining almost 90%.

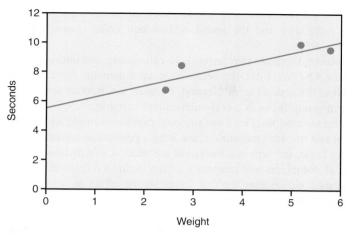

Figure **10.5** Scatterplot showing the relationship between weight (in grams) of different coin types and time (in seconds) it takes them to course through the coin funnel.

Because this was not a true experiment with a real independent variable, we are limited in the conclusions we can draw. Why? Because we did not control the independent variable, and so the groups differ on a number of dimensions (weight, circumference, thickness, type of metal, milling of the edge, etc.). In this situation, I prefer to talk about the percentage of variance *predicted* by the between-group effect rather than the percentage of variance *explained* by the grouping variable. Is it weight that determines speed, circumference, the combination of the two, or some other variable? To know for sure we would have to make our own coinlike disks so that they would vary on only one dimension at a time.

With my psychologist's view of physics, I wondered if it were the weight of the coin that determined run-time. Figure 10.5 is a scatterplot that shows the relation between weight and time. The regression line highlights the linear relationship: as weight increases so does run time.

I've used a scatterplot because I want you to think about correlations. It is reasonable to ask whether weight and run-time are correlated, or whether circumference and run-time are correlated, or thickness and run-time—or any of the other dimensions on which the groups differ. In fact, couldn't we take advantage of the relationship between r and r^2 for ANOVA just as we converted ω^2 to $\hat{r}$ for the t test?* For the coin-funnel

---

*Because of the way it is calculated, $\hat{r}$ will always be positive. So, you'll need to think it through, by examining the means, to decide if it represents a direct or an inverse relationship.

LOOKING CLOSER

data, $\hat{r} = \sqrt{.8948} = .9459 = .95$. The correlation between the group factor of coin type and the speed with which coins course through the funnel is .95.*

However, there are two provisos to calculating and interpreting $\hat{r}$ for a one-way ANOVA. First, the between-group dimension must be measured at least at the ordinal level. Second, $\hat{r}$ makes much more sense when the between-group factor is a real independent variable.

To understand this, let's use my cold pressor example again. The cold pressor test involves measuring how long a person can tolerate the pain of holding his or her arm in a bucket of ice water. Let's imagine that I get a group of volunteers and randomly assign them to receive different doses of the narcotic codeine so that I can see its effect as an analgesic on sudden, intense pain. I have five groups, receiving 0, 15, 30, 45, and 60 mg of codeine. After the medication takes effect, each person performs the cold pressor task, and I time it. No assumptions are violated, I perform the ANOVA, and it is statistically significant. I calculate $\omega^2 = .36$ and turn that into an $\hat{r}$ of .60. There is a straightforward interpretation of this, because we have a real independent variable and it varies in an ordinal fashion. Here's the interpretation: as dose of codeine increases, so does the amount of time that a person can tolerate the ice water.

Let's contrast that with another situation, one where there's also a real independent variable, but it has no ordinal meaning. Suppose that I continue with my cold pressor research but this time I'm investigating which is a more effective analgesic: aspirin, acetaminophen, or ibuprofen. I get a group of volunteers, randomly assign them to three groups, give each group a standard dose of one of the three medications, wait for it to take effect, and then perform the cold pressor test. Again, I violated no assumptions for the ANOVA, so I go ahead and calculate it. Again, it is statistically significant, again I calculate $\omega^2 = .36$, and again I find $\hat{r} = .60$. But, how do I interpret this $\hat{r}$ when there is no logical order to the independent variable? To say that there is a .60 correlation between drug type and analgesic effect seems nonsensical to me. In this scenario, I'm more comfortable going back to ω^2 and saying that drug type predicts 36% of the variability in cold pressor toleration time.

Let's think through our coin-funnel example. We don't have a real independent variable, which means that there are other variables, confounding variables, that are present and that may explain any observed difference between groups. In fact, we've thought of a number of

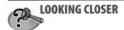

LOOKING CLOSER

*This is an introductory statistics text, and I'm very comfortable with calculating r this way, but be aware that statistical purists may not like it. There is a statistic, called epsilon (Greek letter "ε"), that turns an ANOVA into a correlation coefficient just as we turned a t value into a special correlation called a point biserial correlation. If you apply the epsilon equation to the coin data it turns out to equal .9498. Not very far away from my value of .9459 is it? I think taking the square root of ω^2 will work nicely enough for introductory statistics, don't you?

dimensions (weight, circumference, thickness) on which the coins differ and which may account for the observed effect. We've chosen to focus on weight, which is beyond ordinal, and so it seems sensible to say as the weight of the object increases, the speed with which it traverses the funnel decreases. Ah, but—and this is a big but—it might not be weight that is the relevant factor in determining speed.* Because we don't have a real independent variable, we can't be sure since our grouping variable varies on more than one dimension at a time. So, here's the interpretative statement that I would make, so far, for the coin-funnel data:

"We conducted a study in which we timed how long it took different types of coins to course through a coin funnel. The mean number of seconds that each type of coin took, in increasing order, was dimes (6.82), pennies (8.33), quarters (9.63), and nickels (9.93). By the one-way ANOVA we conducted, there was a statistically significant difference among at least some of the means (F (3, 9) = 37.87, p < .05): different types of coins traverse the funnel in different amounts of time.

The different types of coins differ on a number of physical dimensions (weight, circumference, thickness, etc.), and these factors predict or account for almost 90% of the variability in how long it takes coins to course through a coin funnel.

"There are a number of limitations to the current study. First, only one coin funnel was used; though I don't think it likely that a different coin funnel would provide different results, it is a possibility. Second, the sample of coins was not a random sample of coins from the population of U.S. coinage, and thus there is the possibility that sample was unusual in some way that affected the results. Even if the sample had been a random sample, it is possible to obtain a random sample that is not representative, and thus the conclusion that different coins take different amounts of time may be erroneous. There is a 5% chance that this conclusion is in error. Thus, to have more faith in the results, I suggest replicating this study, ideally with a larger and randomly selected sample.

"Of greater concern is that coin denomination is not a true independent variable, and that the different coins differed on more than one dimension. Dimes, for example, are smaller than the other coins in terms of weight, circumference, and thickness. Thus, it is not possible from this study to determine which physical dimension of a coin influences run-time in a funnel. If one wanted to determine this, one would have to manufacture and test coinlike disks that varied on only one dimension at a time."

> ### Group Practice 10.3
>
> Calculate and interpret ω^2 and $\hat{r}$ for the stroke data introduced in question 7 of Group Practice 10.1.

---

*I consulted some physicists, Bruce Wittmershaus and Jonathan Hall of Penn State Erie, and they explained to me that it was the degree of friction at the point of contact between the coin and the funnel that determined run-time.

LOOKING CLOSER

POST-HOC TESTS

planned comparison

A statistical test, planned in advance of completing the omnibus F of an ANOVA, in which preselected pairs of means are compared to see if a statistically significant difference exists.

post-hoc test

A statistical test, completed only after an omnibus F for an ANOVA is found statistically significant, in which pairs of means are compared to see if there are statistically significant differences between them.

We heard a cheer go up inside the stadium. Thanks to ω^2 we know something big has happened. We even have a rough idea that it is some physical aspect of the coin that influences speed. But now we need to buy a ticket, go in, and find out what happened specifically. This procedure goes by a number of different names. Sometimes a researcher has planned in advance to go in and compare a couple of specified groups, in which case the exploring is called a **planned comparison.** That's not what we're doing here. We don't want to spend our money on a ticket until we're sure that something exciting happened in the stadium. So, we're only going to buy a ticket *after* we've heard the roar of the crowd, after we have found the overall F statistically significant.* Thus, we are doing a **post-hoc test.**

There are a whole variety of post-hoc tests with great names like the Tukey *HSD* or the Fisher *LSD* and it is beyond the scope of this intro text to cover them all.[†] They differ in terms of how conservative they are in determining if a difference between two group means is a statistically significant difference. For example, *HSD* is an abbreviation for "honestly significant difference." If the *HSD* test says that two group means are statistically different, then the difference between the two is probably a real one. Contrast this with the *LSD* test where *LSD* stands for "least significant difference." The *LSD* test is intended to maximize one's chances of finding that two group means are statistically different, and so smaller differences between means will be found as statistically significant differences. Thus, depending on which test you choose, you may end up concluding with one test, the *LSD*, that two means are statistically different and with the other, the *HSD*, that they aren't.[‡]

So, what test should you use? I'm going to make your life easy and just teach you one test so your options will be limited. You'll be surprised to hear that I choose a liberal test, the Fisher *LSD*. One reason that I'm choosing this test is that it maximizes the chance that we'll find something when we go exploring.[§] The other reason is that the Fisher *LSD* goes by other names, the protected t or the multiple t.** Because it is a t test, we'll be able to apply a lot of the interpretative methods that we learned in Chapter 9. And because I first heard it called the protected t, that's the name we'll use for it. Equation 10.5 shows how to calculate it.

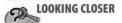
LOOKING CLOSER

*If the overall F is not statistically significant, if there is no roar from the crowd, we'll save our money and not buy a ticket to go inside the stadium.

[†]Want more names? How about Bonferroni-Dunn, or Scheffé, or Newman-Keuls?

[‡]In other words, with one test there is a greater chance of making a Type I error and with the other a greater chance of making a Type II error. Can you figure out which is which?

[§]For just this reason some statisticians don't like it, they think it is likely to result in Type I error. However, with more conservative post-hoc tests, there is a chance of Type II error, of finding that no pairs of means statistically differ even though the omnibus F was statistically significant.

**Why is it called a "protected" t or a "multiple" t? Because it protects, or maintains, the overall alpha level. Thus, though we might be doing multiple t tests, we still have only a 5% chance of making a Type I error.

Protected t Post-Hoc Test Value, with $df_{within} = N - k$

Equation 10.5

$$t = \frac{M_1 - M_2}{\sqrt{MS_{within}\left(\dfrac{1}{n_1} + \dfrac{1}{n_2}\right)}}$$

Where:

t = protected t post-hoc test value being calculated
N = total number of cases in the ANOVA
k = number of groups in the ANOVA
M_1 = mean of one group being compared
M_2 = mean of other group being compared
MS_{within} = mean square within from the ANOVA
n_1 = sample size of one group being compared
n_2 = sample size of other group being compared

In the numerator for the formula, the two means being compared are subtracted from each other. Since it doesn't matter which is which, I always subtract the smaller mean from the larger mean so that I end up with a positive number. For the denominator, MS_{within} is multiplied by the product of the reciprocals of the sample sizes for the two groups being compared.* The t is compared to the critical value of t with $df = df_{within}$.

Now it becomes tedious: with four groups (pennies, nickels, dimes, and quarters), there are six comparisons of pairs we can make.† There are a number of ways to choose which comparison to do first. One option is sequential: pennies vs. nickels, then pennies vs. dimes, then pennies vs. quarters, then nickels vs. dimes, and so on. Another option, the one I prefer, is to start with the two means farthest apart (dimes vs. nickels) and then proceed in descending order of distance. If the sample sizes are the same, which they aren't here, you can stop when you get two means that don't differ statistically. (In fact, in a bit I'll show you a shortcut and a reason why this test is called the *LSD*.) Because there is some variability in sample sizes and because I like to conserve my energy, I will first compare dimes ($n = 4$) to the other three coin types ($n = 3$), and then I'll make comparisons within pennies, nickels, and quarters. That way I only need to calculate the denominator twice. Within each set, I'll go in descending order of the difference between the means.

---

*Here's a heads up. We're going to need the denominator term again, so it would be wise to write it down. And, by the bye, it has a name: the standard error of the difference and is abbreviated $\hat{s}_{M_1-M_2}$, just as it was when we calculated t back in Chapter 9.

† $\dfrac{k(k-1)}{2}$ = the number of pairs comparisons for k groups.

LOOKING CLOSER

First, though, I want to find my t_{cv} so that I know when to stop calculating. $df_{within} = N - k = 13 - 4 = 9$. With 9 degrees of freedom, the critical value of t at the .05 level, two-tailed, is 2.2622 via Appendix Table 9.

OK, let's compare dimes (6.8250 sec) to nickels (9.9333 sec):

$$t_{NvsD} = \frac{9.9333 - 6.8250}{\sqrt{.1875\left(\frac{1}{3} + \frac{1}{4}\right)}} = \frac{3.1083}{.3307} = 9.3992 = 9.40$$

Note several things here. First, I've given this protected t a subscript so that I can keep track of which it is. Also, note that I went back and obtained an MS_{within} value that had more decimal places than the two in the ANOVA summary table. Note that the difference was statistically significant, so I need to go on and calculate t for the next comparison, dimes vs. quarters. Finally, note that if I want to report this in APA format I write this: $t(9) = 9.40$, $p < .05$.

Now let's do the rest. The dimes vs. quarters comparison will be a little easier because the denominator will be the same. Thus, here it is:

$$t_{DvsQ} = \frac{9.6333 - 6.8250}{.3307} = \frac{2.8083}{.3307} = 8.4920 = 8.49$$

This t value is also greater than t_{cv}, so let's go on and compare dimes to pennies:

$$t_{PvsD} = \frac{8.3333 - 6.8250}{.3307} = \frac{1.5083}{.3307} = 4.5609 = 4.56$$

Based on the first three post-hoc tests, the sample of dimes coursed through the coin bank in a time that was statistically faster than any other type of coin.

Now we need to find out if there is any statistical difference between the times for pennies, nickels, or quarters. Our first comparison will be pennies vs. nickels since those two are the furthest apart:

$$t_{PvsN} = \frac{9.9333 - 8.3333}{\sqrt{.1875\left(\frac{1}{3} + \frac{1}{3}\right)}} = \frac{1.6000}{.3536} = 4.5249 = 4.52$$

That difference was statistically significant, so it is on to the next, pennies vs. quarters:

$$t_{PvsQ} = \frac{9.6333 - 8.3333}{.3536} = \frac{1.3000}{.3536} = 3.6765 = 3.68$$

And, finally, we'll need to compare nickels to quarters:

$$t_{NvsQ} = \frac{9.9333 - 9.6333}{.3536} = \frac{.3000}{.3536} = .8484 = .85$$

TABLE **10.9** **Results of Protected *t* Post-Hoc Tests Comparing Mean Times for Different Coin Types**

	Pennies (8.33 sec)	Nickels (9.93 sec)	Dimes (6.82 sec)	Quarters (9.63 sec)
Pennies (8.33 sec)	—	*	*	*
Nickels (9.93 sec)	*	—	*	ns
Dimes (6.82 sec)	*	*	—	*
Quarters (9.63 sec)	*	ns	*	—

NOTE: * = difference is statistically significant at $\alpha = .05$, two-tailed
    ns = difference is not statistically significant at $\alpha = .05$, two-tailed
    — = not applicable

We just did six post-hoc tests, and that is a lot to keep track of. To help, I've arrayed the results in Table 10.9.* As you can see, the time it takes coins to travel through the funnel is statistically different for every type of coin except for the difference between nickels and quarters.

I had promised a shortcut and a reason why this test is called the *least significant difference* test, and here it is. It is possible to do a little algebraic rearranging of Equation 10.5 and calculate a value, called the *LSD* value. If two means differ by that amount or more, then they are significantly different from each other. For the coin data, we only need to calculate two *LSD* values, one for *n*s of 4 and 3 and the other for *n*s of 3 and 3. I think that this is easier than calculating six different *t* values. Here's the formula.[†]

F O R M U L A

LSD Value for Post-Hoc Comparisons for One-Way ANOVA

Equation 10.6

$$LSD = t_{cv} \sqrt{MS_{within} \left(\frac{1}{n_1} + \frac{1}{n_2} \right)}$$

Continued

---

*I've made this table easier to read by making it redundant. With an extra row and column, it contains twice as much information as it needs to. Note that the information above the diagonal is a mirror image of the information below the diagonal.

[†] And if you've been reading these footnotes and saved the standard error of the difference term,

$\sqrt{MS_{within} \left(\frac{1}{n_1} + \frac{1}{n_2} \right)}$, that you calculated earlier, feel free to plug it in.

LOOKING CLOSER

F O R M U L A

LSD Value for Post-Hoc Comparisons for One-Way ANOVA—cont'd

Equation 10.6   Where:

LSD = value if, by which two means differ, the two means statistically differ

t_{cv} = critical value of t, $\alpha = .05$, $df = N - k$

MS_{within} = within-group mean square from the ANOVA

n_1 = sample size for one group being compared

n_2 = sample size for other group being compared

NOTE: N = total number of cases in the ANOVA

k = number of groups in the ANOVA

In English: first sum the reciprocals of the sample sizes of the two groups being compared. Then, multiply this sum by MS_{within}. Finally, take the square root of that product and multiply it by the critical value of t. For comparing the mean of the dimes to the mean of the other three groups, LSD is calculated as follows:

$$LSD = 2.2622 \sqrt{.1875\left(\frac{1}{4} + \frac{1}{3}\right)} = 2.2622 \times .3307 = .7481 = .75$$

Also, for comparing the means for the groups where $n = 3$, this is LSD:

$$2.2622 \sqrt{.1875\left(\frac{1}{3} + \frac{1}{3}\right)} = 2.2622 \times .3536 = .7999 = .80$$

Here's how to use an LSD value. Pennies and nickels differ in their run-times by 1.60 seconds, and the LSD value for samples of size $N = 3$ is .80. Since 1.60 is greater than or equal to .80, the difference between pennies and nickels is a statistically significant one. The easiest way to use these LSD values is to make a table showing the mean differences between the groups and then asterisk the groups that differ statistically. Table 10.10 does so.

Note that this is a stripped-down version of Table 10.9 since it only contains information above the diagonal. If the difference between pennies and nickels is statistically significant, then so is the difference between nickels and pennies. The LSD value tells us that if pennies and nickels differ by .800 or more seconds, then the difference will be statistically significant. Since the actual difference between the two is 1.60 seconds, I have placed an asterisk next to the difference to indicate statistical significance.

TABLE **10.10**   **Absolute Value of Mean Differences between Run-Times for Different Coin Types**

	Nickels	Dimes	Quarters
Pennies	1.60*	1.51*	1.30*
Nickels		3.11*	.30
Dimes			2.81*

NOTE: * = statistically significant difference via Fisher's *LSD* post-hoc test with α set at .05

There is only one more calculation to learn, and then we can wrap up our interpretation of the protected t post-hoc test. Back in Chapter 9, we calculated the 95% confidence interval for the difference between two means after we calculated the t test. We can do the same thing here. And, just as before, we'll glean useful interpretative information from how tight the confidence interval is and how far from zero it lies.

The 95% confidence interval will be calculated using the $\alpha = .05$, two-tailed, critical value of t with $N - k$ degrees of freedom. Thus, the degrees of freedom are the same as the denominator term from the ANOVA, the degrees of freedom for MS_{within}. The formula is shown in Equation 10.7.

F O R M U L A

95% Confidence Interval for the Difference between Two Means for a One-Way ANOVA

Equation 10.7

$$95\% \; CI = (M_1 - M_2) \pm t_{cv} \sqrt{MS_{within}\left(\frac{1}{n_1} + \frac{1}{n_2}\right)}$$

Where:

$95\% \; CI$ = the 95% confidence interval being calculated

M_1 = the mean of one group being compared

M_2 = the mean of the other group being compared

t_{cv} = the critical value of t with $N - k$ degrees of freedom, $\alpha = .05$, two-tailed

MS_{within} = within-group mean square from the ANOVA

n_1 = the sample size of one group being compared

n_2 = the sample size of the other group being compared

NOTE: N = total number of cases in the ANOVA

k = number of groups in the ANOVA

Here's how to calculate this confidence interval. First, find the sum of the reciprocals of the ns for the two groups being compared and multiply the sum by MS_{within}. Take the square root of this product and multiply it by the critical value of t. This product is then subtracted from and added to the difference between the two means to find the lower and upper bounds of the confidence interval.

Again, thinking ahead saves a bit of work. You may have noted that we are encountering the radical term, $\sqrt{MS_{within}\left(\frac{1}{n_1} + \frac{1}{n_2}\right)}$, quite frequently It does have a name, the standard error of the difference, which is the same name that was given to the denominator term for the t test back in Chapter 9 where it was abbreviated $\hat{s}_{M_1-M_2}$. We're going to have to calculate it again, so if you saved this value from either Equation 10.5 or 10.6, we can just plug it in. Because the sample sizes bounce around a little bit, there

TABLE **10.11**   Absolute Value of Observed Differences and 95% Confidence Intervals
for Differences in Run-Times (in Seconds) for Different Coin Types

	Observed Difference	*95% CI*
Pennies vs. nickels	−1.60	.80 to 2.40
Pennies vs. dimes	1.51	.76 to 2.26
Pennies vs. quarters	1.30	.50 to 2.10
Nickels vs. dimes	3.11	2.36 to 3.86
Nickels vs. quarters	.30	−.50 to 1.10
Dimes vs. quarters	2.81	2.06 to 3.56

are two standard errors of the mean that we need: .3307 when our *n*s are
3 and 4, and .3536 when our *n*s are 3 and 3. The critical value of *t*, two-
tailed, with 9 degrees of freedom at the .05 level, is 2.2622. And with that,
we are ready to calculate.

The 95% confidence interval for the difference between run-times for
pennies and nickels is (9.9333 − 8.3333) ± (2.2622 × .3536) = 1.6000
± .7999.* Which means that the difference between the two means ranges
from as little as .80 seconds to as much as 2.40 seconds. In Table 10.11, I
show the confidence intervals for all six comparisons as well as the actual
observed differences.

Note that they are all about the same width, ≈1.5 seconds, which is not
surprising since the two standard errors of the difference that we used
were close to each other and we always used the same critical value of *t*.
Also note that only one, nickels vs. quarters, captures zero. That should
not be surprising since all the protected *t* values but one, nickels vs.
quarters, turned out to be statistically significant. Finally, note that none
of the confidence intervals that fails to capture zero is particularly close to
zero, each one starts at least .5 second away. Two of them in fact, dimes
vs. nickels and dimes vs. quarters, start more than 2 seconds away from
zero. Given that the longest time it took a coin to course through the
funnel was about 10 seconds, a difference of .5 second or a difference of
2 seconds—a difference of 5% or 20%—seems like a meaningful difference to me.

We've done all the calculations, and I'm ready to do some more
interpretation by integrating information from the post-hoc tests into the
statement I made earlier based only on ω^2. So, here's my new, and more
complete, interpretative statement:

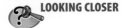
LOOKING CLOSER

*Where do all those numbers come from? The 9.9333 is the mean for the nickels and the 8.3333 is the mean
for the pennies. (As usual, if I can, I prefer to subtract the smaller number from the larger so that I end up
with a positive number.) The 2.2622 is the critical value of *t*, and the 0.3536 was the standard error of the
difference when both *n*s are 3.

Do you want a time-saving shortcut? Note that the *95% CI* can be calculated as the difference between
two means plus/minus the *LSD* value.

"We conducted a study in which we timed how long it took different types of coins to course through a coin funnel. The mean number of seconds that each type of coin took, in increasing order, was dimes (6.82), pennies (8.33), quarters (9.63), and nickels (9.93). Overall, there was a statistically significant difference among the means ($F (3, 9) = 37.87, p < .05$): different types of coins traverse the funnel in different amounts of time.

The different types of coins differ on a number of physical dimensions (weight, circumference, thickness, etc.), and some combination of physical factors predicts or accounts for almost 90% of the variability in how long it takes coins to course through a coin funnel. Specifically, dimes were statistically faster than pennies, which were statistically faster than quarters; the difference in run-time between quarters and nickels was not statistically different from zero. It appears that, in general, smaller coins travel through the funnel more quickly.

"The differences in time seem large and meaningful to me. Based on the 95% confidence intervals that we calculated, the average time that it takes a dime to course through the funnel likely ranges from .75 seconds to 2.25 seconds faster than the time it takes a penny. Given that the average penny took about 8.33 seconds, the average dime is about 9% to 27% faster. This seems to me like a significant increase in speed.

"There are a number of limitations to the current study. First, only one coin funnel was used; though I don't think it likely that a different coin funnel would provide different results, it is a possibility. Second, the sample of coins was not a random sample of coins from the population of U.S. coinage, and thus there is the possibility that the sample was unusual in some way that affected the results. Even if the sample had been a random sample, it is possible to obtain a random sample that is not representative, which would lead to an erroneous conclusion. There is a 5% chance of such an error having occurred. To have more faith in the results, I suggest replicating this study, ideally with a larger and randomly selected sample.

"Of greater concern is that coin denomination is not a true independent variable, and the different coins differed on more than one dimension. Dimes, for example, are smaller than the other coins in terms of weight, circumference, and thickness. Thus it is not possible from this study to determine which physical dimension of a coin influences run-time in a funnel. If one wanted to determine this, one would have to manufacture coinlike disks that varied on only one dimension at a time."

Final Post-Hoc Test Thoughts

We've finished exploring post-hoc tests—and they involved a lot of calculations. Were they worth it? This seems like a particularly appropriate question to ask, because I started the section on ANOVA by saying that ANOVA allows us to do one test rather than a bunch of t tests—and yet I've ended up doing a whole bunch of t tests. What gives?

First, you only do the post-hoc test calculations if the overall F ratio is statistically significant. (I can hear you praying for nonsignificant results.) Second, the post-hoc tests have advantages over a regular independent-sample t test.

As I mentioned, one advantage of doing post-hoc tests is that it maintains our alpha level. If we do six independent sample t tests, we have almost a 30% chance of one of them involving a Type I error. However, by doing them as post-hoc tests, we keep our overall chance of making a Type I error down to 5%.*

This should seem even more amazing when I say that by doing a post-hoc test, we can increase our chances of rejecting the null hypothesis that two population means are equivalent over the chance we have of rejecting the null hypothesis if we use an independent-samples t test. Why? Because the protected t uses a corrected version of MS_{within} as its error term, the denominator for the t test, and the degrees of freedom associated with this are $N - k$. If this comparison is done as an independent-sample t test, the error term has fewer degrees of freedom, $n_1 + n_2$ degrees of freedom. Why does this matter? Because if we compare pennies to quarters, the critical value of t changes from $t_{cv} = 2.262$ for 9 degrees of freedom to $t_{cv} = 2.7764$ for 4 degrees of freedom, making the rare zone smaller and making it harder to reject the null hypothesis. If $t_{observed}$ ends up as, say, 2.50, it is statistically significant for the protected t but not for the independent-samples t. That's a definite advantage for post-hoc tests.

> **Group Practice 10.4**
>
> Calculate and interpret the Fisher *LSD*, or protected *t*, and the 95% confidence intervals for the stroke data introduced in question 7 of Group Practice 10.1.

POWER AND SAMPLE SIZE

For Pearson rs and t tests we ended our interpretative calculations by examining power and sample size. These are concerns for a one-way ANOVA as well. Power, which is equal to $1 - \beta$, or one minus the probability of a Type II error, tells how great the likelihood is that we'll be able to reject the null hypothesis. Since rejecting the null hypothesis is what we usually wish to achieve, we want power to be as high as possible. Power is determined by the alpha level chosen, the size of the effect, and the number of cases. A sad fact of science is that many researchers are destined to fail to reject their null hypotheses because their studies are underpowered—because they don't have enough cases to have a reasonable chance of rejecting H_0. As a result, a researcher may conclude that a treatment is not promising when it really would be beneficial. For ANOVAs as well as for correlations and two-sample tests, researchers should think *in advance of collecting any data* about how many cases they will need to have a reasonable chance of rejecting the null hypothesis if the effect size is of a certain level.

LOOKING CLOSER

*Technically, the α level is maintained only if H_0 is true.

TABLE **10.12** **Travel Times, in Seconds, from My House to a Specified Mile Marker, for Three Different Routes**

Chagrin	595, 619, 679, 722, 723, 750, 767, 780, 793, 849	$M = 727.70$; $s = 74.57$
Cedar	610, 611, 706, 715, 755, 775, 795, 807, 810, 927	$M = 751.10$; $s = 91.06$
Mayfield	707, 719, 776, 800, 800, 810, 816, 826, 889, 975	$M = 811.80$; $s = 73.47$

Calculating power and sample size for ANOVA is daunting enough that many researchers aren't sure how to do it. Teaching you how to do it is beyond the scope of this text.* Yet, we can apply what we learned in previous chapters about power and sample size to the current chapter in order to gain a very rough idea of whether we are in the ballpark in terms of sample size and power. What I am going to advocate is using ω^2 to estimate $\hat{r}$ and then using $\hat{r}$, via Appendix Tables 7 and 8, to approximate power and sample size. My experience has been that doing so *under*estimates power and *over*estimates how many cases one needs. Thus, this is a conservative approach that has the potential cost of collecting data from more cases than necessary.

Let's work with some data to explore this. Since power equals $1 - \beta$ and β is the probability of a Type II error, it makes more sense to explore this with a data set for which I fail to reject the null hypothesis. So, let me describe the data set and follow it through all the steps of Tom and Harry.

My commute to work goes along an interstate highway and I have three places where I can get on the highway. The closest to my house is the Chagrin Boulevard entrance, and to get to it I have to travel south a little bit before I head north on the interstate. The other two entrances are north of my house, with the Cedar Road entrance closer than the Mayfield Road entrance. Each entrance is a different distance from my house, and each is a different combination of roads, traffic, and traffic lights away from my house. Like most people, I want to minimize the time my commute takes, so I decided to investigate whether it was faster to take the nearer entrance (Chagrin) even though it meant heading in the wrong direction for a bit, or whether it was faster to take secondary roads so that I could get on the interstate a little closer to my ultimate destination. So, I got a stopwatch, picked a mile marker beyond the Mayfield entrance— the farthest entrance—used a random number table to decide which route to take on a given day, and then for 30 consecutive commutes I timed how long it took me, in seconds, to get from my house to the specified mile marker. Table 10.12 shows the results.[†]

---

*Daunting? The chapter that explains how to do power analysis for ANOVA, in the major text on the subject (Cohen, 1988), is 134 pages long. (Cohen, J. (1988). *Statistical power analysis for the behavioral sciences.* Hillsdale, NJ: Lawrence Erlbaum Associates.)

[†]And yes, I really did this. "Anything for science," has always been my motto.

LOOKING CLOSER

Inspection of the means shows that there are some differences in travel times. From the Chagrin entrance to the mile marker takes a little over 12 minutes, to Cedar takes about another half minute, and to Mayfield takes an additional minute. The question that I am asking is whether the differences between these three means are statistically significant and this, since I am comparing means among three independent samples, is an ANOVA question.* Specifically, it calls for a one-way ANOVA.

The assumptions for the one-way ANOVA are independent samples, interval- or ratio-level data, random samples, normality, and homogeneity of variance. I know that I've already met the first two assumptions since I chose my route for each day randomly and the dependent variable, seconds, is ratio level. Though I have violated the third assumption—I don't have a random sample of trip times from the entire population of trip days—I don't think that this is a very serious violation. When I checked the 95% confidence intervals for skewness and kurtosis for each of the samples, each *CI* captured zero, so I don't appear to have violated the normality assumption. And, inspection of the standard deviations in Table 10.12 shows that none is twice as large as any other, so the homogeneity of variance doesn't appear to be violated. As a result, I am good to go with the ANOVA.

The null hypothesis is that all population means are equal (H_0: $\mu_1 = \mu_2 = \mu_3$). If any differences are found among sample means, the differences will be small enough that they can be accounted for by sampling error for three samples drawn from the same population. The alternative hypothesis says that all population means are not equal. Thus, at least two of the sample means will differ by an amount that is too large to be plausibly explained by sampling error for samples drawn from a single population.

The easiest way to formulate the decision rule, I find, is to fill out the degrees of freedom section of the ANOVA summary table. Following either Equation 10.1 (for degrees of freedom) or the *df* column in Equation 10.3, Table 10.13 shows a partial ANOVA summary table.

Table 10.13 shows that I will compare $F_{observed}$ to F_{cv} with 2 degrees of freedom in the numerator and 27 degrees of freedom in the denominator. At the .05 alpha level, $F_{cv} = 3.3541$. If $F_{observed} \geq 3.3541$, I'll reject H_0; if $F_{observed} < 3.3541$, I'll fail to reject H_0. In Figure 10.6, I show the sampling distribution of F with the rare and common zones marked off.

The other part of the decision rule involves thinking, in advance, about whether one's sample size is adequate. I have two different ways of

TABLE **10.13** **Partially Completed ANOVA Summary Table for Travel-Time Data**

Source	SS	df	MS	F
Between		2		
Within		27		
Total		29		

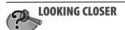

LOOKING CLOSER

*The samples are independent because the route I took one day had no impact on the route I took the next since I used a random number table to decide which route I took on a given day. How did I use a random number table? I assigned Chagrin a value of 1, Cedar 2, and Mayfield 3. I then went through the table and wrote down the 1s, 2s, and 3s as I encountered them, ending up with a sequence like 3, 1, 3, 3, 1, 3, … I wanted to make sure that I ended up with an equal number of 1s, 2s, and 3s, so I played around with where I started my sequence until I achieved my goal.

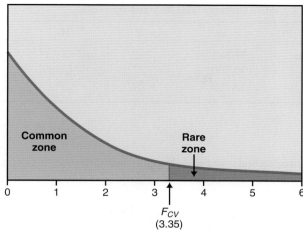

Figure **10.6** Sampling distribution of *F*, at the .05 α level with 2 and 27 degrees of freedom.

thinking about this. One is to speculate about the size of the effect, whether one expects the effect to be small, medium, or large; and the other is to examine the actual means. As we're about to see, they may give very different answers.

Ideally, speculation about the size of the effect is based on previous research. If someone had done a previous study concerning effect of highway entry on commuting time and had found that the size of the effect, ω^2, was, say, .21, I'd take the square root of that as my estimate of r ($\approx$.45) and look up the *N* for $\rho = .45$ in Appendix Table 8. However, no one has done research in this area before and, on my own, I get to engage in idle speculation. I don't think that the effect of where I get on the highway on my commuting time is going to be very large, and Cohen (1988) calls a small effect an *r* of .10.* Based on Appendix Table 8, one needs 784 cases to have an 80% chance of rejecting the null hypothesis if $\rho = .10$, and $\alpha = .05$, two-tailed. With three samples, this works out to more than 250 cases per sample! As I have only 10 cases per sample, my study is more than a bit underpowered if the effect is really that small.

Rather than idly speculate about the size of the effect, why not take advantage of the fact that I do have some information about how big the effect is, since I have means and standard deviations for each of the three samples? Since a statistically significant ANOVA is followed up by a post-hoc test to see which pair(s) of means differ, why not use the rule-of-thumb formula that we used for the *t* test, Equation 9.9, to see how many

---

*Cohen, J. (1988). *Statistical power analysis for the behavioral sciences.* Hillsdale, NJ: Lawrence Erlbaum Associates.

LOOKING CLOSER

TABLE **10.14**   **ANOVA Summary Table for Travel-Time Data**

Source	SS	df	MS	F
Between	37,682.87	2	18,841.43	2.64
Within	192,500.60	27	7129.65	
Total	230,183.47	29		

cases we need to find a statistically significant difference between the pair of means that is farthest apart? This should give a rough estimate of the necessary sample size.

For my highway data, the 84.1 second difference between the Chagrin and Mayfield entrances is the largest difference between samples. Applying Equation 9.9, I find a large effect size of 1.13 and a recommended sample size of $n = 13$ to have an 80% chance of rejecting the null hypothesis. To estimate how many cases to have for the ANOVA, multiply the estimate for n by the number of samples. Thus, I estimate that my ANOVA should be done with 39 cases. I only have 30 cases, and my study is still underpowered, but I need to add only 3 cases per sample in order to approach adequate power if this estimate is right.

Both of these approaches provide rough estimates. One, the estimate of 784 cases, almost certainly overestimates how many cases are needed; and the other, 39 cases, probably underestimates. If I had to pick one at this stage, I'd be more likely to go with the estimate of 39 cases since it is based on actual data and not just idle speculation.* However, if my Appendix Table 8 estimate of the effect size were based on previous research, I'd be more likely to use that.

Whichever estimate you use, remember that more accurately calculating power and sample size for ANOVA is beyond the scope of this introductory statistics text. I'm just taking one of the tools in our toolbox and, since I don't have the correct tool for the job at hand, improvising with it.

Anyway, with all my prep work done, it's time for the calculations. If you want to do them on your own, that's fine by me. (In fact, I recommend it.) In any event, I've done them, and you can see the results in Table 10.14.

$F_{observed}$ is 2.64, which is less than the F_{cv} of 3.3541. Thus the observed F ratio fell into the common zone, and I have failed to reject the null hypothesis. I conclude that there is no statistical difference between any of the sample means, and thus there is not sufficient evidence to conclude

LOOKING CLOSER   *In addition, a sample size of 39 is achievable; 784 cases isn't realistic.

that any of the population means differs from any other. It appears that it doesn't make any difference in travel time which way I drive to work: all ways are statistically equal.

However, before I write my formal interpretative statement, I want to explore the possibility that I have made a Type II error, that I have concluded the population means are the same when they really are different. After all, there is almost a 1.5 minute difference in travel time depending on whether I get on the interstate at Chagrin Boulevard or Mayfield Road. When I calculate the 95% confidence interval for the difference between these two means, I find that it could be as much as just over 2.5 minutes. Maybe there really is a difference, and I had a non-representative sample.

To get a rough idea of power—and remember this is a rough and conservative idea—I need to turn the information from the ANOVA summary table into the correlation between travel time (my dependent variable) and entrance ramp (my independent, or treatment, variable). To do so, I first calculate ω^2 via Equation 10.4:

$$\omega^2 = \frac{37,682.8667 - (3-1)7129.6519}{23,0183.4667 + 7129.6519} = .0987$$

If I take the square root of .0987, I estimate $\hat{r}$ as $\sqrt{.0987}$ or .3142.* Thus I find that there is a .31 correlation between entrance ramp and travel time.[†]

Now comes the rough estimation part. Using Table 7 in the Appendix, I'm going to follow the row with $N = 30$ across until it intersects with the column for $r = .30$, where I'll find power = .36. If power = .36, then $\beta = .64$, or I had almost two chances out of three of making a Type II error. That's a large chance and should make me concerned that it has happened.

Moving to Appendix Table 8 shows that I need a total of 86 cases to have only a 20% chance of making a Type II error (i.e., power = .80) if

---

*There will be situations where the F ratio is small, less than 1, and ω^2 turns out to be less than zero. In such a situation treat the ω^2 value as zero (i.e., the independent variable predicts none of the variability in the dependent variable). But, what about calculating $\hat{r}$ in order to find out what sample size one would need? In this situation I would recommend calculating a different measure of percentage of variance predicted, η^2 (that's "eta squared") and using the square root of η^2 to estimate $\hat{r}$.

[†]I agree that it doesn't make a lot of sense to examine the correlation between the ratio-level variable of travel time and the nominal-level variable of entrance ramp. It makes more sense if I can construe entrance ramp as being at least at the ordinal level, maybe as distance of entrance ramp from my house. Thus, the Chagrin entrance is closest, followed by the Cedar ramp, with the Mayfield entrance being the farthest away.

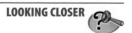

LOOKING CLOSER

ρ is .30 and α is .05. Since I have three groups, that works out to $\approx$ 29 cases per group. Since my ns were 10, not 29, my study was underpowered.*

I want to stress once again that the way I just showed you to estimate power and sample size for ANOVA is a rough and conservative guide. That is, it tends to underestimate power and overestimate the number of cases needed. Using the formulae from Cohen's 1988 book on power, I find power to be .45, not the .36 I calculated, and that I should have 21 cases per cell, not 29. Thus you'll note in my interpretation that I talk about the concepts of power and sample size, but I shy away from giving exact values.[†]

Before I make my interpretation, I want to remind you that with a large enough sample size, even a trivial difference is a statistically significant difference. Is the potential savings in commuting time meaningful enough that it is worthwhile to do the study again, collecting triple the amount of data? For me the answer is no. I'm willing to live with uncertainty about whether it makes a difference where I get on the highway and just pick my entrance ramp based on my whim of the day. I can also accept the fact that interpretations are subjective, and someone else may conclude that it is worthwhile do redo the study with a larger sample size.

Here's my interpretation:

"I conducted a study in which I compared three different routes for the initial stage of my commute to work to determine whether one route was faster than another. I measured the time it took to travel from my home to a specific point on the interstate highway that I take to work. I found that the route that used the Chagrin Boulevard entrance ramp took a little over 12 minutes, the route using the Cedar Road on-ramp took about 12.5 minutes, and the Mayfield Road entrance took about 13.5 minutes. I subjected my data to a one-way analysis of variance and found that there was no statistically significant difference in travel time among the three routes ($F (2, 27) = 2.64, p > .05$). From these results it appears that I can choose whichever route I wish to get to work, that one route is not better or worse than another in terms of the time it takes to traverse a set distance.

There are a number of limitations to this study. First, the data were collected only during my morning commute, and thus I cannot generalize the results to different times of day. It is possible that traffic patterns are different during the afternoon rush hour and that, if I did the study at that time, I would find different results.

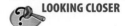

LOOKING CLOSER

*And I'd need a total of 140 cases to have a 95% chance of rejecting the null hypothesis.

[†]You can find out how to use SPSS to compute an analysis of variance, and how an SPSS option allows you to calculate power, on the accompanying Evolve website (www.elsevier/evolve). For the travel time data, SPSS calculates power $= .48$.

"Of greater concern to me, however, is that my study was underpowered, making it unlikely that I would find a statistically significant difference among the routes. My rough calculation of power showed that, with the number of cases I had (10 per group) I had less than a 40% chance of being able to reject the null hypothesis and find a statistically significant difference among the means. To have an 80% chance of finding a statistically significant difference among the groups, I would need close to 30 cases per group.

"Thus, before I conclude that which route I choose to drive to work does not matter in terms of how long my travel time is, I would need to replicate this study with a much larger sample size. Finally, even if I redid the study with a larger sample size and found a statistically significant difference between two of the routes, that does not mean that the savings in time would be meaningful. Given that my entire commute is close to 2 hours long, I don't think saving a minute or two has much impact. Thus I can choose where I get on the interstate each day based on a whim without worrying that it is increasing the time it takes me to get to work."

Note that I reported the means in my interpretation even though the differences were not statistically significant. I did this so that the reader could get some idea of the size of the observed differences, and because my study was underpowered. Note also that I change the metric in which I reported the means from seconds to the more easily understood minutes.

Before I finish with one-way ANOVA, let's apply what we've learned about power and sample size to the coin data and see if there is anything that I would like to change in the interpretation as a result. For the coin data, we had calculated $\hat{r}$ as a whopping .95. Consulting the power and sample size tables in the Appendix, I find that power is greater than .99 and that with that level of relationship we need only a total of six cases to have an 80% chance of rejecting the null hypothesis. Since we had a total of 13 cases I'm not worried about being underpowered. In my interpretation, I had mentioned that I would prefer that the study be done with random samples of coins from the population of coins in circulation, and with larger ns. Now, after doing my quick and dirty sample size calculation, I know that our ns were adequate. Nonetheless, sample sizes of three or four do not provide very robust estimates of population parameters. So, even though an N of six is all that is necessary for power, I still would feel more comfortable with larger sample sizes. Bottom line: my power analysis of the coin data has had no impact on my interpretation.

I am done with the one-way ANOVA! As a conclusion to this chapter, Table 10.15 outlines the interpretation options that are available.

Group Practice 10.5

Write a complete interpretative statement for the stroke data from question 7 of Group Practice 10.1. Be sure to address power and sample size as well as to use material calculated for previous group practice exercises.

TABLE **10.15**   **Interpreting One-Way ANOVA**

I. State, briefly, the objective of the study and report the results (means, standard deviations, APA format results)

II. If fail to reject H_0:
  A. Report that sample means did not statistically differ from each other (difference was not statistically significant)
  B. Report that evidence is insufficient to conclude that there is a mean difference between any two of the populations
  C. Calculate confidence intervals, power, and sample size. (Some statisticians recommend calculating and reporting effect sizes (e.g., ω^2) even when H_0 is not rejected.)
  D. Discuss possibility of Type II error
  E. Discuss strengths/limitations and suggestions

III. If reject H_0
  A. Report that difference between at least two sample means is statistically greater than zero (i.e., at least two means have a statistically significant difference)
    1. Conduct post-hoc tests to determine which means differ
    2. Calculate confidence intervals to learn size of difference(s)
    3. Report the direction of the difference(s)
  B. Calculate the overall effect size
    1. ω^2
    2. $\hat{r}$
  C. Calculate power and sample size
  D. Discuss the possibility of Type I error
  E. Discuss the strengths and limitations and make suggestions

SUMMARY

Multiple-sample difference tests are used when central tendency is being compared among three or more groups. The multiple-sample test chosen depends on (1) the number of independent or grouping variables, (2) whether the samples are independent or dependent, and (3) the level of measurement of the dependent variable. One-way ANOVA is used to compare means for three or more independent samples that differ on one grouping (independent) variable.

One-way ANOVA is called an omnibus test since it tells if, overall, there is a statistically significant difference between one or more of the pairs of means being compared. Its advantage over doing several two-sample tests is that the omnibus test tells if there is a difference while maintaining the overall alpha level where originally set. If one analyzes the data by using several two-sample tests, the overall probability of a Type I error increases, causing a run-away alpha

problem. The downside of using analysis of variance is that if the results are statistically significant you need follow-up tests, called post-hoc tests, to determine which pair(s) of means differ.

The assumptions, hypotheses, and decision rule for the one-way ANOVA are extensions of those we encountered for the independent-samples t test. What we end up calculating for ANOVA is called an F ratio, and it is the ratio of variability between groups divided by variability within groups. This partitioning of variability in individual scores to the sources from which it derives is why ANOVA is called analysis of variance.

Though all cases in a group receive the same level of the independent variable, the same treatment, each case will respond differently on account of individual differences and random error. As a result, there is variability within groups. Between-group variability has the same sources of variability plus a new one: differences between groups due to the effect, if any, of the treatment. Thus, the more variability there is due to treatment, the more the independent or grouping variable leads to groups ending up with different means. The larger the F ratio, the more likely it is to fall in the rare zone of the sampling distribution of F ratios, and the more likely we are to conclude that there is a statistically significant effect of the treatment on the outcome variable.

Once the F ratio has been computed, the interpretation of the one-way ANOVA results begins. ω^2, the percentage of variability in the dependent variable accounted for or predicted by the independent or grouping variable, can be calculated and turned into a correlation that estimates the degree of relationship between the two variables. A post-hoc test like the Fisher *LSD*, also known as the protected t, can be used to find out which pairs of means caused the overall F to fall in the rare zone and to calculate 95% confidence intervals for differences between pairs of means. Of course, the possibility that the results are in error, either Type I or Type II, has to be addressed.

Calculating power and sample size for ANOVA is more complex than is reasonable for an introductory statistics textbook, so I teach a short-cut that makes use of $\hat{f}$. My shortcut is conservative in that it usually underestimates power and overestimates how many subjects one needs.

Review Exercises

1. A psychologist measured the effectiveness of treatment for spider phobia by measuring how close, in inches, patients could come to touching a large and scary-looking spider. Patients with severe spider phobias were randomly divided into four different groups: (1) a no-treatment control group, (2) an education treatment that involved learning more about spiders through reading and videos, (3) a modeling treatment in which the therapist modeled spider handling, and (4) an anxiety-reduction treatment in which relaxation techniques were learned. After treatment was concluded a live, large, and scary-looking spider was placed 36″ away from the patient and how close the patient came to the spider was measured. Smaller distances indicate less fear. Here are the data:

Control: 36, 28, and 30 ($M = 31.3333, \hat{s} = 4.1633$)
Education: 31, 28, and 24 ($M = 27.6667, \hat{s} = 3.5119$)
Modeling: 27, 29, and 33 ($M = 29.6667, \hat{s} = 3.0551$)
Relaxation: 21, 27, and 22 ($M = 23.3333, \hat{s} = 3.2146$)

Assuming that approach distance is normally distributed for each group, complete and interpret the analysis of variance using the six-step null hypothesis significance testing procedure.

2. An education researcher wished to evaluate three different ways of improving writing in sixth-graders. He selected one classroom in one elementary school in his district as a test classroom and, not using random assignment, divided students into three groups. The control group received the classroom instruction regularly used in the researcher's school district. One experimental group, the reading group, learned writing indirectly by *reading* more advanced material. The second experimental group, the writing group, was directly taught advanced writing skills. At the end of the year, each student took a writing test that is scored on an interval level so that scores reflect grade level. A score of 6.0, for example, represents the beginning of sixth grade, and 6.5 represents a score halfway through sixth grade. Here are the data collected:

Control group: 6.5, 6.3, 6.6, and 6.5
                    ($M = 6.4750, \hat{s} = .1258$)
Advanced reading: 7.1, 6.8, 7.0, 6.9, and 7.2
                    ($M = 7.0000, \hat{s} = .1581$)
Advanced writing: 6.6, 6.8, 6.5, and 6.7
                    ($M = 6.6500, \hat{s} = .1291$)

Assuming that the variables are normally distributed, analyze and interpret the data using the six-step procedure for null hypothesis significance tests.

3. Dutch elm disease has been in the United States since the 1930s and has been estimated to have

destroyed about half of the elm trees in the United States since then. Imagine that a town completed a tree survey and found that 11% of the trees within city limits were elm trees. Further, imagine that they found a U.S. Forest Service estimate that in their region in the early 1900s, 18% of the trees were elm trees. What statistical test should they do to see if the number of elm trees in their city is statistically different from 18%?

4. A fruit farmer decided to find out if size of apples is related to the size of the tree that is bearing the fruit. He measured the diameters of all of the trees in his orchard and classified the trees into three types: small, medium, and large. He obtained a random sample of trees in each of the three categories, obtained a random sample of apples from each of these trees, and weighed each of the apples. What statistical test should he do to see if apple size, as measured by weight, varies as a function of tree size, as measured by diameter?

5. The best way to cook a hamburger is a very personal decision. Nonetheless, a food science researcher decided to put it to the test. She recruited 10 cooks who believed that using a charcoal grill was the best way to cook a hamburger, 10 who believed that a gas grill was the best way, and 10 who swore by the George Foreman grill. Each person cooked one hamburger by each method, resulting in 30 hamburgers cooked on charcoal, 30 cooked on a gas grill, and 30 cooked on George Foreman grills. (The order in which each cook used each of the three appliances was randomly determined for each cook.) After the hamburgers were cooked, a blind taste-test panel rated each one as (1) poor, (2) good, (3) very good, (4) excellent, or (5) superlative. What statistical test should be used to analyze the data?

6. A researcher with the Florida Department of Relocation was curious to ascertain what the impact of weather was on the perception of Florida. She contacted, at three different times, a group of retirees who were living in Minnesota. Each time she contacted them she asked whether they viewed Florida as a desirable place to live (+1) or an undesirable place to live (−1). The first time she contacted the participants was right after a blizzard had occurred in Minnesota. The second time was right after a major hurricane had struck Florida. The third time was when there had not been a blizzard or a hurricane for the previous 3 months. What statistical test should she use to see if these meteorological factors have an influence on the perception of Florida?

7. Many colleges believe that internships are a good way for their students to explore potential careers and make better-informed decisions about their futures. A faculty member at such a university decided to collect some data that addressed this issue. He obtained a sample of students who had had internships and a sample of students who had not had internships. Just before they graduated, he asked them what career they planned to pursue and, on an interval-level scale, how sure they were that this career was a good fit for them. What statistical test should he use to see if having an internship has any impact on certainty about career choice?

Homework Problems

1. Buffy chooses to perform a post-hoc test and is trying to decide between an *LSD* test and an *HSD* test. If she wants to minimize her chances of making a Type II error, which should she pick?
   a. *HSD*
   b. *LSD*
   c. It doesn't matter since both are equivalent in terms of Type I error.
   d. It doesn't matter since both are equivalent in terms of Type II error.

2. Which of the following is in descending order of size?
   a. SS_{total}, SS_{within}, MS_{within}
   b. SS_{within}, SS_{total}, MS_{within}
   c. MS_{within}, SS_{within}, SS_{total}

3. If treatment has an effect, then there is
   a. More variability between groups than there is in total.
   b. More variability within groups than there is in total.

c. More variability between groups than within groups.

d. More variability within groups than between groups.

4. Between-group variability is built of
   a. Treatment effect.
   b. Individual differences.
   c. Random error.
   d. All of the above.
   e. None of the above.

5. If one uses the rough guide to power/sample size outlined in this chapter and finds that for $k = 3$, $N = 39$, that means that one needs
   a. Exactly 13 subjects per group.
   b. Exactly 39 subjects per group.
   c. Approximately 13 subjects per group.
   d. Approximately 39 subjects per group.

For questions 6 through 11, (a) write out the research question and (b) select the appropriate statistical test.

6. According to a national study, the mean level of satisfaction with one's health insurance is 47.38 on an interval-level scale where scores can range from 0 to 80 and the standard deviation is 12.00. The administrator of a small health care insurance company wishes to advertise that use of his company's health care insurance is associated with increased satisfaction. He conducts a survey of a random sample of 1000 of his customers and finds that their mean level of satisfaction is 63.28.

7. A nutritionist is curious whether body mass index (BMI) remains constant over time. She measures BMI in the same people at birth, age 10, age 20, and age 30.

8. A teacher asks students to rate, on an interval-level scale, how well they think they know the material on which they are about to be tested. After testing, she compares these scores with the percentage of items correct on the multiple choice test.

9. A sport researcher compares the win/loss percentages for left-handed and right-handed professional baseball pitchers.

10. Knowledge of current events, scored as the percentage of items right on a multiple choice test, is compared for adults who (a) read newspapers, (b) watch the news on commercial TV, or (c) listen to the news on National Public Radio.

11. An ordinal-level measure of sociability is used to compare the degree of sociability of children in the same family. Families with three children are selected so that the sociability of the firstborn can be compared to the second- and third-born. Families with twins or triplets are excluded.

12. I've developed a test of understanding of principles of physics that has $\mu = 12$ and $\sigma = 3$, and is normally distributed in the general population. (a) I've given this test to recent college graduates who majored in physics, and their average score was 17.5. They understand physics better, on average, than what percentage of the general population? (b) I've given the same test to college physics professors, and their average score was 23.45. They understand physics better than what percentage of the general population? (c) In the general population, what is the interquartile range?

13. An orthopedic surgeon wanted to know if a patient's weight affected his or her recovery after surgical repair of the anterior cruciate ligament in the knee. The surgeon divided her patients into three categories: (a) underweight or normal weight, (b) overweight, and (c) obese, and then measured how many days it took after surgery until the patient was sufficiently pain-free to begin the physical therapy program. Here are the data she collected:

a: 3, 5, 6, 7, and 3 ($M = 4.8000$, $\hat{s} = 1.7889$)
b: 6, 11, 6, 7, and 8 ($M = 7.6000$, $\hat{s} = 2.0736$)
c: 11, 14, 18, 15, and 12 ($M = 14.0000$, $\hat{s} = 2.7386$)

Trusting me that skewness and kurtosis for each group fall within normal limits, analyze and interpret these data using the six-step null hypothesis significance testing procedure.

11

Multiple Sample Difference Tests II

Factorial and Repeated-Measures
Analysis of Variance

Learning Objectives

After completing this chapter, you should be able to do the following:

1. Understand, when there are multiple grouping variables, how factorial ANOVA partitions variability into that due to each grouping variable separately and that due to the interaction between the grouping variables.
2. Graph the effects for a two-way factorial ANOVA, speculate whether an interaction exists, and realize that when an interaction exists it is less reasonable to interpret the main effects for a factorial ANOVA.
3. Recognize repeated-measures ANOVA, ANOVA for dependent samples, as a form of factorial ANOVA in which the subjects factor partitions out variability due to individual differences.
4. Evaluate the assumptions, explain the hypotheses, and formulate a decision rule for repeated measures ANOVA.
5. Given the sums of squares, complete an ANOVA summary table for repeated-measures ANOVA.

(Continued)

6 Complete a full interpretation of repeated-measures ANOVA results, making use of ω^2, post-hoc tests, and confidence intervals.

7 Explain why a dependent-samples difference test has more power than an independent-samples difference test, and explain the advantage of repeated-measures ANOVA over dependent-samples *t* test when comparing the means of two dependent samples.

8 Evaluate the assumptions, explain the hypotheses, and formulate a decision rule for a dependent-samples *t* test/repeated-measures ANOVA.

9 Given the sums of squares, complete an ANOVA summary table for a dependent-samples *t* test/repeated-measures ANOVA.

10 Write an interpretative statement for the results of a dependent-samples *t* test/repeated-measures ANOVA, making use of confidence intervals, ω^2, $\hat{r}$, *d*, power, and sample size.

Chapter Roadmap

In this chapter we will apply the ANOVA concept of partitioning the variability in scores to more complex experimental situations where a researcher investigates the effects of more than one grouping variable at a time. Thus, we'll see how factorial ANOVA tests (a) whether the effect of each factor (or grouping variable) is statistically significant separately *and* (b) whether the effect of factors combined, the interaction of the grouping variables, is statistically significant. If the interaction is statistically significant—which means that the effect one independent or grouping variable has depends on the level of the other—we'll be less concerned about interpreting the effect of any independent or grouping variable by itself.

Knowing how factorial ANOVA works, by partitioning out variability, we will apply the concept to repeated-measures ANOVA where we partition out the variability due to individual differences between subjects. In that way, we can have an uncontaminated measure of the effect of the independent or grouping variable that was measured at two or more points in time. Though I teach how to use repeated-measures ANOVA when comparing three or more groups, I will focus on using it in two-sample situations in place of the dependent-samples *t* test. (The dependent-samples *t* test, because it does not partition out the variability due to subjects, gives an inflated view of the size of the effect of the grouping variable.) Thus, we'll learn how to complete and interpret a dependent-samples *t* test/repeated-measures ANOVA, including how to calculate power and find an appropriate sample size.

I n Chapter 9 we learned how statisticians compare two groups to determine if there is a statistically significant difference between them. In Chapter 10, we moved to a more complex topic, how comparisons are made between three or more groups. Now we are going to move to an even more complex topic, how researchers find out if groups differ when there is more than one independent or grouping variable. I'm going to use our understanding of this technique, factorial ANOVA, as a springboard to exploring repeated-measures ANOVA, an analysis of variance used with dependent samples.

THE FACTORIAL ANOVA

Often the questions raised by researchers are more complex than the examples we've been dealing with. Until now, we've analyzed situations in which there is one independent or grouping variable. For example, we might ask what the effect of math anxiety is on learning statistics and compare the performance on a standardized statistics exam of two groups of students, one high on math anxiety and the other low on math anxiety. You should recognize this as an independent-samples *t* test question with two levels of the grouping variable, high and low math anxiety. Another question that a researcher might ask could involve different ways of teaching. For example, do students learn more in a statistics class if they take it online, take it in a traditional classroom setting, or just read the textbook on their own? You should recognize this as a one-way ANOVA question in which there is one grouping variable, type of instruction, with three levels (online, classroom, and textbook).

An inquisitive researcher might begin to wonder about combining the two studies into one, about combining the two factors (type of student and type of instruction) into one **factorial design.** Such a design would have six cells (see Table 11.1) and goes by a variety of names. As I've already mentioned, it is called a factorial ANOVA because it has more than one factor, or grouping variable and is comparing means. It is also called a two-way ANOVA because it has two "ways," or independent variables. (There can also be three-way ANOVAs, four-way ANOVAs, etc.) It is also called a 3 × 2 or 2 × 3 ANOVA to indicate that there are three levels of one factor and two levels of the other.

Using a factorial ANOVA instead of calculating two separate one-way ANOVAs, one for the type of student factor and one for the type of

factorial design

An experimental design in which there are two or more independent or grouping variables that are crossed with each other.

TABLE **11.1** **Factorial Design for Influence of Two Factors, Type of Student and Type of Instruction, on Learning**

	Online Course	Classroom Course	Textbook Only
High math anxiety	80	60	80
Low math anxiety	83	85	83

main effect

A term for the impact of a single independent or grouping variable on the dependent variable in a factorial experimental design.

row effect

A term for the impact of the independent or grouping variable that is in the rows of the matrix that displays the experimental design.

column effect

A term for the impact of the independent or grouping variable that is in the columns of the matrix that displays the experimental design.

interaction

A term for the combined impact of two or more independent or grouping variables on the dependent variable in a factorial experimental design.

learning factor, has certain advantages. The major advantage of such a design is that it allows us to look at the effect of *three* different factors at once. That's right, I said three, not two. Two of the factors are obvious and are called **main effects** because they represent the effects of the main variables under investigation, the independent or grouping variables. Thus, one main effect is the **row effect** of level of math anxiety and the other is the **column effect** of type of instruction. The third factor that is being investigated is the **interaction** between the two main effects. An interaction is what occurs if the impact of one independent variable on the dependent variable depends on the level of the other independent variable. For example, if people with low math anxiety did equally well in all types of instruction but people with high math anxiety only did well with online and textbook instruction, that would be an interaction because type of student and type of instruction *interact* to determine how well one does. This interaction is shown graphically in Figure 11.1.

When an interaction exists, our interest in the main effects diminishes, because the conclusion is no longer simply that the main effects by themselves make a difference. Does type of instruction affect how much statistics one learns? It depends. It depends on whether one is a high–math anxiety or a low–math anxiety student. Is level of math anxiety related to how much statistics a person learns? It depends on the type of instruction you are talking about.

Though the number of "ways" an ANOVA can take is unlimited (e.g., 3 × 2 × 4 × 3), you'll be pleased to know that I am going to limit our exploration of factorial ANOVA to two-way ANOVA. That is, we won't

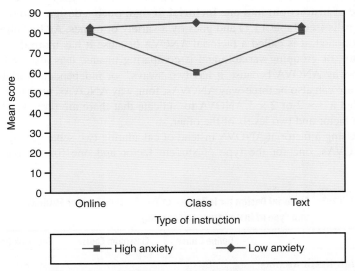

Figure **11.1** Effect of type of student and type of instruction on amount of statistics learned.

have more than two independent or grouping variables to work with and interpret.

With a one-way ANOVA, we partitioned the variability in the dependent variable into variability due to between-group effects and variability due to within-group effects. With factorial ANOVA we will do the same, but we are going to further partition the between-group variability into (a) variability due to the row effect, (b) variability due to the column effect, and (c) variability due to the interaction effect. Then, we'll compute an F ratio for each one to find out if each explains a statistically significant amount of the variability in the dependent variable.

You'll also be pleased to know that we won't be doing many computations for the factorial ANOVA. With factorial ANOVA, I'm more concerned that you understand the concept than I am with having you learn to do the calculations. My objective in introducing factorial ANOVA is to make you familiar with the idea of partitioning variance so that the move to repeated-measures ANOVA later in this chapter will be smooth.

Let's start with a simple example without an interaction. Imagine getting samples of 14 teenage boys and 14 teenage girls, dividing each group in half, and then measuring their hand strength on some machine where higher numbers equal more hand strength. For half of the boys we test hand strength on the dominant hand, and for half we test hand strength on the nondominant hand; ditto for the girls. The mean results for the seven people in each cell are shown in Table 11.2.

First, we calculate the **marginal means,** the means for each row and column. Because the n for each cell is the same, we can simply add the relevant cell means together and divide by the number of cells in order to find the marginal means. Table 11.3 shows the marginal means and the grand mean.

Inspection of the marginal means shows that, in general, dominant hands are stronger than nondominant hands (row marginals of 40 vs. 20) and that, in general, boys are stronger than girls (column marginals of 40 vs. 20). These are called main effects for hand dominance and gender.*

TABLE 11.2 Mean Hand Strength for Dominant and Nondominant Hands for Boys and Girls

	Boys	Girls
Dominant hand	50	30
Nondominant hand	30	10

marginal means

The means for the row and column effects in a factorial design.

TABLE 11.3 Cell Means and Marginal Means for Hand Strength by Gender and Hand Dominance

	Boys	Girls	
Dominant hand	50	30	40
Nondominant hand	30	10	20
	40	20	30

*Of course, we can't be sure if these main effects are statistically significant until we complete the ANOVA.

LOOKING CLOSER

Let me use these marginals, and the grand mean of 30 in the lower right-hand corner, to show why there is no interaction in this example. The question raised by the interaction is whether the value in a cell depends on more than the simple additive effects of the levels of the independent variables that intersect at that cell. Let's look at the cell in the upper left hand corner, the cell for the seven boys who had the strength of their dominant hand tested. Comparing the row marginal mean for dominant hands, 40, to the grand mean of 30, we see that having the dominant hand tested appears to add 10 points to one's score. Similarly, the marginal mean for boys is 10 points higher than the grand mean. (Being a boy adds, on average, 10 points to a score.) If we add 10 points for having the dominant hand tested and 10 points for being a boy to the grand mean of 30, we end up with 50, which is the cell mean. In fact, every cell mean can be calculated exactly—predicted—if one knows the grand mean and the marginal means. If you can predict the cell means exactly from knowing the marginal means and the grand mean, there is no interaction. Phrased alternatively, there is some interaction if the cell means can't be predicted from the marginal means and the grand mean.

This method is not the most common way to decide if there is an interaction. The usual way to determine if there is an interaction is to graph the results and see whether the two lines are parallel. If the lines are parallel, then there probably isn't an interaction; if the lines aren't parallel, then there may be a statistically significant interaction. (Officially, we can't decide if there is a statistically significant interaction until we have completed the factorial ANOVA and examined the F ratio for the interaction effect.) Figure 11.1, showing the type-of-student-by-type-of-instruction data, is a nice example of the nonparallel lines of an interaction. Figure 11.2, which shows the data for hand strength as a function of gender and which hand is tested, has parallel lines, indicating no interaction.

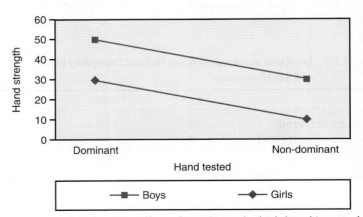

Figure **11.2** Graph showing effect of gender and which hand is tested on hand strength.

TABLE **11.4** **ANOVA Summary Table for Influence of Gender and Hand Dominance on Hand Strength**

Source	SS	df	MS	F
Between	5600.00	3	1866.67	
Rows	2800.00	1	2800.00	600.00*
Columns	2800.00	1	2800.00	600.00*
Interaction	.00	1	.00	.00
Within	112.00	24	4.67	
Total	5712.00	27		

Note: * $= p < .05$

This graph shows three things clearly: (1) boys have more hand strength than girls, (2) dominant hands are stronger than nondominant hands, and (3) there is no interaction between gender and hand dominance in terms of hand strength.

As promised, we're not going to worry about doing the calculations for a factorial ANOVA. Nonetheless, I completed the two-way ANOVA on the gender and hand dominance data, and the results are shown in Table 11.4.

The ANOVA summary table should seem familiar to the ones from the last chapter. The column headings are the same, but extra rows have been added. The extra rows partition the sum of squares for the between-groups factor into the effects for rows (which hand is tested), columns (gender), and interaction.* Note that $SS_{rows} + SS_{columns} + SS_{interaction} = SS_{between}$. This means that $SS_{between}$ tells the overall effect of both treatments combined. We are not interested in this combined effect, or overall effect, which is why we partition it into its subcomponents. Similarly $df_{between}$ is parceled out to the three subfactors. As with a one-way ANOVA, MS_{within} is the error term, or the denominator, for the F ratio.

Two of the F ratios, F_{rows} and $F_{columns}$, in Table 11.4 are statistically significant, indicating that there is a main effect for the rows and the columns. $F_{interaction}$ is not statistically significant, indicating that there is no interaction. There are post-hoc tests for the factorial ANOVA, but I'm not going to go into them here.[†] Similarly, it is possible to calculate the percentage of variance in the dependent variable predicted by each main effect and by the interaction.

---

*Sometimes the interaction term is written as R × C or RC to indicate that it is the interaction of the row effect by the column effect.

[†]Indeed, there is not much need for post-hoc tests when one has only two levels of each independent variable and there is no statistically significant interaction. The only explanation for the main effects are that boys are stronger than girls and dominant hands are stronger than nondominant hands.

LOOKING CLOSER

TABLE **11.5**   **Mean Scores on Physical and Verbal Aggression for Boys and Girls**

	Boys	Girls	
Physical	52	20	*36*
Verbal	23	51	*37*
	37.5	*35.5*	**36.5**

So what is the story that these data tell—that is, what would my interpretation be? It would be something along the lines that regarding the hand strength of teenage boys and girls, boys are stronger, in general, than girls. In addition, to compare the strength of the dominant to the nondominant hand: the dominant hand is stronger, in general, than the nondominant.

Let's see another example, this one with an interaction. Again we use boys and girls, and this time we measure level of aggression. For half the 18 boys in the sample we measure physical aggression and for the other half we measure verbal aggression; ditto for the 18 girls. The two aggression measures we use, one for verbal and one for physical, are scored on the same metric so that we can compare scores. On both measures, higher scores indicate greater levels of aggression. The results are shown in Table 11.5.

Though the cell means differ dramatically, the marginal means don't differ very much. In fact, overall it doesn't look like there is much difference in aggression between boys ($M = 37.5$) and girls ($M = 35.5$) or between the two types of aggression. In statistics-speak, we would say that there does not appear to be a main effect for gender or for aggression.

Trying to predict cell means from the marginal means is our first hint that there is an interaction. The row mean for physical aggression (36) is .5 below the grand mean of 36.5, and the column mean for boys (37.5) is 1.0 above the grand mean. Thus, if there were no interaction, we'd predict that the cell mean for physical aggression and boys is 36.5 minus .5 plus 1.0, or 37.0. We'd be wrong, since the actual cell mean is 15 points higher, 52, than our no-interaction prediction of 37. The graph for the aggression data is shown in Figure 11.3 and this, since the lines are not parallel, suggests there is an interaction.

The graph shows an interaction between gender and type of aggression: boys are more aggressive physically, and girls are more aggressive verbally. If asked whether boys are more aggressive than girls, the only reasonable answer is, "It depends on the type of aggression you are talking about." Similarly, if asked whether kids are more aggressive physically or verbally, one needs to say, "It depends on the gender of the child." When an interaction plays a role, as it does here, our interest in the main effects diminishes.

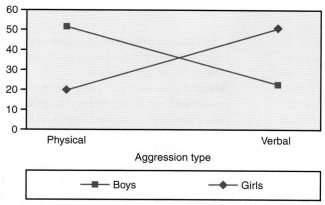

Figure **11.3** Graph showing influence of gender and type of aggression on level of aggression.

The ANOVA summary table is shown in Table 11.6. Note that the *F* ratio for the interaction is quite large and will certainly fall in the rare zone of the sampling distribution. Though the main effect of gender (the column variable) is also statistically significant, it does not make much sense to conclude that gender by itself predicts degree of aggression. We must know whether physical or verbal aggression is being referred to in order to comment on how gender relates to aggression.

Thus my interpretation of the results would run along the lines of: "When measuring aggression in children it is important to note what type of aggression one is concerned with, physical aggression or verbal aggression. If one combines the two it will appear that boys and girls are equally aggressive, but that is not true. Boys are more aggressive than girls physically, but girls are more aggressive than boys verbally."

TABLE **11.6** **ANOVA Summary Table for Influence of Type of Aggression (Row Effect) and Gender (Column Effect) on Aggression Level**

Source	SS	df	MS	F
Between	8145.00	3	2715.00	
Rows	9.00	1	9.00	1.62
Columns	36.00	1	36.00	6.47*
Interaction	8100.00	1	8100.00	1456.18*
Within	178.00	32	5.56	
Total	8323.00	35		

NOTE: * = $p < .05$

Group Practice 11.1

1. I have six 5-year-old boys, six 5-year-old girls, six 15-year-old boys, and six 15-year-old girls. For each one I measure muscle mass using a scale where higher numbers represent more muscles. The four means, respectively, are 20, 20, 50, and 35. Put the data into a 2 × 2 matrix, calculate marginal and grand means, graph the data, and *speculate* about main effects and/or interactions in an interpretative statement.

2. For each scenario that follows, write out the research question and choose the appropriate statistical test to analyze the data.

   a. A university president wants to investigate whether cheating is viewed differently by different majors. She obtains random samples of pre-med majors, English majors, business majors, and engineering majors, and has each complete an interval-level measure, the Cheating Acceptability Scale (CAS).

   b. Intrigued by the results, the university president now plans a different study. She will obtain a random sample of accepted students and administer to them the CAS at first-year orientation, at the end of the first semester, and at the end of the second semester.

   c. Hearing rumors about fraternity and sorority members condoning cheating, the college president obtains yet another sample of students, divides them into Greek/non-Greek, and compares their CAS scores.

   d. Confused by the results she obtained in Study A and Study C, the university president consults with an education professor. He recommends doing the study one more time, this time classifying each student both in terms of major and in terms of Greek status.

   e. The university president does one last study. She obtains yet another sample, administers the CAS, and classifies each student as scoring in the top third or the bottom third of scores on the CAS. She calls the top third "Pro cheating students" and the bottom third "Anti cheating students." She's curious if the two groups differ in terms of gender.

THE REPEATED-MEASURES ANOVA

I introduced factorial ANOVA in order to introduce the idea of partitioning variability into two factors, a row effect and a column effect. For the rest of this chapter, I will leave factorial ANOVA behind and move on to repeated-measures ANOVA, or analysis of variance with dependent samples.

Back in Chapter 9, when we first encountered difference tests, I explained the difference between independent and dependent samples. With independent-samples difference tests the samples that are being compared are independent of each other: how the cases are gathered for one sample has no impact on how the cases are gathered for the other sample(s). For dependent-samples difference tests, also called matched-samples tests or paired-samples tests, the cases in one sample are tied to the cases in the other sample(s). An example should make this clear.

Imagine that I have developed a new treatment for depression and I want to evaluate it. I obtain four people with severe depression who desire treatment for their depression, and before I give them my new treatment I measure their levels of depression. The interval-level depression scale

TABLE **11.7** **Depression Scores at Three Points in Time**

	Pretreatment	Post-treatment	Follow-up
Case 1	24	16	18
Case 2	21	11	17
Case 3	17	10	15
Case 4	28	13	23
M	22.50	12.50	18.25
$\hat{s}$	4.65	2.65	3.40

used measures six symptoms of depression on a scale where $0 =$ not at all, $1 =$ slightly, $2 =$ moderately, $3 =$ considerably, and $4 =$ extremely. Scores can range from zero to 24; higher scores indicate a greater level of depression. I call this first measurement the Time 1 (T1) measurement, or the pre-test measurement. I then give the participants my new treatment, and after it is over, at Time 2 (T2)—the post-test measurement—I measure their levels of depression again. Each participant now has a pair of scores, T1 and T2. Because I want to make sure that the effects of my treatment are long-lasting, I wait 6 months after treatment and then administer a follow-up assessment at Time 3. For each participant I now have scores at three points in time (T1, T2, and T3; or pretreatment, post-treatment, and follow-up), and my study is over. You can see the data collected in Table 11.7. I hope that it is clear that this longitudinal study involves dependent samples, or repeated measures, since the same cases are followed over time.

Please pay careful attention to how the data are arrayed in Table 11.7. Note that each case takes a row, and each assessment point takes a column. If you want to think of individual differences as the row effect, and the effect of treatment (or time) as the column effect, that's fine by me. In fact, I want you to think of them this way because that should remind you of partitioning the variability into two factors, as we just saw for factorial ANOVA. A person's score at each point of the treatment depends on both (1) the row effect, or his or her individual factors (genetics, recent events, life history, how he or she interprets the test questions), and (2) the column effect, or the effect of treatment over time. Note, for example, that case number three obtains a score lower than the other cases at each point in time.

We know that individual differences exist, that cases start off different and these differences may persist over time, so we are not very much interested in the row factor. What we *are* interested in with repeated measures is the effect that treatment has over and above these individual differences. In other words, how much of the total variability in scores is left to be explained by the treatment effect, the column effect, once we partition out the variability due to the row factor of individual differences?

Repeated-measures ANOVA, then, is a form of factorial ANOVA where we are not interested in either the row effect or the interaction, but only in the main effect of columns. With this understanding of repeated-measures ANOVA, let's move on to hypothesis testing with Tom and Harry.

Test

Looking at the column means in Table 11.7, the data appear to tell a story: "The new treatment decreases depression scores but over the 6 months after treatment, depression level starts to climb back up." However, simply eyeing the scores can't tell us if the differences are statistically significant differences, if they represent real differences between the populations of people pretreatment, post-treatment, and 6 months later. We find out if we should consider these differences real differences by doing a statistical test. If we want to compare the means of three dependent samples, then (via Table 10.1) the test to choose is the repeated-measures ANOVA.

Assumptions

These are assumptions for the repeated-measures ANOVA:
- Dependent samples (repeated-measures ANOVA is not robust to violations of this assumption)
- Interval- or ratio-level data (repeated-measures ANOVA is not robust to violations of this assumption)
- Random samples (repeated-measures ANOVA is robust to violations of this assumption, but mention of the violation must be made in the interpretation)
- Normality (repeated-measures ANOVA is robust to violations of this assumption if n is large)
- Sphericity (if this assumption is violated, the F ratio for the repeated-measures ANOVA can be corrected)

The first four assumptions should be familiar to you by now, but the fifth is new. The sphericity assumption is an extension of the homogeneity of variance assumption with which we are already familiar. Briefly, the sphericity assumption holds that the variances of the difference scores for all possible pair combinations are equal. For the current data set, for example, here is what we would do: (1) find the difference scores for T1 vs. T2, for T1 vs. T3, and for T2 vs. T3; (2) for each set of difference scores compute the variance; and then (3) compare these three variances to determine whether they are close enough to each other that we think it reasonable that they came from the same population. This, clearly, is a lot of work, and I'm not going to ask that you do it. It is rare that a person calculates a repeated-measures ANOVA by hand, and the computer programs that do the calculations also spit out sphericity information. In addition, the computer programs report information that allows you to make corrections to the overall F ratio if sphericity is violated. So, all that I am going to do for this assumption, for the moment, is bring it back to its roots as a homogeneity of variance assumption, and compare the standard deviations of the groups.

With that background, let's examine the assumptions for the depression-treatment data. I know that neither of the first two assumptions was violated: they can't have been violated or I wouldn't have chosen the repeated-measures ANOVA to compare the means of dependent samples. The third assumption, that the sample is a random one, was certainly violated since I did not obtain a random sample from the population of people in the world with severe depression. This will limit the degree to which I can generalize my results, but it won't stop me from doing the ANOVA. The fourth assumption is the normality assumption, and it was not violated: when I calculated the 95% confidence intervals for skewness and kurtosis for depression scores at T1, T2, and T3, each confidence interval captured zero, suggesting that each variable is normally distributed in its population. Similarly, no standard deviation was twice another, so my simple approximation to sphericity suggests that we are OK with this assumption as well.*

Since the only assumption that appears to have been violated is the assumption of random samples, and the ANOVA is robust to that, I can proceed to the next step.

Hypotheses

ANOVA compares sample means to help us determine if we think it likely that the samples come from the same or different populations. The null hypothesis, which we want to reject, maintains that all the samples come from the same population. The alternative hypothesis, which can't be true if the null hypothesis is true, maintains that at least one sample comes from a different population. Thus the null hypothesis, written in symbolic notation, is H_0: $\mu_1 = \mu_2 = \mu_3$, for as many populations as one has. The alternative hypothesis is more complex in symbolic notation, so most researchers just state it as "not all μs are equal."

The null hypothesis for the depression data says, in English, that treatment has no effect on level of depression; that, in essence, the three samples all come from the same population. As a result, the mean depression scores at T1, T2, and T3 should be close enough to each other that sampling error can explain any discrepancy among them. The alternative

---

*I'm willing to play a little fast and loose with the sphericity assumption and treat it as homogeneity of variance, because I can almost guarantee that when you do a repeated-measures ANOVA in the future it will be via computer and that the computer program you use will allow you to test the sphericity assumption. In the SPSS application at the Evolve website (www.elsevier/evolve), I'll show how SPSS does this.

LOOKING CLOSER

hypothesis says that treatment has an effect at some point in time, that at least one observed difference between the means for T1, T2, and T3 is so large that it is unlikely that sampling error for samples drawn from the same population is a viable explanation for the difference.

Decision Rule

The decision rule involves finding the critical value of F so that we can determine if our observed value of F falls in the rare zone or the common zone of the sampling distribution of F. To find the critical value of F we need to know the degrees of freedom for the numerator and denominator terms that go into calculating the F ratio. The easiest way to know these is to calculate them for the ANOVA summary table, so let me introduce the ANOVA summary table for a repeated-measures ANOVA.

The summary table for a repeated-measures ANOVA is similar to the summary table for a one-way ANOVA in its columns, but is different in its rows. That is, the *sources* of variability will be different, but we'll still be interested in calculating sums of squares, degrees of freedom, mean squares, and the F ratio. One of the sources of variability will be labeled "Total" to indicate that it represents all the variability in the scores. It is this total variability that is partitioned into variability due to subjects (individual differences) and variability due to treatment. The final source of variability consists of all the variability that is not accounted for by either individual differences or treatment. Since it is equivalent to the variability that is left after the other sources of variability have been removed, it is called **residual variability.*** It is this residual variability that will be used as the denominator term, the error term, in the repeated-measures ANOVA.

Now that you know what to expect, here's an initial ANOVA summary table for repeated-measures ANOVA (Table 11.8).

For the depression data where $n = 4$ (there are four cases per cell), $k = 3$ (there are three cells), and $N = 12$ (there are a total of 12 observations made as each of the four cases is observed 3 times), $df_{subjects} = 3$, $df_{treatment} = 2$, $df_{residual} = 6$, and $df_{total} = 11$. Note that $3 + 2 + 6 = 11$, that $df_{total} = df_{subjects} + df_{treatment} + df_{residual}$. This makes sense since we partition the total variability into those three components.[†]

Table 11.8 shows that the F ratio that is calculated is for the effect of treatment, so the numerator degrees of freedom for our depression data is 2.

residual variability

Variability that remains in a set of scores after variability due to individual differences and treatment has been removed.

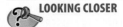

LOOKING CLOSER

---

*In a sense, this is an interaction term, the variability that is due to the unique interaction of subjects by treatments.

[†] Note that I abbreviate degrees of freedom residual as $df_{residual}$ not as df_{res}. I use these longer abbreviations to make the referents for the abbreviations crystal clear. Please be careful if you use shorter abbreviations since there are two different sources of variability, treatment and total, that can be abbreviated with the same letter and thus can be mistaken for each other.

TABLE **11.8** **Summary Table for Repeated-Measures ANOVA Showing How to Calculate Degrees of Freedom**

Source	SS	df	MS	F
Subjects	—	$n - 1$	—	
Treatment	—	$k - 1$	—	—
Residual	—	$(n - 1)(k - 1)$	—	
Total	—	$N - 1$		

Where:
  n = sample size per group
  k = number of groups
  N = total number of observation (i.e., $n \times k$)
  — = cell to be completed later

As I've mentioned, the error term—the denominator term—for the F ratio for repeated-measures is the residual term, so the denominator degrees of freedom for the depression data is 6. Thus the critical value will be for an F with 2 and 6 degrees of freedom. Using the same table of critical values of F that we used for the one-way ANOVA, Appendix Table 10, which only has values for $\alpha = .05$, we find that F_{cv} (2, 6) = 5.1433. I've put this critical value into a sampling distribution of F in Figure 11.4, which I have marked off into common and rare zones. Our decision rule is the same as for the one-way ANOVA: if $F_{observed} \geq F_{cv}$, we reject the null hypothesis; if $F_{observed} < F_{cv}$, we fail to reject the null hypothesis.

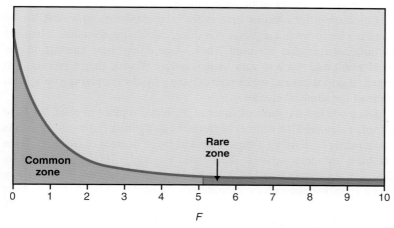

Figure **11.4** Sampling distribution of F with 2 and 6 degrees of freedom. (From Lowry, R. [2006]. *Concepts and applications of inferential statistics* [online]. Available: http://faculty.vassar.edu/lowry/webtext.html)

The decision rule also involves deciding how often one wants to make a Type I error. I want this to be a conscious decision where you weigh the costs of a Type I error, of erroneously rejecting the null hypothesis. At the same time, I present a streamlined table of critical values of F by presenting in it only critical values for $\alpha = .05$. As a beginning student of statistics, please use this default value of $\alpha = .05$, but justify it by saying that you are willing to run the risk of having a 5% chance of making a Type I error.

Luckily, with F, unlike with r or t, you don't need to worry about whether you are doing a one-tailed or a two-tailed test. The F ratio is a nondirectional test for differences among means.

Finally, the decision step also involves power, deciding if one has enough cases to have a reasonable chance of rejecting the null hypothesis if the null hypothesis should be rejected. Just as for the previous statistical tests, I will leave that in the background until we discuss power in the interpretation section.

Calculations

The calculations for the repeated-measures ANOVA involve calculating four sums of squares, $SS_{subjects}$, $SS_{treatment}$, $SS_{residual}$, and SS_{total}. SS_{total} represents the total variability in the scores, the variability that we'll partition into other factors. Stating this another way: $SS_{total} = SS_{subjects} + SS_{treatment} + SS_{residual}$.

$SS_{subjects}$ represents the variability in scores that is due to variability among individuals, $SS_{treatment}$ represents the variability due to differences among the treatment factors, and $SS_{residual}$ represents the variability in scores that has not been accounted for by either of these other two factors. Thus, $SS_{total} - SS_{subjects} - SS_{treatment} = SS_{residual}$. If you know any three of the sums of squares, you can figure out the fourth.

Calculating the sums of squares for a repeated-measures ANOVA by hand is a lot of work and, when it is done, calculating formulae instead of definitional formulae are used. Thus, since doing these calculations by hand won't add much to your understanding of what they represent, I'm going to skip them and make your life easy by always giving you at least three of the sums of squares.

Once one has the sums of squares, the rest is a piece of cake. We have already calculated the degrees of freedom, so figuring out mean squares is just a matter of dividing a sum of squares by its degrees of freedom. Once we have the mean squares, the F ratio is simply $MS_{treatment}$ divided by $MS_{residual}$. As always, the ANOVA summary table is laid out in such a way that it leads you through the calculations as shown in Equation 11.1. Note that no mean square is calculated for total variability and, following APA format, values are reported only to two decimal places.*

LOOKING CLOSER

*This means that at times we will need to go back and calculate values more exactly for some of our interpretative activities.

F O R M U L A E

The Repeated-Measures ANOVA

Source	SS	df	MS	F	Equation 11.1
Subjects	provided	$n-1$	$\dfrac{SS_{subjects}}{df_{subjects}}$		
Treatment	provided	$k-1$	$\dfrac{SS_{treatment}}{df_{treatment}}$	$\dfrac{MS_{treatment}}{MS_{residual}}$	
Residual	provided	$(n-1)(k-1)$	$\dfrac{SS_{residual}}{df_{residual}}$		
Total	provided	$N-1$			

Where:

$provided$ = the sum of squares value is provided

n = sample size per group

k = number of groups

N = total number of observations (i.e., $n \times k$)

For the depression data, $SS_{subjects} = 94.2500$, $SS_{treatment} = 201.5000$, $SS_{residual} = 26.5000$, and $SS_{total} = 322.2500$. Applying the formulae in Equation 11.1 to these sums of squares yields the summary table seen in Table 11.9.

$F_{observed}$ is 22.81, and F_{cv} was 5.14. Since $F_{observed} \geq F_{cv}$, the results fall in the rare zone of the sampling distribution and are considered statistically significant. Thus the results are written as $F(2, 6) = 22.81$, $p < .05$.

Whether the results fall in the rare or the common zone, all the decision rule conclusion options for the one-way ANOVA that were outlined in Table 10.4 apply here to the repeated-measures ANOVA.

TABLE **11.9**   **ANOVA Summary Table for Depression-Treatment Data**

Source	SS	df	MS	F
Subjects	94.25	3	31.42	
Treatment	201.50	2	100.75	22.81*
Residual	26.50	6	4.42	
Total	322.25	11		

NOTE: $*=p<.05$

Group Practice 11.2

If appropriate, complete the repeated-measures ANOVA for these data and report the results in APA format.

A health care researcher was interested in whether the costs of having a child varied as a function of how many children one had. Excluding women who gave birth via cesarean section and women with multiple births (twins, etc.), she obtained a sample of women who had had three or more children and obtained the hospital bills for the first three births. She converted the hospital bills to constant dollars so that inflation would not play a role. Below are the data she obtained from her large, university-affiliated hospital in Dallas, Texas.

The table below shows the data, in thousands of dollars, that each birth cost.* *Below the table are sums of squares.*

Child 1	Child 2	Child 3
7.6	6.9	5.4
11.8	9.8	7.4
5.6	4.8	4.3
5.7	4.8	3.7
8.3	8.5	7.9
4.7	4.2	3.9
6.3	6.3	7.3
11.4	10.0	9.9
6.6	7.6	5.4
10.9	10.8	8.9
4.4	4.2	3.7
5.8	4.3	3.9
7.3	7.8	7.1
3.8	3.6	3.3

Child 1	Child 2	Child 3
$M = 7.5190$	$M = 6.9952$	$M = 6.2048$
$s = 2.3066$	$s = 2.2338$	$s = 1.9759$
$\hat{s} = 2.3636$	$\hat{s} = 2.2890$	$\hat{s} = 2.0247$
skewness = .2008	skewness = .0180	skewness = .0336
kurtosis = −.9817	kurtosis = −1.3811	kurtosis = −1.3242

$(SE_{skewness} = .5345; SE_{kurtosis} = 1.0690)$
$SS_{subjects} = 281.2708, SS_{treatment} = 18.3860,$
$SS_{residual} = 17.2406.$

Child 1	Child 2	Child 3
7.5	5.3	5.2
8.9	7.9	8.1
9.3	8.9	7.3
9.6	9.0	7.3
9.5	9.8	8.5
4.6	4.6	4.2
8.3	7.8	7.6

Interpretation

Calculating the F ratio is just our entrée to the world of interpretation. The omnibus F simply tells us that at least two of the means being compared are statistically different. So, if the overall F is statistically significant we can (a) calculate an overall effect size and (b) use post-hoc tests to find which pairs of means have a difference that is statistically nonzero. Let's start with the effect size.

Percentage of Variance Predicted

The percentage of variance predicted tells the amount of variability in the dependent variable that is accounted for by the grouping variable. Obviously, it can range from 0 to 100, with the effect of the independent variable on the dependent variable being larger as the percentage

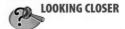
LOOKING CLOSER

*Reporting the data as 7.5 thousand, not 7500, makes the calculations for the ANOVA less cumbersome. However, it does present a little more challenge when it comes time to interpretation. I suggest that you add the zeros back in at that point to make the results easier to understand.

of variance predicted increases. For Pearson r we calculated r^2 as the percentage of variance predicted, and for independent-samples t tests and one-way ANOVA we calculated ω^2.* For the repeated-measures ANOVA we will also calculate ω^2. The formula is shown in Equation 11.2.

FORMULA

ω^2, Percentage of Variance in the Dependent Variable Predicted by the Grouping Variable, for a Repeated-Measures ANOVA

Equation 11.2

$$\omega^2 = \frac{SS_{treatment} - (k-1)\,MS_{residual}}{SS_{total} + MS_{residual}}$$

Where:

ω^2 = omega squared; the percentage of variance in the dependent variable that is predicted by the independent (grouping) variable

$SS_{treatment}$ = sum of squares for treatment

k = the number of groups being compared

$MS_{residual}$ = mean square residual

SS_{total} = sum of squares total

In this formula the numerator is the sum of squares for treatment minus the product of mean square residual multiplied by the number of groups minus one. This numerator is then divided by the denominator, the sum of sum of squares total plus mean square residual.

Just as with omega squared for the one-way ANOVA, the formula finds how much of the total variability sum of squares is accounted for by one of the other sums of squares, in this case the variability due to the treatment effect. Then it is "shrunk" by applying some correction factors, by subtracting something from the numerator and adding something to the denominator. Thus ω^2 provides an estimate, *for the population*, of the percentage of variance accounted for by the independent variable

Applying Equation 11.2 to the depression-treatment data, this is what we find:

$$\omega^2 = \frac{201.5000 - (3-1)4.4167}{322.2500 + 4.4167} = \frac{192.6666}{326.6667} = .5898 = .59$$

As we did for one-way ANOVA, we're going to use the square root of ω^2 as an estimate of the degree of relationship between the grouping variable and the dependent variable. In this case, $\hat{r} = \sqrt{.5898} = .7680 = .77$. That's a strong relationship.

For the depression data, here is what my interpretation would sound like so far: "I conducted a study in which I examined the effectiveness of a new treatment for depression. I took four people with depression and,

---

*In case you've forgotten, that's omega squared.

LOOKING CLOSER

using a depression scale where higher scores indicate more depression, examined their level of depression at three points in time: before treatment started ($M = 22.50$, $\hat{s} = 4.65$), at the end of treatment ($M = 12.50$, $\hat{s} = 2.65$), and at a follow-up 6 months later ($M = 18.25$, $\hat{s} = 3.40$). I found a statistically significant effect of treatment ($F (2, 6) = 22.81$, $p < .05$). Treatment status (pre, post, or follow-up) predicted almost 60% of the variability in depression scores. Though this new treatment seems to have a large impact on depression, there is a chance that this conclusion is in error, and the study should be replicated with a larger sample in order to have more faith that the effect exists."

Post-Hoc Tests

The F test, which compares the means of three or more groups, is an omnibus test. This means that if the results fall into the rare zone—if the results are statistically significant—all we know is that at least two of the means are statistically different from each other. In our current example, the depression data, there are three pairs of means (T1 vs. T2, T1 vs. T3, and T2 vs. T3), and so we don't know if the significant F ratio indicates a change in depression score from pretreatment to post-treatment, from pretreatment to follow-up, or from post-treatment to follow-up. As we saw when we first encountered ANOVA in the last chapter, it is the role of the post-hoc test to go in and find out which pair(s) of means are statistically different.

A variety of post-hoc tests can be used, but I am going to continue with the Fisher *LSD* test. *LSD* stands for "least significant difference," so this is a liberal test. It finds the *minimum* amount by which two means must differ for us to conclude that the difference is statistically significant at the α level selected. To phrase that in a different way: if the difference between two means is greater than or equal to the Fisher *LSD* value, it is a statistically significant difference.

F O R M U L A

Fisher *LSD* Value for Post-Hoc Test for a Repeated-Measures ANOVA

Equation 11.3

$$LSD = t_{cv} \sqrt{\frac{2MS_{residual}}{n}}$$

Where:

LSD = Fisher *LSD* (least significant difference) value: if the difference between two means is greater than or equal to this amount, the two means differ at the specified α level

t_{cv} = the critical value of t, two-tailed, with $df = df_{residual}$ and α set at the desired level (usually .05)

$MS_{residual}$ = mean square residual calculated via Equation 11.1

n = sample size per group in the repeated-measures ANOVA

TABLE **11.10**   **Comparison of Means for Depression-Treatment Data**

M_1	M_2	|Dif|	$\geq$ *LSD*?	95% CI
PRETREATMENT VS. POST-TREATMENT				
22.50	12.50	10.00	Yes	6.36 to 13.64
PRETREATMENT VS. FOLLOW-UP				
22.50	18.25	4.25	Yes	.61 to 7.89
POST-TREATMENT VS. FOLLOW-UP				
12.50	18.25	5.75	Yes	2.11 to 9.39

The formula for calculating the Fisher *LSD* value involves multiplying the critical value of *t* by the square root of the product of $2 \times MS_{residual}$ divided by the sample size per group. There will only be one *LSD* value for our repeated-measures ANOVA since all the groups in this repeated-measures ANOVA have the same *n*.* Let's use Equation 11.3 to calculate the *LSD* value for the depression data. Inspection of the ANOVA summary table (Table 11.9) shows that $df_{residual} = 6$. Applying these degrees of freedom to the table of critical values of *t* (either Appendix Table 3 or Appendix Table 9) shows that, for $\alpha = .05$, $t_{cv} = 2.4469$. The ANOVA summary table also shows a value of $MS_{residual}$, 4.42. But this is only to two decimal places, so we recalculate to obtain more decimal places. Thus, the more exact value of $MS_{residual}$ is $\dfrac{SS_{residual}}{df_{residual}} = \dfrac{26.5000}{6} = 4.4167$. Finally, we need to know *n*. Because we have four cases in each group, $n = 4$. We can now plug these numbers into the formula, and we find this:

$$LSD = 2.4469 \sqrt{\frac{2(4.4167)}{4}} = 2.4469 \times 1.4861 = 3.6363$$

If the absolute value of the difference between any two pairs of means is greater than or equal to 3.6363, then it is, at the .05 level, a statistically significant difference. Results are shown in Table 11.10.

Once the *LSD* value has been calculated, it is easily used to calculate a confidence interval (Sheskin, 2004).[†] As shown in Equation 11.4, all you need to do is subtract and add the *LSD* value to the difference between

---

*In fact, having the same *n* per group is a requirement for repeated-measures ANOVA.

[†]Sheskin, D. J. (2004). *Handbook of parametric and nonparametric statistical procedures.* Boca Raton, FL: Chapman & Hall/CRC.

LOOKING CLOSER

the two sample means. The 95% confidence interval for the 10-point pre- to post-treatment difference is calculated as 10.0000 ± 3.6363, the interval ranging from 6.36 to 13.64.

F O R M U L A

95% Confidence Interval for the Difference between a Pair of Means in a Repeated-Measures ANOVA

Equation 11.4 $95\% \ CI = |M_1 - M_2| \pm LSD$

Where:
M_1 = mean of one group
M_2 = mean of other group
LSD = Fisher LSD value calculated via Equation 11.3

When there are multiple means being compared, the easiest way to keep track of them is to make a table such as Table 11.10.

It is apparent from Table 11.10 that each pair of means shows a statistically significant difference using the Fisher LSD test, and, via the confidence intervals, it is clear that in some cases (e.g., pretreatment vs. follow-up) that difference, though statistically significant, may be small. For the next step in interpretation, let's think about the direction of the differences and the size of the differences.

Inspection of the means shows us the direction. Remember, we used a depression scale on which higher values indicate a greater degree of depression. Thus, the 10-point decrease from pretreatment to post-treatment and the 4.25-point decrease from pretreatment to follow-up are statistically significant *decreases* in depression. The 5.75-point increase from post-treatment to follow-up is a statistically significant *increase* in depression. Thus, we know direction, but how meaningful are the changes? Are the changes clinically significant?

For this we have to think. Our work would be easier if we knew more about the depression scale, if there were cut-off points for different levels of depression. However, even without this we can reach some reasonable conclusions in this human endeavor of interpretation. Let's look at the 4.25-point change from the pretreatment to follow-up, which shows that 6 months after treatment, people are significantly less depressed than they were at the start of treatment. This sounds like a good thing, no? But the confidence interval ranges from as little as a .61 decrease to as much as a 7.89 decrease. A .61 decrease means that the depression score could have gone down from 22.50 at the start of treatment to 21.89 at the follow-up. If the change is that small, although it might be statistically signifi-cant, I don't think it makes much difference in the quality of a person's life: I don't think it is clinically significant. Of course, it is also pos-sible that the change is almost 8 points, from 22.50 to 14.61, and that might be a clinically significant change. Given the present study, we don't know which extreme—a .61 decrease, a 7.89 decrease, or somewhere in between—is the population reality. As you already might be guessing, I'm going to call for a replication with a larger sample to help resolve this uncertainty.

Another method to make sense of results is to change the metric of the scores. In the last chapter, we took a dependent variable, travel time, that was scored in seconds and transformed it into the easier-to-grasp metric of minutes (e.g., 727 seconds is 12 minutes, 7 seconds). The depression scale is made up of six questions, each one answered on a 5-point scale ranging from 0 (not having that symptom of depression at all) to 4 (having that symptom of depression to a severe degree). Thus, if we divide the total score by six (the number of questions asked), we'll put the score back into the 5-point metric on which the questions were answered. Thus the pretreatment score of 22.50 becomes 3.75 (almost extreme symptoms), the post-treatment score of 12.50 becomes 2.08 (moderate symptoms), and the follow-up score of 18.25 becomes 3.04 (considerable symptoms). The 95% confidence interval for the difference between pretreatment and 6-month follow-up of .61 to 7.89 becomes a change of from .10 to 1.32 points. A change of over a point means moving down a whole symptom severity level, and that would probably be clinically meaningful. However, a change of .10 in symptom severity level probably would not be clinically significant to an individual. The real difference between the pretreatment population and the follow-up population is likely within that 95% confidence interval, so either of those options could be true. Before I make a big deal of the potential 1.32-point change for the better, I'd like to have more evidence that it is not a little deal, only a .10 change. I want replication. So, here's my interpretation:

"I conducted a study in which I examined the effectiveness of a new treatment for depression. I took four people with depression and examined, using a depression scale where higher scores indicate more depression, their level of depression at three points in time: before treatment started (M = 22.50, ŝ = 4.65), at the end of treatment (M = 12.50, ŝ = 2.65), and at a follow-up 6 months later (M = 18.25, ŝ = 3.40). I found a statistically significant effect of treatment (F (2, 6) = 22.81, p < .05). Overall, treatment status (pre, post, or follow-up) predicted almost 60% of the variability in depression scores.

"The decrease in depression over the course of treatment was statistically significant and seems to represent a meaningful change in depression level from the start to the end of treatment. At the start of treatment the average patient reported almost extreme levels of depression symptoms, and by the end of treatment the reported level of symptoms was down at the moderate range.

"Unfortunately, there was also a statistically significant increase in depression level from the end of treatment to the 6-month follow-up, suggesting that the effect of treatment was relatively short-lived. Though the amount of relapse was statistically significant, it is

worthwhile pointing out that there was some long-term effect of treatment since the degree of depression experienced 6 months after treatment was statistically less than existed before treatment. However, the 95% confidence interval calculated for this difference shows that the difference could be small, meaning that the change in depression level from pretreatment to follow-up was trivial (less than a point on a 24-point scale), or it could be clinically meaningful (almost 8 points on a 24-point scale).

"Though this new treatment seems to be promising, there is a 5% chance that the conclusion is in error and that the treatment has no real effect. Thus, the study should be replicated in order to have more faith that the effect is real. When replicating, I suggest using more participants, both to increase the generalizability of the results and to provide better estimates of the treatment effect. If the results replicate, future research should be directed at (a) making the treatment even more effective, that is, finding ways to reduce end-of-treatment symptomatology below the moderate symptom level, and (b) making the effects of treatment last longer."

Power and Sample Size

Power, remember, is the probability of being able to reject the null hypothesis when the null hypothesis should be rejected. In general, dependent-sample designs (i.e., repeated-measures) are more powerful than independent-sample designs. This means that to achieve the same degree of power for a dependent-samples test as for an independent-samples test, one needs fewer cases. For example, for an *independent-samples, one-way ANOVA*, one needs 237 cases to yield a power of .80 with a small-to-moderate effect size according to Murphy and Myors (2004).* You need fewer cases for a repeated-measures ANOVA, but how many fewer depends on how highly correlated the variables are in the different groups. Variables are correlated from group to group because when the same case is measured at different points in time or under different conditions, it is likely to maintain its relative standing in the group over time. Case 3 in the depression data, for example, had the lowest score in the pretreatment group, the lowest score in the post-treatment group, and the lowest score in the follow-up group. For the depression data there was a correlation of .65 between T1 and T2 scores, a correlation of .96 between T1 and T3 scores, and a correlation of .43 between T2 and T3 scores. The scores in the groups were correlated.

The more correlated the scores, the greater the power. Murphy and Myors (2004) report that for a repeated-measures ANOVA with three groups and that same small-to-moderate effect size, only 65 cases, not

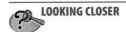
LOOKING CLOSER

Murphy, K. R. and Myors, BH. (2004). Statistical power analysis: a simple and general model for traditional and modern hypothesis tests, (2nd ed.). Mahwaw, NJ: Lawrence Erlbaum Associates.

237, are needed to achieve a power of .80 if the scores in the groups correlate at the .20 level. If the correlation is greater, say $r = .40$, the number of cases required drops even more, to $N = 50$.

A repeated-measures ANOVA offers a big savings in power and sample size. Unfortunately, calculating power and sample size for a repeated-measures ANOVA is hard to do, and the calculations are beyond the scope of an introductory statistics text. Having the statistical software product SPSS do the calculations for the depression data shows that power equaled .996.* Though I don't need to worry about Type II error, since I have successfully rejected the null hypothesis, $\beta = 1 - .996 = .004$. Thus, there is a very, very small chance of making a Type II error, of failing to reject H_0, when the effect size is at the present level and with four observations per group. Frankly, having so much power is surprising to me because the effect ($\omega^2 = .59$) is large but not *that* large. But, that's the power of dependent samples.

Though we're not calculating power and sample size for a repeated-measures ANOVA with multiple samples, we're not going to abandon common sense. Even though power was more than adequate, I feel that an *n* of four is too small to have confidence in the robustness of the results. Without SPSS I may not know exactly what my power was or how many cases I should have had, but I feel that more cases would be better. In my interpretative statements so far, I've advocated for a larger (albeit unspecified) sample size to yield a better estimate of population values.

Group Practice 11.3

For the cost-of-birth data introduced in Group Practice 11.2, calculate ω^2, the Fisher *LSD* value, and 95% confidence intervals for the differences between group means, and complete a table like Table 11.10.

Then, write a complete interpretative statement. (Be sure to read the footnote in Group Practice 11.2 before completing your interpretation.)

USING REPEATED-MEASURES ANOVA INSTEAD OF DEPENDENT-SAMPLES *t* TESTS

Back in Chapter 9 when we discussed the difference between independent-sample and dependent-sample tests, we compared prices at two grocery stores. If we had the same items in our shopping carts at the two stores, then we had dependent samples; on the other hand, if we had a random sample of the items from store A and a random sample of the items from store B, we had independent samples. The questions addressed by these two techniques are the same, yet different. They are the same since each test is asking if there is a difference between the two stores. Yet, they are different, because the dependent-samples grocery store

---

*Visit the Evolve website at www.elsevier/evolve to see how to use SPSS to calculate power.

LOOKING CLOSER

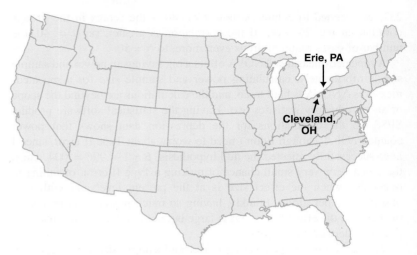

Figure **11.5** Map showing the locations of Cleveland, Ohio and Erie, Pennsylvania.

comparison asks if the two grocery stores differ in prices *for the same items* whereas the independent-samples comparison asks *if one store stocks more expensive items, in general*, than the other.

The technique chosen should be dictated by the question being asked. Yet, there are times that either technique can be used: whether aspirin or ibuprofen is more effective in treating headache pain can be answered with either technique. In such a case, the decision should be guided by which technique is more powerful, which has a smaller chance of leading to a Type II error. And the winners in this competition, as I noted above, are the dependent-sample tests.

Let me give an example that will explain why this is so. Though I teach at Penn State in Erie, Pa., I live in Cleveland, Ohio, over 100 miles away.* In the larger scheme of the United States, as seen in Figure 11.5, the cities aren't that far from each other, and they share the characteristic of being cities at the same latitude along the shore of Lake Erie.

One problem about living so far from work is that the weather in the two locations may differ, and what I decide to wear based on the forecast at home in Cleveland may be inappropriate when I get to work in Erie. So, being an empirical kind of guy, I might decide to collect data comparing the temperatures in the two cities to see if the difference between the two is statistically significant or practically meaningful.

LOOKING CLOSER

*Yes, that is one heck of a commute. But still, I like where I work, and I like where I live, so... And, that explains why I was collecting data to see if I could shave some time off my commute.

One way to do this is with an *independent*-samples *t* test: gathering data about a random sample of days from Cleveland and a random sample of days from Erie, and dividing the difference between the two means by the standard error of the difference to yield a *t* value.

I hope that you remember from Chapter 9 that the standard error of the difference for an independent-samples *t* test is the standard deviation of the sampling distribution of the difference scores. So, let's think about how much variability there will be in the sampling distribution of the difference scores, or about how large the standard error of the difference may be. To make it simple, let's say that the sample size is 2, that $n = 2$. With a random sample from each population, it is possible that the sample of days from Cleveland will be from one season—say, summer—and the sample of days from Erie will be from another season—say, winter. Clearly the difference in temperature between these two means would be large. Of course the samples will also include summer days in Cleveland to be compared to summer days in Erie, but the occasional disparate comparison should lead to more variability in the sampling distribution, resulting in a relatively larger standard error of the difference.

We haven't learned how to calculate a *dependent*-samples *t* test, but the basic format is the same. The difference between two sample means is divided by the standard deviation of the sampling distribution of difference scores, which is also called the standard error of the difference. So, let's think what the denominator looks like if I use *dependent* samples to compare the temperature in Cleveland to the temperature in Erie.

If I use dependent samples, then I "match" the day selected to measure the temperature for Cleveland to the same day in Erie: if I find the temperature for January 28 for Cleveland, I also find the temperature for January 28 for Erie. Thus, if I have two winter days for my sample in Cleveland, I have two winter days for my sample in Erie. As a result, there will be less difference between the sample means, resulting in less variability in the sampling distribution of difference scores, resulting in a smaller standard error of the difference. This is an important point, so if it doesn't make sense, please read it over again.

What is the point? My point is that the *denominator* for a dependent-samples *t* test is smaller than the denominator for an independent-samples *t* test. This has important implications. Given the same size difference between the means (given the same *numerator*), $t_{observed}$ for a *dependent*-samples *t* test will be *larger* than $t_{observed}$ for an *independent*-samples *t* test. Since a larger *t* value is more likely to fall in the rare zone of the sampling distribution, one is more likely to be able to reject the null hypothesis with a dependent-samples *t* test! If the difference between two means is small, it is more likely to be found to be a statistically significant difference if one uses a dependent-samples test than if one uses an independent-samples test. Dependent-samples *t* tests have more power than independent-samples *t* tests.

Since dependent-samples tests have more statistical power than independent-samples tests, using a dependent-samples test means that one needs fewer cases. Thus it is to your advantage, when you can, to plan your research so that you can use a dependent-samples test.*

The dependent-samples test explored earlier in this chapter, the repeated-measures ANOVA, is an analysis of variance, and so it was developed for use with more than two samples. But, you *can* use it with just two samples, and there are certain advantages to using a repeated-measures ANOVA instead of a dependent-samples *t* test when one has two dependent samples.

When there are just two samples, an ANOVA and a *t* are the same test. Back in Chapter 9, we used the *t* test to compare maze-running speeds of mice under a control and an experimental condition and found $t(8) = 3.78$, $p < .05$. If we take those same data and subject them to a one-way ANOVA, we find $F(1, 8) = 14.28$, $p < .05$. Now the numbers 3.78 and 14.28 may not look the same, but the square root of 14.28 is 3.78. When there are only two groups, $t^2 = F$. So, there is no reason, except that the computations are a bit more tedious, that one couldn't use an ANOVA instead of a *t* test when one has two samples.

There's no practical reason to use ANOVA instead of *t* when the samples are independent, but there *is* a reason to do so with *dependent* samples. The reason is that the dependent-samples *t* test doesn't partition the total variability into its components, and as a result it ends up over-estimating the percentage of variability in the dependent variable that is predicted (accounted for) by the grouping variable. Trust me on this for a while, but I'll provide plenty of examples.

Here's our first example. Imagine being a nutritionist at an elementary school. You are concerned that the children aren't consuming enough milk at lunch. You think that if the teachers ate lunch with the students and drank milk while doing so, then this modeling would increase milk consumption. So, you obtain a random sample of five students from the population at the school and observe how many ounces of milk each drinks at lunch. You then have the teachers eat lunch with the students and observe how much milk the students drink on this occasion. Thus you have data for milk consumption on five students at two points in time, at Time 1 (T1) with no teacher present and at Time 2 (T2) with teachers present. The data are shown in Table 11.11. Does the presence of teachers modeling milk consumption have an impact on milk consumption? Milk consumption increases over four ounces, from 9.0 to 13.2 ounces; but is the increase statistically significant, is the variability between groups greater than the variability within groups?

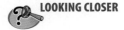
LOOKING CLOSER

*Not all questions lend themselves to dependent-samples tests, and sometimes there are practical reasons not to use dependent-samples tests. For example, if one were investigating which method of teaching reading was more effective for first-graders one couldn't first teach a student to read using method A, and then teach him or her to read using method B, because the student already knows how to read thanks to method A.

TABLE **11.11**   **Lunchtime Milk Consumption, in Ounces, at Two Points in Time**

	No Teachers Present (Control)	Teachers Present (Experimental)
Student 1	12	16
Student 2	0	9
Student 3	16	16
Student 4	10	15
Student 5	7	10
M	9.00	13.20
ŝ	6.00	3.42

As I noted before, the arrangement of the data is very important for a dependent-samples test since the integrity of the paired samples must be maintained. Each case takes a row, and each time point takes a column. I hope that arranging the data this way makes you think of *subjects* as the row effect and *time* as the column effect, that it makes you think back to the factorial ANOVA. And that, I hope, reminds you of partitioning the variability in the individual cells into variability due to treatment and variability due to subjects. Analysis of variance is designed to partition variability, and that is exactly what a repeated-measures ANOVA does. A dependent-samples *t* test, though it ends up at the same answer as does the ANOVA, does not partition the variance. As a result, when one calculates the percentage of variance predicted for a dependent-samples *t* test, the variability due to subjects and the variability due to treatment are mixed together, leading to a spuriously high percentage of variance appearing to be explained by the grouping variable. Because a repeated-measures ANOVA subtracts out the variability due to subjects, it provides a more honest measure of the variability due to treatment than does the dependent-samples *t* test. For this reason, I prefer the repeated-measures ANOVA over a dependent-samples *t* test. So, let me quickly march through the first five steps of Tom and Harry for these milk-consumption data. Then we'll spend more time on the sixth step, interpretation, where we venture into some new ground for power and sample size.

Test

What test are we doing? We're comparing the means of two dependent samples, and we could use either a dependent-samples *t* test or repeated-measures ANOVA to do so. I'm going to choose a repeated-measures analysis of variance because it will provide a better estimate of the effect of the grouping variable on the dependent variable.

Assumptions

These are the assumptions for the repeated-measures ANOVA when it is a two-sample test:
- Dependent samples (not robust to violations)
- Interval- or ratio-level data (not robust to violations)
- Random samples (robust to violations)
- Normality (robust to violations if n is large)
- Homogeneity of variance (robust to violations if n is large)

Note that the last assumption has changed. When a repeated-measures ANOVA is a multiple (more than 2) sample test, the last assumption is sphericity, that the variances of the difference scores are equal. When there are only two samples, this assumption drops back to the old, familiar homogeneity of variance.

The samples are dependent, since the same participants are observed at two points in time, so the first assumption is not violated. The dependent variable is ratio-level, so the second assumption is not violated. The participants are a random sample from the school but not from the larger population of all elementary school children, so we can generalize the results to the school but not beyond. The n is not large—we're only following five kids—so neither of the last two assumptions is robust to violations. I calculated the confidence intervals for skewness and kurtosis at both points in time and did not violate the normality assumption. Also, neither standard deviation is more than twice the other, so we are OK in terms of homogeneity of variance as well.

Hypotheses

These are the two hypotheses:

$$H_0: \mu_1 = \mu_2$$
$$H_1: \mu_1 \neq \mu_2$$

The null hypothesis states that the two population means, milk consumption at T1 and milk consumption at T2, are equal, that the two populations are really one and the same population. Even so, because of sampling error we don't expect that the means of two samples drawn from one population will be exactly equal. However, they should be close enough to each other that sampling error is a credible explanation for the observed difference.

The alternative hypothesis says that the two populations have different means. As a result, when comparing the mean of a sample drawn from one population to the mean of a sample drawn from the other population, we'll find a difference between the two sample means. This difference reflects the reality of the difference between the two populations and should be so large that sampling error for two samples drawn from the same population is not a credible explanation.

Decision Rule

There are five cases ($n = 5$) in two groups ($k = 2$), so, via Equation 11.1, the degrees of freedom for treatment is 1 and for residual it is 4. Let's set α at .05, meaning we are willing to make a Type I error 5% of the time. Consulting the table of critical values of F, Appendix Table 10, F_{cv} (1, 4) = 7.7086. If $F_{observed} \geq 7.7086$, then the results fall in the rare zone of the sampling distribution of F and we'll reject H_0. If $F_{observed} < 7.7086$, then the results fall in the common zone of the sampling distribution of F and we'll fail to reject H_0. Another part of this step involves calculating the necessary sample size, and I'll address that in a bit.

Calculations

For repeated-measures ANOVA, I provide the sums of squares. For the milk-consumption data, SS_{total} = 234.9000, $SS_{subjects}$ = 169.4000, and $SS_{treatment}$ = 44.1000. Though we were not given $SS_{residual}$, we can easily calculate it by subtracting $SS_{subjects}$ and $SS_{treatment}$ from SS_{total}. Thus, $SS_{residual}$ = 234.9000 – 169.4000 – 44.1000 = 21.4000. Since we now have all the sums of squares, we can complete the ANOVA summary table by applying the formulae in Equation 11.1 (Table 11.12).

Since our observed F of 8.24 is $\geq F_{cv}$ of 7.71, we shall reject the null hypothesis. Written in APA format, the results are F (1, 4) = 8.24, $p < .05$.

Interpretation

Interpreting a repeated-measures ANOVA when there are only two groups is simpler than when there are multiple groups. We don't have to worry about post-hoc tests when only one pair of means is being compared. If the overall F is indicative of a statistically significant difference, as it is in the current example, then the only pair of means that can differ is the T1 vs. T2 comparison. Thus we can conclude that the difference between the T1 mean (9.00 ounces of milk consumed) and the T2 mean (13.20 ounces consumed) is statistically significant. We can go a step further and look at the direction of the difference, and conclude that having a teacher present at lunch and modeling milk consumption leads to *increased* milk consumption by children.

TABLE **11.12**   **ANOVA Summary Table for Milk-Consumption Data**

Source	SS	df	MS	F
Subjects	169.40	4	42.35	
Treatment	44.10	1	44.10	8.24*
Residual	21.40	4	5.35	
Total	234.90	9		

NOTE: * = $p < .05$

Effect Size I: 95% Confidence Interval

There are a number of ways of looking at how strong the effect is, so let's start with my favorite, the 95% confidence interval for the difference between the two population means. The formula for this is shown in Equation 11.5, and it is simply a combination of Equations 11.3 and 11.4 so that you can avoid the intermediate step of having to calculate an unnecessary *LSD* value.

F O R M U L A

The 95% Confidence Interval for the Difference between Two Means for a Repeated-Measures ANOVA Used in Place of a Dependent-Samples *t* Test

Equation 11.5

$$95\% \; CI = |M_1 - M_2| \pm t_{cv} \sqrt{\frac{2MS_{residual}}{n}}$$

Where:
$95\% \; CI$ = the 95% confidence interval for the difference between two means being calculated
M_1 = the mean of the first sample
M_2 = the mean of the second sample
t_{cv} = the critical value of *t*, two-tailed, with $df_{residual}$
$MS_{residual}$ = the mean square residual value from the repeated-measures ANOVA
n = sample size per group

Working from right to left, this formula says first multiply the mean square residual by two and divide this product by the sample size. Take this quotient and find the square root of it. (This is the *LSD* value.) Take the square root and multiply it by the critical value, two-tailed, of *t* with $df_{residual}$ degrees of freedom. This product is then subtracted from and added to the absolute value of the difference between the two means to yield the confidence interval. For the milk-consumption data the formula looks like this:*

$$95\% \; CI = |9.0000 - 13.2000| \pm 2.7764 \sqrt{\frac{2 \times 5.3500}{5}}$$
$$= 4.2000 \pm (2.7764 \times 1.4629) \; = \; 4.2000 \pm 4.0616$$

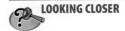 **LOOKING CLOSER**   *Note that I am using a more exact value for $F_{observed}$ than was in my ANOVA summary table, one with more decimal places.

Thus the 95% confidence interval ranges from a difference of .14 ounces of milk between the two populations to a difference of 8.26 ounces of milk between the two populations. Under the experimental condition, having a teacher present, children probably drink from .14 to 8.26 more ounces of milk.

We know that there is a difference, we know the direction of the difference, and we have some sense of the size of the difference thanks to the confidence interval. Let's look at a couple of other measures of the size or meaningfulness of the difference, specifically ω^2 and d.

Effect Size II: ω^2

It is because of ω^2 that we are using a repeated-measures ANOVA instead of the dependent-samples t test as our preferred difference test with two dependent samples and an interval- or ratio-level dependent variable. Omega squared is calculated via Equation 11.2 from earlier in this chapter. For the milk-consumption data, this is ω^2:

$$\omega^2 = \frac{44.1000 - (2 - 1)5.3500}{234.9000 + 5.3500} = .1613 = .16$$

Thus, about 16% of the variability in milk consumption is predicted by knowing whether there are teachers modeling milk consumption present in the lunchroom.

One could also calculate $\hat{r}$ by taking the square root of ω^2. In this case, I estimate that the relationship between teacher presence/absence and milk consumption is .40, a substantial degree of relationship.

If we analyze these data using a dependent-samples t test and then calculated ω^2 for the dependent-samples t test, we would find that 42% of the variability in milk consumption was predicted by the independent, or grouping, variable. There is a large discrepancy between the independent variable accounting for 42% of the variability in the dependent variable or its accounting for 16%. Frankly, the dependent-samples t test ω^2 value of 42% is an unreasonably large amount of variability to be accounted for, and a real-life example should help to make that point.

Remember my temperature comparison for Cleveland and Erie? You won't be surprised that I actually collected some data about this. I randomly selected 1 day from each of the 12 months in the year and found the high temperature in each of the two cities on those days. On average, the temperature in Cleveland was 3.17° warmer (60.25 vs. 57.08), and the difference was statistically significant. Table 11.13 displays the data for the two cities as well as the difference scores.

If you take a look at the 12 pairs of temperatures, I think you'll note how similar they are. In fact, the correlation between the temperature in the two cities is .99: when it is summer and hot in Cleveland, it is summer and hot in Erie; the same holds true for the winter temperatures in the two cities.

What factors do you think influence temperature? I think that the major influence on temperature is seasonal, how the earth is tilted in

TABLE **11.13** **High Temperatures in Cleveland, Ohio, and Erie, Pennsylvania**

	Cleveland	Erie	Difference Score
	36	35	1
	40	37	3
	44	39	5
	49	47	2
	54	49	5
	55	49	6
	69	66	3
	70	69	1
	73	67	6
	73	69	4
	77	75	2
	83	83	0
M	60.25	57.08	3.17
$\hat{s}$	15.81	16.25	2.04

relation to the sun. When part of the earth is closer to the sun (i.e., when it is summer in that region), the temperatures are warmer. Next in order of priority are things like cloud coverage and geographic features like lakes and mountains. When two cities are at about the same latitude, longitude, and altitude and both are next to the same Great Lake (as seen in Figure 11.5), and there is no mountain range separating the two cities, to what extent do you think slight differences in location influence temperature?

In such a situation I don't think that slight differences in location influence temperature very much, and looking at the values in Table 11.13 supports this. Look at these values, and at the variability *between* cities and the variability *within* cities, and decide which factor shows the greater variability.* Contrast the almost 50-point seasonal fluctuations in temperature for each city (from 36° to 83° for Cleveland and from 35° to 83° for Erie) with the maximum difference in temperature of 6° between the cities for any given month. Clearly, the greater variability is the within-city variability, with within-city standard deviations of approximately 16 compared to a standard deviation for the difference scores of approximately 2. So, when we apportion the variance in temperature, you shouldn't expect very much to be attributable to location, to city.

Yet, if one analyzes these data using a dependent-samples t test and goes on to calculate ω^2, one finds that almost 54% of the variability in the dependent variable can be attributed to the grouping variable, to city. Contrast that with an ω^2, when calculated from a repeated-measures ANOVA, of 1%. This 1% is a truer estimate of the effect that the grouping variable of location has on the temperatures in these two cities: not very much effect. When the variability that is due to individual differences, to the seasonal tilting of the planet in this case, is removed, we get an accurate accounting of the degree to which the grouping variable affects the dependent variable.[†] And that—the more honest accounting of the effect of the grouping variable—is why I prefer a repeated-measures ANOVA over the dependent-samples t test when there are only two dependent samples.

Effect Size III: *d*

The last method that I want to use to judge the effect of the grouping variable involves calculating d, what often is simply called the effect size. We first encountered d with the independent-samples t test, where it transformed differences between sample means by standardizing them, by dividing the difference between means by the pooled standard deviation.

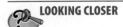

LOOKING CLOSER

*Bye the bye, independent-samples designs are often called **between-subject** designs. Dependent-samples designs are called **within-subject** designs.

[†]Here's another way to think about this. The correlation between the temperatures in Erie and the temperatures in Cleveland is .99. The coefficient of determination, r^2, for .99 is .98, indicating that we can predict 98% of the variability of the temperature in one city by knowing the temperature in the other city. With 98% of the variability accounted for, there's not much variability left to be predicted, is there?

We're going to do something similar here, but we will use a different denominator, the standard deviation of the difference scores. Even if the null hypothesis is true, there will be variability in difference scores, which will allow us to calculate a standard deviation for the difference scores. By converting the difference between two means into these standard deviation units, we standardize it. Thus a difference of 5 points and a difference of 15 points is equivalent, if the first came from a population with a standard deviation of 10 and the second from a population with a standard deviation of 30.

The formula for d for dependent-samples t test/repeated-measures ANOVA is given in Equation 11.6. Note that I am using the estimated population value of the standard deviation of the difference scores, not the sample standard deviation, as the denominator. This is for two reasons. First, we are working with inferential statistics and so are interested in population values. Second, $\hat{s}$ is bigger than s, which means that it will yield a smaller, more conservative estimate of d, a shrunken d if you will.

FORMULA

Effect Size, d, for Difference between Means of Two Dependent Samples

$$d = \frac{|M_1 - M_2|}{\hat{s}_D}$$

Equation 11.6

Where:
d = the effect size for two dependent samples being calculated
M_1 = the mean of one group
M_2 = the mean of the other group
$\hat{s}_D$ = the estimated population standard deviation for the difference scores

Here's what one does: find the absolute value of the difference between the two means, and then divide it by the estimated population standard deviation of the difference scores. It's been a while since we've calculated a standard deviation, so let me demonstrate how to do so with the milk-consumption data in Table 11.14.

We're going to find $\hat{s}$ for the final column, for the *difference scores* for milk consumption. The formula for $\hat{s}^2$ (Equation 4.8) finds the sum of the squared deviations from the mean for the difference scores and then divides this by the number of scores minus one. Thus we calculate:

$$\hat{s}_D^2 = \frac{(4 - 4.2)^2 + (9 - 4.2)^2 + (0 - 4.2)^2 + (5 - 4.2)^2 + (3 - 4.2)^2}{(5 - 1)}$$

$$= \frac{42.8}{4} = 10.70$$

TABLE **11.14**   **Lunchtime Milk Consumption (in Ounces) at Two Points in Time**

	No Teachers Present (Control)	Teachers Present (Experimental)	Difference Score (E – C)
Student 1	12	16	4
Student 2	0	9	9
Student 3	16	16	0
Student 4	10	15	5
Student 5	7	10	3
M	9.00	13.20	4.20

The square root of this, $\hat{s}_D$, is 3.2711, and we use that to calculate d:

$$d = \frac{|9.00 - 13.20|}{3.2711} = \frac{4.20}{3.2711} = 1.2840 = 1.28$$

The mean of the experimental group, the group that is eating lunch with teachers present, has milk consumption that is 1.28 estimated population standard deviations of the difference score (that's quite a mouthful) above that of the control group. Cohen (1988), speaking only of research in the social and behavioral sciences, offered a rough frame of reference for effect sizes that has become reified and treated as gospel. He said that a small effect size was $d \approx .2$, a medium effect size was $d \approx .6$, and a large effect size was $d \approx 1.2$. By these standards a d of 1.28 is large.

But, before overinterpreting this effect size, be aware that effect sizes are calculated differently for independent-samples tests and dependent-samples tests. For independent-samples t tests, the mean difference is divided by either the standard deviation of the control group or the pooled standard deviation for the two groups. For the dependent-samples t test, the mean difference is divided by the standard deviation of the difference scores. Almost always the standard deviation of the difference scores is smaller than the standard deviations of the groups individually, so $d_{dependent}$ will be larger than $d_{independent}$ and Cohen's guide to effect sizes doesn't apply to d for dependent samples. (Note that I am now differentiating between d calculated for independent samples, $d_{independent}$, and for dependent samples, $d_{dependent}$.)

Here's an example of how Cohen's guide to effect sizes doesn't apply to d for dependent samples. Suppose I take 40 people, randomly divide them into two groups, and do something to one group to increase intelligence. I then administer an IQ test to everyone and analyze the data with an independent-samples t test. The control group has a mean IQ of 100.60, and the experimental group mean of 105.20. Given that $\sigma = 15$ for IQ, $d_{independent} = .31$. Now, imagine that I do the study a different way. I take 20 people, measure their IQs, administer my intelligence-increasing treatment, and then measure their IQs again. This time I use a dependent-samples t test to analyze the data. The means of the two groups are the same, so the difference between them is the same; but $\hat{s}_D = 3.75$, which is a lot smaller than 15.* As a result, $d_{dependent}$ is 1.24.

Note the difference between the two ds. The mean difference between the two samples is the same, but the effect size is very different depending on whether I use an independent-samples or a dependent-samples design. You can't interpret $d_{dependent}$ using the same standards as for $d_{independent}$.

The bottom line is that an effect size ($d_{dependent}$) of 1.24 is large, and you can say so; but you can't interpret it by saying that it will lead to an 18.6-point increase in IQ as we could do if it were a $d_{independent}$.[†] Thus, d for dependent-samples t tests is less intuitive than it is for independent-samples t tests, and it is harder to interpret. Would it make much sense to an intelligent but not statistically savvy adult to say that the effect of teacher presence on milk consumption leads to a mean increase of 1.28 standard deviations of the difference scores? Heck, I'm a statistically savvy guy, and it doesn't make much intuitive sense to me other than that I know that a d of 1.28 is large. So, why calculate d for a dependent-samples t test/repeated-measures ANOVA? Because as well as giving a measure of effect size, $d_{dependent}$ is useful for calculating power and sample size.

Power and Sample Size

Moving from a repeated-measures ANOVA with multiple samples to a repeated-measures ANOVA with only two samples allows us to explore power and sample size more easily. If the null hypothesis is true, then the sampling distribution of the difference scores will be centered around zero. We just learned how to calculate the standard deviation of the difference scores, $\hat{s}_D$. For the milk-consumption data, $\hat{s}_D$ was 3.27. Panel A of Figure 11.6 shows a sampling distribution of the difference scores for the milk data. Note that I centered the distribution at a difference score of zero and marked off each standard deviation unit from it, each 3.27 ounces of milk.

When teachers were present the children consumed, on average, 4.20 more ounces of milk, and that difference score (13.20 − 9.00) is shown in Panel B of Figure 11.6. In Panel B, I've also superimposed another sampling distribution of the difference scores, one drawn with a dotted line, that has the same standard deviation (3.27) but that is centered about the value of 4.20.

---

*There's no way to know that $\hat{s}_D = 3.75$ from the information I've presented above. But, trust me that this is the correct value for the data set that I am using.

[†]How do I get that value of 18.6? Well, if a standard deviation is 15 and the effect is an increase of 1.24 standard deviations, then $15 \times 1.24 = 18.6$.

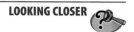

LOOKING CLOSER

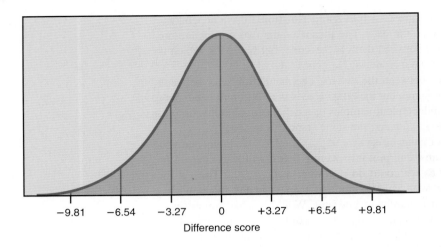

−9.81   −6.54   −3.27   0   +3.27   +6.54   +9.81

Difference score

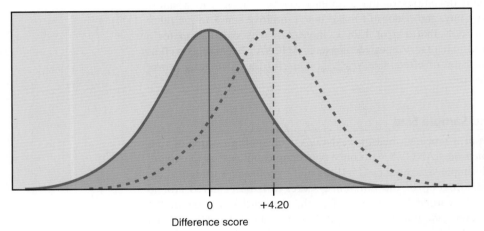

0   +4.20

Difference score

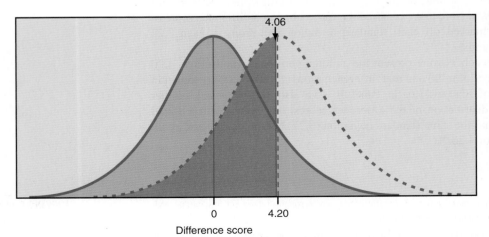

4.06

0   4.20

Difference score

Figure **11.6** Graphs showing sampling distributions of the difference score for H_0 and H_1.

Look at Panel B of Figure 11.6 and think about this for a second: if the null hypothesis is true, then the sampling distribution drawn with the unbroken line should occur. But what if the null hypothesis is not true? If the null hypothesis is not true, our best guess is that the sampling distribution should be centered about the observed difference of 4.20, since that is the only information we have. Thus, if H_1 is true, the sampling distribution drawn with the dotted line should occur. We're going to use these two sampling distributions to get an estimate of power, and Panel C will lead us through that.

First, let me remind you of what power is. Power is the likelihood of rejecting the null hypothesis if the null hypothesis *should* be rejected. So the question is, how likely are we to conclude that the dotted line sampling distribution is the true sampling distribution if it *is* the true sampling distribution?

However, we judge whether the dotted line sampling distribution represents reality by seeing whether the observed difference score falls in the common zone or the rare zone of the *unbroken line* sampling distribution, the sampling distribution that should occur if the null hypothesis is true. So, if we can figure out where *on the dotted line distribution* the critical value *for the unbroken line distribution* falls, we can use this to find out the area *of the dotted line distribution* above and below this point. As a result, we'll know power and β.

Believe it or not, we calculated this critical value when we calculated the 95% confidence interval for the difference. The 95% confidence interval for the milk-consumption data was 4.20 ± 4.06, and that 4.06 is our critical value.*

A moment's reflection should convince you that this is the critical value we need. If the difference score were greater than 4.06—say, 4.07—then the confidence interval would not capture zero, indicating that the null hypothesis should be rejected. To phrase that just a bit differently: as long as the difference score is 4.06 or bigger, we'll reject the null hypothesis.

In Panel C of Figure 11.6, I marked the value of 4.06 on the abscissa and shaded in the portion of the dotted line sampling distribution that falls at or below this point. If the dotted line distribution were really true—that is, if we should reject H_0—and if the observed difference is less than 4.06, we wouldn't reject H_0: so we'd make a Type II error. The shaded portion of the dotted line sampling distribution, the sampling distribution for H_1, represents β, the probability of Type II error. The unshaded portion of the sampling distribution for H_1, the dotted line sampling distribution, represents power—our probability of rejecting H_0 when it should be rejected.[†]

---

*Remember, this value is the product of t_{cv} times the *LSD* value.

[†]Though I didn't go into this explanation of power for independent-samples t tests, it is true for them as well.

LOOKING CLOSER

I've represented both of the sampling distributions with normal distributions, and I hope that this puts you in the mindset of z scores, of using the table of area under the normal curve, Appendix Table 1, to figure out power and/or β for a two-sample repeated-measures ANOVA/dependent-samples t test.

Let's use the milk-consumption data as an example. If H_1 is true, then its sampling distribution has a mean of 4.2000. The critical value for the confidence interval that we calculated with Equation 11.5 is 4.0615. Further, we calculated the standard deviation of the sampling distribution, $\hat{s}_D$, as 3.2711. We have everything we need to calculate a z score, an observed score (4.0615), a mean (4.2000), and a standard deviation (3.2711):

$$\frac{4.0615 - 4.2000}{3.2711} = -.0423 = -.04$$

This z score represents the distance, in standard score units, between the cutoff point for the rare zone of the sampling distribution of difference scores if the *null* hypothesis is true, and the mean of the sampling distribution of difference scores if the *alternative* hypothesis is true. That last sentence was a mouthful, so reread it while referring back to Figure 11.6. Does it make sense that a score of 4.06 is .04 standard score units below 4.20?

If we take this value, –.04, and look it up in Appendix Table 1, we'll find that 48.40% of the area under the normal curve falls below it, and 51.60% of the area under the normal curve falls above it. Thus, $\beta = .48$ and power = .52 for the milk data.

I went through this long explanation because I thought that you were ready for a deeper understanding of power and β. This procedure works to give a rough estimate of β and power, especially when n is large, but it is a bit tedious. Most researchers and statisticians use computer programs and/or tables to find power and/or β. The power table I provided before, Appendix Table 7, does not work with a dependent-samples t test/repeated-measures ANOVA, so I am going to provide you with a new one, Appendix Table 11, and a small piece of it here, Table 11.15.

TABLE 11.15   Section of Appendix Table 11, Power for Dependent-Samples *t* Test

	EFFECT SIZE (*d*)					
n	1.0	1.1	1.2	1.3	1.4	1.5
5	.40	.46	.53	.59	.65	.71
6	.50	.58	.65	.72	.78	.83
7	.60	.68	.75	.81	.86	.90
8	.68	.76	.82	.88	.92	.95

The columns in Appendix Table 11 represent the effect size $d_{dependent}$, calculated via Equation 11.6 and the rows represent different ns. The entries in the cell represent the power, with $\alpha = .05$, two-tailed, for the intersection of the effect size with the n. For example, if the population value of the effect size, δ, is 1.0 and one has a sample size of 5, one has a 40% chance of rejecting the null hypothesis.

Looking at the table, several things about power become apparent. Looking across the rows, it is clear that as the effect size increases, so does power. And, looking down the columns one can see that as sample size increases, power increases.

For the five students in the milk-consumption experiment, $d = 1.28$. Since the exact value of $d = 1.28$ is not in the table, I'm going to continue with my conservative, "Price is Right" approach of using the closest value without going over, and use the column where $d = 1.2$. Following $n = 5$ over, I find power $= .53.$* Our milk-consumption study was underpowered, and we were lucky to reject the null hypothesis.

The final topic to address for the dependent-samples t test/repeated-measures ANOVA is sample size. We just saw that the power of our test of the effect of teacher-models on milk consumption was only .53, less than the minimum standard of .80. Since power is heavily dependent on sample size, how many cases would we need to have an 80% or a 95% chance of being able to reject the null hypothesis?

You'll be pleased to know that the answer to this question is straightforward: I have made a table, Appendix Table 12, that displays the sample sizes necessary to have powers of .80 and .95 for a two-tailed dependent-samples t test/repeated-measures ANOVA with α set at .05. Table 11.16 displays a section of this table.

To use this table, one finds the row for d, the effect size (calculated via Equation 11.6), and then reads n from the column for the power that one wants. For the milk-consumption data, I had calculated $d = 1.28$. That value is not in the table, so we'll continue our "Price is Right" tradition, be conservative, and use the next lower value, 1.25. Reading across, I see

TABLE 11.16 Section of Appendix Table 12, Sample Size Needed for a Dependent-Samples t Test (Repeated-Measures ANOVA) for Power $= .80$ and $.95$, $\alpha = .05$, Two-Tailed

	POWER	
d	.80	.95
.80	15	23
.85	13	21
.90	12	19
.95	11	17
1.00	10	16
1.05	10	14
1.10	9	13
1.15	9	12
1.20	8	12
1.25	8	11
1.30	7	10

*Before you remark that the value of .53 is remarkably close to the value of .52 that I calculated via the overlapping distributions method, I should tell you that when I calculate power for this example using the exact d value of 1.28, it turns out to be .58. So, I was in the ballpark and even in the section close to my seat, but I wasn't in my exact seat.

Also, as 1.28 is closer to 1.30 than it is to 1.20, I'll admit that I let my eye wander down that column and power turns out to be .59. The value of .59 is closer to the real value of .58 and so is a better estimate. Why, then, do I use the "Price is Right," closest-without-going-over approach? Because it is conservative and gives a lower estimate of power. If, for example, you use this estimate of power to decide how many subjects you need for a replication, you'll *over*estimate the number and end up with more cases than you need. If you underestimate, you might not have enough cases when you redo the study and will be wasting your effort.

LOOKING CLOSER

that to have a power of .80, you would need eight subjects, three more than we had. If the cost of making a Type II error were greater and you wanted to have power = .95, you would need to measure 11 children under the two conditions.

Putting the Interpretation Together

It's time to write an interpretative statement for the milk-consumption experiment. We have seven facts:

1. $F (1, 4) = 8.24, p < .05$
2. $M_1 = 9.00, M_2 = 13.20$
3. 95% confidence interval: .14 to 8.26 ounces
4. $\omega^2 = .16$ (and $\hat{r} = .40$)
5. $d = 1.28$
6. $\beta = .47$ (power = .53)
7. Sample size needed to have power of .80 = 8; for power of .95, $n = 12$.

You will probably not be surprised that I focus my interpretation on the confidence interval. Though the effect size is large, the confidence interval is quite wide and comes close to representing a trivial effect on one side. Thus, I'll end up suggesting a replication of the study with a larger sample size:

> *"We conducted a study examining the effect on the milk consumption of students of having teachers eat lunch with them and model milk drinking. I obtained a random sample of five students from a single school and found that they consumed, on average, 9 ounces of milk ($\hat{s} = 6.00$) while eating lunch with no teachers present. When teachers ate lunch with these students and modeled milk consumption, the students' average milk consumption climbed to 13.20 ounces ($\hat{s} = 3.42$). I used a repeated-measures ANOVA to analyze these data and found that the increase in milk consumption with the teachers' presence was statistically significant ($F (1, 4) = 8.24, p < .05$).*
>
> *"Though the effect of teachers' presence on milk consumption was large in the present study, I want to caution against making too much of these results until they have been replicated with a larger sample. The 95% confidence interval for the size of the increase in milk consumption was quite wide, ranging from a low of only a .14-ounce increase in milk consumption to a high of over an 8-ounce increase in milk consumption. Thus, the effect could be either trivial (less than a quarter of an ounce increase) or meaningful (more than a cup more milk consumed). Having a larger sample size would provide a better estimate of the population value, narrowing the confidence interval. It would also address the 5% chance that my conclusion is in error—that I obtained an unusual sample of cases and that teacher modeling actually has no impact on milk consumption.*

"I would also suggest that the sample be more representative of the population of elementary-age children. All the children in the present study came from the same school, and it is possible that there is something special about this school, such as the type of students who attend or the relationship between the teachers and the students, that could affect the results.

"Finally, I am concerned that the observed effect may be a 'novelty' effect: that either the children are responding to the novelty of having teachers present by being on their best behavior, including drinking more milk, or the teachers are responding to the novelty of the situation by being more adamant about milk consumption. To see how powerful, and long-lasting, this effect really is, I recommend measuring the effect of teacher presence on milk consumption after several months of teacher presence, not on the first day."

PRACTICING DEPENDENT-SAMPLES *t* TEST/ REPEATED-MEASURES ANOVA

For practice, let's go through one more dependent-samples *t* test/repeated-measures ANOVA, and this time let's see what happens when the results are not statistically significant. Imagine that a pharmaceutical company has developed a new cholesterol-lowering medication and has hired our research firm to analyze the data obtained from a clinical trial. They tested the new drug, the experimental condition (E), by comparing its effectiveness to an already established drug, the control condition (C). The design of the study consisted of placing an ad in the newspaper looking for people who had elevated cholesterol and would be willing to take an experimental drug to treat it. There were 103 people who responded to the ad, but only 47 were interested after learning what the study entailed. Of these 47, only 19 met the criteria to participate. (They couldn't be taking any other medications, couldn't be cigarette smokers, couldn't be pregnant, had to be in good health otherwise, etc.) Of these 19, only 13 actually completed the study. The 13 participants were randomly assigned to receive one drug, either E or C, for 2 months. At the end of those 2 months the total cholesterol level was checked. (Cholesterol is measured in blood as mg/dL. Higher scores indicate more cholesterol, and scores above 200 are considered to indicate an elevated risk of heart attacks.) At this point everyone switched conditions and remained on the other medication for 2 months, after which the total cholesterol level was checked again. The study was then complete, and the participants were told of their cholesterol levels on both medications and allowed to choose which treatment, if any, they wished to continue. Oh, one more thing: the study was double blind, which means that while the study was underway neither the participants nor the researchers knew who was taking which medication. The results of the experiment are shown in Table 11.17.

TABLE **11.17**   **Data for Study Comparing New Treatment for Elevated Cholesterol (Experimental Group) to Standard Treatment (Control Group)**

Case	Experimental	Control	Difference
1	176	187	11
2	183	204	21
3	185	185	0
4	188	194	6
5	198	216	18
6	210	205	−5
7	210	212	2
8	211	202	−9
9	214	216	2
10	221	215	−6
11	234	243	9
12	256	270	14
13	264	258	−6
n	13	13	13
M	211.54	215.92	4.38
$\hat{s}$	27.16	26.10	9.73

NOTE: Values in table represent total cholesterol level in mg/dL.

Test

The question being asked is whether one medication, the experimental one or the control, is more effective than the other. Inspecting the means, 211.54 vs. 215.92, shows that the experimental medication does appear to work a little better than the control medication. Still, does the difference between these sample means represent a real difference between the two populations, or is it a small enough difference that sampling error could account for it?* An appropriate test to choose to answer this question, comparing the means of two dependent samples, is a dependent-samples t test. However, because the repeated-measures ANOVA apportions the variance in a way that is more useful, I'll use that instead.

Assumptions

The assumptions for the repeated measures ANOVA with only two samples are (a) dependent samples, (b) interval- or ratio-level data, (c) random samples, (d) normality, and (e) homogeneity of variance. The

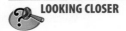

LOOKING CLOSER

*You could also think of the question being asked as whether the variability between groups is greater than the variability within groups. Makes it sound like an ANOVA, no?

first two assumptions are not violated since the samples are dependent samples and the dependent variable is measured at the ratio level. The third assumption, of random samples, pretty clearly is violated. All participants came from only one city, they were readers of newspapers, they self-identified as having high cholesterol, they were willing to receive an experimental treatment, they were not cigarette smokers, they were in good health, and they actually completed the study. This seems to be a very select group from the larger population of people with elevated cholesterol, and we must bear that in mind when it is time to interpret the results. Though the third assumption has been violated, repeated-measures ANOVA is robust to this as long as we remember the limitations.

The fourth and fifth assumptions, normality and homogeneity of variance, are not violated. I calculated the 95% confidence intervals for skewness and kurtosis for cholesterol level for both treatments, and all the confidence intervals capture zero, suggesting that the underlying populations are normally distributed. And, as the two standard deviations are very close to each other, the homogeneity of variance assumption does not appear violated.

Hypotheses

$$H_0: \ \mu_E = \mu_C$$
$$H_1: \ \mu_E \neq \mu_C$$

The null hypothesis says that, in the populations, there is no difference in the average effectiveness of the experimental and control treatments. There might be a difference between samples drawn from these populations, but the difference should be small enough that it can be accounted for by sampling error for two samples drawn from the same population. The alternative hypothesis says that the two treatments are differentially effective, that one is more effective than the other. That difference will be reflected in the means of samples drawn from the populations, and the difference between sample means will be too large to be explained by sampling error.

Decision Rule

We are willing to make a Type I error 5% of the time, so the critical value of F with 1 and 12 degrees of freedom is 4.7472. If $F_{observed} \geq 4.7472$, we'll reject H_0; if $F_{observed} < 4.7472$, we'll fail to reject H_0.

Before proceeding further with the study we want to check whether the sample size provides adequate power. The difference between the two means of 4.38 can be used as an estimate of the distance between the two population means. We can divide this by the standard deviation of the

TABLE **11.18** **ANOVA Summary Table for Cholesterol Data**

Source	SS	df	MS	F
Subjects	16,458.62	12	1371.55	
Treatment	124.96	1	124.96	2.64
Residual	567.54	12	47.29	
Total	17,151.12	25		

difference scores to find the effect size, *d,* for these results. Table 11.16 shows the difference scores for the 13 cases and that $\hat{s}_D$ is 9.7257. Thus,

$$d = \frac{4.3846}{9.7257} = .4508 = .45.$$

Using Appendix Table 11, we find that with *n* = 13 and *d* set at .40 (I'm using *d* = .40 because the actual value, .45, is not in Table 11), the power is .26. If the effect size in the population is .40 and we have only 13 cases, we have only about a 25% chance of drawing a sample that will yield enough of a difference to result in rejecting the null hypothesis. Looking *d* = .45 up in Appendix Table 12, we see that to have an 80% chance of finding this 4.38 point difference a statistically significant difference, the client needs more participants in the study, *n* should be 41. If I want to have a 95% chance of rejecting the null hypothesis, then *n* should be 67.

Unfortunately, the pharmaceutical company did not consult us in advance of doing the study; they have already collected all the data, and they do not want to reopen enrollment. We warn the client that this study is underpowered and that unless the sample size is dramatically increased they stand a good chance of finding that the new medication is no more effective than the standard treatment even if it really is more effective.*

Calculations

Here are the sums of squares for the data: SS_{total} = 17,151.1154, $SS_{subjects}$ = 16,458.6154, $SS_{treatment}$ = 124.9615, $SS_{residual}$ = 567.5385. The ANOVA summary table is shown in Table 11.18.

Since $F_{observed}$ of 2.64 is less than F_{cv} of 4.75, I'll fail to reject the null hypothesis and report my results as *F* (1, 12) = 2.64, *p* > .05.

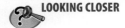 **LOOKING CLOSER**

*Note, that the question of sample size is a question of statistical significance, not of practical significance. If the researcher were to increase the sample size and maintain the 4.38 difference between the two means, there is a reasonable chance that the researcher would find statistical significance. But, that does not mean that the 4.38 point increase in effectiveness of the experimental medication over the control medication is a clinically meaningful improvement, that it would be worth the extra cost or side effects if the new treatment were more costly or had a different side effect profile.

Interpretation

I know that we failed to reject the null hypothesis, that we found that the difference between the two sample means is not statistically significant; however, now I need to interpret, or explain this. Before I start doing any calculations, let me think about what I'll want to know. Given a lack of statistical significance, I'll still want to calculate a 95% confidence interval so that I can get some idea of how far from zero it reaches (i.e., how big the effect might be) and how tight the interval is. In Step 4 we calculated how many cases were needed, and I already calculated power. So, if I add the 95% confidence interval to what I've done, I think I'll have enough for an interpretation.

Using Equation 11.5, I calculate:

$$95\% \ CI \ = \ |211.5385 - 215.9231| \pm 2.1788 \sqrt{\frac{2 \times 47.2945}{13}}$$
$$= \ 4.3846 \pm (2.1788 \times 2.6974) \ = \ 4.3846 \pm 5.8771$$

Thus, the confidence interval ranges from −1.49 to 10.26. I already calculated power as .26, which means that we had a 74% chance of making a Type II error. I think that I have everything I need to write my interpretation.

"We analyzed the data for a study in which the effectiveness of a new cholesterol-lowering medication was investigated by comparing it to a standard treatment. Thirteen participants with elevated cholesterol were solicited via newspaper advertisements, met criteria for participation, and completed the study. In a double-blind study, each participant took one medicine for 2 months and then switched to the other medicine for 2 months. Cholesterol level was measured at the end of each 2-month period.

"Though the study showed that there was no statistically significant difference between the two treatments (F [1, 12] = 2.64, p < .05), the results are inconclusive since the study had too few subjects and was underpowered. If the observed effect of the new drug (an additional 4-point reduction in cholesterol level) were real, then a study with this few subjects would have only a 26% chance of finding the effect statistically significant. To phrase that a different way, there are almost three chances out of four that the conclusion from the current study is in error.

"Before concluding that the new treatment offers no increase in effectiveness over the old treatment, I suggest replicating the study with a larger sample size. Following 41 cases instead of 13 would give the study less than a 20% chance of failing to find a statistically significant difference if one at the current level existed. If one wishes to reduce the chance of error to 5%, then 67 cases should be followed. Of course, finding that an effect is statistically significant does not mean it would be a clinically meaningful effect.

"In addition, though this may not be feasible, I recommend that the researchers try to increase the representativeness of the sample to the population of people with elevated cholesterol levels. In order to participate in this study a person had to see the advertisement in the newspaper, call to learn more about the study, come in for an interview, meet the screening criteria (e.g., not smoke cigarettes, be in good health otherwise), wish to continue with the study, and actually complete the study. I understand why the researchers used this methodology and I'm not sure how else to proceed, but I do want to point out that these constraints limit the generalizability of the results to other healthy, motivated, organized people with high cholesterol."

Group Practice 11.4

Every year, especially in rural areas of the United States, people are killed by trains at railroad crossings. A public health researcher decided to try to reduce these deaths by increasing driver safety at railroad crossings. He decided to focus his efforts on 20 small towns throughout America, small towns that he selected because there was a nearby railroad crossing. For a 1-week period he hid a camera near the rail crossing and tallied the percentage of cars that came to a full stop at the rail crossing before proceeding. He then initiated a public safety campaign advocating greater railroad crossing safety that used billboards, newspaper articles and ads, radio ads, speakers at the high school, and increased police presence at the rail crossing. The intervention lasted for 6 months. Then, for a second 1-week period, 1 year after the first, he positioned his camera near the rail crossing and again tallied the percentage of cars that came to a full stop at the crossing before proceeding. His data, which he planned to analyze with a dependent-samples *t* test/repeated-measures ANOVA are shown below. Complete and interpret the analysis. (NOTE: Sums of squares are given below the table.)

Time 1	Time 2	Difference score
88	90	
54	67	
66	73	
78	80	
59	66	
89	90	
93	92	
69	73	
78	81	
91	90	
67	73	
68	75	
78	81	
84	86	
77	83	
79	84	
$M = 75.7500$	$M = 79.9500$	$M = 4.2000$
$s = 11.1887$	$s = 8.2005$	$s = 3.4000$
$\hat{s} = 11.4794$	$\hat{s} = 8.4135$	$\hat{s} = 3.4883$
skewness = −.3624	skewness = −.2364	skewness = .7520
kurtosis = −.7920	kurtosis = −1.0644	kurtosis = .3688

$SE_{skewness} = .5477$, $SE_{kurtosis} = 1.0954$
$SS_{subjects} = 3733.1000$, $SS_{treatment} = 176.4000$, and $SS_{residual} = 115.6000$.

Time 1	Time 2
76	78
87	90
56	66
78	81

SUMMARY

Researchers often ask complex questions, questions that involve more than one independent or grouping variable. When such questions involve a dependent variable that is measured at the interval or ratio level, the statistical test used to answer them is the factorial analysis of variance. Factorial ANOVA partitions the variability found in the dependent variable into (a) that due to each independent or grouping variable by itself, and (b) that due to the interaction of the independent or grouping variables. When the interaction has a statistically significant effect, our interest in the effect of each independent or grouping variable by itself, each main effect by itself, diminishes, since the effect of each variable depends on the other. Using an example from this chapter, the answer to the question of whether boys are more aggressive than girls depends on whether you are talking about physical or verbal aggression.

The concept of partitioning variance into components that I introduced with factorial ANOVA can be applied to situations with dependent samples, where, for example, a dependent variable is measured at multiple points in time for a sample of cases. In such a situation, we are not interested in variability due to individual differences among the cases since we already know that individual differences exist. Rather, we want a measure of the variability due to changes over time (commonly called the treatment effect) that is uncontaminated by individual differences. This statistical technique, when applied to an interval- or ratio-level dependent variable, is called repeated-measures ANOVA.

When interpreting a repeated-measures ANOVA, focus first on whether there is a statistically significant treatment effect and then on the size of the effect (ω^2). If the effect is statistically significant, explore, using a post-hoc test, to find out which pair(s) of means differ. Confidence intervals can also be calculated to show how large (or small) the effect may be in the population. Unfortunately, when there are three or more samples in the repeated-measures ANOVA, calculating power and sample size are beyond our scope.

Independent-samples tests and dependent-samples tests often address slightly different questions (does one store have items that are more expensive than another vs. do these two stores have comparable prices for the same items), but sometimes they can be used to address the same question. In situations in which either test can be used, dependent-samples tests have the advantage of being more powerful, of making it easier to reject the null hypothesis, because they generate sampling distributions of the test statistic that have less variability.

In situations in which there are two dependent samples and an interval- or ratio-level dependent variable, most statisticians' thoughts turn to a dependent-samples t test. However, you can use a repeated-measures ANOVA instead, and I advocate doing so. Doing so has an important advantage: repeated-measures ANOVA provides an estimate of the amount of variance in the dependent variable that is accounted for by the independent or grouping variable that is not inflated by the variability due to individual differences.

Assumptions, hypotheses, and the decision rule must all be considered when using dependent-samples t tests or repeated-measures ANOVA. The interpretation of a dependent-samples t test/repeated-measures ANOVA is simpler than the interpretation of a repeated-measures ANOVA with three or more samples, since there is only one pair of means about which to be concerned. Thus, if the F ratio is statistically significant there is no need for post-hoc tests to decide which pair of means account for the statistically significant difference when using repeated-measures ANOVA in place of a dependent-samples t test. We learned how to calculate the 95% confidence interval for the difference, how to calculate the percentage of variance accounted for by the grouping variable, how to calculate the effect size d, and how to use d to calculate power, as well as the sample size needed to have adequate power. But remember that d calculated for a dependent-samples test cannot be interpreted the same way as d can be for an independent-samples test.

Review Exercises

1. For each scenario, write out the research question and select the appropriate statistical test.

   a. An orthopedic surgeon classifies his patients with chronic back pain into two categories, those with and those without an apparent physical cause for their pain. He randomly divides each group in half and then conducts either surgery A or surgery B on their backs. He measures the outcome of the different types of surgeries on the different types of patients by administering an interval-level scale, the Level of Back Pain Inventory, after they have recovered from surgery.

   b. A researcher divides first-graders into three groups: those whose families never or almost never eat dinner together, those whose families almost always eat dinner together, and those whose families fall somewhere in the middle. She then waits 12 years and finds out whether the first-graders completed high school.

   c. A researcher finds out how many of a child's biological parents and grandparents attended college and, based on this, divides the children into three groups. The groups are (a) zero biological parents or grandparents attended college, (b) one or two attended college, or (c) three to six attended college. He then compares high-school grade point averages (GPAs) for the three groups.

   d. To see how lung capacity affects exercise endurance, a researcher measures the lung capacity (how much air the lungs can contain) of a random sample of young adults and measures how many steps they can climb on a step climber before they feel out of breath.

   e. A researcher finds second-generation Americans, first-generation Americans, and recent immigrants and matches them in terms of age, gender, and IQ. She then examines each person's tax return to find his or her adjusted gross income from the previous year.

2. A researcher interviews people regarding their perception of the degree of racism in the United States. He uses an interval-level scale, where higher scores indicate a greater perceived level of racism in U.S. society. The samples are randomly chosen from people of European descent, African descent, and Mexican descent. Half of each group hold white collar jobs, and half hold blue collar jobs. With all ns equal, here are the data:

	European Descent	African Descent	Mexican Descent
Blue Collar	12	24	22
White Collar	10	28	26

   Calculate marginal and grand means, graph the data, and speculate about main effects and interactions in an interpretative statement.

3. A gastroenterologist obtains a sample of people with gastroesophageal reflux disease (GERD) from her own practice and matches them into quadruplets in terms of symptom severity. She then randomly assigns each of the four people in each group to receive either (a) dietary change therapy, (b) medication, (c) acupuncture, or (d) a waiting-list control status. (Waiting-list control group members are told that the treatment groups are filled and that they will receive treatment when room opens up.) After 8 weeks of treatment (or 8 weeks of waiting-list time), the gastroenterologist measures symptoms using the GERD Symptom Severity Scale (GERD SSS). The GERD SSS is an interval-level scale that measures symptom severity for gastroesophageal reflux disease on a scale running from 0 (no symptoms) to 50 (extremely debilitating symptoms).

   Here is the information from the four groups. Using the six-step hypothesis testing procedure, complete the analysis and write an interpretative statement.

Diet	Medication	Acupuncture	Waiting List
M			
33.5556	28.2222	38.7778	40.0000
$\hat{s}$			
9.2751	6.4957	4.7376	5.6569
n			
9	9	9	9
Skewness			
−.5529	−.2269	−.0177	−.7866
Kurtosis			
−.8239	−1.1824	−1.2128	.5140

$SS_{subjects} = 1051.5556$, $SS_{treatment} = 784.9722$,
$SS_{total} = 2246.3056$

4. A political scientist is interested in the impact that college has on the political beliefs of children of conservative parents. He obtains a sample of adults who (a) define themselves as politically conservative and (b) are large donors to conservative causes. When the children of these parents are seniors in high school, she administers to them (the children) the Political Beliefs Inventory (PBI). The PBI consists of 75 items that a person can agree with or disagree with. The items are scored so that each item a person endorses in a conservative direction scores 1 point. Thus, scores on the PBI can range from 0 (ultraliberal) to 75 (ultraconservative). Four years later, she readministers the PBI as the 25 students are about to graduate from college.

The means (and estimated population standard deviations) at T1 and T2, respectively, are as follows: 61.7600 (9.4529) and 60.480 (10.7243) and $\hat{s}_D$ =2.4583. $SS_{subjects}$ is 4832.2800, $SS_{residual}$ is 72.5200, and SS_{total} is 4925.2800. (By the bye, at T1 skewness [SE] and kurtosis [SE] are −.638 [.464] and −.688 [.902]; at T2 they are −.673 [.464] and −.415 [.902] as calculated by SPSS.)

Analyze and interpret these data using the six-step hypothesis testing procedure.

Homework Problems

1. A researcher is analyzing some data using dependent-samples t tests. For one set of data the correlation between the T1 and T2 variable is .6, and for another set of data the correlation is .4. Assuming that everything else remains the same, for which data set is power greater?
   a. $r = .4$
   b. $r = .6$
   c. If the two variables are correlated, then a dependent-samples t test should not be used.
   d. Degree of correlation does not affect power.
2. When conducting a factorial ANOVA, a researcher finds that the row effect is statistically significant and the column effect is statistically significant. Regarding the interaction effect, this
   a. Means that it must be statistically significant.
   b. Means that it must not be statistically significant.
   c. Gives no information about the statistical significance of the interaction effect.
3. When a repeated-measures ANOVA is used in place of a dependent-samples t test, the amount of variability in the dependent variable that is accounted for by the independent variable (the grouping variable) is
   a. The effect size d
   b. Contaminated by the row effect of individual differences
   c. Larger than it should be
   d. All of the above
   e. None of the above
4. The Fisher LSD is a liberal post-hoc test. This means that if two means are found to be statistically different by the Fisher LSD,
   a. The omnibus F is not significant.
   b. The omnibus F is significant.

c. A conservative post-hoc test would also find the two means to have a statistically significant difference between the two means.

d. A conservative post-hoc test would not find the two means to have a statistically significant difference.

e. A conservative post-hoc test might find a statistically significant difference between the two means.

5. If the interaction effect in a factorial ANOVA is statistically significant, then
   a. The main effects should not be interpreted, whether they are statistically significant or not.
   b. The effect of the row variable depends on the level of the column variable.
   c. The effect of the column variable depends on the level of the row variable.
   d. All of the above hold.
   e. None of the above hold.

6. A psychologist obtains random samples of 15 alcoholics and of 15 people who have never touched a drop of alcohol and randomly divides each sample into thirds. He tells one of the three groups that they will receive no alcohol and gives them a nonalcoholic beverage. He tells the second group that they will receive a small dose of alcohol (equivalent to the amount of alcohol in 12 ounces of beer), but gives them a non-alcoholic beverage. He tells the third group that he will give them a small dose of alcohol and actually does give them a dose of alcohol equivalent to 12 ounces of beer. Thus, he manipulates two things: what people expect to receive and what they actually do receive. After the manipulation, he waits a sufficient time for the alcohol to take effect and then measures the dependent variable (how much effect the alcohol has had) by measuring postural stability—having participants walk along a narrow, straight line. The more they fall off the line, the worse their postural stability and the higher their scores. Scores can range from 0 to 100 where 0 represents a perfect score (they did not fall off the line at all) and 100 represents not being able to stay on the line at all. Below are the data. Calculate marginal and grand means, graph the data, and speculate about main effects and interactions in an interpretative statement.

	Expect No Alcohol, Receive No Alcohol	Expect Alcohol, Receive Placebo	Expect Alcohol, Receive Alcohol
Alcoholics	6	8	10
Teetotalers	4	30	50

7. For each scenario, write out the research question and select the statistical test appropriate to analyze the data.
   a. A political scientist takes a sample of undecided voters and after the presidential election is over classifies them as having voted for the Democratic or Republican candidate for president of the United States. He is curious as to the impact on subsequent voting behavior of having made a decision about which party to support. Thus, 4 years later, after the next presidential election, he contacts these voters again and finds out which candidate, Democratic or Republican, they supported.
   b. A researcher from the National Highway Traffic Safety Administration (NHTSA) takes a sample of motorcyclists and administers to them an ordinal scale that measures the personality dimension of obedience to authority. She compares their scores on this scale to the known value for the U.S. population.
   c. She takes her sample of motorcyclists and divides them into two groups: those who wear helmets and those who don't. She compares the two groups in terms of scores on the obedience-to-authority scale.
   d. The NHTSA researcher takes her motorcyclists and divides them into two groups, high vs. low scorers on the obedience-to-authority scale. Using this dichotomy and the

dichotomy of helmet wearing, she ends up with four groups (high obedience and helmet, high obedience and no helmet, etc.) She compares the four groups in terms of scores on an interval-level IQ scale.

e. Finally, the traffic safety researcher divides the motorcyclists into four groups based on the size of the engines on their motorcycles: small, medium, large, and very large. She compares the groups in terms of obedience to authority.

8. For each scenario, write out the research question and select the statistical test appropriate to analyze the data.

a. A nutritionist asks people what their favorite food is and divides them into three categories: protein (e.g., steak), carbohydrates (e.g., bread), and sweets (e.g., ice cream). He compares people in the three groups in terms of body mass index.

b. A nurse gets a group of overweight adults and matches them into groups of three based on body mass index. She then randomly assigns them into three groups, making sure that one member of each triplet is assigned to each group. One group serves as the control group, and two groups are experimental groups. She encourages one experimental group to lose weight; the other experimental group is encouraged to exercise. Six months later she measures systolic blood pressure in all subjects.

c. A teacher takes a group of third-graders, matches them in terms of IQ, and then randomly assigns them either to (a) first-year teachers, (b) experienced teachers, or (c) teachers who are about to retire. At the end of the year, he compares the third-graders for the different teachers in terms of an interval-level measure of academic achievement.

d. At the end of the year this teacher-researcher asks the third-graders to rank, on an ordinal-level scale, how much they liked their teachers. He's curious as to how this affects the amount the students learned as measured on the interval-level measure of academic achievement. (For this analysis the researcher is lumping all the students together into one group and disregarding what type of teacher each had.)

e. Continuing with those third-graders... Before the school year started, the teacher-researcher had asked the students' previous teachers to classify them into three groups (poised to take off and do really well, likely to continue as before, likely to get into trouble) so that he could see how that predicts future performance. Based on how much the students learned during the next year (the third grade), he puts them into three categories: those who blossomed, those who were unchanged, and those who fell behind. What is the relation between the teachers' predictions and the students' actual performance?

9. Reporters at a college newspaper decide to investigate bookstore prices at the on-campus bookstore vs. at an on-line bookstore. They obtain typical courses for first-semester students, randomly select books from these courses, and find the prices for the books at the two stores. For the on-line store, they include the price of shipping and handling, dividing it equally among the 12 books purchased.

Below are the data they obtain. Analyze these data using the six-step hypothesis testing procedure, and write a complete interpretative statement.

On-Campus	On-Line
49.95	39.83
7.89	6.76
89.95	85.43
35.95	34.78
19.95	12.78
27.95	25.13
104.99	78.96

On-Campus	On-Line
79.99	54.78
45.49	44.67
13.95	9.95
35.89	33.34
65.95	55.87
$M = 48.1583$	$M = 40.1900$
$\hat{s} = 31.0599$	$\hat{s} = 25.4327$
skewness (SE) = .563 (.637)	skewness (SE) = .454 (.637)
kurtosis (SE) = −.740 (1.232)	kurtosis (SE) = −.546 (1.232)

$SS_{subjects} = 17,296.5239$, $SS_{treatment} = 380.9660$, $SS_{total} = 18,107.8930$, $\hat{s}_D = 8.8462$.

NOTE: Skewness and kurtosis were calculated in SPSS.

10. A researcher wants to know how the price of gas and the fuel economy of cars affects driving behavior. She gets a large sample of adults from a metropolitan area and matches them into triplets based on (a) the score on an environmental-consciousness scale, (b) their age, (c) their gender, and (d) annual mileage driven. She then randomly assigns them, within each triplet, to receive either (1) a fuel-efficient hybrid (Toyota Prius, estimated miles-per-gallon [est mpg] 60 city/51 highway, (2) a normal sedan (Toyota Camry, est mpg 24/34), or (3) a fuel-inefficient SUV (Toyota 4Runner, est mpg 17/21). (Yes, this research is funded by Toyota.) Each person is given use of the car for a year, but must pay for the gas and routine maintenance. At the end of the year, the researcher notes how many miles each person has driven. To make the data easier to work with, she reports them as thousands of miles (i.e., the first person in the Prius column, for example, with a value of 17.189, drove 17,189 miles.) Here are the data:

Prius	Camry	4Runner
17.189	17.123	15.679
13.234	12.989	11.231
7.896	8.123	6.876
11.175	10.932	9.812
23.145	22.134	19.341
13.145	14.811	9.861
12.452	12.348	11.234
17.834	17.683	15.121
13.452	12.678	9.871
17.638	17.123	14.321
12.381	11.678	9.836
9.542	8.995	7.619
$M = 14.0902$	$M = 13.8848$	$M = 11.7335$
$s = 4.0144$	$s = 3.8689$	$s = 3.4989$
$\hat{s} = 4.1929$	$\hat{s} = 4.0410$	$\hat{s} = 3.5645$
skewness (SE) = .742 (.637)	skewness (SE) = .552 (.637)	skewness (SE) = .774 (.637)
kurtosis (SE) = .636 (1.232)	kurtosis (SE) = .010 (1.232)	kurtosis (SE) = .086 (1.232)

$SS_{subjects} = 510.1248$, $SS_{treatment} = 40.8975$, $SS_{total} = 560.8129$.

NOTE: Skewness and kurtosis were calculated in SPSS.

Analyze and interpret these data using the six-step hypothesis testing procedure. (Reporting the data in terms of thousands of miles driven makes them easier to work with for calculating an ANOVA, but it makes the interpretation of results a little trickier.)

12

The Chi-Square Test for Contingency Tables

Learning Objectives

___

After completing this chapter, you should be able to do the following:

1 Decide when to select a chi-square test for contingency tables and differentiate between the chi-square test of association and the chi-square difference test.

2 Evaluate the assumptions, explain the hypotheses, state the decision rule, and evaluate the adequacy of the sample size for the chi-square test for contingency tables.

3 Calculate and report a chi-square value for the chi-square test for contingency tables.

4 Interpret the results from a chi-square test for contingency tables, including the direction, size (*95% CI, r, d*), and power of the effect.

5 For clinical research studies, be able to calculate and interpret the relative risk ratio and the number needed to treat.

I've mentioned the chi-square test both in Chapter 7 as a relationship test and in Chapter 9 as a difference test. Now, at last, we get to calculate and interpret it, to see how one test wears two hats.

The chi-square test has a generic name, the chi-square test for contingency tables, and is used in two different situations. In one situation, when it is called the chi-square test of association, there is one sample of cases on which two nominal variables are measured to see if they are related. For example, we may compare grades (passing vs. failing) on the first and second tests in a class, to see if performance on the first test predicts performance on the second. In another situation, when it is called the chi-square difference test, we have two or more groups being compared to see if they differ in the proportion of each group that possesses some nominal variable. For example, we may compare final grades in a class, passing vs. failing, for males and females, to see if one gender performed better than the other. In the first scenario, the chi-square is a nominal-level corollary to the Pearson r, and in the second it is a nominal-level corollary to the independent-samples t test. The chi-square test, whether a difference test or a relationship test, is called a nonparametric test, a test that makes no assumptions about normality or homogeneity of variance, a test that can be used with a nominal-level dependent variable.

I like the chi-square and have placed it in this chapter because it reminds us that statistics compares what is actually observed to what would be expected if the null hypothesis were true. The chi-square is more transparent in this regard than the other tests, because in the process of calculating a chi-square value we actually compute the expected values and directly calculate how discrepant they are from the observed values.

Here are a few sights to pay special attention to as we proceed through this chapter:

- Note that the chi-square test for contingency tables can be either a difference test or a relationship test. This fluidity leads into the next chapter when I further blur the lines between relationship tests and difference tests.
  - One new interpretative device we'll encounter turns a correlation coefficient into the effect size d.
    - We'll also encounter two clinically relevant interpretation options: the relative risk ratio (*RR*) and the number needed to treat (*NNT*). The *RR* tells how much more likely a bad outcome is for the control group than for the experimental group. The *NNT* is a measure of improvement in outcome for the treatment group over the control group.

I've always had a soft spot in my heart for the chi-square test for contingency tables, what is almost always just called chi-square, because it was the first statistical test that I understood. The chi-square was clear to me because to arrive at it we calculate the expected values and compare them to observed values, and then use the discrepancy between the two as the test statistic. The bigger the discrepancy between observed and expected, the bigger the chi-square value and the more likely we are to reject the null hypothesis. Thus, the whole notion that statistics is about comparing observed to expected, about comparing what you *actually have* to what you would *expect to have* if the null hypothesis were true, became clear to me with the chi-square test.

I also like chi-square because it is a wallflower. It is a less powerful test and stands around the periphery of the statistical dance floor, hoping that someone will ask it to dance. Most people don't see its beauty and don't ask it out. But it sits there patiently, and when the flashier tests fail, when their assumptions aren't met, you can always count on chi-square to step in and help you safely navigate the dance floor. For a dependable good time, call chi-square.

Most textbooks relegate chi-square to the final chapter, grouped with other **nonparametric statistical tests.*** It is not placed at the back as a capstone, but as an oh-by-the-bye-we're-out-of-time-but-here-are-a-bunch-of-other-less-important-tests-you-should-know-about section. So, when I set out to write a statistics text, my number-one rule was that I would put chi-square in its rightful spot, in the place of honor, right up front as the first null hypothesis significance test taught. And yet, here we are with chi-square in the next-to-last chapter. What happened?

You'll be pleased to know that chi-square has not fallen out of my favor. (It is the only statistical test whose formula I have memorized.) But, as I wrote the text, I realized that covering correlation first was a good idea, and that focusing on the Pearson product moment correlation coefficient as my example would provide a base for the interpretation of the other tests that we would encounter. When I moved to difference tests, it made more sense to focus on the *t* test, not the chi-square, since the *t* is one of the most commonly used tests in statistics. After two sample tests it made sense to move to multiple-sample tests like analysis of variance—and once again chi-square was usurped. Chi-square just wasn't fitting in, and that wasn't acceptable.

I've resolved this by putting chi-square in the penultimate chapter, not as an oh-by-the-way sort of thing, but in fact as a capstone. Chi-square provides a fresh way of looking at statistics, a clear way of seeing the logic of comparing observed to expected and deciding if the discrepancy between them is too great to be due to sampling error. In addition, chi-square nicely blurs the line between relationship tests and difference tests. So, you'll be prepared in the next chapter, when I provide a

nonparametric statistical test

A statistical test that does not require assumptions about the normality of the distribution of the dependent variable in the population.

parametric statistical test

A statistical test that does require assumptions about the normality of the distribution of the dependent variable in the population.

---

*A nonparametric test is one for which assumptions about the shape of the distribution of the dependent variable don't have to be met. As used here, a parameter concerns the distribution of a set of data, like whether it is normally distributed. All of the tests that I've mentioned that are used when the dependent variable is ordinal- or nominal-level, tests like the Spearman *r* or the Mann Whitney *U*, are nonparametric tests. Nonparametric tests used to be called "assumption-free" tests, but that is a misnomer. They do have assumptions that must be met before they can be used, but fewer and less restrictive assumptions than **parametric statistical tests.** They just don't require that the data set be normally distributed.

LOOKING CLOSER

flowchart that leads you through the "what test when" decision making process, a flowchart that does not distinguish between relationship tests and difference tests. Without further ado, then, let's move to the test that I've been wanting to write about since I started thinking about this book: the statistical love of my life, chi-square.

DEFINING AND USING THE CHI-SQUARE TEST FOR CONTINGENCY TABLES

The "chi-square test for contingency tables" is a mouthful of a name. It gets even more confusing since almost no one ever uses the formal name, preferring just to call it chi-square. Further, even though there are two versions of the chi-square test for contingency tables, a difference test and a relationship test, the actual statistic is calculated via the same formula. So, let me first explain what a contingency table is, and then explain the two different versions of chi-square.*

A contingency table is a matrix that displays the frequency with which two variables *co-occur*. For example, imagine conducting a study in which you randomly assign students to read the textbook either before or after the lecture and then measure whether the students pass or fail the course. Table 12.1 shows the co-occurrence of a passing grade for the class with when the students read the text. This is called a contingency table because the frequency in each cell is *contingent on*, depends on, both of the variables. The 15 people in the upper left-hand corner cell are in that cell because they *both* read the text before the lecture *and* passed the course.

I trust that you recognize this situation—is there a difference in performance based on when the text is read—as a difference test, with the independent variable being when the text is read (before vs. after lecture) and the dependent variable being whether the course is passed or failed. These data should be analyzed with a chi-square test, since the dependent variable is measured at the nominal level. We'll call this kind of chi-square a **chi-square difference test.** The chi-square difference test is analogous to an independent-samples *t* test, but with a nominal-level dependent variable.

The other type of chi-square is analogous to a Pearson product moment correlation coefficient, but with both the predictor and criterion variables measured at the nominal level. We'll call this a **chi-square test of association.** For the chi-square test of association there is *one* sample of cases, whereas for the chi-square difference test there are *two independent* samples. An example of data appropriate for a chi-square association test would be looking at the relationship between performance on the first

TABLE **12.1**   **Example of a Contingency Table for a Chi-Square Difference Test**

	Pass Course	Fail Course
Read text before	15	6
Read text after	17	3

chi-square difference test

A chi-square test for contingency tables used when comparing two or more independent samples on a nominal-level dependent variable.

chi-square test of association

A chi-square test for contingency tables used when examining the relationship, in a sample, between two nominal-level variables.

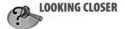 **LOOKING CLOSER**

*And to confuse things even more, there is another chi-square test called the chi-square goodness-of-fit test, abbreviated χ^2 GOF. The χ^2 GOF is a one sample test that compares how a nominal-level variable is distributed in a sample to how it is distributed in a population.

exam in a class, scored as pass or fail, and final grade in the class, scored as pass or fail. Such a contingency table is shown in Table 12.2.

The difference between the two chi-square tests lies in their assumptions. The chi-square difference test requires independent samples whereas the chi-square test of association does not (Sheskin, 2004).* Beyond that, the two tests are calculated in exactly the same fashion and are, in a sense, interchangeable. We could interpret the chi-square test that asks if course outcome differs depending on when a person reads the text, before vs. after lecture, as asking if there is a *relationship* between when one reads the text and how much one learns. We could interpret the chi-square test that asks if there is a relationship between performance on the first test and course grade, as asking if there is a difference in final course grade between people who passed and those who failed the first test.

The chi-square test for contingency tables is used with nominal-level variables or with variables that have been scaled back to the nominal level. For the chi-square test of association, both variables are at the nominal level. For the chi-square difference test, the dependent variable is at the nominal level. The variable other than the dependent variable for chi-square difference test can be a real independent variable, one where the researcher controls the experimental manipulation, or it can be a grouping variable (like gender), or it can be a predictor variable as in a correlation. For simplicity's sake, I'm going to call it an independent variable when I am speaking in general.

Theoretically the independent variable or the predictor variable is not limited in terms of how many levels it can have; but practically, chi-square works better when there are a small number of categories. Thus, though the chi-square could be used to compare outcome (good vs. bad) for 20 different doses of a drug, it is very likely that such an analysis would run into sample size problems for some of the cells. In addition, the results could be hard to interpret. If it made sense to collapse the categories of dose into a smaller number (e.g., zero, low, medium, and high) the chi-square would proceed more smoothly.[†]

TABLE **12.2** **Example of a Contingency Table for a Chi-Square Test of Association**

	Pass Course	Fail Course
Pass first test	14	2
Fail first test	4	4

NULL HYPOTHESIS SIGNIFICANCE TESTING WITH CHI-SQUARE FOR CONTINGENCY TABLES

Let's come up with some data to use in exploring the chi-square test. I'm going to use data appropriate for a chi-square difference test, but except for one assumption the chi-square difference test is exactly the same as the

---

*Sheskin, D. J. (2004). *Handbook of parametric and nonparametric statistical procedures*. Boca Raton, FL: Chapman & Hall/CRC.

[†]There are a number of different ways that these data could be analyzed without losing information by reducing the number of dose levels. One option would be to turn the outcome variable (good vs. bad) into the grouping variable and then compare the mean dose for the two groups with a *t* test. Another option would be to use a test mentioned in passing in the *t* test chapter, the point biserial correlation coefficient.

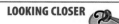

LOOKING CLOSER

chi-square test of association. This sounds more confusing than it is, so trust me and read on.

Lung cancer is a disease for which, at present, there is not a particularly effective treatment. The mortality rate for lung cancer is high; fewer than 15% of lung cancer patients survive 5 years after diagnosis. Let's imagine that a researcher has developed a new treatment that he hopes will improve outcomes. The researcher contacts 200 people in his medical center who were recently diagnosed with lung cancer and, after being informed of the risks and benefits of the study, 150 agree to participate. For each person the researcher flips a coin, and 81 are assigned to receive the experimental treatment. The other 69 are in the control condition and receive the current standard treatment. Thus treatment, experimental vs. control, is the independent variable. A year later the researcher finds out which patients are alive; in other words, his dependent variable is mortality. The outcome data, arrayed in a two-by-two matrix, are shown in Table 12.3.

Looking at the table it looks like more people who have the experimental treatment are alive a year later than are people who receive the control treatment (60% vs. 42%). However, by now I hope you recognize that random sampling error could account for such a distribution even if there were no difference in the population. We need to do a statistical test to figure out what is going on. So, let's march through Tom and Harry.

TABLE **12.3**   **One-Year Outcome Data, Lung Cancer Treatment Study**

	Alive	Dead
Experimental treatment	49	32
Control treatment	29	40

Test

Our research question is whether there is a *difference* in survival rate between experimental and control treatments for lung cancer. We have two independent groups, experimental treatment and control treatment, and since we are comparing these groups on a nominal-level dependent variable, we'll use a chi-square difference test. Functionally, this is the same as a chi-square test of association, and we could phrase the research question thus: Is there a *relationship* between type of treatment and survival? However, because we have two independent groups and because our research question has the word difference in it, let's consider this a chi-square difference test.

Assumptions

For the chi-square difference test we don't worry about normality or homogeneity, but there are other assumptions with which we need to be concerned. These are the assumptions:

1. Nominal-level dependent variable (not robust to violations)
2. Independent samples (not robust to violations)
3. Random samples (robust to violations)
4. Expected frequencies in all cells ≥ 5 (not robust to violations, but fallback options exist if a violation occurs)

The first three assumptions should be familiar, but the fourth is a new one for us. Let's do the old ones first. The first assumption, that the dependent variable is measured at the nominal level, is a no-brainer since the nominal level is the lowest level of measurement. If a variable is measured, it is at least at the nominal level. For our lung cancer data, mortality is measured at the nominal level.

The second assumption sounds like an assumption from the independent-samples difference tests. In any event, the groups based on the independent variable, or the grouping variable, should be independent of each other. For the lung cancer study, the researcher randomly assigned people to receive the control or the experimental treatment, so the samples are independent.

The third assumption is a familiar one—the samples are random samples from their respective populations. And, as with previous tests, though this is an ideal for which we strive, we can still go ahead with the statistical test if we don't reach that goal. For the lung cancer data this assumption was probably violated since I gave little information about how the original 200 potential participants were obtained. Even if the original 200 had been a random sample from the medical center, the fact that not all of them agreed to participate can call into question the representativeness of the sample. And even if we could be sure that the sample of 150 was representative of lung cancer patients at the medical center, that is no guarantee that it is representative of lung cancer patients in the city, country, continent, or world. Thus, the third assumption was almost certainly violated. We can go ahead with the analyses, but when it comes time for interpretation we will need to bear these limitations in mind.

The fourth assumption says that the expected frequencies in each of the cells should be five or greater. Exactly how one determines this won't be clear until we get to the calculation step, so trust me for the moment when I say that this assumption hasn't been violated for the lung cancer data.

But, if the assumption were to be violated, there are a couple of fallback options. The lung cancer data fit in the format of a two-by-two matrix since there are two levels of the independent variable (experimental vs. control) and two levels of the dependent variable (alive vs. dead). If the no-cell-has-less-than-five-observations assumption were violated for a two-by-two matrix, then something called Yates' correction for continuity (sometimes just called Yates' correction or just the correction for continuity) could be applied.

A two-by-two matrix, or a two-by-two contingency table, is the smallest table that can be analyzed by a chi-square test for contingency tables. If one has a larger matrix, say a three-by-two—or example, three doses of a drug (high, medium, and low) by two outcomes (good vs. bad)—and the expected frequencies assumption was violated, one could collapse categories of the independent variable to yield expected frequencies greater than five in each cell. Thus, one might merge the small and medium dose categories, turning a three-by-two matrix into a two-by-two matrix.

The assumptions for the chi-square test of association are simpler than they are for the chi-square difference test. Since the chi-square test of association involves only one sample, there is no need for an assumption about independent samples. That is the only difference between the two tests! Everything else is exactly the same.

Hypotheses

Technically, the way in which you phrase your hypotheses for the chi-square depends on how you conceptualize the test, as a relationship test or a difference test.* For null hypothesis significance tests the null hypothesis, H_0, says that there is no difference between the populations or that there is zero relationship between the two variables. Even though this is the case in the *population*, when *samples* are examined a difference or a relationship may be found; however, the difference or relationship should be small enough that it can be explained by sampling error.

I find it more straightforward to conceptualize the lung cancer data as a difference test, as asking if there is a difference in mortality between the two populations. Since the dependent variable is nominal, we're not examining a mean difference (interval- or ratio-level variable) or a rank difference (ordinal-level variable), but a difference in proportion. That is, is the proportion of people who survive 1 year in the experimental group the same as the proportion of people who survive 1 year in the control group? We could write this as $p(Alive_E) = p(Alive_C)$, where p is the abbreviation for probability and the subscripts E and C stand, respectively, for experimental and control. Thus, that statement says that the probability of being alive in the experimental group is the same as the probability of being alive for the control group.

Though it would be possible to write the null and alternative hypotheses as $p(Alive_E) = p(Alive_C)$ and $p(Alive_E) \neq p(Alive_C)$, respectively, most statisticians don't do so. Instead, they avoid symbolic notation and just use English to write out the null hypothesis, saying either that one variable is independent of the other or the two variables are unrelated; the alternative hypothesis is that the two variables are not independent or the two variables are related.[†]

The null hypothesis states that in the population there is independence, or a lack of relationship, between the two variables, X and Y. For the lung

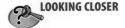

LOOKING CLOSER

*Whenever I see the word "technically," I think that the author means "this is the way things should be, but you won't get in much trouble if you ignore what you are supposed to do." And, as you are about to see, that's the case here.

[†] Another option for writing the null hypothesis of independence is as $\rho_{xy} = 0$. This should look familiar as the null hypothesis for a correlation coefficient. This works well for a chi-square test for contingency tables as long as the contingency table is a simple two-by-two matrix, but it falls apart with larger matrices unless both variables can be scaled ordinally.

cancer data X (the independent or predictor variable) is group status, and Y (the dependent variable) is mortality. Thus the null hypothesis states that in the population of lung cancer patients there is no relationship between having or not having the experimental treatment and being alive a year later, that the cases' outcomes are independent of the treatment received. This is the same as saying that there is no difference in mortality level between the two treatments and that could be the null hypothesis as well. Though either no relationship or no difference, is true in the population, it is possible that in a sample some relationship or difference would be observed; but the degree of observed relationship or difference should be small enough that it can be explained as a deviation from zero due to sampling error.

The alternative hypothesis says that there is a lack of independence, in the population, between treatment and outcome, that there is a relationship, or difference in outcome, between these two variables: the outcome one has depends, at least to some degree, on the treatment one receives. All this nondirectional hypothesis says is that the relationship is different from zero; it says nothing about the direction or the strength.* In any event, it says that there is a relationship between the two variables in the population. So, when we take a sample from the population we should expect to find a relationship between the two variables in the sample. The lack of independence, or the size of the difference, found in the sample should be far enough away from absolute independence that sampling error deviation from a population where there is independence or zero difference is not a reasonable explanation.

Decision rule

The decision rule is just like all the other decision rules we've encountered so far. We will calculate a chi-square value, $\chi^2_{observed}$, and compare it to the critical value of chi-square, χ^2_{cv}, that we have obtained from the sampling distribution of chi-square values. If $\chi^2_{observed}$ falls in the rare zone of the sampling distribution, if $\chi^2_{observed} \geq \chi^2_{cv}$, then we'll reject the null hypothesis. If $\chi^2_{observed}$ falls in the common zone of the sampling distribution, if $\chi^2_{observed} < \chi^2_{cv}$, we'll fail to reject the null hypothesis.

---

*Thus, the alternative hypothesis would be true even if there were only an infinitesimally small relationship between treatment and outcome. We're near the end of the book now, and so I want to let you in on some concerns with null hypothesis significance testing. In point of fact, the alternative hypothesis is almost always true! It is very, very rare that two variables have exactly a zero relationship in the population, and it is very, very rare that populations have means that are exactly the same. Thus, the alternative hypothesis is actually almost always true. As a result, you can think of power not just as the probability of rejecting the null when the null should be rejected, but as the probability of making the right decision. Of course, whether the effect is big enough to be meaningful is a separate question.

LOOKING CLOSER

Remember, our decisions are probabilistic, so our decision *probably* is true. But, α percentage of the time when H_0 is true, $\chi^2_{observed}$ will be greater than or equal to χ^2_{cv}, resulting in the wrong conclusion, a Type I error. And β percent of the time when H_1 is true, we'll find $\chi^2_{observed} < \chi^2_{cv}$ and we'll make a different wrong conclusion, we'll make a Type II error.

All we need to find the critical value of chi-square are the degrees of freedom and the alpha level; we don't need to worry about whether we are doing a one-tailed or a two-tailed test. Chi-square is a *squared* value, and so it is always positive. The sampling distribution starts at zero and tails off to the right. As a result, it includes both tails of the distribution in one tail; it is always a two-tailed test.

Degrees of freedom are easy to calculate for a chi-square test for contingency tables, and they don't depend on sample size. Rather, one simply counts the number of rows and columns in the contingency table, subtracts one from each, and then multiplies the two values together. This is shown in Equation 12.1.

FORMULA

Degrees of Freedom for Chi-Square Test for Contingency Tables

Equation 12.1 $df = (R - 1) \times (C - 1)$

Where:
df = degrees of freedom being calculated
R = number of rows in the contingency table
C = number of columns in the contingency table

Thus, for the lung cancer data where there are two rows (experimental vs. control) and two columns (alive vs. dead), $df = (2 - 1) \times (2 - 1) = 1$. If, for example, the dependent variable were more complex and had three options (Alive/healthy, Alive/sick, and Dead), degrees of freedom would equal $(2 - 1) \times (3 - 1) = 2$.

As always, the alpha level chosen depends on how concerned the researcher is with making a Type I error. The more concerned, the smaller the rare zone and the smaller the alpha level. My table of critical values of chi-square in the back of the book, Appendix Table 13, has five different levels of α, but the column for $\alpha = .05$ is bolded because that is the most commonly used. Table 12.4 is a section of the table of critical values of chi-square.

This table is used like the other tables of critical values. Find the critical value of chi-square, χ^2_{cv}, at the intersection of the α level column and the degrees of freedom row. Thus, for the lung cancer data where $df = 1$ and α is set at .05, $\chi^2_{cv} = 3.8415$. Figure 12.1 displays a sampling distribution of chi-square on which I have marked the critical value.

TABLE **12.4** **Section of Appendix Table 13, Critical Values of Chi-Square**

df	ALPHA LEVEL				
	.100	.050	.025	.010	.001
1	2.7055	**3.8415**	5.0239	6.6349	10.8276
2	4.6052	**5.9915**	7.3778	9.2103	13.8155
3	6.2514	**7.8147**	9.3484	11.3449	16.2662
4	7.7794	**9.4877**	11.1433	13.2767	18.4668

Notice how it separates the sampling distribution into common and rare zones.

There are a couple of observations I want to make about the table of critical values of χ^2. As in other tables, when alpha gets smaller—when the rare zone gets smaller—the critical value gets larger. This makes sense since when the rare zone is smaller, the critical value is further away from zero. What is unusual about χ^2, however, is that as the degrees of freedom become larger, the critical value becomes larger. For r, t, and F, as sample sizes got larger and df increased, the critical value became smaller. Chi-square is different. For chi-square the degrees of freedom depend on how many *cells* there are, not on how many *cases* there are. Chi-square, as we are about to see, is calculated by adding up values calculated for each cell, so as the number of cells increases, the potential sum of the values increases as well. Thus, as df increases for chi-square, χ^2_{cv} becomes larger.

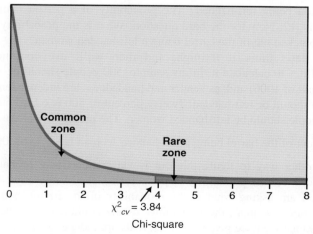

Figure **12.1** Sampling distribution of chi-square with one degree of freedom. (From Lowry, R. [2006]. *Concepts and applications of inferential statistics* [online]. Available: http://faculty.vassar.edu/lowry/webtext.html)

There is one other factor that is part of Step 4, the decision rule: think about power and whether the sample size is adequate. As with previous tests, I am going to let this lie fallow until the interpretation stage.

Calculations

For the chi-square we actually calculate the expected values to which we compare the observed values in the cells. For this to make sense, let's make a little excursion back to the world of conjunctional probability, a topic we covered in Chapter 6 when we used the example of tossing a coin multiple times to explore hypothesis testing. I hope you remember that the probability of a heads on any one toss of a fair coin is .5, and if a coin is tossed twice and the tosses are independent of each other, the probability of two heads is .25. That value of .25 is a conjunctional probability, the conjunction of the probability of a heads on the first toss and a heads on the second toss. When two events are *independent,* the probability of their conjunction is the probability of the first outcome *times* the probability of the second outcome. For a fair coin turning up heads twice in a row, this is .5 × .5 = .25.

Let me give you another example. Let's say that a person's dominant hand, left or right, and that person's gender are independent. That is, men are neither more nor less likely to be right-handed than are women. Further, let's say that exactly 50% of the people in the United States are men and 50% are women. In addition, let's say that 12% of the people in the United States are left-handed and 88% are right-handed. Now, let's imagine a random sample of 1000 people from the United States placed in a big barrel. We shake up the barrel, reach in, and pluck someone out at random. What is the probability that the person chosen is a woman? The probability of the person being a woman is .5. What is the probability of the person being left-handed? The probability of a person being left-handed is .12. Now for the hard question: What is the probability of the person plucked out of the barrel being a left-handed woman?

First let's think it through, and then we'll use conjunctional probabilities to calculate it. In my sample, 500 people should be women (that's half of 1000) and, as gender and handedness are independent, 12% of these should be left-handed. Twelve percent of 500 is 60, so 60 of the 1000 people should be left-handed women. The probability of the person I pluck out of the barrel being a left-handed woman is $\frac{60}{1000}$ or .06.

The other way to figure this out is via conjunctional probabilities. When I ask for the probability of the person picked being a left-handed woman, I am asking what is the probability of the person being left-handed *and* a woman, the probability of the conjunction of these two events. Since we were given that the events are independent, we can find the conjunctional probability by multiplying the probability of one, being a woman, by the probability of the other, being left-handed: .50 × .12 = .06.

TABLE **12.5** **Lung Cancer Data Showing Marginal Frequencies and Probabilities**

	Alive	Dead	
Experimental	49	32	$81, p = .54$
Control	29	40	$69, p = .46$
	$78, p = .52$	$72, p = .48$	$N = 150$

Just as we figured out above, via logic, we find, via conjunctional probabilities, that the probability of picking a left-handed woman is .06.

Conjunctional probabilities can be calculated by multiplying together the individual probabilities *as long as the factors are independent.* Remember our null hypothesis that the two variables are independent? Let's look at the lung cancer data again and see how we can use conjunctional probabilities to calculate frequencies expected for the cells if and when the null hypothesis is true. To do so, I'm going to put marginal frequencies and marginal probabilities into the contingency table (Table 12.5).

Looking at Table 12.5 we can see that 81 patients, or 54%, received the experimental treatment. Thus, if we put all 150 people into a barrel, stirred them up, and picked one out at random, the probability that the person picked had received the experimental treatment would be .54. Similarly, there were 78 people, or 52% of the 150, who were alive a year later. If we picked a person at random from these 150, the probability that the person picked would be a person who was alive a year later would be .52.

My null hypothesis says that presence or absence of the experimental treatment is unrelated to mortality, that these two variables are independent. Null hypothesis significance tests are based on developing a model of the world that would exist if H_0 were true, and then comparing the observed results to the results expected if H_0 were true. If H_0 is true, which we are assuming it is, then we can calculate the probability of a person being picked at random from the 150 being *both* alive *and* having received the experimental treatment as the product of those two individual, and presumably independent, probabilities. Thus, the probability, if the two variables are independent, of a person picked at random from the 150 people of being both alive and having received the experimental treatment is .52 (the probability of being alive) × .54 (the probability of being in the experimental group), or .2808. Phrased another way, if the two variables are independent, then 28.08% of the cases should be alive–experimental-treatment recipients. We can use this conjunctional probability to calculate the expected frequency in a cell: 28.08% of the cases is .2808 of 150, or 42.12 cases. Although we *observed* 49 cases in the cell on the upper left of the matrix, the cell where experimental treatment intersects with a positive outcome, we would *expect* only 42.12 cases if H_0 were true. In

observed frequency

The actual number of cases in each cell of a contingency table.

expected frequency

The number of cases expected in each cell of a contingency table if the null hypothesis is true.

the terminology that is used with chi-square, the **observed frequency** ($f_{observed}$) is 49 and the **expected frequency** ($f_{expected}$) is 42.12. (By the bye, don't be bothered by the fact that there are fractional cases in the expected frequency.)

For the chi-square we will compare the observed frequency for each cell to its expected frequency to yield the χ^2 statistic. My calculated expected frequency demonstrates how the logic of conjunctional probabilities applies to chi-square for contingency tables. However, Equation 12.2 is a shortcut way of calculating expected frequencies that I would like you to use.

F O R M U L A

Expected Frequencies for Chi-Square Tests for Contingency Tables

Equation 12.2

$$f_{expected} = \frac{f_{row} \times f_{column}}{N}$$

Where:

$f_{expected}$ = the expected frequency for a specific cell
f_{row} = the marginal frequency for the cell's row
f_{column} = the marginal frequency for the cell's column
N = the total number of cases in the contingency table

This formula says that we calculate the expected frequency for a cell by finding the product of the marginal frequencies for the cell's row and the column divided by the total number of cases in the table. For the upper left cell in our lung cancer data set, this would be $\frac{81 \times 78}{150} = 42.12$, exactly the same value that we calculated earlier. Following the same procedure, we would end up with expected frequencies for the four cells as shown in Table 12.6.

There's one very important thing to note in the matrix of expected frequencies seen in Table 12.6: the marginal frequencies haven't changed. The marginal frequencies, and the marginal probabilities, for the contingency

TABLE **12.6**   **Expected Frequencies for the Lung Cancer Data Set**

	Alive	Dead	
Experimental	42.12	38.88	81
Control	35.88	33.12	69
	78	72	$N = 150$

table of *expected* frequencies are exactly the same as they are for the contingency table of *observed* frequencies.*

Now, having both the observed and the expected frequencies for the four cells, we're ready to calculate χ^2 via the formula shown in Equation 12.3.

F O R M U L A

χ^2 for the Chi-Square Test for Contingency Tables

Equation 12.3

$$\chi^2 = \sum \frac{(f_{observed} - f_{expected})^2}{f_{expected}}$$

Where:

χ^2 = the chi-square value being calculated

$f_{observed}$ = the observed frequency for a cell

$f_{expected}$ = the expected frequency for a cell

This equation says (a) take the observed frequency for a cell, subtract from it the expected frequency, and square that difference. (b) Take the squared difference and divide it by the expected frequency. (c) Do this for all the cells and add up all the quotients to yield the chi-square value. For the lung cancer data this is how it looks:

$$\chi^2 = \frac{(49 - 42.12)^2}{42.12} + \frac{(32 - 38.88)^2}{38.88} + \frac{(29 - 35.88)^2}{35.88} + \frac{(40 - 33.12)^2}{33.12}$$

$$= 1.1238 + 1.2174 + 1.3192 + 1.4292 = 5.0896 = 5.09$$

Thus $\chi^2_{observed} = 5.09$. Since $\chi^2_{cv} = 3.84$, the observed value falls in the rare zone of the sampling distribution, and we reject the null hypothesis.

---

*The fact that the marginal frequencies don't change allows, if you're willing to take your chances on another Dirty Harry moment, a shortcut that takes advantage of the degrees of freedom for the chi-square. Feeling lucky? This two-by-two contingency table has one degree of freedom. That is, if you know the marginal frequencies *and* if you know the frequency for one cell, then you can figure out the frequencies for the other three cells. Similarly, for a two-by-three contingency table, which has six cells and two degrees of freedom, if you know the marginal frequencies and the frequencies for two of the cells, you can figure out the frequencies of the other four cells.

Using the lung cancer data as our example, here's how it works. If the marginal frequency for the first row is 81 and the expected frequency for one of the two cells in that row is 42.12, then the frequency for the other cell in that row is determined, it must be 81 − 42.12, or 38.88. Similarly, if the marginal frequency for the first column is 78 and the expected frequency for one of the two cells in that column is 42.12, then the expected frequency for the other cell in the column must be 78 − 42.12, or 35.88. Thus, we can move around the matrix, filling in the expected frequencies for the empty cells based on the expected frequencies we have already calculated until all the cells are filled.

LOOKING CLOSER

Chi-square is reported, in APA format, as: χ^2 (df, N = nn) = $\chi^2_{observed}$, $p >/< \alpha$. Substitute the actual degrees of freedom for "df", the actual N for "nn", and the actual observed chi-square value for "$\chi^2_{observed}$". For "$>/<\alpha$" substitute the actual alpha level chosen and the correct sign indicating whether the results are common ($>$) or rare ($<$) under the null hypothesis. Thus, the lung cancer data results, in APA format, look like this: χ^2 (1, N = 150) = 5.09, $p < .05$.

Group Practice 12.1

1. For each scenario, write the research question and select the appropriate statistical test.

   a. A CEO of a large company has heard that organizing offices along principles of feng shui leads to increased productivity. (Feng shui is a Chinese system in which furniture and decorations are placed in such a way as to maximize harmony and energy.) He brings a feng shui practitioner to the corporate headquarters and has her redecorate offices either to bring about good feng shui or bad feng shui. The workers know that their offices are redecorated, but are blind to whether it was to help or hinder harmony and energy. The workers' supervisors are also blind to the manipulation. One year later, the CEO compares the raises, which are based on supervisor ratings of performance, of the people who had their offices redecorated for positive and negative feng shui.

   b. Some adults like dogs; others like cats. I get a large sample of adults and have them classify themselves as "dog people" or "not dog people." From each person I also learn if his or her family had dogs as pets when they were children. Is there a relationship between such childhood experience with a dog and adult classification as a dog person?

   c. In tennis matches, the person who serves has an advantage and has an increased likelihood of winning the point. A tennis coach wondered if the server's advantage "wore off" as the point was played. He observed the men's final match at Wimbledon, where he figured that the two players should be reasonably evenly matched. For each point he noted (a) who won, the server or the receiver, and (b) how many times the ball

was hit. A "1" would indicate that the only person who hit the ball was the server, a "2" would mean both the server and the receiver hit the ball, a "3" that the ball was hit by the server, the receiver, and again the server, etc. If the number of times the ball was hit was 4 or less, he classified it as a short rally, from 5 to 8 was a medium rally, and 9 or more was a long rally. Does who wins the point, the server or the receiver, differ as a function of whether the rally was short, medium, or long?

   d. I have a colleague who believes that students who take classes early in the morning are more serious students. Curious as to whether this was true, I had the college registrar draw a random sample of graduating seniors and calculate the percentage of classes they took that started before 10 AM. I also had the registrar find the grade point average (GPA) for each of these students. Do students who take more early classes do better in college?

   e. Some of my statistics students have fancy graphing calculators, and some have much simpler (and cheaper) calculators. No matter what calculator they have, I have discovered that some students know and understand the features of their calculator (e.g., how to put data into memory and how to recall it), and some don't. Curious as to how these two variables affected a student's final point total in my class, I classified students as (a) fancy calculator vs. simple calculator and (b) understand calculator vs. not understand calculator. What statistic should I use to analyze these data and answer my question?

Group Practice 12.1—cont'd

2. A first-grade teacher has developed a theory that she can predict success in school by behavior in first grade. At the end of a school year she takes a list of all the first-grade students to the principal and has her note which ones were discipline problems during the year. She then takes the list and locks it away in a file cabinet. Eleven years later, after the students had had enough time to graduate from high school, she gets out the list and finds out whether each student finished high school or dropped out. She even tracked down people who moved out of the district to find out their status. Using the data she collected, go through the first five steps of the six-step hypothesis testing procedure.

	Graduated	Dropped Out
1st grade discipline problem yes	10	17
1st grade discipline problem no	186	43

3. You may be aware that there are three ranks for college professors. In ascending order they are assistant professor, associate professor, and full professor. Assistant professors don't have tenure, whereas associate and full professors do. It usually takes about 6 or 7 years to move from assistant professor to associate, and then another 6 or 7 before one can try to get the promotion to full professor. A labor organizer came to a college campus and asked professors whether they were satisfied with their salaries. Using the data he collected, go through the first five steps of the six-step hypothesis testing procedure.

	Satisfied with $	Not satisfied with $
Assistant professor	10	20
Associate professor	8	4
Full professor	2	3

Interpretation

How you interpret the results depends on whether you view the completed chi-square test for contingency tables as a difference test or a relationship test. Either way, we will follow the same order of interpretation we've used previously, first seeing if we consider the results statistically significant and then investigating the direction of the difference or relationship and the size of the effect. In other words, the interpretation proceeds the same way whether you have completed a chi-square difference test or a chi-square test of association.

Direction

Our first task for the lung cancer data is to address whether the difference between the two groups is statistically significant and, if so, in what direction the difference lies. Both of these tasks are easy since all the work has already been done. We know, thanks to the decision rule generated in Step 4, that the difference in mortality between the patients who received the experimental and control treatments is statistically significant, so the first task is complete. Then, just like we looked at the means for a t test to determine the direction of the difference, we can look at the observed frequencies to determine which group has more satisfaction. Table 12.5

shows that 49 of the 81 people who received the experimental treatment, or 60.49%, were alive a year later. This is in contrast to 42.03% (or 29 of 69) of the people who received the control treatment being alive a year later. Since 60% is greater than 42% and we know that the difference is statistically significant, my interpretation will note the statistically significant difference in survival between patients based on type of treatment received and will mention that those who were in the experimental group were statistically more likely to be alive a year later.*

Size of the Effect

There are a number of ways to determine the size of the effect, and we're going to examine four of them: calculating a confidence interval, turning the χ^2 into an r (which gives us access to all the interpretative options we used for correlations), and, for clinical data, calculating relative risk and number needed to treat.

Confidence Intervals

Just as for a t test we found the mean difference between the groups and then calculated the confidence interval for this difference, we can do something similar for the χ^2, albeit with proportions. For the lung cancer data, the proportion of people in the experimental treatment who were alive a year later was .6049, and the proportion of people in the control group who were alive was .4203. Thus the difference in proportions between them is .6049 minus .4203, or .1846.† This probability of .1846 can be transformed into a percentage, indicating that the percentage of people in the experimental group who were alive a year later is 18.46% higher than in the control group.

This .1846 represents the proportional difference between the two samples, and we know, thanks to sampling error, that it is probably not an exact representation of the population value. The confidence interval, which we are about to calculate, will give us the range within which it is likely that the population value for the proportional difference falls. As with other confidence intervals we have calculated, the narrower the interval the better, and the further away the lower bound of the interval falls from zero, the larger the effect.

Calculating a confidence interval is based on the concept of a sampling distribution. Say we take repeated random samples of $N = 150$ from the population of lung cancer patients who received the experimental or

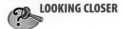

LOOKING CLOSER

*Direction is not as easy to figure out for a chi-square test of association as for a Pearson r because there is no sign that reveals whether the relationship is direct or inverse. So, one must look at the contingency table and see, for example, if the larger dose of a drug is associated with a better or a worse outcome.

†Since I am going to use the absolute value of the difference score, I always subtract the smaller value from the larger.

control treatments. If each time we calculate the difference between the proportions of patients alive in the two groups, we would end up with a sampling distribution of the difference in proportions that centers around the population value of the difference in proportions. This sampling distribution has a standard deviation, called the standard error of the difference between proportions, abbreviated as $s_{p_1-p_2}$. For any single observed sample value (e.g., .1846 for our lung cancer data), there is a 95% chance that if we add and subtract 1.96 $s_{p_1-p_2}$ to the sample value that the calculated interval would contain the population value.* Since we already have the sample value, we need only to calculate the standard error of the difference between proportions, the formula for which (Sheskin, 2004) is found in Equation 12.4.

F O R M U L A

Standard Error of the Difference between Proportions ($s_{p_1-p_2}$)

Equation 12.4

$$s_{p_1-p_2} = \sqrt{\frac{p_1 q_1}{n_1} + \frac{p_2 q_2}{n_2}}$$

Where:

$s_{p_1-p_2}$ = the standard error of the difference between the proportions
p_1 = the proportion of the first group that possesses the attribute
q_1 = the proportion of the first group that does not possess the attribute (equivalent to $1 - p_1$)
n_1 = the number of cases in the first group
p_2 = the proportion of the other group that possesses the attribute
q_2 = the proportion of the other group that does not possess the attribute (equivalent to $1 - p_2$)
n_2 = the number of cases in the other group

NOTE: for chi-square test of association, use the predictor variable to divide cases into groups

---

To calculate this standard error: (1) for each group find the proportion of the group that possesses the attribute under question and the proportion that does not possess the attribute, multiply them together, and divide this by the number of cases in the group. (2) These two quotients are then added together, and the square root of the sum is the standard error of the difference between the proportions. For the lung cancer data, the attribute

---

*I'm trusting that you recognize the value 1.96 as the z score associated with the middle 95% of the observations in the normal distribution.

LOOKING CLOSER

that I am focusing on is survival. There are 81 people in the experimental group, and 49 of them survived 1 year. Thus p_1 equals $\frac{49}{81}$ or .6049. I can find q_1, the proportion of people in the experimental group who did not survive two ways: either by $\frac{32}{81}$ or by $1 - .6049$.* In either event, I'll end up with $q_1 = .3951$. Similarly, I'll find $p_2 = .4203$ and $q_2 = .5797$. With $n_1 = 81$ and $n_2 = 69$, I have everything I need to plug into the formula to find the standard error of the difference between proportions:

$$\sqrt{\frac{.6049 \times .3951}{81} + \frac{.4203 \times .5797}{69}} = \sqrt{.0030 + .0035} = .0806 = .08$$

Now that we have $s_{p_1-p_2}$ we can calculate the confidence interval around the sample value, .1846, of the difference between the proportions. Although it is possible to calculate an interval for any level of confidence, I am going to show the formula for the most common confidence interval, the 95% confidence interval, in Equation 12.5.

FORMULA

The 95% Confidence Interval for the Difference between Two Proportions

Equation 12.5 $95\% \; CI = |p_1 - p_2| \pm 1.96 s_{p_1-p_2}$

Where:

$95\% \; CI$ = the 95% confidence interval for the difference between two proportions

p_1 = the proportion of cases in one group that possess the attribute

p_2 = the proportion of cases in the other group that possess the attribute

$s_{p_1-p_2}$ = the standard error of the difference between proportions, calculated via Equation 12.4

According to this formula, 1.96 standard errors of the difference between proportions are subtracted from and added to the observed difference in proportions between the two samples in order to calculate the 95% confidence interval. For the lung cancer data the formula becomes the following:

$$|.6049 - .4203| \pm 1.96(.0806) = .1846 \pm .1580$$

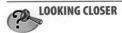 **LOOKING CLOSER**

*Where did that 32 come from? If there are 81 in the group and 49 survived, then 81 − 49, or 32, did not survive.

The confidence interval is reported as a range, from low to high, of .0266 (.03) to .3426 (.34). This confidence interval means that there is a reasonable certainty, a 95% chance, that *in the population* the increase in survival rate of the experimental group over the control group could be as little as a 3% increase or as much as a 34% increase. This is not a particularly wide interval, but it does come close to a zero increase in survival. If being in the experimental group led to a 3% increase in survival—say, a change from 42% to 45%—that would not seem to me to be a very meaningful effect.* However, if the increase in survival were an increase of 34%—say, a change from 42% to 76%—I would consider that a meaningful increase. Given our current results, we don't know which of these—a 3% increase or a 34% increase, or anywhere in between, or the 5% chance that it is less than 3% or more than 34%—reflects reality, though the odds are that it is somewhere between 3% and 34%.

Given this uncertainty and given that it could be as low as a 3% increase, I am uncomfortable concluding that the effect is a strong one. So, I will suggest that the study be replicated before implementing any changes in the treatment of lung cancer. If, on replication, the increase in survival is still around the 18% level, even though the lower limit of confidence interval still approaches zero, I'd be more likely to consider the effect to be meaningful.

The sample size, $N = 150$, seems large in the present instance. Sample size certainly has some impact on the width of the confidence interval, with larger sample sizes leading to smaller confidence intervals. However, the impact of an increase in sample size is not huge for chi-square for contingency tables. In the present instance if the sample doubles in size with no change in mortality rate, the confidence interval shrinks to .07 to .30 from .03 to .34. The other factor that influences the width of the confidence interval is the discrepancy between p and q; the more p and q deviate from a 50/50 split, the narrower the confidence interval.

The new information that can be used in the interpretative statement for the lung cancer results is the confidence interval for the distance between two proportions, from .03 to .34. Confidence intervals provide a lot of fodder for interpretative statements with both their width and their distance from zero. Using the proportion in the control group as a standard, and adjusting the proportion found in the experimental group on the basis of the confidence interval, is a good way to put a confidence interval into a comprehensible context.

> ## Group Practice 12.2
>
> Calculate and interpret 95% confidence intervals for questions 2 and 3 from Group Practice 12.1.

---

*I chose 42% as the survival rate for comparison because that was the 1-year survival rate for the control group.

Interpretation is not black and white, it is subjective. I don't consider a change in survival rate from 42% to 45% particularly strong. But, for people with lung cancer or a loved one with lung cancer, even this slight increase in the likelihood of survival would be desirable.

LOOKING CLOSER

Turning χ^2 into *r*

A chi-square test for contingency tables can be construed as a relationship test, and so it is possible to convert a chi-square into an *r*. Doing so has certain advantages, for we can then apply many of the techniques we used for interpreting a Pearson product moment correlation coefficient to interpreting a chi-square.

Back in the days before computers, statisticians developed specialized versions of correlation coefficients to speed calculations. One, which we've already encountered, was the point-biserial correlation, used when one variable is dichotomous and the other variable continuous. Another, called the phi coefficient,* was developed to calculate the correlation between two dichotomous variables. The phi coefficient, abbreviated ϕ, is really just a Pearson product moment correlation calculated for two dichotomous variables. Please do not be bothered by the fact that I told you earlier that Pearson *r*s are to be calculated only when the data are measured at the interval or ratio level. What I am about to do is legitimate.

It is easy to transform a χ^2 value into ϕ, as shown in Equation 12.6.

F O R M U L A

Transforming χ^2 from a Chi-Square Test for Contingency Tables into a Phi Coefficient, ϕ, a Form of Pearson *r*

Equation 12.6

$$\phi = r = \sqrt{\frac{\chi^2}{N}}$$

Where:

ϕ = the phi coefficient being calculated (equivalent to *r*)
χ^2 = the chi-square value calculated via Equation 12.3
N = number of cases in the chi-square

The formula says that one divides the observed chi-square value by the total number of cases and then takes the square root of this to find the phi coefficient. For the lung cancer data this is calculated as follows:

$$\sqrt{\frac{5.0896}{150}} = \sqrt{.0339} = .1841 = .18$$

This can be interpreted as indicating that the correlation between treatment status and survival status is .18.[†] (Note that the phi coefficient

---

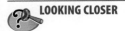
LOOKING CLOSER

*Phi is pronounced with a long i, as in "fee, fi, fo, fum."

[†] If you took the lung cancer data, assigned a value of 0 to people in the control group, 1 to people in the experimental group, 0 to people who had not survived, 1 to people who were alive, and then calculated the Pearson *r* for these data, it would equal .18.

is always positive and so is mum about the direction of the correlation.) You may recognize this correlation, using Cohen's rough guide to effect sizes for the social and behavioral sciences (1988), as a small to moderate correlation.* This correlation can be interpreted on its own, but we can also use it to calculate r^2, a binomial effect size display, power, sample size, and even d.[†]

The percentage of variance in one variable predicted by or accounted for by the other, the coefficient of determination or r^2, was first encountered in Chapter 8 (Equation 8.3) as a measure of the strength of an effect. For the lung cancer data we would calculate it so:[‡]

$$.1841^2 = .0339 = .03$$

This can be interpreted as indicating that 3% of the variability in survival is accounted for—is predicted by—treatment status. Three percent does not sound like much, so this suggests that the effect size is not very large. Though, as noted earlier, the interpretation of the size of the effect depends on one's perspective. There are scenarios where a 3% improvement in prediction is huge. A gambler who could improve his or her chances of knowing whether a poker hand would win or lose by 3% would be heading to Las Vegas and retiring young.

Speaking of effect sizes puts me in mind of d, and it is possible to transform r into d.[§] We didn't do this for correlations back in Chapter 8, because we had not yet encountered d. But, now that we know what it is, we'll do so for chi-square, and you can add Equation 12.7 to your interpretative armamentarium for correlations.

FORMULA

Transforming a Pearson r into an Effect Size (d)

Equation 12.7

$$d = \frac{2r}{\sqrt{1 - r^2}}$$

Where:
d = the effect size being calculated
r = the Pearson r value (or ϕ)

---

*Cohen, J. (1988). *Statistical power analysis for the behavioral sciences*. Hillsdale, NJ: Lawrence Erlbaum Associates.

[†] It makes sense to interpret r for a two-by-two matrix, and it is OK to interpret r for a larger matrix, as long as there is an ordinal meaning for both the row and column variables. You can even calculate a 95% confidence interval for r if you follow the procedures outlined in Chapter 8.

[‡] If you have a good memory this value, .0339, should look familiar. We took the square root of it to find $\phi = .1841$. So, if you plan ahead you can save yourself some calculations.

[§] To continue with the distinction introduced in the last chapter, this is interpreted as $d_{independent}$ not $d_{dependent}$.

LOOKING CLOSER

This formula says, (1) multiply the Pearson r value (or the phi coefficient) by two, and (2) divide this by the square root of one minus r squared. For the lung cancer data this is as follows:

$$\frac{2 \times .1841}{\sqrt{1 - .1841^2}} = \frac{.3682}{\sqrt{.9661}} = \frac{.3682}{.9829} = .3746 = .37$$

Remember, d represents how far, in standard score units, the mean of one group is from the mean of another group when both are normally distributed. Back when we first encountered d in Chapter 9, we interpreted it either by thinking of it in terms of a familiar variable (e.g., IQ or blood pressure) or by calculating the amount of overlap in two normal distributions. Neither makes much sense with nominal-level dichotomous data. So, why convert χ^2 to d? For two reasons: (1) to gain a sense of how large the effect size is, and (2) to have a common metric to compare disparate studies.

Cohen (1988) suggested that, for the social and behavioral sciences, a correlation of .10 represents a small effect, a correlation of .30 is a medium effect, and a correlation of .50 is a large effect.* Thanks to Equation 12.7, we can transform these into effect sizes and find that a d of $\approx .20$ is a small effect, $d \approx .60$ is a medium effect, and $d \approx 1.20$ is a large effect. Thus, I would conclude that the effect of being assigned to the experimental treatment, $d = .37$, is small to moderate.

The other use of the effect size d is comparing disparate studies. Suppose someone else conducted a study comparing some other new treatment for lung cancer to the standard treatment, but measured survival in terms of days and used a t test to analyze her data. If both of us converted our results to the effect size d, we'd be able to compare results. In fact, there is a statistical technique, meta-analysis, that combines results from multitudes of studies in order to synthesize disparate research findings. Meta-analysis depends on transforming different statistics into a common metric like d or r.

We've looked at converting χ^2 into r, r^2, and d; now let's think about converting it into a binomial effect size display. The bottom line is that though you can do so, I don't recommend it.

The binomial effect size display (Equation 8.4) displays a correlation in terms of the relationship between two dichotomous variables. In some sense, there's no need to transform chi-square into a binomial effect size display because, if it is based on a two-by-two matrix as is the lung cancer data, it is already a binomial display. For the lung cancer data, I can report that approximately 60% of the people in the experimental group survived for a year, compared to approximately 42% of the people in the control group.

LOOKING CLOSER

*Cohen, J. (1988). *Statistical power analysis for the behavioral sciences.* Hillsdale, NJ: Lawrence Erlbaum Associates.

The advantages of the binomial effect size display over the observed sample percentages are minimal. First, with our actual data we have different ns for the two groups, 81 in the experimental group and 69 in the control group. The binomial effect size display recasts the correlation of $r = .18$ into how it would look with equal sample sizes. Thus, it shows that 59% of the experimental group would survive, compared to 41% of the control group.

The binomial effect size display also smoothes out disparities. Whereas based on the actual sample frequencies the experimental patients were 10 percentage points above 50 and the control cases were 8 percentage points below 50, now both are the same amount, 9 percentage points, above and below 50. Is this a good thing? It depends.

Suppose that the chi-square was still statistically significant but the frequencies looked different—that approximately 75% of the experimental cases survived whereas for the control group it was approximately 50%. The phi coefficient is then about .26, and the binomial effect size display shows a 63% survival rate with the experimental treatment, compared to only a 37% chance of survival for the control group. This makes it sound like being in the control group leads to worse odds of survival than a coin flip, whereas the actual data show that being in the control group does lead to a 50/50 chance of survival. For this reason, because the effect is equalized for both groups, I don't recommend converting a chi-square from a two-by-two matrix into a binomial effect size display.

Though it doesn't make sense to apply the binomial effect size display to a two-by-two chi-square test for contingency tables, it does make sense to think about power and sample size. The simplest way to do so is to, as we have already done, convert χ^2 into r and then use Appendix Tables 7 and 8. For the lung cancer data we had $N = 150$ and found $r = .1841$. Looking at the intersections of both $r = .15$ and $r = .20$ with $N = 150$ in Appendix Table 8, we find that power falls somewhere in the interval from .44 to .69. In either case, our study was underpowered, and we were lucky to reject the null hypothesis. Appendix Table 9 shows how many cases we would need for the study, depending on the power we desire. To have power of .80—that is, a 20% chance of making a Type II error—with a real correlation between the two variables of .175, we would need about 256 cases. If we are concerned about the dangers of making a Type II error and wish to set power at .95, we need about 420 cases. That's a lot of people with lung cancer to find and to persuade to participate in a research project.

When a chi-square is transformed into a correlation, there are a lot of options that can be added to the interpretation. For the lung cancer data, $r = .18$, $r^2 = .03$, $d = .37$, power was in the range from .44 to .69, and the sample size needed for an 80% chance of rejecting the null hypothesis was greater than 250 cases. Which of these, if any, you choose to add to an interpretation depends on your audience and what you wish to stress. I'm going to hold off on writing an interpretation until we've considered the next set of interpretative options.

Group Practice 12.3

For questions 2 and 3 from Group Practice 12.1, calculate and interpret r, r^2, d, power, and sample size required if $\beta = .80$ or .95.

Relative Risk Ratio (RR) and Number Needed to Treat (NNT)

As with my example, two-by-two tables are commonly used to examine outcomes in clinical or medical research where a treatment group is compared to a control group in terms of good outcome (e.g., alive) vs. bad outcome (e.g., dead). There is a very basic question involved here—to what degree is this treatment helpful?—and statisticians have developed a number of ways to quantify it with a single number. In this section we will look at some clinically relevant ways of interpreting two-by-two tables with nominal data. We'll see, later on, that these techniques may on occasion profitably be applied to nonclinical data sets as well.

Though the techniques that I am going to address here—risk ratio and number needed to treat—do not need to be preceded by a significant chi-square test, I usually calculate them only when preceded by statistical significance. You've heard my reasoning before: without a statistically significant test we haven't found sufficient evidence to conclude that an effect exists. So, why worry about how big the effect is if we aren't even sure that there is one? However, there are occasions—when a study is underpowered and I think that there is reason to believe that an effect exists—that I will calculate measures of effect size.*

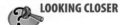

relative risk ratio

How much greater the likelihood of an adverse outcome is for a case in the control group than it is for a case in the treatment group.

The **relative risk ratio**[†] compares the risk of an adverse outcome under two conditions. The *relative* and the *ratio* parts of its name indicate that it involves a comparison. The *risk* part shows that it focuses on the likelihood of a bad, or adverse, outcome. The way the risk ratio is calculated, it tells how much more likely the risk of a bad outcome is for cases that are at higher risk (usually the control cases) than for cases at lower risk (usually the experimental treatment cases). For our lung cancer example, people in the control group have a .5797 probability of having an adverse outcome (dying) compared to a .3951 probability of an adverse outcome for the people in the experimental group. As Equation 12.8 shows, we compute the risk ratio as the ratio of the two:

$$\frac{.5797}{.3951} = 1.4672 = 1.47$$

LOOKING CLOSER

*There are statisticians who advocate calculating effect sizes as a matter of course when the null hypothesis is not rejected. They argue that an effect size can be viewed as a descriptive statistic, and so it simply describes the size of the effect observed in the sample. In addition, they argue that by focusing on null hypothesis significance testing and ignoring effect sizes, we run the risk of making a Type II error in situations in which the effect is large but power is low. Finally, they argue that by aggregating results from a number of statistically nonsignificant studies, all of which had small effect sizes, we can conclude that a small, but perhaps meaningful, effect exists. All of these arguments are legitimate, and if you choose to calculate effect sizes when you fail to reject the null hypothesis, I won't stand in your way.

[†] Though the formal name has three *r*s in it and it seems like it should be abbreviated as *RRR*, the tradition is to abbreviate it as *RR*. Perhaps because of this it is often just called a risk ratio and sometimes it is called the relative risk.

F O R M U L A

Relative Risk Ratio (*RR*)

Equation 12.8

$$RR = \frac{p\,(AdverseOutcome_{control})}{p\,(AdverseOutcome_{treatment})}$$

Where:

RR = the relative risk ratio being calculated

$p(AdverseOutcome_{control})$ = the probability of an adverse outcome occurring for the group with the higher percentage of adverse outcomes, usually the control group

$p(AdverseOutcome_{treatment})$ = the probability of an adverse outcome occurring for the group with the lower percentage of adverse outcomes, usually the treatment group

The beauty of the relative risk ratio is that it is intuitively easy to interpret. The value of 1.47 that I calculated above indicates that a bad outcome is almost 1.5 times more likely in the control group than in the treatment group. If 2 out of 10 people in the experimental group had an adverse outcome, then almost 3 out of 10 people in the control group would be expected to have an adverse outcome. Which group would you rather be in?*

Though relative risk ratios were developed for situations with two groups, they can be applied to chi-square tests of association with predictor and criterion variables as well. In such an instance, for example when looking at the relationship between performance on the first test (pass vs. fail) with final grade in the class (pass vs. fail), one simply treats the predictor variable (outcome on the first test) as a grouping variable. Thus the risk ratio addresses the question of how much greater the risk is of failing the second exam if one failed instead of passed the first exam.

It is also possible to use risk ratios to examine positive outcomes, and if one does so it shows that the "risk" of a good outcome for the lung

---

*The advantage of comparing the group with the more common bad outcome to the group with the less common bad outcome is that the risk ratio will be greater than zero, which is easier to interpret. We can calculate the relative risk as the ratio of bad outcomes in the treatment group to bad outcomes in the control group, and the answer is the reciprocal of 1.47, .68. This is interpreted as indicating that the probability of having a bad outcome if one were in the treatment group is .68 times as likely as it was for the control group. I don't know about you, but I find it harder to know what that means.

LOOKING CLOSER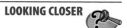

relative benefit ratio

How much greater the likelihood of a positive outcome is in the treatment group than the control group.

cancer patients was 1.44 times higher in the experimental group than in the control group.* This should more properly be called a **relative benefit ratio.**

I like relative risk ratios, but as I mentioned at the top of this section, I recommend using them only if the initial data showed statistically significant results. Why? Because if the chi-square was not statistically significant, then there is not sufficient evidence to conclude that the relationship between the two variables, between treatment and outcome, is anything but zero. And if there is no relationship between treatment and outcome, there is no reason to speculate about relative risk or benefit.

Relative risk ratios are easy to calculate and interpret, and they are commonly used in clinical and/or epidemiological research. If the ratio is one, then there is no additional risk to being in the control group. Ratios below one (and they can't drop below zero) indicate a reduction in the likelihood of the outcome for the numerator group compared to the denominator group. Ratios above one (and they are, theoretically, unlimited in how high they can go) indicate an increased likelihood of the outcome for the numerator group compared to the denominator group. Later on in this chapter, in Table 12.7, I present a number of different outcome matrices for which I have calculated risk ratios. This should help to give you some sense of what different risk ratios mean.

Confidence intervals can be, and should be, calculated for risk ratios since their width and their distance from a value of 1 provide valuable information about where the population value falls. Why deviation from a value of 1 and not 0 as we used for the other confidence intervals we've encountered? Because a risk ratio of 1 indicates no increased risk of being in the control group over being in the treatment group.

Though the official calculation of a confidence interval for a risk ratio is more complex than is appropriate for an introductory statistics text, I do have a shortcut technique that takes advantage of the 95% confidence interval for the difference between proportions we learned to calculate earlier. If you remember, we focused on the difference between the *positive* outcome, survival rate, of 60.49% in the experimental group vs. 42.03% in the control group, and built a confidence interval around the observed difference in proportion of .1846, a confidence interval that ranged from a difference as small as .0266 to a difference as large as .3426. If we turn that around and examine the difference in proportions for the *negative* outcome, mortality rate, of .5797 (control group) and .3951 (experimental group), we find that the difference remains .1846 with a confidence interval from .0266 to .3426. Thus, the difference in mortality between the control group and the experimental group could be as small as 3% or as great as 34%.

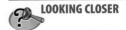 **LOOKING CLOSER**

*Want to calculate that "risk"? The probability of a good outcome in the treatment group is .6049 and in control group it is .4203, so .6049/.4203 = 1.4392.

To approximate a 95% confidence interval for the relative risk ratio we can calculate, as shown in Equation 12.9, the relative risk ratio for the two endpoints of the confidence interval.

Estimating the 95% Confidence Interval for a Relative Risk Ratio

$$95\% \, CI_{RR_{LB}} = \frac{\dfrac{p(AdverseOutcome_{control}) + p(AdverseOutcome_{treatment})}{2} + \dfrac{LB_{95\% \, CI}}{2}}{\dfrac{p(AdverseOutcome_{control}) + p(AdverseOutcome_{treatment})}{2} - \dfrac{LB_{95\% \, CI}}{2}}$$

Equation 12.9

$$95\% \, CI_{RR_{UB}} = \frac{\dfrac{p(AdverseOutcome_{control}) + p(AdverseOutcome_{treatment})}{2} + \dfrac{UB_{95\% \, CI}}{2}}{\dfrac{p(AdverseOutcome_{control}) + p(AdverseOutcome_{treatment})}{2} - \dfrac{UB_{95\% \, CI}}{2}}$$

Where:

$95\% \, CI_{RR_{LB}}$ = the lower bound of the 95% confidence interval for the relative risk ratio

$95\% \, CI_{RR_{UB}}$ = the upper bound of the 95% confidence interval for the relative risk ratio

$p(AdverseOutcome_{control})$ = the probability of an adverse outcome occurring for the group expected to have a higher percentage of adverse outcomes, usually the control group

$p(AdverseOutcome_{treatment})$ = the probability of an adverse outcome occurring for the group expected to have a lower percentage of adverse outcomes, usually the treatment group

$LB_{95\% \, CI}$ = the lower bound of the 95% confidence interval for the difference between two proportions, the value closer to zero, expressed as a proportion, calculated via Equation 12.5

$UB_{95\% \, CI}$ = the upper bound of the 95% confidence interval for the difference between two proportions, the value further away from zero, expressed as a proportion, calculated via Equation 12.5

Those equations may look a little daunting, but all they do is split the difference in proportions from the confidence interval between the control and experimental groups. To use an equation, first find the mean of the probability of an adverse outcome for the treatment and control groups. This mean value is put into both the numerator and denominator. Before finding the ratio of the numerator and denominator, add to the numerator half of one of the ends of the 95% confidence interval for the difference between proportions and subtract from the denominator the same value. For example, the first equation finds the average probability of an adverse outcome for two groups $\left(\text{that's } \dfrac{p(AdverseOutcome_{control}) + p(AdverseOutcome_{treatment})}{2}\right)$. Then add to the numerator, and subtract from the denominator, half of one side of the lower bound of the confidence interval, $\dfrac{.0266}{2}$, or .0133. For the lung cancer data these are what the proportions become:

$$\frac{\dfrac{.5797 + .3951}{2} + \dfrac{.0266}{2}}{\dfrac{.5797 + .3951}{2} - \dfrac{.0266}{2}} = \frac{.4874 + .0133}{.4874 - .0133} = 1.0561 = 1.06$$

$$\frac{\dfrac{.5797 + .3951}{2} + \dfrac{.3426}{2}}{\dfrac{.5797 + .3951}{2} - \dfrac{.3426}{2}} = \frac{.4874 + .1713}{.4874 - .1713} = \frac{.6587}{.3161} = 2.0838 = 2.08$$

Thus, for the lung cancer study, we can conclude that the risk ratio for the population lies in the range from 1.06 to 2.08. That is, the likelihood of death for members of the control group ranges from almost equal to that of the experimental group (1.06) to a little more than double (2.08).

There is another statistical technique used to compare the likelihood of an outcome between two groups, the **odds ratio.** Notice, this is a ratio between odds, not between probabilities. Unless you are a bookmaker, you probably don't have an intuitive understanding of odds, and so most people find the interpretation of odds ratios less comprehensible than of risk ratios. For that reason, I have left the details out of this book, though it is important that you have heard of them and can recognize, roughly, what they do.

Our final interpretative technique is called **number needed to treat,** abbreviated *NNT. NNT* is an increasingly common statistic used in clinical research. The number needed to treat is usually described as telling how many cases must be treated to yield one additional positive outcome. For *NNT* the closer the value is to 1, the better. Number needed to treat takes a little while to get used to, so stick with me for just a few paragraphs.

NNT is not hard to calculate, but it takes a little thought, so let's think about the lung cancer data, where we saw that positive outcomes occurred 60.49% of the time for the experimental treatment group and 42.03% of the time for the control group. One way to think about this is that if

odds ratio

A comparison of the odds of an adverse outcome in the control group to the odds of an adverse outcome in the treatment group.

number needed to treat

How many cases must be given the treatment in order to yield one additional positive outcome over what would be achieved if the cases received the control treatment.

we were to give 100 people the control treatment, 42.03 of them would have a positive outcome, whereas if we gave 100 people the experimental treatment, 60.49 of them would have a positive outcome. Thus, for every 100 people receiving the experimental treatment, an extra 18.46 people can be expected to stay alive, as $60.49 - 42.03 = 18.46$.* If I turn that percentage into a proportion and divide one by it, I get $\frac{1}{.1846} = 5.4171$, which rounds to 5.42.

5.42 is the number needed to treat for the lung cancer data, so let me explain what it means and how it works. We know that 42.03% of the control treatment cases have a positive outcome, so if 5.42 people were in the control group, 2.28 of them would have a positive outcome ($.4203 \times 5.4171 = 2.28$). If those 5.42 people were in the treatment group, which has a 60.49% success rate, then 3.28 would have a positive outcome ($.6049 \times 5.4171 = 3.28$). Note that the difference between 2.28 and 3.28 is one, that *one* more person had a positive outcome! And that is what the number needed to treat represents: the number of people one would need to treat with the experimental treatment to yield one more positive outcome than would be obtained from just administering the control treatment. This is important, and confusing, so note it well: The number needed to treat is *not* the number that must be treated in order to get one positive outcome, it is the number that must be treated so that *one more* positive outcome will occur than would occur if the control treatment were used.

Numbers needed to treat are rounded up to the next larger integer since one can't, in real life, treat fractional people. So, in this scenario, I would report the number needed to treat as six: the experimental treatment works well enough that for every six people who receive it there will be one more positive outcome than would occur under the control condition for those six people.

What is a good *NNT* value? The ideal *NNT* for a treatment technique is one, which means that for every case treated there is one more positive outcome than would occur under the control condition. This happens if the experimental treatment helps everyone and the control treatment has a positive impact on no one. As *NNT*s climb above one, the return of treatment, the effectiveness of the experimental treatment relative to the control condition, gets lower. An *NNT* of 10, for example, means that 10 cases must receive the experimental treatment in order for there to be an increase in one positive outcome over what would happen if those 10 cases had received the control treatment. If a treatment has no improvement at all over the control, then *NNT* equals one divided by zero, it is incalculable. If a treatment leads to a worse outcome than the control condition, *NNT* is a negative number. Table 12.7 shows risk ratios and number needed to treat for a number of different outcome matrices so that

---

*That number, 18.46, should sound familiar to you. It is the observed difference in proportion between the two groups expressed as a percentage.

LOOKING CLOSER

TABLE **12.7**   **Risk Ratios (*RR*) and Number Needed to Treat (*NNT*) for Examples of Different Outcome Matrices, Ranging from Treatment Always Leads to a Good Outcome and Control Always Leads to a Bad Outcome (Panel A) to Treatment Has No Impact (Panel H)**

A.	Good Outcome	Bad Outcome	RR	NNT
Treatment	100	0	*nc*	1.00
Control	0	100		

B.	Good Outcome	Bad Outcome	RR	NNT
Treatment	99	1	99.00	1.02
Control	1	99		

C.	Good Outcome	Bad Outcome	RR	NNT
Treatment	90	10	9.00	1.25
Control	10	90		

D.	Good Outcome	Bad Outcome	RR	NNT
Treatment	80	20	4.00	1.67
Control	20	80		

E.	Good Outcome	Bad Outcome	RR	NNT
Treatment	70	30	2.33	2.50
Control	30	70		

F.	Good Outcome	Bad Outcome	RR	NNT
Treatment	60	40	1.50	5.00
Control	40	60		

G.	Good Outcome	Bad Outcome	RR	NNT
Treatment	51	49	1.04	50.00
Control	49	51		

H.	Good Outcome	Bad Outcome	RR	NNT
Treatment	50	50	1.00	*nc*
Control	50	50		

NOTE: *nc* = not calculable

you can see the inverse relationship between these two and you can begin to get a sense of perspective for them.

One commonly cited scenario to help think about *NNT* values is the risk of infection after a dog bite. Dogs' mouths are not particularly clean, so when a person is bitten by a dog, he or she runs the risk of infection. A reasonable preventative response by emergency room personnel is to administer prophylactic antibiotics to dog-bite victims. Cummings (1994) investigated the effectiveness of this and found an *NNT* value of 15 for this practice.* In other words, every 15 dog-bite victims treated prophylactically with antibiotics yielded one fewer infection than would have occurred if no antibiotics had been administered to these 15 people. Is this prophylactic antibiotic treatment of dog bites worth it? Well, it depends. It depends on how expensive the antibiotics are, on the side effects of the antibiotics, on how difficult it is to treat a dog bite infection once it emerges, and so on. If the cost of antibiotics is high and the side effects of prophylactic antibiotics severe, and it is not problematic to treat a dog bite after it becomes infected, then it may not be worthwhile to treat dog bites prophylactically.[†] However, if antibiotics are inexpensive, they have minimal side effects, and the infection is difficult to treat, then it may be reasonable to treat dog bites prophylactically. Interpretation is a human endeavor!

I've spent so much time explaining and interpreting number needed to treat that I've neglected to give you a formula. Here it is:

F O R M U L A

Number Needed to Treat (*NNT*)

Equation 12.10

$$NNT = \frac{1}{p(PositiveOutcome_{treatment}) - p(PositiveOutcome_{control})}$$

Where:

NNT = the number needed to treat being calculated; the number of people who need to be treated in the experimental condition for each additional positive outcome over what would occur as a result of receiving the control treatment

$p(PositiveOutcome_{treatment})$ = the probability of a positive outcome in the experimental treatment condition

$p(PositiveOutcome_{control})$ = the probability of a positive outcome in the control condition

---

In English, number needed to treat is calculated by putting one in the numerator and dividing that by the difference between the probability of a positive outcome for a case in the treatment group and for a person in the control group.

---

*Cummings, P. (1994). Antibiotics to prevent infection in patients with dog bite wounds: a meta-analysis of randomized trials. *Annals of Emergency Medicine*, 23(3), 535-540.

[†]There is even a corollary to the number needed to treat, the number needed to harm. This looks at the side effects due to treatment vs. those due to the control condition.

LOOKING CLOSER

As with the risk ratio, I favor calculating number needed to treat only if the chi-square was statistically significant. My reasoning is the same: if the chi-square is not significant then there is not sufficient evidence to support the notion that treatment makes a difference, and so number needed to treat may be irrelevant. Though, if the original study was under-powered and there seems to be some positive impact of treatment, *NNT* would give some sense of the size of the effect.

Calculating a 95% confidence interval for *NNT* is easier than for the *RR*. The denominator for *NNT* for the lung cancer data was .1846, and that should sound familiar to you as the difference in proportions between the two groups. I hope that this makes you wonder about using the upper and lower bounds of the 95% confidence interval for the difference between two proportions in order to approximate the 95% confidence interval for *NNT*. The 95% confidence interval for the lung cancer data ranged from .0266 to .3426, so we conclude the 95% confidence interval for number needed to treat would range from $\dfrac{1}{.0266}$ to $\dfrac{1}{.3426}$, or from 37.59 to 2.92. (Since higher numbers are "bad" for *NNT*, I report the confidence interval from higher number to lower.) Though I reported earlier that *NNT* for the lung cancer sample was 6, the confidence interval shows that it could be, in the population, as good as 3 or as bad as 38. (Remember, *NNTs* are rounded up to the next higher integer.) Thus the effect of treatment could be as strong as for every three people treated one additional person has a positive outcome, or it could be as weak as 38 people must be treated to yield one additional positive outcome over what would happen for 38 people receiving the control treatment.

Again, don't forget the subjective aspect of interpretation, the per-spective of the interpreter. For a fatal disease like lung cancer, where treatment is not yet very effective, an *NNT* of 38 can still be viewed as providing some hope, though it is not as low (good) as we would like.

Here is the formula for approximating a 95% confidence interval for number needed to treat.*

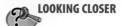

LOOKING CLOSER

*An odd thing happens when you calculate a *95% CI* for *NNT* for a nonsignificant chi-square: the confidence interval won't capture the observed *NNT* value! This is because *NNT* gets larger as the denominator (the difference in positive outcomes between treatment and control) gets smaller. For example, if the probability of a positive outcome for the treatment group is .51 and for the control group it is .49, then the difference is .02 and *NNT* = 50. But, when we cross the equator of no difference between treatment and control and start heading toward the control treatment working better, the *NNT* value turns negative. For example, if the probability of a positive outcome for the treatment group is .49 and it is .51 for the control group, then *NNT* = −50. Think about it: as the difference in positive outcome between the two groups moves from .02 to −.02, the *NNT* value jumps from 50 to −50. Thus, we can end up with a situation—as you'll see in one of the group practice problems—where *NNT* is 4 but the *95% CI* ranges from −30 to 2. Is the observed value of 4 captured by the confidence interval? Read the answer to the group practice problem to learn what to do in such a situation.

Approximating the 95% Confidence Interval for Number Needed to Treat

$$95\% \ CI_{NNT} = from \ \frac{1}{LB_{95\% \ CI}} \ to \ \frac{1}{UB_{95\% \ CI}}$$

Equation 12.11

Where:

$95\% \ CI_{NNT}$ = the 95% confidence interval for the number needed to treat that is being calculated

$LB_{95\% \ CI}$ = the lower bound of the 95% confidence interval for the difference between two proportions; the value closer to zero, expressed as a proportion, calculated via Equation 12.5

$UB_{95\% \ CI}$ = the upper bound of the 95% confidence interval for the difference between two proportions; the value further away from zero, expressed as a proportion, calculated via Equation 12.5

We've covered all the interpretative options that I want to present for a chi-square test of association. Before writing a complete interpretative statement for the lung cancer results, let's make a list of all the calculations we've done so that we can pick and choose what to interpret:

- $\chi^2 \ (1, N = 150) = 5.09, p < .05$
- Survival rate = 60.49% vs. 42.03% (experimental vs. control)
- Difference in proportions between the two groups: .1846
- 95% confidence interval for difference in proportions: .03 to .34
- $r = .18 \ (r^2 = .03, d = .37)$
- Power $\approx .44$ to .69; $\beta = .31$ to .56; $N = 256/420$ for power of .80/.95
- Risk ratio = 1.47 (approximate 95% CI from 1.06 to 2.08)
- Number needed to treat = 6 (approximate 95% CI from 38 to 3)

And, let's list our goals for these statistically significant results:

1. Explain the purpose and the methods of the study
2. Report the results in APA format and report the direction of the results
3. Report, in a clear fashion, how meaningful the results are—how strong the effect is
4. Report the strengths and limitations of the study, including the type of error that might have occurred and any concerns about generalizability

Note that in the following interpretation I am careful not to oversell the meaningfulness of this new treatment, and that I do not feel compelled to include all of the interpretation options that we calculated:

"We analyzed the data for a study of the efficacy of a new treatment for lung cancer using a chi-square test. In the study, 150 patients who were recently diagnosed with lung cancer were randomly assigned either to

the control group where they received the current standard treatment, or to the experimental group, where they received a new treatment. The outcome variable was mortality, whether the patients were alive or dead a year later.

"There was a statistically significant difference in mortality between the treatment and control groups (χ^2 (1, N = 150) = 5.09, p < .05). Of those who received the experimental treatment, 60% were alive a year later compared to only 42% of those who received the standard treatment. Based on this sample, it appears that the experimental treatment statistically increases survival for lung cancer.

"However, when we calculated the 95% confidence interval for the difference between the two samples it showed that the size of the difference between the two populations (experimental treatment vs. standard treatment) could be as small as a 3% increase in survival or as large as a 34% increase in survival. Given that the group receiving the standard treatment had a survival rate of 42%, the confidence interval suggests that the effect of the experimental treatment might be as small as leading to a survival rate of 45% or as large as leading to a survival rate of 76%. Clearly one change, from 42% to 45%, is small and the other, from 42% to 76%, is large. It is impossible to tell from the present study which one reflects reality and so I recommend replicating the study before deciding to adopt this new treatment for lung cancer. Replication would also address the 5% chance that the conclusions from the current study are in error—that the new treatment does not really lead to increased survival.

"In addition, as all participants in the study came from the same medical center, there is a possibility that there is something unique about this medical center that led to these results. Thus, when the study is replicated one might want to include patients from a variety of medical centers and regions for a more representative sample. In any event, when the study is replicated the sample size should be increased to about 250 to achieve an accepted standard of statistical power.

"In summary, the results of the present study suggest that the new treatment is a promising one that has the potential of increasing the lung cancer survival rate. However, until the results of this study are replicated it is unclear how large the effect is, and it would be premature to offer this treatment in clinical practice."

Group Practice 12.4

For questions 2 and 3 from Group Practice 12.1, calculate and interpret the risk ratio and the number needed to treat, as well as their 95% confidence intervals.

PRACTICING CHI-SQUARE

Let's do one more chi-square test for contingency tables for practice, this time with results that are not statistically significant. The data involve fast food restaurants that have playrooms. Having been harassed by my children to go to fast food restaurants that have playrooms, I wondered whether restaurants with playrooms were more likely to attract families with young children. I found two fast food restaurants that were right next door to each other, one with a playroom and one without, and observed

TABLE **12.8** **Data for Use of Fast Food Restaurants with and without Playrooms by Patrons with and without Young Children**

	Playroom Yes	Playroom No	
Young children yes	12	8	20
Young children no	6	9	15
	18	17	35

each at lunchtime on a Saturday to see whether the people who dined there had young children. Here, in Table 12.8, are the data I collected.

Test

I am exploring whether the presence or absence of young children has an impact on fast food restaurant choice, one with or without a playroom. From the data I've collected it looks like it does, since 60% of patrons with young children chose the restaurant with a playroom, compared to 40% of patrons without young children making such a choice. However, I know that to answer the question of whether one variable affects the other, I should do a statistical test.

In this study I had two independent groups of cases, fast food patrons with or without young children, and for each case I measured whether the restaurant patronized had a playroom. The question that I am asking is whether there is a difference in restaurant choice between patrons with and without young children, and this is answered with a chi-square difference test.*

Assumptions

The assumptions for the χ^2 difference test are (1) nominal-level dependent variable, (2) independent samples, (3) random sample, and (4) adequate expected frequencies. As I've already noted, the dependent variable, choice of restaurant, is nominal, so the first assumption was not violated. There is no apparent way that the selection of cases for one sample influences the other, so I consider my samples independent of each other. The samples were not random samples from the populations of fast food patrons, and so the third assumption was violated. I'm going

---

*Note that I could phrase my research question as a relationship question, "Is there a relationship between restaurant choice and presence/absence of young children?" In this case I would conceptualize my sample as one group of cases where, for each case I would measure its standing on two different nominal-level variables: restaurant choice and young child presence/absence.

LOOKING CLOSER

TABLE **12.9**   **Expected Frequencies for Fast Food Data**

	Playroom Yes	Playroom No	
Young children yes	10.2857	9.7143	20
Young children no	7.7143	7.2857	15
	18	17	35

to be leery of generalizing my results since it is not clear to me to what population they apply, but I can go ahead with the chi-square even though this assumption was violated. Finally, using Equation 12.2 I calculated the expected frequencies shown in Table 12.9. As no cell had an expected frequency less than 5, the fourth assumption was not violated.

Hypotheses

The null hypothesis is that there is no relationship between young child status and restaurant choice status and the alternative hypothesis is that there is a relationship between the two variables. This is written as:

H_0: Restaurant choice is independent of child presence or absence
H_1: Restaurant choice is not independent of child presence or absence

The null hypothesis says that though the two variables are independent in the population, there may be a lack of independence observed between the two variables in a sample. The observed relationship should be small enough, close enough to zero in correlation coefficient terms, that sampling error can explain its deviation from zero. In my scenario, where I am treating the chi-square as a difference test, the null hypothesis says that the likelihood of patronizing a fast food restaurant that has a playroom is the same whether the patron does or doesn't have young children.

The alternative hypothesis says that the two variables are not independent of each other in the population, and that the observed relationship in the sample is reflective of that reality. There is enough deviation from independence in the sample that sampling error from a population with independence is not a plausible explanation. For my current scenario, this means that fast food patrons without children have a different likelihood of choosing to patronize a restaurant with a playroom than do patrons with young children.

Decision rule

I set my α level at .05 because I am willing to make a Type I error 5% of the time. By Equation 12.1, I calculate that the chi-square has one degree of freedom. Thus my $\chi^2_{cv} = 3.8415$. If my $\chi^2_{observed}$ is ≥ 3.8415, then I'll reject the null hypothesis; if $\chi^2_{observed} < 3.8415$, I'll fail to reject H_0.

TABLE **12.10** **New, Larger, More Representative Data Set for Fast Food Data**

	Playroom Yes	Playroom No	
Young children yes	65	49	114
Young children no	39	51	90
	104	100	204

This is also the time to think about sample size, whether the study is underpowered. I'm not aware of any other research in this area, so I have no previous research to use as a guideline to estimate the effect size. My guess is that the effect of presence of young children on choice of restaurant at lunch time is not a major one. That is, there are probably other factors (e.g., food preference, restaurant preference, convenience) that play a more major role. I would guess that at best presence of young children has a small to moderate effect. Using Cohen (1988) as a guide, a small effect is a correlation of .10 and a moderate effect is a correlation of .30. Splitting the difference, a small-to-moderate effect is equivalent to a correlation of .20. Looking at Appendix Table 8, I see that with α set at .05, if I want to have an 80% chance of rejecting H_0 when $\rho = .20$, I should have 195 cases in my sample. Since I only have 35, my study is underpowered if the effect in the population is the level I think it is.

At this point, I should stop my analyses until I have collected more data. Ideally, I should address my generalizability question by collecting data from a variety of fast food restaurants, with and without playrooms, at a variety of locations, at a variety of times of day.

So, I did that. I made a list of all the fast food restaurants, for chains that had playrooms in some of their restaurants, within a 5-mile radius of my office and then noted whether each had a playroom. I filled one hat with the addresses of the different restaurants and the other with times of day (lunch vs. dinner) and days of the week. I then drew slips of paper until I had a schedule of which restaurant to observe at which time on which day (e.g., the McDonalds on Upper Peach Street at noon on Friday) and went out to collect my data. Here is my new data set (Table 12.10).

I will still analyze these data with a chi-square test for contingency tables, though I am in better shape with regard to assumptions. My dependent variable is still nominal, I still view my samples as independent, and all cells have expected frequencies greater than five, as shown in Table 12.11. I still don't have random samples from the populations of people with and without young children who go to fast food restaurants, but such a random sample isn't attainable. All things considered, I have about as good a sample, albeit only from one city in the United States, as one is likely ever to have.*

---

*By the bye, I made these data up, I didn't really collect them. So, don't take my results too seriously.

LOOKING CLOSER

TABLE **12.11**   **Expected Frequencies for New Fast Food Data Set**

	Playroom Yes	Playroom No	
Young children yes	58.1176	55.8824	114
Young children no	45.8824	44.1176	90
	104	100	204

My null and alternative hypotheses have not changed, and neither has my decision rule. Though now, with $N = 204$, I have adequate power, an 80% chance, to reject the null hypothesis if the degree of relationship between the two variables in the population is at the level of $\rho = .20$. So, let me go on to the calculation stage.

Calculations

Using Equation 12.3, we calculate as follows:

$$\chi^2 = \frac{(65 - 58.1176)^2}{58.1176} + \frac{(49 - 55.8824)^2}{55.8824} + \frac{(39 - 45.8824)}{45.8824} + \frac{(51 - 44.1176)}{44.1176}$$

$$= .8150 + .8476 + 1.0324 + 1.0737 = 3.7687$$

As the observed chi-square value of 3.7687 is less than the critical value of 3.8415, I'll fail to reject the null hypothesis and report the results, in APA format, as $\chi^2 (1, N = 204) = 3.77, p > .05$.

Interpretation

Before I start my interpretation, let me think about what I want to do with these results that are not statistically significant. First, I need to explain why the study was done, what was done, and what was found. Then, I must comment on the lack of difference between the two groups. Since I run the risk of making a Type II error, I need to calculate power; and I should make sure that my sample size was adequate. Then, especially if my study was underpowered, it makes sense to calculate the 95% confidence interval for the difference between two proportions in order to gain some idea of how large the effect might be, even though it was not statistically significant. I feel no need to calculate r^2 or d, because the effect is not statistically significant, and I'll be using the confidence interval to speculate about the effect size. Similarly, the risk ratio and number needed to treat don't need to be calculated. However, if my study were underpowered, I might calculate the 95% confidence interval for the risk ratio (what is the "risk" of choosing a restaurant with a playroom if one has young children) because this might be a useful way to express the possible strength of the apparently-not-statistically-significant relationship. I will not choose number needed to treat for this because the interpretation wouldn't be sensible: how many families would you need to "treat" with young children in order to achieve one more family dining at a restaurant with a playroom? With my interpretation planned, let's turn to the calculations.

Difference between Groups

Since the results are not statistically significant, there is no reason to conclude that a real difference is indicated by the difference in percentages of patrons with and without young children choosing a fast food restaurant with or without a playroom (57% vs. 43%). Thus, there is no reason to talk about the direction of the difference: our results say there is not sufficient evidence to conclude that there *is* a difference.*

95% Confidence Interval for the Difference between Proportions

The probability of going to a fast food restaurant with a playroom is .5702 if the patron has young children, compared to .4333 if there are not young children present. Though it is not a statistically significant increase, there is a .1369 increase in the probability of choosing a restaurant with a playroom for patrons with young children. Not being statistically significant means that we are without reason to question the hypothesis that there is no difference in proportion between the two groups, that we have no reason to question that the real difference in proportions is zero. However, calculating the confidence interval, especially if power turns out to be low, gives some idea of how large the effect might be and whether the study deserves replication.

The first step in calculating the 95% confidence interval is to calculate the standard error of the difference for proportions ($s_{p_1-p_2}$) via Equation 12.4:

$$\sqrt{\frac{.5702 \times .4298}{114} + \frac{.4333 \times .5667}{90}} = \sqrt{.0021 + .0027} = .0692$$

Then, via Equation 12.5, we find the 95% confidence interval for the difference between two proportions:

$$.1369 \pm 1.96(.0692) = .1369 \pm .1356$$

Thus, the 95% confidence interval ranges from the proportion of patrons with young children choosing to eat at fast food restaurants with playrooms being .0013 *lower* than the proportion of patrons without young children choosing such restaurants, to the proportion being .2725

---

*I know that this seems wrong. The observed difference—57% vs. 43%—appears large, yet we are saying it is not a difference. But, those were the rules by which we agreed to play the game of null hypothesis significance testing—if the results are not statistically significant, we conclude that there is not sufficient evidence to conclude there is a difference.

LOOKING CLOSER

higher. It is not surprising that the confidence interval captures zero since the chi-square value is not statistically significant. Note that the confidence interval is lopsided, that it barely captures zero on one side and extends a reasonable distance above zero on the other side. This suggests to me that there may be an effect but that this study failed to find it.

Power and Sample Size

When one fails to reject the null hypothesis there is the possibility that one has made a Type II error, and the probability of this needs to be calculated. I had assumed that the degree of correlation, in the population, between presence or absence of young children and choice of restaurant was .20 and had calculated that I would need 195 cases in order to have an 80% chance of getting a sample that would allow me to find a statistically significant relationship. Now I need to calculate the actual degree of correlation observed in the study. Using Equation 12.6 we can calculate ϕ, a form of r:

$$\sqrt{\frac{3.7687}{204}} = \sqrt{.0185} = .1360 = .14$$

Via Appendix Table 7, where I would use $r = .10$ and $N = 200$, I find that my actual power was not the .80 I desired, but rather was .29.* Using Appendix Table 8, I find that I would need 502 cases to have an 80% chance of finding statistically significant results when $\rho = .125$. Put simply, my study was still underpowered, and I will have to be careful to raise the possibility that there really is some relationship between the two variables, I just didn't have enough cases for it to be statistically significant.[†]

Risk Ratio

When the results of a statistical analysis are not statistically significant, I don't advocate calculating either a risk ratio or the number needed to treat. Ahh, but... Just as the 95% confidence interval for the difference between two proportions may provide useful interpretative information even when the chi-square is not statistically significant, the 95% confidence interval for either the risk ratio or number needed to treat may help put not-statistically-significant results in perspective, especially when power is low as it was in this study.

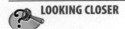 **LOOKING CLOSER**

*Since my observed r of .14 is closer to $\rho = .15$ than .10, I did let my eye wander down that column. In which case power would rise from .29 to .56. Beta, then, would range from .44 to .71.

[†] We're entering a bit of a hall of mirrors here, with the possibility that each time I complete a study that has nonstatistically significant results I can claim that there really is a relationship—the study was just underpowered. Since it is very unlikely that the relationship, in the population, between the two variables is really *exactly* zero, I can keep claiming that if only I had some more subjects... But, at some point one has to say that though there may be a statistically significant relationship it is so small as to be meaningless.

Risk ratios and number needed to treat were designed for use with clinical data, but they can sometimes meaningfully be applied to other data sets. For example, it might be reasonable to talk about how much greater the "risk" of dining at a fast food restaurant with a playroom is for patrons with young children than it is for patrons without young children. On the other hand, talking about the number of patrons needed to "treat" with young children in order to get one more family to dine at a restaurant with a playroom doesn't make much sense. Therefore I'll only calculate the relative risk ratio for these data.

The risk ratio, calculated by Equation 12.8, for the "risk" of eating at a fast food restaurant with a playroom for people with young children compared to those without is this:

$$\frac{.5702}{.4333} = 1.3159 = 1.32$$

In other words, diners with young children are 1.32 times more likely to eat at a restaurant with a playroom.

The chi-square was not significant, so I'm not going to interpret the risk ratio. I am, however, going to calculate a 95% confidence interval for it in case I want to use the upper bound when, in the context of low power and Type II error, I talk about how strong the relationship between the two variables might have been. Via Equation 12.9, the 95% confidence interval for the risk ratio ranges from this low:

$$\frac{\frac{.5702 + .4333}{2} + \frac{-.0013}{2}}{\frac{.5702 + .4333}{2} - \frac{-.0013}{2}} = \frac{.5018 + .0001}{.5018 - .0001} = 1.0002 = 1.00$$

to this high:

$$\frac{\frac{.5702 + .4333}{2} + \frac{.2725}{2}}{\frac{.5702 + .4333}{2} - \frac{.2725}{2}} = \frac{.5018 + .1363}{.5018 - .1363} = \frac{.6381}{.3665} = 1.7458 = 1.75$$

The risk, for patrons with young children compared to diners without young children, of eating at a fast food restaurant ranges from no increased risk ($RR = 1.00$) to it being 1.75 times more likely. So, with all the pieces in place, here's my interpretation:

"I conducted a study in which I investigated whether fast food patrons with young children, compared to patrons without young children, differed in their choice of whether to dine at a fast food restaurant that had a playroom. I listed all the fast food restaurants within a 5-mile radius of my office, noted whether each had a playroom, and then randomly selected the days and times that each restaurant would be observed. All told, 204 patrons were observed. For each patron it was

noted whether the restaurant had a playroom and whether the purchaser was with young children.

"Though it appeared that patrons with young children were more likely to choose restaurants with playrooms than were patrons without young children (57% vs. 43%), the difference was not statistically significant (χ^2 (1, N = 204) = 3.77, p > .05). Thus I am forced to conclude that there is not enough evidence to conclude that the presence or absence of young children has an impact on restaurant choice.

"This conclusion is called into question by the fact that my study was underpowered. Given the degree of relationship that I observed between presence or absence of young children and choice of a restaurant with or without a playroom, and given my sample size, there is a 44% to 71% chance that this conclusion is in error, that there really is a relationship between child presence or absence and restaurant choice.* Before concluding that such a relationship is unlikely to exist, the study should be replicated with a sample size that is 2.5 times as large.

"Though the observed difference was not statistically significant, I calculated the 95% confidence interval for the difference between proportions and found that the population difference could be as large as .27. In other words, if the percentage of patrons without young children who chose to dine at fast food restaurants with playrooms remained steady at 43%, the percentage with young children that dined at restaurants with playrooms could be as high as 70%. Though the results of the present study argue against the difference being that large, it could be. For this reason, as well as to have adequate power, the results should be replicated before I would feel comfortable concluding that there is no difference in playroom restaurant utilization between patrons with and without young children.

"One of the strengths of the current study was the way that the sample was obtained. Though it was not a random sample from the population of all the patrons from all the fast food restaurants in the whole world, it was gathered in such a way that there was no obvious bias in the selection of cases. In the most narrow sense, my sample seems representative of fast food consumers who frequent the restaurants within a 5-mile radius of my office, but I would be comfortable in generalizing the results to the city in which they were obtained. Whether the results generalize to other cities that differ in socioeconomic status or ethnic and cultural make-up is unknown. If that is of concern, then it should be addressed when the results are replicated."

Group Practice 12.5

Write a complete interpretative statement for questions 2 and 3 of Group Practice 12.1.

With that, this chapter is over. Table 12.12 lists the interpretative options for a chi-square test of association.

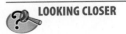 **LOOKING CLOSER**

*Note that there is flexibility in what one does in an interpretation, and I chose to violate my "Price is Right" rule regarding calculating power. As my observed r was .14 and Appendix Table 7 reports power for rs separated by .05 points, I chose to look at the power both for $\rho = .10$ and for $\rho = .15$ and reported the probability of Type II error as a range.

TABLE **12.12**   **Interpreting a chi-square test for contingency tables**

I. Report, briefly, objective of study and results (e.g., proportions and χ^2 value)

II. If fail to reject H_0:

  A. Report (a) no statistical difference in proportion between samples, or (b) statistical relationship between predictor and criterion variables in the sample is not different from zero

  B. Conclude (a) not sufficient evidence to conclude is a difference in proportions between the populations, or (b) not sufficient evidence to conclude is a nonzero relationship, in the population, between predictor and criterion variables

  C. Calculate confidence interval, power, and sample size. (Many statisticians recommend reporting a measure of effect size, such as d or r, when one fails to reject the null hypothesis.)

  D. Discuss possibility of Type II error

  E. Strengths/limitations/suggestions

III. If reject H_0:

  A. Report (a) difference in proportions between samples is statistically different from zero, or (b) relationship between predictor and criterion variables is statistically different from zero in the sample

  B. Conclude (a) there is likely a difference in proportions between the populations, or (b) is likely a nonzero relationship between predictor and criterion variable in the population

  C. Report direction of difference/relationship

  D. Report size of difference/relationship

    1. Confidence interval

    2. Effect size

      a. $r\ (\phi)$, r^2, or d

      b. If clinical study (or if appropriate), relative risk ratio and/or number needed to treat

  E. Calculate power and sample size

  F. Discuss possibility of Type I error

  G. Strengths/limitations/suggestions

SUMMARY

The chi-square test for contingency tables is a relationship test or a difference test that is used with a nominal-level dependent variable. It is called a nonparametric test because one doesn't need to make assumptions about the parameters of a distribution, the normality of the distribution, in order to use it. Thus, chi-square test for contingency tables is often used as a test of last resort, turned to when tests that use more information in numbers, tests that work with ordinal or interval and ratio numbers, have failed because their assumptions were not met.

The chi-square test directly compares the observed outcome to the outcome that would be expected if the null hypothesis were true. If the discrepancy between observed and expected is too great to be explained by sampling error, the null hypothesis is rejected. The two versions of the chi-square test for contingency tables, the chi-square difference test and the chi-square test of association, differ only in their assumptions, with the difference test version requiring independent samples.

Interpretation of a chi-square test for contingency tables follows along the lines seen for r, t, or ANOVA. If the null hypothesis is rejected, one should first explore the direction of the difference or relationship and then the size of the difference/relationship. The size of the effect can be explored via a 95% confidence interval for the difference between proportions, by converting χ^2 to r (technically, a ϕ coefficient), or by converting r into the effect size d. If you fail to reject the null hypothesis, use r to calculate power and necessary sample size.

Also explored in this chapter are two new interpretative options, ones seen in clinical research: the relative risk ratio (*RR*) and the number needed to treat (*NNT*). The risk ratio tells how much more likely a bad outcome is if a case is in the control group instead of being in the treatment group. The larger the *RR* value, the more it is above one, the more treatment helps relative to the control group. Number needed to treat tells how many more people must given the treatment condition in order to have one additional positive outcome. The closer *NNT* is to one, the more efficient the treatment is in leading to positive outcomes. For both *RR* and *NNT*, the 95% confidence interval for the difference between proportions can be used to estimate a 95% confidence interval to suggest how effective (or ineffective) a treatment might be in the larger population.

Review Exercises

1. Given χ^2 (3, $N = 57$) = 4.52, $p > .05$: (a) what is the power of the test? (b) What sample size is required to have a 95% chance of rejecting the null hypothesis? An 80% chance?

2. Given χ^2 (1, $N = 37$) = 3.80, $p > .05$: (a) what is the power of the test? (b) What sample size is required to have a 95% chance of rejecting the null hypothesis? An 80% chance? (c) What is the best estimate of ρ? (d) What is the best estimate of *RR*? (You'll have to think a bit to figure out parts c and d.)

3. For each scenario, (a) state the research question and (b) select an appropriate statistical test.

   a. A researcher wonders if a full moon makes it more likely that people will have a psychiatric or a medical emergency. She classifies the 7 days of the 28-day lunar month that are on or around the full moon as "full moon days," and the other 21 days as "non–full moon days." She then goes to emergency rooms and classifies people admitted to the hospital as having either a psychiatric or a medical emergency. Further, she notes whether they arrived at the emergency on a full moon day or a non–full moon day.

   b. The makers of a gel cushion for the feet want to find out if it decreases fatigue. They randomly assign nurses to wear the gel cushion, a foam cushion, or no cushion for an 8-hour shift. At the end of the shift they have the nurses, on an interval-level scale, report how fatigued they feel.

   c. Curious about the relationship between astrological sign and intelligence, an astrologer gets a large and representative sample of people from the United States, divides them according to the 12 astrological signs, and gives each one an ordinal measure of intelligence.

   d. A public health researcher wants to know if college students who get flu shots differ from those who don't in terms of how much risk they take with their physical health. He obtains a representative sample of college students from across the nation and finds out whether each has had a flu shot. He also administers to each student an interval-level physical-health–risk scale. (The physical-health–risk scale measures things like not washing hands after going to the bathroom, not getting enough sleep, etc. Higher scores indicate engaging in more behaviors that put one's health at risk.)

   e. A researcher at a specific college wants to find out if high-school class rank is associated with whether a person completes college in 4 years. She obtains the class ranks of a random sample of first-year students at her college, then waits 4 years to see whether these students graduate on time.

4. A graphologist (that's a person who analyzes handwriting) claims that he can tell a lot about a person from his or her handwriting. Being a suspicious sort, I obtain a sample of people and have them copy out the Gettysburg Address. I give the samples to the graphologist and ask him to tell me whether the person who wrote the sample was a male or a female. Below are the results. Analyze these data using the six-step hypothesis testing procedure, and draw a conclusion about his forecasting abilities.

	Graphologist Says "Male"	Graphologist Says "Female"
Samples from males	29	22
Samples from females	20	27

5. A researcher is comparing the standard treatment to a new treatment for an illness. She has 60 people with this illness who she randomly assigns to the two groups. After each person receives treatment, his or her outcome is classified as good, neutral, or bad. Two different good outcomes are possible: Outcome A or Outcome B. Similarly, there are two bad outcomes: Outcome X or Outcome Y. Here are the data that the researcher collects and that she plans to analyze with a chi-square test for contingency tables:

Outcome A	Outcome B	Neutral	Outcome X	Outcome Y
New treatment				
8	3	10	4	5
Standard treatment				
6	3	12	5	4

Why can't she do the test that she was planning, and what is a solution for this problem?

6. A health teacher takes a group of ninth-graders in a suburban school district who are deemed at risk to start smoking cigarettes and randomly divides them into two groups that receive different messages in their health classes. One group, called the control group, received standard health class material about the dangers of smoking. The other group, called the experimental group, received a new antismoking curriculum. Three years later, he tracked down each student and found out whether the student was smoking cigarettes. Here are the data:

	Not Smoking	Smoking
Experimental	56	18
Control	47	33

No assumptions were violated and, with α set at .05, he found χ^2 (1, $N = 154$) = 4.97, $p < .05$. (The exact chi-square value was 4.9720, if you care to know.)

Calculate: (a) the 95% confidence interval for the difference between two proportions, (b) r (i.e., ϕ), (c) d, (d), RR, (e) NNT, (f) α, (g) β, and (h) the sample size necessary to have power of .80 and .95. Then, pick and choose from a-h in writing a complete interpretative statement.

Homework Problems

1. If you were comparing string players (violinists, cellists, etc.) to brass players (trumpeters, trombonists, etc.) in terms of gender (male vs. female), the test to use would be
   a. Chi-square test for contingency tables.
   b. Chi-square difference test.
   c. Chi-square test of association.
   d. Any of the above.
   e. None of the above.

2. A podiatrist develops a new treatment to remove warts on the sole of the foot. She tests the new treatment by comparing it to a no-treatment control group. People with warts are randomly assigned to receive the new treatment or no treatment and then, a month after treatment, the podiatrist measures whether the wart is gone.

She has a large sample size and calculates the relative risk ratio as $RR = .50$. This means that
   a. The new treatment works better than the no-treatment control.
   b. There is no difference in outcome between the two control and experimental groups.
   c. The control treatment works better than the new treatment.

3. You calculate two different chi-square tests for contingency tables and find that χ^2_{cv} for test A is greater than χ^2_{cv} for test B. This means
   a. Test A has more cells than Test B.
   b. Test A has fewer cells than Test B.
   c. Test A has more cases than Test B.
   d. Test A has fewer cases than Test B.
   e. None of the above.

4. Which of these can't be converted into the others?
   a. χ^2
   b. r
   c. ϕ
   d. d
   e. t
   f. They can all be converted.

5. If X and Y are independent, then the probability of X and Y occurring together is
   a. Less than the probability of either happening by itself.
   b. Greater than the probability of either happening by itself.
   c. The probability of X happening *plus* the probability of Y happening.
   d. None of the above.

6. You conduct a clinical research study and find $NNT = 4$. This means that
   a. The treatment should be implemented on a larger scale.
   b. The study should be replicated.
   c. The treatment does not work.
   d. Interpretation of NNT depends on a cost/benefit analysis.

7. Given a standard, interval-level IQ test ($\mu = 100$ and $\sigma = 15$), and assuming that intelligence is normally distributed, answer the following questions.
   a. If anyone with an IQ greater than 135 is considered a genius, what percentage of people in the world should be geniuses?
   b. If Desdemona's IQ score is 67, what is her score as a percentile rank?
   c. Buffy was told that her IQ score, as a percentile rank, was a 67. What is her IQ score?
   d. Skip is exactly of average IQ and realizes that he needs a life partner who is smarter than he is. However, he realizes that someone who is too smart may—how shall I phrase this delicately?—find him a little "dull." Thus, he decides that his eligible pool of life partners consists of people who are from 10 to 25 IQ points smarter than he is. What percentage of people in the world, purely on the basis of IQ, are potential life partners for Skip?
   e. You want to do a study that involves people whose IQs are in the "normal" range, from 70 to 130. How many people must you screen with IQ tests in order to find a sample of 50 people with IQs in this range?

8. One way to divide up computer users is into those who prefer Windows-based machines and those who prefer Apple-based machines. Another way people are divided is into those whose left brain hemispheres are more dominant vs. those whose right brain hemispheres are more dominant. (Left brain–dominant people are described as being more logical and analytical, whereas right brain–dominant people are described as being more intuitive and creative.) I've always had the impression that people in the visual and creative arts prefer Apple computers. Since being more creative is considered a hallmark of having the right hemisphere of the brain be dominant, I wondered if there were a relation between brain hemisphere dominance and computer preference. I obtained a representative sample of adult computer users in the United States and had them tell me which type of computer they used: Apple or Windows. I also administered to them a brain hemisphere test that classified them as being left brain– or right brain–dominant. Below are the data. As you can see, I found that while only 23% of Windows users were right hemisphere–dominant, 40% of Apple users were. Analyze these data using the six-step hypothesis testing procedure.

	Left Hemisphere–Dominant	Right Hemisphere–Dominant
Windows user	90	27
Apple user	12	8

9. For each scenario, (a) state the research question, and (b) select the appropriate statistical test.
   a. A home economist decides to find out if it is true that one bad apple spoils the bunch. He gets 50 bushels of apples, each with 100 unspoiled apples in it and randomly divides them into two groups. In each bushel in one of the groups, he inserts a "bad" apple and in each bushel in the other group he inserts a

"good" apple. He then stores the bushels in a climate-controlled chamber for a month, after which he counts the number of spoiled apples per bushel.

b. A health outcomes research was curious to see how health status changed over time. She obtained a representative sample of people from the state in which she lived and had each person indicate his or her health status as 1, "good," or 2, "not good." Five years later, she contacted the people and again had them rate their health status on this two-point scale. Five years after the second assessment she contacted the people for a third and final time and again had them rate their health status on the two-point scale.

c. Though most of the people to whom I have taught statistics have been psychology majors, my impression is that some of my best statistics students have been non–psychology majors. And, contrary to the idea that men are better at math than women, I've been struck by how well women do in my stats class. So, I've decided to investigate how gender and/or major affect performance in my statistics class. I obtain a random sample of students from the hundreds to whom I have taught statistics and for each person I note three facts: (a) his or her gender, (b) whether he or she was a psychology major, and (c) his or her total accumulated points in my class.

d. A college administrator is concerned that grade inflation has been occurring over the years. He picks a "GenEd" class, first-year English composition, and finds out the distribution of grades (A, B, C, D, or F) for a random sample of students in 1976 and for a random sample of students in 2006.

e. At one university the top 5% of the class is supposed to graduate with honors. A university official had reason to believe that the university, suffering from the Lake Wobegon effect, an effect named after a mythical Minnesota town where "all the children are above average," was awarding more honors diplomas than it should. At a recent graduation there were 535 graduates, of whom 35 graduated with honors.

10. A sociologist was concerned that children who repeated a grade in elementary school were at increased risk for failing to graduate from high school, which put them at increased risk for engaging in criminal behavior. He devised an intervention program that was designed to get these kids back onto the academic track and help them graduate on time. To evaluate this program, he took 150 kids from a large urban school district who repeated a grade in elementary school, and randomly assigned them either to be in the control group, which received no special treatment, or to receive his experimental intervention. He then waited the appropriate number of years and found out whether the children graduated on time. Using the data below, analyze them using the six-step hypothesis testing procedure.

	Graduated on Time	Did Not Graduate on Time
Experimental	55	25
Control	30	40

13

What Test When

Choosing the Appropriate Statistical Test

Learning Objective

After completing this chapter you should be able to do the following:

Choose the correct statistical test to use in analyzing a data set.

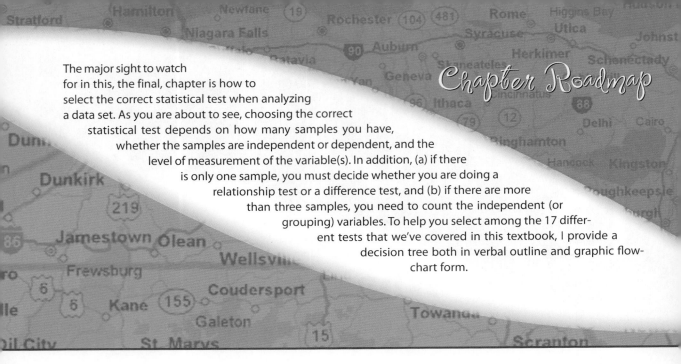

Chapter Roadmap

The major sight to watch for in this, the final, chapter is how to select the correct statistical test when analyzing a data set. As you are about to see, choosing the correct statistical test depends on how many samples you have, whether the samples are independent or dependent, and the level of measurement of the variable(s). In addition, (a) if there is only one sample, you must decide whether you are doing a relationship test or a difference test, and (b) if there are more than three samples, you need to count the independent (or grouping) variables. To help you select among the 17 different tests that we've covered in this textbook, I provide a decision tree both in verbal outline and graphic flow-chart form.

W hen the semester comes to an end, I usually discover that my statistics students are better at doing calculations than interpretations. That is, if I give them some data and ask them to calculate a *t* value, the vast majority of them accurately do so. As I grade a calculation question on the final, I feel pretty good as most students seem to have "gotten" the course. However, when I give a *t* value and ask what it means… Well, let's just say that I am more likely to get discouraged when grading this question on the final.

It is not new news that interpreting a statistical test is harder than calculating the value of a statistic. Interpretation is harder because it is less objective: there is not a formula that you can plug into and churn out just one correct answer. Interpretation takes perspective. It means standing back and seeing the big picture. This is hard to do for statistical newcomers.

Interpretation is subjective, and I call the subjective aspects of statistics the human side of statistics in order to emphasize the role of humans, not computers, in statistics. SPSS is great at calculating a *t* value, but it does not tell you the meaning of the calculated *t* value. For that, we need *us*, human beings with both a cerebral cortex *and* common sense.

Human decision making comes into play in most of the steps of the six-step hypothesis testing procedure that we've used since Chapter 7. The first step in the procedure—picking the appropriate test to analyze one's data, whether from the hundreds that exist or the 17 mentioned in this book—requires stepping back, figuring out the question being asked, and weighing options. This is a subjective, human endeavor.

Part of the second step in Tom and Harry is subjective as well. The second step involves listing the assumptions for the statistical test, deciding if they have been violated, and determining if the test can proceed. This, too, is a human endeavor: the decisions here are not cut and dried. One of the assumptions underlying the Pearson product moment correlation coefficient, for example, is that the relationship between the predictor and the criterion variable is linear. We learned to evaluate this assumption by making a scatterplot and observing it for nonlinearity. There is judgment involved here, and reasonable people may disagree, when viewing the same scatterplot, as to whether it represents a nonlinear relationship. Similarly, an independent samples t test is robust to violations of the normality assumption when N is large and the sample sizes are about equal. Different statisticians define "large" differently, and sample sizes that are "about" equal to one statistician may be unequal to another. Similarly, another statistician may decide that, even though N is large and the sample sizes are equal, the deviation from normality is too large to be forgiven.

The third step in the six-step null hypothesis testing procedure, stating the null and alternative hypotheses, is relatively rote. If you are doing a correlation, the null hypothesis is $\rho_{xy} = 0$, and the mutually exclusive alternative hypothesis is $\rho_{xy} \neq 0$. Similarly, the null and alternative hypotheses for other statistical tests are determined. Most beginning students of statistics find this a manageable step.

The decision rule, Step Four, also involves human decision making. As a beginning student of statistics I want you to make your life easy and set alpha at .05, two-tailed. However, I also want you to be aware that this should be a thoughtful decision, that one's alpha level should be based on one's willingness to avoid Type I error. If the costs of a Type I error—of erroneously rejecting the null hypothesis—are high, then set the alpha level to make it harder to reject the null hypothesis. Similarly, the decision about the possible size of the effect, the desired power, and the required sample size should be thoughtful decisions, decisions based on prior research and/or educated guesswork. These are not things that a computer can know or decide.

The least subjective, the most machine-like aspect of statistics, is Step Five, the actual calculations. It is at this that computers excel. As long as you have entered the data correctly, and as long as the machine has been programmed correctly, the computer will spit out the right answer. Unfortunately, if you've made a data entry error or if you've chosen the wrong statistical test, the computer will still quickly give you an answer.*

Finally, as I've been hammering home since Chapter 8, the last step of Tom and Harry, the interpretation of results, is a human endeavor. It is to

---

*Statistical programs can use different formulae, resulting in different answers. SPSS, for example, calculates ŝ not s when it calculates a standard deviation.

LOOKING CLOSER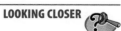

answer a question that we use a statistical test, but a single statistical value, whether it is t, r, F, or χ^2 is not an answer by itself. It takes our big brains and our common sense to understand the size, the meaning, and the limitations of an effect.

CHOOSING STATISTICAL TESTS

We've learned about 17 different statistical tests, though we've only learned to calculate five (the Pearson product moment correlation coefficient, the independent-samples t test, one-way ANOVA, repeated-measures ANOVA, and the chi-square test for contingency tables). Choosing the appropriate test to analyze your data—or recognizing that none of them is appropriate—is the most important step in statistics because it is the first step. If you choose the wrong path at the beginning, then you are not taking the most direct route to an answer, and there is a possibility that you might become lost. There is even the possibility, and this is a scary outcome, that you might think you have reached your destination and not recognize that you are at the wrong place.

I've likened statistical tests to tools, and that metaphor still holds. Imagine that you are a handyman and that I call on you to install some blinds on a window. To work most efficiently, you have to recognize what tools are needed and pack them in your toolbox. Once you are on the jobsite, if you are lacking a necessary tool, do you have the time to go back and get it? Or, do you not have one back at the shop and so need to go buy one? Or, is there a creative way that you can adapt an existing tool so that it will work? Clearly, with practice and experience you'll know what tools are needed, have them at hand, and know how you can adjust your existing tools to do things for which they were not originally intended.

Choosing the right tool helps you do the job more accurately, quickly, cleanly, and efficiently. If you don't have a drill and a screwdriver to attach the blinds, you can still manage to get them up with a hammer and nails. It is not optimal, and it won't look pretty—but it will work. If your task is comparing two independent samples on an interval-level variable, then a t test is the right tool to use. However, if you left your t test at home today and only have your chi-square test for contingency tables in the toolbox, you can use that. It is not ideal, but it will work in a pinch.

Though I hope that I made it clear that this is not a hard and fast distinction, earlier I separated null hypothesis significance tests into two broad categories: relationship tests and difference tests. The overlap between difference and relationship tests was especially clear in the last chapter with the chi-square test for contingency tables, which could be construed as a relationship test ("Is there a relationship between treatment received and survival?") or as a difference test ("Does the treatment group have a better survival rate than the control group?"). Whether a test is a relationship test or a difference test depends in good part on how one interprets the results. In this chapter, in providing you with a procedure for selecting the appropriate statistical test, I am not going to divide tests into relationship tests and difference tests.* Rather, I will focus on the number of samples, and use a five-question procedure:

1. How many samples do you have?
2. If there is only one sample: are you comparing the sample to a population or looking at the relationship between two variables in the sample?
3. If you have two or more samples: are the samples independent or dependent?
4. If you have more than three samples: how many independent or grouping variables are there?
5. And, always: what is the level of measurement of the variable(s) being analyzed?

HOW MANY SAMPLES?

The first question asked in the "What Test When" decision tree is, "How many samples do you have?" A sample is a group of cases, a "cell," and the possible answers to this question for purposes of deciding what test to choose are "one," "two," or "three or more." There is one sample when one is doing either a one-sample difference test (comparing a sample to a population) or a correlation coefficient, two samples when doing a two-sample difference test like an independent-samples t test, and three samples when doing a multiple-samples difference test like an analysis of variance.

The same set of data may be conceptualized as different numbers of samples, depending on how the research question is phrased. Imagine that my sample consists of students in a sixth-grade class. If I am studying these students to see if there is a relationship between their heights and the distances they can long jump, then I have one sample. If I change my question to ask if there is a difference in long jump ability between boys and girls, then I have two samples. And, if I change my question to ask if there is a difference in long jump ability between people who are left-handed, right-handed, and ambidextrous, then I have three samples.

One-Sample Tests

If there is one sample, then there are two types of statistical tests that come into play: (a) one-sample difference tests in which a sample is compared to a population to see if the two are similar on some attribute, or (b) a correlation coefficient that examines the degree of relationship between two variables in the sample. So, if you have determined that there

---

*SPSS, with its statistics "coach" that helps you figure out what test to do, uses the relationship vs. difference test distinction.

LOOKING CLOSER

is one sample, then the next question is whether you are asking (a) if the sample differs from a population, or (b) about the degree of relationship between two variables measured on cases in the sample.

Let's continue with my long jump example. As mentioned, I've collected my data from one sixth-grade class. If I want to make the case that these data apply to other sixth-graders, then I need to make the case that my sample is similar to sixth-graders in general. If, for example, I collect data about physical characteristics of my cases (e.g., height and weight), and if there are national data available about the mean height and weight of sixth-graders, then I can compare sample values to population values for the variables. If I find that there is no statistically significant difference between the values, then I feel more comfortable generalizing from my results to the larger sixth-grade population.

The next question is, Which one-sample difference test should be selected? This question depends on the level of measurement (nominal, ordinal, interval, or ratio) of the dependent variable. If the variable is measured at the interval or ratio level, as it is for height and weight in my long jump example, then a one-sample *t* test is called for. For an ordinal variable, the Kolmogorov-Smirnov goodness-of-fit test would be used; if the variable is nominal, a chi-square goodness-of-fit test is appropriate.*

When there is one sample, the other type of data analysis question used is a relationship question, one that addresses the degree of relationship between two variables measured in a sample of cases. If, for example, I examine my sample of sixth-graders to determine whether height is predictive of length of long jump, then I am asking a relationship question. The statistical test used to address the relationship question depends on the level of measurement of the variables. (Remember, with relationship questions we talk about predictor and criterion variables, not about independent and dependent variables.) If both variables are measured at the interval or ratio level, then the Pearson product moment correlation coefficient can be used. If both are measured at the ordinal level, or one is ordinal and the other interval or ratio, then the test used is the Spearman rank order correlation coefficient. If both variables are measured at the nominal level, then the chi-square test of association should be used. Things become a bit more complex when one variable is nominal and the other is not. In this instance, treat the nominal-level variable as a categorical or grouping variable, that is, as one that divides the one group of cases into samples. For example, suppose that I ask if there is a relationship between gender and long jump ability in the sample of sixth-graders. Gender is nominal, with two levels, and long jump distance is ratio. I recast my one sample as two samples, a sample of males and a sample of females, and then move on to select a statistical test from the two-sample test options.

LOOKING CLOSER

*I do need to mention that statistical tests have assumptions other than level of measurement that must be met before the test can be used. So, one needs to assess more than just the level of measurement.

Two-Sample Tests

Two-sample tests can be construed either as relationship tests ("Is there a relationship between gender and long jump ability?") or difference tests ("Do boys and girls differ in long jump ability?") and are used when two samples or categories are being compared on some dependent variable. Whether the dependent variable is being measured at the nominal, ordinal, interval, or ratio level will, of course, be important; but first you must decide if the samples are dependent or independent.

Samples are independent when the selection of cases for one sample has no influence over how the cases are selected for the other. For example, if I take a random sample of girls from the population of girls in the world, and a random sample of boys from the population of boys, then there is no relationship between the two samples: the samples are independent.* However, if I took a random sample of girls from the population of girls in the world, and asked each girl to bring along a boy, then my samples would be dependent since how the cases were selected for one sample was influenced by, or determined by, how the cases were selected for the other sample.† In my long jump example, even though each sample is not randomly selected from its respective population, and even though I can't use random assignment to divide my sample into a group of boys and a group of girls, I consider the samples of boys and girls to be independent samples since there is no apparent connection between how the cases were selected for the two samples.‡

There are three different two-sample difference tests for independent samples, and which one you choose depends on the level of measurement of the dependent variable. If the dependent variable is measured at the interval or ratio level and the other assumptions are met, then opt for an independent-samples t test. For an ordinal-level dependent variable, use the Mann Whitney U test; for a nominal-level dependent variable, use the chi-square difference test. When the samples are dependent and the variable is measured at the interval or ratio level, I prefer, as you know, repeated-measures ANOVA over a dependent-samples t test. For an ordinal-level dependent variable, the binomial sign test should be used, and for a nominal-level variable, use the McNemar test.

---

*Another way to achieve independent samples is to use random assignment to divide one group of cases into multiple samples.

†A variety of names are used to describe dependent samples: matched samples, pre-post samples, longitudinal samples, paired samples, and yoked samples are ones of which I am aware.

‡"Wait," I hear you saying, "the boys and girls are from the same class. Of course there is a connection between how the two samples were gathered—they're from the same environment. These are dependent samples!" Would you consider them dependent samples if I took a sample of boys and a sample of girls from the same city? From the same country? From the same planet? In each case they are coming from the same environment, but I doubt you would want to call them dependent samples. Dependent samples have to be yoked together in some way. Have I matched the boys and girls together into pairs? No. So, independent samples it is.

LOOKING CLOSER

Three or More Sample Tests

Finally, consider the tests used when there are three or more samples. Again, these could be construed as relationship tests or as difference tests. Along with asking whether the samples are independent or dependent, and along with asking about the level of measurement of the dependent variable, there is one new question to ask: How many independent or grouping variables are there?

An independent variable is a variable manipulated by the researcher, and a grouping variable is a naturally occurring characteristic on the basis of which cases are sorted into samples, groups or categories. If my sixth-graders are randomly divided into two groups, with the experimental group receiving special long jump training and the control group not, then type of training received is an independent variable. Dividing them up by gender means using a grouping variable, since gender is a naturally occurring characteristic and we can't assign people to be male or female.

All the tests that we have learned to calculate are used when there is only one independent or grouping variable, but there are a variety of situations with multiple independent and/or grouping variables. For example, a researcher might be interested in seeing if the impact of long jump instruction differed on the basis of gender. Thus, the sixth-graders would end up classified into four groups or samples: experimental group boys, control group boys, experimental group girls, and control group girls. If you ever take a more advanced statistics course you'll find a lot of specific tests available for analyzing such data. I'm just going to give them a generic name for now: factorial multiple-samples difference test.*

When there are three or more samples and only one independent or grouping variable, then we ask the same questions we did with two samples. If the samples are independent and the dependent variable is nominal, the test of choice is the chi-square test for contingency tables. For ordinal data, choose the Kruskal-Wallis one-way ANOVA by ranks, and for interval- or ratio-level data choose a one-way ANOVA. With dependent samples, the choices for nominal-, ordinal-, and interval- or ratio-level dependent variables are, respectively, Cochran's Q test, the Friedman two-way ANOVA by ranks, and repeated-measures ANOVA.

PRACTICE CHOOSING A STATISTICAL TEST

Choosing the statistical procedure takes practice and sometimes takes looking beyond the language used in describing the problem to the deeper question being posed. For example, take the following scenario, differentiating good teachers from bad teachers. Suppose, I take a sample of recent high-school graduates and ask them to think of their best and worst high school teachers. I then ask each to describe, using a series of

---

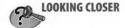 **LOOKING CLOSER**

*In Chapter 11 we saw examples of a specific version of a factorial multiple-samples difference test, one used with an interval- or ratio-level dependent variable: factorial ANOVA.

interval-level scales, the characteristics of those teachers. Each former student describes his or her best high-school teacher and his or her worst high-school teacher on scales that measure the student's perception of (a) the teacher's knowledge of the subject matter being taught, (b) the teacher's degree of excitement about the subject matter, (c) the teacher's degree of fairness, (d) how challenging the teacher's class was, and (e) how well organized the teacher was. What test should I use to analyze these data?

First, note, but don't be confused by, the fact that there are five dependent variables. Each is measured at the interval level, so when I figure out what test to use to analyze one, I'll know what test to use to analyze the other four.*

Second, note that I said that I have one sample of cases. This probably has started you down the one-sample tests path, but that would be a mistake. Step back and think. I want to compare students' ratings of good teachers to their ratings of bad teachers. Thus, I have two samples: a set of ratings of good teachers and a set of ratings of bad teachers. Further, since each pair of ratings is being made by the same person, so the samples are dependent. Thus, I'll end up analyzing these data with repeated-measures ANOVA.

Selecting the appropriate statistical test is challenging, but it does get easier with practice and experience. Here, as an aid in the test-selection decision, are two representations of a "What Test When" decision tree. One, Table 13.1, is in outline format for those who like words, and the other, Figure 13.1, is a flow chart for those who like pictures.

FINAL THOUGHTS ON EFFECT SIZES

I have just one more thing to offer you before this book draws to a close. In 1988, Jacob Cohen, writing about statistical power in the social and behavioral sciences, used the terms "small," "medium," and "large" effect sizes.[†] He offered his definitions of these, well aware that they were arbitrary and, I think, well aware that his definitions would be misused. Because he was a well-respected statistician and because researchers were eager to have different effect sizes defined, his definitions have become codified and employed in research outside the realm of the social and behavioral sciences. I'm as guilty as anyone of promoting Cohen's definitions. From Chapter 8 on, I've used them in interpreting results and helping to decide how large a sample size should be.

---

*There are statistical tests, called multivariate tests, that are used to analyze several dependent variables in one pass. That's a whole different, and more advanced, topic. In this book, I've just focused on univariate tests. Multivariate tests have the advantage, just like ANOVA does over multiple t tests, of keeping the overall α level lower.

[†]Cohen, J. (1988). *Statistical power analysis for the behavioral sciences.* Hillsdale, NJ: Lawrence Erlbaum Associates.

LOOKING CLOSER

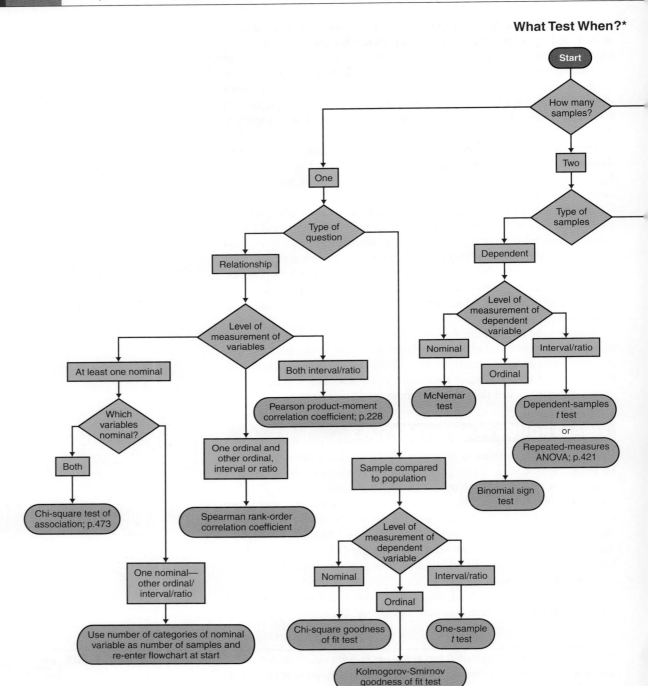

*Only proceed with the selected test if the assumptions on which it is based are not violated.

Figure **13.1** Flowchart of decision tree for choosing a statistical test.

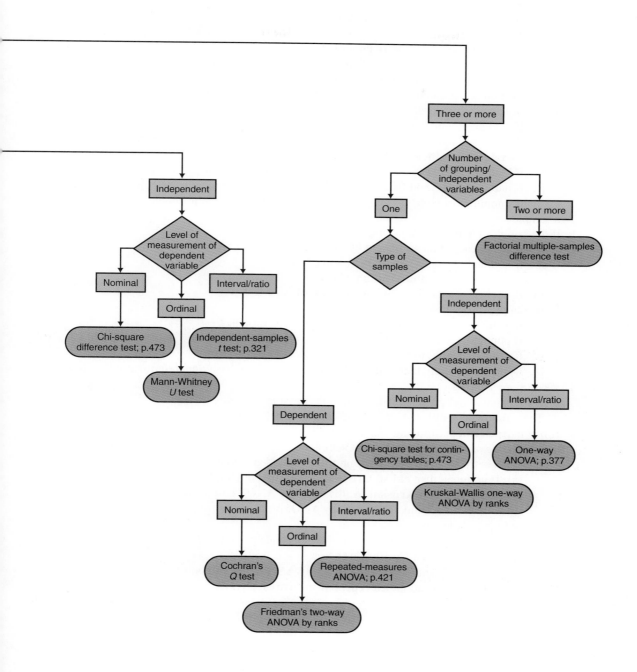

TABLE **13.1**   **Outline of Decision Tree for Choosing a Statistical Test**

I. How many samples of cases are there?
  A. One sample
    1. Is the question being asked if the sample differs from a population?
      a. If yes, what is the level of measurement of the dependent variable?
        i.   If nominal, then **chi-square goodness-of-fit**
        ii. If ordinal, then **Kolmogorov-Smirnov goodness-of-fit test**
        iii. If interval or ratio, then **one-sample *t* test**
    2. Is the question being asked about a relationship between two variables?
      a. If yes, what are the levels of measurement of the predictor and criterion variables?
        i.   If both are nominal, then **chi-square test of association**
        ii. If one is ordinal and the other is ordinal, interval, or ratio, then **Spearman rank order correlation coefficient**
        iii. If both are interval or ratio, then **Pearson product moment correlation coefficient**
        iv. If one is nominal and the other is ordinal, interval, or ratio, then see how many categories the nominal variable has and go to the tests for that number of samples
  B. Two samples
    1. If the samples are independent samples
      a. What is the level of measurement of the dependent variable?
        i.   If nominal, then **chi-square difference test**
        ii. If ordinal, then **Mann Whitney *U* test**
        iii. If interval or ratio, then **independent-samples *t* test**
    2. If the samples are dependent samples
      a. What is the level of measurement of the dependent variable?
        i.   If nominal, then **McNemar test**
        ii. If ordinal, then **binomial sign test**
        iii. If interval or ratio, then **repeated-measures ANOVA** (or a **dependent-samples *t* test**)
  C. Three or more samples
    1. If more than one independent and/or grouping variable
      a. Then, **factorial multiple-samples difference test**
    2. If one independent or grouping variable…
      a. … *And* the samples are independent samples
        i.   What is the level of measurement of the dependent variable?
          (a) If nominal, then **chi-square test for contingency tables**
          (b) If ordinal, then **Kruskal-Wallis one-way ANOVA by ranks**
          (c) If interval or ratio, then **one-way ANOVA**
      b. … *And* the samples are dependent samples
        i.   What is the level of measurement of the dependent variable?
          (a) If nominal, then **Cochran's Q test**
          (b) If ordinal, then **Friedman's two-way ANOVA by ranks**
          (c) If interval or ratio, then **repeated-measures ANOVA**

Note: Only proceed with the selected test if the assumptions on which it is based are not violated.

TABLE **13.2** **Cohen's Rough Guide to Effect Sizes for Correlations and Independent Sample Difference Tests in The Social and Behavioral Sciences**

	r	r^2 or ω^2	d	N (power of .80 / power of .95)
Small effect	$\approx.10$	$\approx.01$	$\approx.20$	784 / 1295
Medium effect	$\approx.30$	$\approx.10$	$\approx.60$	86 / 140
Large effect	$\approx.50$	$\approx.25$	≈1.20	30 / 47

Cohen offered definitions of effect size for, among others, r and d, in his book. Though r may be converted to d, and vice versa, Cohen was not entirely consistent in his definitions since he made a large effect larger for r than for d. I've focused on his effect sizes for r, partly because we encountered correlations first, but also because his effect sizes for correlations set a higher standard: they made it harder to call an effect large.

Because Cohen's definitions are so useful—but never forget that they are his arbitrary definitions meant as rough guides for research in the social and behavioral sciences—I've summarized them in Table 13.2. Use it advisedly, remembering that common sense, experience, and attention to context—in short, human decision making—will trump a slavish following of arbitrary, reified, rules.

PARTING THOUGHTS

You've reached the end of the book, and I feel the need to say something to mark this moment. I hope that you've enjoyed this journey through statistics, or at least found it less onerous than you feared at the outset. But, more important than enjoying it, I hope that you've gained some understanding of what statistics are and how statisticians think.

I also hope that you'll take another statistics course sometime. Some of the truest words I ever read about statistics were written by Robert Abelson (1995), a professor at Yale*:

"It has been my observation that most students do not really understand statistical material until they have been through it three times—once for exposure, once for practice, and once for the dawn of genuine insight."

Abelson is mostly right, though it has been my experience that it takes more than 3 times. I find that the best way to realize how little one knows *and* to come to understand more deeply what one does know, is to teach.

---

*Abelson, R. P. (1995). *Statistics as principled argument*. Hillsdale, NJ: Lawrence Erlbaum Associates, Publishers.

LOOKING CLOSER

Every time I teach this course I learn something new and/or gain a deeper understanding of something I thought I understood. If I thought teaching was an educational experience—well, it has nothing on writing a textbook. Thanks for coming on this journey of discovery with me. I hope that you've learned as much about statistics from reading this textbook as I have from writing it.

Group Practice 13.1

An infectious disease specialist at the Centers for Disease Control has, he believes, developed a vaccine for the common cold. To test its efficacy, he designs a study. In this double-blind study, a group of volunteers will agree to be inoculated either with the active vaccine or a placebo. They will then be monitored for a year, during which he will record whether they contract a cold. If they contract a cold, the researcher will note the number of days elapsed between inoculation and onset of the cold. In addition, the researcher will assess the severity of the cold on two dimensions: (a) measuring how many days the cold lasts, and (b) having the cold sufferers report, on an ordinal scale, how sick they were. I also want to mention that when potential participants called in to learn about the study, the researcher collected demographic information (age, race, gender) from them and administered an interval-level measure of general physical health.

1. The researcher wants to show that his sample is comparable to the U.S. population in terms of age, race, and gender. What statistical tests should he use?

2. Not everyone who called in to learn about the study volunteered to participate once they learned about the potential side effects and that, as it was a double-blind study, they might not receive the active vaccine. The researcher wants to show that people who volunteered for the study did not differ from those who chose not to participate. What statistical tests should he use?

3. The primary measure of the vaccine's effectiveness is whether people in the experimental group, compared to the control group, contracted a cold during the year after the vaccine. What statistical test should he use to answer this question?

4. Secondary measures of the vaccine's effectiveness were, for those who contracted colds, (a) how many days after the vaccination the cold occurred, (b) how long the cold lasted, and (c) how sick they were. What statistical tests should he use to answer these questions?

5. For the control group participants, the researcher was interested in the relationship between general physical health and contracting a cold. What statistical test should he use to answer this question?

6. For the control group participants who contracted a cold, the researcher was interested in the relationship between general physical health and the severity of the cold. What statistical test should he use?

SUMMARY

The five-question decision process introduced in this chapter can be used to select the correct statistical test for analyzing a set of data. The first step is counting the number of samples (one, two, or three or more). If there is only one sample, decide whether you are conducting a relationship test or a difference test. For two samples, decide if the samples are dependent or independent and the level of measurement of the dependent variable. If there are more than three samples, count the independent or grouping variables, and then decide whether the samples are independent or dependent and determine the level of measurement of the dependent variable.

Review Exercises

1. A political scientist is interested in familial consistency in terms of voting patterns. She gets three generations of the male members of families (grandfathers, fathers, and sons) and asks each if he supported the Democratic or the Republican candidate in the most recent presidential election. What statistical test should the researcher use to analyze these data?

2. As a college professor, I am aware that there are often two versions of a textbook, the full version and a briefer "fundamentals" version. I am also aware that some students read the text and others don't. I do a study in which students are assigned (a) to have either the full or the brief version of an introductory psychology textbook and (b) to take or not take on-line quizzes that cover the assigned chapters. What statistical test should I use to see how these two factors influence performance on an interval-level standardized exam at the end of the semester?

3. The American Civil Liberties Union has asked you to investigate whether people of minority status are more likely to be stopped by police for driving violations. You obtain, from a representative sample of police departments in the United States, records of the status (minority or not) of drivers stopped for violations. What statistical test will you use to compare the frequency with which people of minority status are stopped to data from the U.S. Census Bureau regarding the percentage of people in the United States who are of minority status?

4. Some teenagers have access to phones and instant messaging (IM) software while they are working on their homework, and others don't. Those who don't often complain to parents that their popularity will suffer as a result of lack of contact. A teacher at a particular school finds out which kids have access to phones and IM software while doing homework (Group A) and which don't (Group B). He also has all the kids in the school write down the names of their friends. Thus he can calculate, for each person, how many others list that person as a friend. This count is his measure of a person's popularity. What statistical test should he use to see if Group A kids differ from Group B kids in level of popularity?

5. A principal was curious as to the degree to which class rank was consistent over time. He obtains class rank when children were in sixth, ninth, and twelfth grades. What statistical test should he use to analyze these data?

6. Metal fatigue is a concern for airplanes. An engineer develops an ordinal-level metal fatigue scale that can be used to assess the degree to which the metal in an airplane is at risk of failing. The scale ranges from 0 to 50; higher numbers indicate more metal fatigue. She gets 40 airplanes that are currently in service and classifies them as (a) being built by European or American manufacturers, and (b) being in service for 5 or fewer years or more than 5 years. Below are the data she collects. Analyze them using the six-step hypothesis testing procedure.

	≤ 5 years in service	> 5 years in service
American-built	3, 5, 7, 1, 6, 6, 7, 8, 11, 1	5, 8, 11, 12, 13, 8, 7, 10, 9, 15
European-built	4, 6, 2, 2, 12, 3, 3, 4, 2, 3	9, 8, 13, 11, 10, 9, 8, 7, 12, 14

7. I like to do crossword puzzles, and my favorite puzzles come from *The New York Times*. The *New York Times* puzzles get harder as the week progresses: Monday puzzles are the easiest, and Saturday puzzles are the hardest. I decided to figure out what made one puzzle harder than another, whether it was some physical dimension of the puzzle. One that occurred to me was the length of the answers: maybe longer or shorter answers are harder to figure out. So, I obtained a random sample of puzzles from the population of Monday puzzles, a random sample of puzzles from the population of Wednesday puzzles, and a random sample of puzzles from the population of Friday puzzles, all from the past 10 years, and calculated the mean length (in letters) of the answers for each puzzle. Below are the data. Trusting me that they are normally distributed,

analyze them using the six-step hypothesis testing procedure.

	Monday	Wednesday	Friday
Mean answer length	2.31, 2.27, 2.37, 2.37, 2.39, 2.40, 2.42, 2.42, 2.43, 2.48	2.31, 2.38, 2.40, 2.41, 2.42, 2.45, 2.46, 2.49, 2.53, 2.59	2.75, 2.63, 2.64, 2.64, 2.67, 2.69, 2.84, 2.86, 2.90, 2.92
Mean	2.3860	2.4440	2.7540
s	.0575	.0754	.1139
$\hat{s}$	.0606	.0795	.1201

(The grand mean is 2.5280.)

8. A medical researcher has developed a treatment for the common cold. To measure its effectiveness, he obtains a sample of people with colds and randomly assigns them to receive his new treatment (the experimental group) or a placebo treatment (the control group). He measures outcome by measuring how long, in hours, it takes after receiving treatment before each participant reports being symptom-free. Below are the data he collects. Assuming that they are normally distributed, analyze them using the six-step hypothesis testing procedure.

	Experimental	Control
Hours until cold goes away	36, 32, 20, 22, 24, 30, 32, 24, 20, 26, 30, 28	25, 17, 12, 32, 30, 18, 12, 16, 14, 18
M	27.0000	19.4000
s	4.9329	6.8000
$\hat{s}$	5.1522	7.1678

Homework Problems

1. For the statistical tests that you have learned to calculate in this text, what is the correlation between the observed value of the test statistic and the probability of the observed value occurring if the null hypothesis is true?
   a. It is a positive correlation.
   b. It is a negative correlation.
   c. It is a zero correlation.
   d. The direction of the correlation is different for the different statistical tests.

2. A nurse practitioner takes people who have elevated cholesterol and randomly assigns them to (a) exercise, (b) eat sensibly, (c) take a cholesterol-lowering medication, or (d) do nothing. She plans to use analysis of variance to analyze the data. How many independent variables does she have?
   a. One
   b. Two
   c. Three
   d. Four

3. You are measuring a variable. The numbers that you assign to cases indicate whether they have the same or a different degree of the attribute being measured. You are measuring the variable at least at the _____ level.

   a. Nominal
   b. Ordinal
   c. Interval
   d. Ratio

4. An independent-samples t test
   a. Is a difference test.
   b. Is a relationship test.
   c. Can be interpreted either as a difference test or a relationship test.

5. I am doing a study in which I am looking at the relationship between the profession of parents (blue-collar vs. white collar) and the tuition price of the college that their child plans to attend. Profession of parents (blue-collar vs. white-collar) is best conceptualized as which of the following?
   a. A criterion variable
   b. A predictor variable
   c. An independent variable
   d. A dependent variable
   e. A grouping variable
   f. a and d
   g. b and e
   h. b, c, and e

6. I've never been convinced that weather forecasts are very accurate. Being an empirically minded guy, I decide to collect some data to see if my

hunch is correct. I randomly select 72 cities from throughout the United States, find their local newspapers for April 14, 2005, and note whether the weather forecast for the next day predicts any precipitation. I then check the newspapers from April 16 and note whether any precipitation occurred on April 15. Below are my results. Analyze them using the six-step hypothesis testing procedure.

	No Precipitation Occurred	Some Precipitation Occurred
No precipitation forecast	40	12
Some precipitation forecast	14	6

7. Recently it has been reported that daily consumption of flavonoid-rich dark chocolate promotes physical health. Although certainly in favor of physical health, a psychologist wondered about the impact of regularly eating chocolate on psychological health. To explore this he obtains a sample of adults who are not regular eaters of chocolate and gives them a hassle scale to measure their current mental outlook. The hassle scale consists of 50 annoying things that can happen (like misplacing one's keys), and a person completing the scale is asked to indicate if the hassle has occurred in the past 7 days. All hassles are considered equal; thus scores can range from 0 (no hassles were experienced in the past week) to 50 (all possible listed hassles occurred in the past week). After completing the hassle scale, each participant consumes 2 ounces of flavonoid-rich dark chocolate per day for 30 days. At the end of the month, each participant completes the hassle scale again. Here are the pairs of data (Time 1, Time 2) for each participant:

17, 13   12, 10   13, 9   8, 8   6, 8   12, 11
23, 18   4, 5   5, 4   10, 8   11, 11   10, 8

The mean at Time 1 is 10.9167, and at Time 2 it is 9.4167. The standard deviation ($\hat{s}$) at Time 1 is 5.2822, and at Time 2 it is 3.5227; $\hat{s}_{M_1-M_2} = 2.1106$. $SS_{subjects} = 431.3333$, $SS_{treatment} =$

13.5000, and $SS_{residual} = 24.5000$. Assuming that normality was not violated, analyze the data using the six-step hypothesis testing procedure.

8. In Ohio, they "grade" school districts by reporting how many of 18 possible state standards each district meets or exceeds, based on standardized testing. A teacher is curious how student/teacher ratio affects schools' performances. She randomly selects 15 suburban school districts from the county in which she lives. For each school district she finds the student/teacher ratio and also how many standards, out of a possible 18, it met. (Lower student/teacher ratios indicate smaller class size—which is generally considered good—and more standards met indicate better school performance.) Here are the data:

Ratio	Standards Met
17.8	18
16.0	14
17.8	18
16.8	10
16.2	9
15.2	15
19.5	12
16.0	4
16.4	5
19.0	13
15.7	6
15.8	15
18.4	17
14.6	3
18.0	16
$M = 16.8800$	$M = 11.6667$
$s = 1.4010$	$s = 5.0155$

Assuming that each variable is normally distributed, analyze the data using the six-step hypothesis testing procedure. (In your interpretation, talk about the difference in expected outcome for a school district with a 12:1 student/teacher ratio vs. a 20:1 ratio.)

9. Read each scenario and then select the appropriate statistical test to answer the question.

a. A waitress decides to do an experiment to see if she can increase tips. Before giving the check to a customer she flips a coin. If the coin turns up heads, she draws a smiley face on the check; if the coin turns up tails, she does not draw a smiley face. She does this for a week and keeps track of how much of a tip each customer leaves her. What statistical test should she use to see if drawing a smiley face has an impact on tipping?

b. An etiquette researcher is interested in knowing whether first or second children have better social skills. From the population of families with two—and only two—children he draws a random sample of families. To each child in the families in the sample he administers an interval-level measure of social skills. The mean for one group is 72.34 with a standard deviation of 17.45. For the other group the mean is 83.46 with a standard deviation of 3.47. What statistical test should he use to decide if one group differs from the other in terms of level of social skills? (This one is not what it first appears, so think it through carefully.)

c. A researcher is interested in seeing if Catholics, Jews, and Muslims have different views on abortion. She develops the Abortion Attitude Scale (AAS), a normally distributed, interval-level measuring device on which scores can range from –50 (very antiabortion) to +50 (very proabortion). She then obtains random samples from the populations of Catholics, Jews, and Muslims and gives each person the AAS. What statistical test should she use to analyze the data?

d. A health researcher is interested in whether nurses and physicians have different views on assisted suicide. He obtains random samples from both populations and asks each case in his sample a single yes-no question. The question is, "Can you envision a situation in which you would assist one of your patients in committing suicide?" What statistical test should be used to see if nurses and physicians differ in their answers?

e. A psychologist believes that the more direct experience a person has with handicapped people, the more positive a person's attitude is to handicapped people. She obtains a random sample of people and from each one learns two facts: (a) how many times the person has interacted with handicapped people, and (b) how the person feels about handicapped people in general. The latter item is measured on an interval-level scale. What statistical test should be done to see what the relationship is between the two variables?

10. Again, select the appropriate statistical test for each scenario.

a. I believe that the development of physical coordination affects mental development. I get a group of 16-year-olds and find out from their parents whether they were normal, early bloomers, or late bloomers in terms of physical coordination as children. I then administer an interval-level measure of IQ to each 16-year-old. Is there a relationship between age of development of physical coordination and degree of intelligence?

b. When my children were younger and took naps, I was very focused on trying to determine what influenced how long their naps were. With one of my children, it seemed that if he started his nap before 1 PM he took a longer nap than if he started after 2 PM. Further, it seemed that he took a longer nap when a babysitter was watching him than when I was. Being a statistician, I designed an experiment in which half the time he was put down before 1 PM and half after 2 PM. Further, each naptime option was equally divided into me or a babysitter putting him down. What statistical test should I use to see the degree to which start of naptime and/or me vs. babysitter putting him down affects how long he naps, as measured on an ordinal-level scale?

c. A psychologist is interested in examining power in male/female relationships. She has come up with a novel way to determine who has the upper hand in the relationship: by watching a couple hold hands and seeing whose hand is on the top. She gets a large sample of handholding couples and for each couple randomly picks whether she will observe the male or the female member of the couple. (She does this so that she will have independent samples of males and females.) Then, for each couple she determines whether the person she is observing is the upper or the lower handholder when the couple is holding hands. What statistical test should she do to determine if men or women are more likely to have the upper hand in relationships?

d. A researcher knows that in the general population about 2% of people have IQs in the genius range. He is curious to know if college professors mirror the general population in the frequency with which they can be classified as geniuses. He obtains a random sample of college professors and administers to them a standard IQ test. He uses this IQ test to classify them as "genius" or "not genius." What statistical test should he use to see if more (or fewer) college professors are geniuses than are found in the general population?

e. A psychologist uses classical conditioning to teach dogs to salivate to the sound of a bell. (She measures salivation in milliliters of saliva produced.) She puts each dog back in its home cage and tests each to see how much it salivates to the sound of the bell 24 hours after conditioning, 48 hours after conditioning, and 72 hours after conditioning. What statistical test should she use to see if there are differences in the level of salivation at those three points after conditioning?

APPENDIX

TABLE 1 Area under the Normal Curve

z Score	Below +z Above −z	From Mean to z	Above +z Below −z	z Score	Below +z Above −z	From Mean to z	Above +z Below −z
.00	50.00%	.00%	50.00%	.50	69.15%	19.15%	30.85%
.01	50.40%	.40%	49.60%	.51	69.50%	19.50%	30.50%
.02	50.80%	.80%	49.20%	.52	69.85%	19.85%	30.15%
.03	51.20%	1.20%	48.80%	.53	70.19%	20.19%	29.81%
.04	51.60%	1.60%	48.40%	.54	70.54%	20.54%	29.46%
.05	51.99%	1.99%	48.01%	.55	70.88%	20.88%	29.12%
.06	52.39%	2.39%	47.61%	.56	71.23%	21.23%	28.77%
.07	52.79%	2.79%	47.21%	.57	71.57%	21.57%	28.43%
.08	53.19%	3.19%	46.81%	.58	71.90%	21.90%	28.10%
.09	53.59%	3.59%	46.41%	.59	72.24%	22.24%	27.76%
.10	53.98%	3.98%	46.02%	.60	72.57%	22.57%	27.43%
.11	54.38%	4.38%	45.62%	.61	72.91%	22.91%	27.09%
.12	54.78%	4.78%	45.22%	.62	73.24%	23.24%	26.76%
.13	55.17%	5.17%	44.83%	.63	73.57%	23.57%	26.43%
.14	55.57%	5.57%	44.43%	.64	73.89%	23.89%	26.11%
.15	55.96%	5.96%	44.04%	.65	74.22%	24.22%	25.78%
.16	56.36%	6.36%	43.64%	.66	74.54%	24.54%	25.46%
.17	56.75%	6.75%	43.25%	.67	74.86%	24.86%	25.14%
.18	57.14%	7.14%	42.86%	.68	75.17%	25.17%	24.83%
.19	57.53%	7.53%	42.47%	.69	75.49%	25.49%	24.51%
.20	57.93%	7.93%	42.07%	.70	75.80%	25.80%	24.20%
.21	58.32%	8.32%	41.68%	.71	76.11%	26.11%	23.89%
.22	58.71%	8.71%	41.29%	.72	76.42%	26.42%	23.58%
.23	59.10%	9.10%	40.90%	.73	76.73%	26.73%	23.27%
.24	59.48%	9.48%	40.52%	.74	77.04%	27.04%	22.96%
.25	59.87%	9.87%	40.13%	.75	77.34%	27.34%	22.66%
.26	60.26%	10.26%	39.74%	.76	77.64%	27.64%	22.36%
.27	60.64%	10.64%	39.36%	.77	77.94%	27.94%	22.06%
.28	61.03%	11.03%	38.97%	.78	78.23%	28.23%	21.77%
.29	61.41%	11.41%	38.59%	.79	78.52%	28.52%	21.48%
.30	61.79%	11.79%	38.21%	.80	78.81%	28.81%	21.19%
.31	62.17%	12.17%	37.83%	.81	79.10%	29.10%	20.90%
.32	62.55%	12.55%	37.45%	.82	79.39%	29.39%	20.61%
.33	62.93%	12.93%	37.07%	.83	79.67%	29.67%	20.33%
.34	63.31%	13.31%	36.69%	.84	79.95%	29.95%	20.05%
.35	63.68%	13.68%	36.32%	.85	80.23%	30.23%	19.77%
.36	64.06%	14.06%	35.94%	.86	80.51%	30.51%	19.49%
.37	64.43%	14.43%	35.57%	.87	80.78%	30.78%	19.22%
.38	64.80%	14.80%	35.20%	.88	81.06%	31.06%	18.94%
.39	65.17%	15.17%	34.83%	.89	81.33%	31.33%	18.67%
.40	65.54%	15.54%	34.46%	.90	81.59%	31.59%	18.41%
.41	65.91%	15.91%	34.09%	.91	81.86%	31.86%	18.14%
.42	66.28%	16.28%	33.72%	.92	82.12%	32.12%	17.88%
.43	66.64%	16.64%	33.36%	.93	82.38%	32.38%	17.62%
.44	67.00%	17.00%	33.00%	.94	82.64%	32.64%	17.36%
.45	67.36%	17.36%	32.64%	.95	82.89%	32.89%	17.11%
.46	67.72%	17.72%	32.28%	.96	83.15%	33.15%	16.85%
.47	68.08%	18.08%	31.92%	.97	83.40%	33.40%	16.60%
.48	68.44%	18.44%	31.56%	.98	83.65%	33.65%	16.35%
.49	68.79%	18.79%	31.21%	.99	83.89%	33.89%	16.11%

TABLE 1   Area under the Normal Curve—cont'd

z Score	Below +z Above −z	From Mean to z	Above +z Below −z	z Score	Below +z Above −z	From Mean to z	Above +z Below −z
1.00	84.13%	34.13%	15.87%	1.60	94.52%	44.52%	5.48%
1.01	84.38%	34.38%	15.62%	1.61	94.63%	44.63%	5.37%
1.02	84.61%	34.61%	15.39%	1.62	94.74%	44.74%	5.26%
1.03	84.85%	34.85%	15.15%	1.63	94.84%	44.84%	5.16%
1.04	85.08%	35.08%	14.92%	1.64	94.95%	44.95%	5.05%
1.05	85.31%	35.31%	14.69%	1.65	95.05%	45.05%	4.95%
1.06	85.54%	35.54%	14.46%	1.66	95.15%	45.15%	4.85%
1.07	85.77%	35.77%	14.23%	1.67	95.25%	45.25%	4.75%
1.08	85.99%	35.99%	14.01%	1.68	95.35%	45.35%	4.65%
1.09	86.21%	36.21%	13.79%	1.69	95.45%	45.45%	4.55%
1.10	86.43%	36.43%	13.57%	1.70	95.54%	45.54%	4.46%
1.11	86.65%	36.65%	13.35%	1.71	95.64%	45.64%	4.36%
1.12	86.86%	36.86%	13.14%	1.72	95.73%	45.73%	4.27%
1.13	87.08%	37.08%	12.92%	1.73	95.82%	45.82%	4.18%
1.14	87.29%	37.29%	12.71%	1.74	95.91%	45.91%	4.09%
1.15	87.49%	37.49%	12.51%	1.75	95.99%	45.99%	4.01%
1.16	87.70%	37.70%	12.30%	1.76	96.08%	46.08%	3.92%
1.17	87.90%	37.90%	12.10%	1.77	96.16%	46.16%	3.84%
1.18	88.10%	38.10%	11.90%	1.78	96.25%	46.25%	3.75%
1.19	88.30%	38.30%	11.70%	1.79	96.33%	46.33%	3.67%
1.20	88.49%	38.49%	11.51%	1.80	96.41%	46.41%	3.59%
1.21	88.69%	38.69%	11.31%	1.81	96.49%	46.49%	3.51%
1.22	88.88%	38.88%	11.12%	1.82	96.56%	46.56%	3.44%
1.23	89.07%	39.07%	10.93%	1.83	96.64%	46.64%	3.36%
1.24	89.25%	39.25%	10.75%	1.84	96.71%	46.71%	3.29%
1.25	89.44%	39.44%	10.56%	1.85	96.78%	46.78%	3.22%
1.26	89.62%	39.62%	10.38%	1.86	96.86%	46.86%	3.14%
1.27	89.80%	39.80%	10.20%	1.87	96.93%	46.93%	3.07%
1.28	89.97%	39.97%	10.03%	1.88	96.99%	46.99%	3.01%
1.29	90.15%	40.15%	9.85%	1.89	97.06%	47.06%	2.94%
1.30	90.32%	40.32%	9.68%	1.90	97.13%	47.13%	2.87%
1.31	90.49%	40.49%	9.51%	1.91	97.19%	47.19%	2.81%
1.32	90.66%	40.66%	9.34%	1.92	97.26%	47.26%	2.74%
1.33	90.82%	40.82%	9.18%	1.93	97.32%	47.32%	2.68%
1.34	90.99%	40.99%	9.01%	1.94	97.38%	47.38%	2.62%
1.35	91.15%	41.15%	8.85%	1.95	97.44%	47.44%	2.56%
1.36	91.31%	41.31%	8.69%	1.96	97.50%	47.50%	2.50%
1.37	91.47%	41.47%	8.53%	1.97	97.56%	47.56%	2.44%
1.38	91.62%	41.62%	8.38%	1.98	97.61%	47.61%	2.39%
1.39	91.77%	41.77%	8.23%	1.99	97.67%	47.67%	2.33%
1.40	91.92%	41.92%	8.08%	2.00	97.72%	47.72%	2.28%
1.41	92.07%	42.07%	7.93%	2.01	97.78%	47.78%	2.22%
1.42	92.22%	42.22%	7.78%	2.02	97.83%	47.83%	2.17%
1.43	92.36%	42.36%	7.64%	2.03	97.88%	47.88%	2.12%
1.44	92.51%	42.51%	7.49%	2.04	97.93%	47.93%	2.07%
1.45	92.65%	42.65%	7.35%	2.05	97.98%	47.98%	2.02%
1.46	92.79%	42.79%	7.21%	2.06	98.03%	48.03%	1.97%
1.47	92.92%	42.92%	7.08%	2.07	98.08%	48.08%	1.92%
1.48	93.06%	43.06%	6.94%	2.08	98.12%	48.12%	1.88%
1.49	93.19%	43.19%	6.81%	2.09	98.17%	48.17%	1.83%
1.50	93.32%	43.32%	6.68%	2.10	98.21%	48.21%	1.79%
1.51	93.45%	43.45%	6.55%	2.11	98.26%	48.26%	1.74%
1.52	93.57%	43.57%	6.43%	2.12	98.30%	48.30%	1.70%
1.53	93.70%	43.70%	6.30%	2.13	98.34%	48.34%	1.66%
1.54	93.82%	43.82%	6.18%	2.14	98.38%	48.38%	1.62%
1.55	93.94%	43.94%	6.06%	2.15	98.42%	48.42%	1.58%
1.56	94.06%	44.06%	5.94%	2.16	98.46%	48.46%	1.54%
1.57	94.18%	44.18%	5.82%	2.17	98.50%	48.50%	1.50%
1.58	94.29%	44.29%	5.71%	2.18	98.54%	48.54%	1.46%
1.59	94.41%	44.41%	5.59%	2.19	98.57%	48.57%	1.43%

Continued

TABLE 1 Area under the Normal Curve—cont'd

z Score	Below +z Above −z	From Mean to z	Above +z Below −z	z Score	Below +z Above −z	From Mean to z	Above +z Below −z
2.20	98.61%	48.61%	1.39%	2.80	99.744%	49.744%	.256%
2.21	98.64%	48.64%	1.36%	2.81	99.752%	49.752%	.248%
2.22	98.68%	48.68%	1.32%	2.82	99.760%	49.760%	.240%
2.23	98.71%	48.71%	1.29%	2.83	99.767%	49.767%	.233%
2.24	98.75%	48.75%	1.25%	2.84	99.774%	49.774%	.226%
2.25	98.78%	48.78%	1.22%	2.85	99.781%	49.781%	.219%
2.26	98.81%	48.81%	1.19%	2.86	99.788%	49.788%	.212%
2.27	98.84%	48.84%	1.16%	2.87	99.795%	49.795%	.205%
2.28	98.87%	48.87%	1.13%	2.88	99.801%	49.801%	.199%
2.29	98.90%	48.90%	1.10%	2.89	99.807%	49.807%	.193%
2.30	98.93%	48.93%	1.07%	2.90	99.813%	49.813%	.187%
2.31	98.96%	48.96%	1.04%	2.91	99.819%	49.819%	.181%
2.32	98.98%	48.98%	1.02%	2.92	99.825%	49.825%	.175%
2.33	99.01%	49.01%	.99%	2.93	99.831%	49.831%	.169%
2.34	99.04%	49.04%	.96%	2.94	99.836%	49.836%	.164%
2.35	99.06%	49.06%	.94%	2.95	99.841%	49.841%	.159%
2.36	99.09%	49.09%	.91%	2.96	99.846%	49.846%	.154%
2.37	99.11%	49.11%	.89%	2.97	99.851%	49.851%	.149%
2.38	99.13%	49.13%	.87%	2.98	99.856%	49.856%	.144%
2.39	99.16%	49.16%	.84%	2.99	99.861%	49.861%	.139%
2.40	99.18%	49.18%	.82%	3.00	99.865%	49.865%	.135%
2.41	99.20%	49.20%	.80%	3.01	99.869%	49.869%	.131%
2.42	99.22%	49.22%	.78%	3.02	99.874%	49.874%	.126%
2.43	99.25%	49.25%	.75%	3.03	99.878%	49.878%	.122%
2.44	99.27%	49.27%	.73%	3.04	99.882%	49.882%	.118%
2.45	99.29%	49.29%	.71%	3.05	99.886%	49.886%	.114%
2.46	99.31%	49.31%	.69%	3.06	99.889%	49.889%	.111%
2.47	99.32%	49.32%	.68%	3.07	99.893%	49.893%	.107%
2.48	99.34%	49.34%	.66%	3.08	99.896%	49.896%	.104%
2.49	99.36%	49.36%	.64%	3.09	99.900%	49.900%	.100%
2.50	99.38%	49.38%	.62%	3.10	99.903%	49.903%	.097%
2.51	99.40%	49.40%	.60%	3.11	99.906%	49.906%	.094%
2.52	99.41%	49.41%	.59%	3.12	99.910%	49.910%	.090%
2.53	99.43%	49.43%	.57%	3.13	99.913%	49.913%	.087%
2.54	99.45%	49.45%	.55%	3.14	99.916%	49.916%	.084%
2.55	99.46%	49.46%	.54%	3.15	99.918%	49.918%	.082%
2.56	99.48%	49.48%	.52%	3.16	99.921%	49.921%	.079%
2.57	99.49%	49.49%	.51%	3.17	99.924%	49.924%	.076%
2.58	99.51%	49.51%	.49%	3.18	99.926%	49.926%	.074%
2.59	99.52%	49.52%	.48%	3.19	99.929%	49.929%	.071%
2.60	99.53%	49.53%	.47%	3.20	99.931%	49.931%	.069%
2.61	99.55%	49.55%	.45%	3.21	99.934%	49.934%	.066%
2.62	99.56%	49.56%	.44%	3.22	99.936%	49.936%	.064%
2.63	99.57%	49.57%	.43%	3.23	99.938%	49.938%	.062%
2.64	99.59%	49.59%	.41%	3.24	99.940%	49.940%	.060%
2.65	99.60%	49.60%	.40%	3.25	99.942%	49.942%	.058%
2.66	99.61%	49.61%	.39%	3.26	99.944%	49.944%	.056%
2.67	99.62%	49.62%	.38%	3.27	99.946%	49.946%	.054%
2.68	99.63%	49.63%	.37%	3.28	99.948%	49.948%	.052%
2.69	99.64%	49.64%	.36%	3.29	99.950%	49.950%	.050%
2.70	99.65%	49.65%	.35%	3.30	99.952%	49.952%	.048%
2.71	99.66%	49.66%	.34%	3.31	99.953%	49.953%	.047%
2.72	99.67%	49.67%	.33%	3.32	99.955%	49.955%	.045%
2.73	99.68%	49.68%	.32%	3.33	99.957%	49.957%	.043%
2.74	99.69%	49.69%	.31%	3.34	99.958%	49.958%	.042%
2.75	99.702%	49.702%	.298%	3.35	99.960%	49.960%	.040%
2.76	99.711%	49.711%	.289%	3.36	99.961%	49.961%	.039%
2.77	99.720%	49.720%	.280%	3.37	99.962%	49.962%	.038%
2.78	99.728%	49.728%	.272%	3.38	99.964%	49.964%	.036%
2.79	99.736%	49.736%	.264%	3.39	99.965%	49.965%	.035%

TABLE 1 **Area under the Normal Curve—cont'd**

z Score	Below +z Above −z	From Mean to z	Above +z Below −z	z Score	Below +z Above −z	From Mean to z	Above +z Below −z
3.40	99.966%	49.966%	.034%	3.75	99.9912%	49.9912%	.0088%
3.41	99.968%	49.968%	.032%	3.76	99.9915%	49.9915%	.0085%
3.42	99.969%	49.969%	.031%	3.77	99.9918%	49.9918%	.0082%
3.43	99.970%	49.970%	.030%	3.78	99.9922%	49.9922%	.0078%
3.44	99.971%	49.971%	.029%	3.79	99.9925%	49.9925%	.0075%
3.45	99.972%	49.972%	.028%	3.80	99.9928%	49.9928%	.0072%
3.46	99.973%	49.973%	.027%	3.81	99.9931%	49.9931%	.0069%
3.47	99.974%	49.974%	.026%	3.82	99.9933%	49.9933%	.0067%
3.48	99.975%	49.975%	.025%	3.83	99.9936%	49.9936%	.0064%
3.49	99.976%	49.976%	.024%	3.84	99.9938%	49.9938%	.0062%
3.50	99.9767%	49.9767%	.0233%	3.85	99.9941%	49.9941%	.0059%
3.51	99.9776%	49.9776%	.0224%	3.86	99.9943%	49.9943%	.0057%
3.52	99.9784%	49.9784%	.0216%	3.87	99.9946%	49.9946%	.0054%
3.53	99.9792%	49.9792%	.0208%	3.88	99.9948%	49.9948%	.0052%
3.54	99.9800%	49.9800%	.0200%	3.89	99.9950%	49.9950%	.0050%
3.55	99.9807%	49.9807%	.0193%	3.90	99.9952%	49.9952%	.0048%
3.56	99.9815%	49.9815%	.0185%	3.91	99.9954%	49.9954%	.0046%
3.57	99.9822%	49.9822%	.0178%	3.92	99.9956%	49.9956%	.0044%
3.58	99.9828%	49.9828%	.0172%	3.93	99.9958%	49.9958%	.0042%
3.59	99.9835%	49.9835%	.0165%	3.94	99.9959%	49.9959%	.0041%
3.60	99.9841%	49.9841%	.0159%	3.95	99.9961%	49.9961%	.0039%
3.61	99.9847%	49.9847%	.0153%	3.96	99.9963%	49.9963%	.0037%
3.62	99.9853%	49.9853%	.0147%	3.97	99.9964%	49.9964%	.0036%
3.63	99.9858%	49.9858%	.0142%	3.98	99.9966%	49.9966%	.0034%
3.64	99.9864%	49.9864%	.0136%	3.99	99.9967%	49.9967%	.0033%
3.65	99.9869%	49.9869%	.0131%	4.00	99.9968%	49.9968%	.0032%
3.66	99.9874%	49.9874%	.0126%	4.10	99.99793%	49.99793%	.00207%
3.67	99.9879%	49.9879%	.0121%	4.20	99.99867%	49.99867%	.00133%
3.68	99.9883%	49.9883%	.0117%	4.30	99.99915%	49.99915%	.00085%
3.69	99.9888%	49.9888%	.0112%	4.40	99.99946%	49.99946%	.00054%
3.70	99.9892%	49.9892%	.0108%	4.50	99.99966%	49.99966%	.00034%
3.71	99.9896%	49.9896%	.0104%	4.60	99.99979%	49.99979%	.00021%
3.72	99.9900%	49.9900%	.0100%	4.70	99.99987%	49.99987%	.00013%
3.73	99.9904%	49.9904%	.0096%	4.80	99.99992%	49.99992%	.00008%
3.74	99.9908%	49.9908%	.0092%	4.90	99.99995%	49.99995%	.00005%
				5.00	99.99997%	49.99997%	.00003%

TABLE **2**   **Random Number Table**

	A	B	C	D	E	F
1	4963	4775	6746	1453	6349	3103
2	3538	8169	4029	8333	6806	4925
3	9475	6997	8843	5435	2479	3814
4	4783	3087	6777	8001	9582	9193
5	6985	7743	5185	7611	2279	2830
6	8161	8409	7758	5150	4970	8791
7	5774	9914	2316	2101	2619	4515
8	5688	5767	2666	5917	5068	7054
9	8748	6072	1734	1284	8886	1281
10	3269	4133	6507	6175	1750	5840
11	5790	9899	3923	7204	2029	6989
12	2282	6307	8442	1343	8086	9895
13	9666	5097	8935	3598	2207	2418
14	9318	6080	9228	2373	7685	5302
15	2614	9617	8101	4184	4816	8265
16	3295	6504	7092	4989	8638	3551
17	1839	2316	1863	4471	8142	1323
18	6462	9582	5235	4053	6974	5042
19	1337	2366	5503	4636	7233	3466
20	7380	9733	5088	2914	6181	9839
21	1272	5275	6133	1212	1713	6028
22	9567	9432	9156	3531	9550	1187
23	3639	6086	8733	2846	6003	3612
24	7494	7700	4691	4940	7143	6093
25	1889	7576	5388	4217	5838	5567
26	4806	7227	5587	5601	7407	7878
27	6520	1532	1592	4420	9718	2877
28	4777	2102	4480	9239	5643	5009
29	9070	4634	3349	4308	9023	5130
30	3564	7566	2637	5036	2122	2332
31	2789	7317	2392	2750	5413	7336
32	1096	1797	7287	5855	2855	9051
33	9472	2187	2406	2486	4514	2722
34	4371	9117	9556	7544	7562	8233
35	3422	2250	2399	8074	5683	6461
36	6101	6675	2729	7183	8008	2091
37	1909	6260	8709	5327	5782	5006
38	6774	5649	2832	7279	5077	3066
39	2640	6204	2949	7634	9488	5073
40	1816	1829	4270	6152	5381	6812

Generated via Lotus 123

TABLE 3 **Critical Values of *t* for 95% Confidence Intervals ($\alpha = .05$, Two-Tailed)**

df	t	df	t	df	t	df	t
1	12.7062	36	2.0281	71	1.9939	160	1.9749
2	4.3027	37	2.0262	72	1.9935	170	1.9740
3	3.1824	38	2.0244	73	1.9930	180	1.9732
4	2.7764	39	2.0227	74	1.9925	190	1.9725
5	2.5706	40	2.0211	75	1.9921	200	1.9719
6	2.4469	41	2.0195	76	1.9917	210	1.9713
7	2.3646	42	2.0181	77	1.9913	220	1.9708
8	2.3060	43	2.0167	78	1.9908	230	1.9703
9	2.2622	44	2.0154	79	1.9905	240	1.9699
10	2.2281	45	2.0141	80	1.9901	250	1.9695
11	2.2010	46	2.0129	81	1.9897	260	1.9691
12	2.1788	47	2.0117	82	1.9893	270	1.9688
13	2.1604	48	2.0106	83	1.9890	280	1.9685
14	2.1448	49	2.0096	84	1.9886	290	1.9682
15	2.1314	50	2.0086	85	1.9883	300	1.9679
16	2.1199	51	2.0076	86	1.9879	320	1.9674
17	2.1098	52	2.0066	87	1.9876	340	1.9670
18	2.1009	53	2.0057	88	1.9873	360	1.9666
19	2.0930	54	2.0049	89	1.9870	380	1.9662
20	2.0860	55	2.0040	90	1.9867	400	1.9659
21	2.0796	56	2.0032	91	1.9864	420	1.9656
22	2.0739	57	2.0025	92	1.9861	440	1.9654
23	2.0687	58	2.0017	93	1.9858	460	1.9651
24	2.0639	59	2.0010	94	1.9855	480	1.9649
25	2.0595	60	2.0003	95	1.9853	500	1.9647
26	2.0555	61	1.9996	96	1.9850	600	1.9639
27	2.0518	62	1.9990	97	1.9847	700	1.9634
28	2.0484	63	1.9983	98	1.9845	800	1.9629
29	2.0452	64	1.9977	99	1.9842	900	1.9626
30	2.0423	65	1.9971	100	1.9840	1000	1.9623
31	2.0395	66	1.9966	110	1.9818	2000	1.9612
32	2.0369	67	1.9960	120	1.9799	3000	1.9608
33	2.0345	68	1.9955	130	1.9784	4000	1.9606
34	2.0322	69	1.9949	140	1.9771	5000	1.9604
35	2.0301	70	1.9944	150	1.9759	infinity	1.9600

Calculated via Microsoft Excel 2004

TABLE **4** **Critical Values of _r_ for Pearson Product Moment Correlation Coefficients When $\rho = 0$**

	Level of Significance (α), One-Tailed Test						Level of Significance (α), One-Tailed Test			
	.05	.025	.01	.005			.05	.025	.01	.005
	Level of Significance (α), Two-Tailed Test						Level of Significance (α), Two-Tailed Test			
_df_ = _N_ − 2	.10	.05	.02	.01		_df_ = _N_ − 2	.10	.05	.02	.01
1	.9877	**.9969**	.9995	.9999		39	.2605	**.3081**	.3621	.3978
2	.9000	**.9500**	.9800	.9900		40	.2573	**.3044**	.3578	.3932
3	.8054	**.8783**	.9343	.9587						
4	.7293	**.8114**	.8822	.9172		41	.2542	**.3008**	.3536	.3887
5	.6694	**.7545**	.8329	.8745		42	.2512	**.2973**	.3496	.3843
						43	.2483	**.2940**	.3458	.3801
6	.6215	**.7067**	.7887	.8343		44	.2455	**.2907**	.3420	.3761
7	.5822	**.6664**	.7498	.7977		45	.2429	**.2876**	.3384	.3721
8	.5493	**.6319**	.7155	.7646						
9	.5214	**.6021**	.6851	.7348		46	.2403	**.2845**	.3348	.3683
10	.4973	**.5760**	.6581	.7079		47	.2377	**.2816**	.3314	.3646
						48	.2353	**.2787**	.3281	.3610
11	.4762	**.5529**	.6339	.6835		49	.2329	**.2759**	.3249	.3575
12	.4575	**.5324**	.6120	.6614		50	.2306	**.2732**	.3218	.3542
13	.4409	**.5140**	.5923	.6411						
14	.4259	**.4973**	.5742	.6226		55	.2201	**.2609**	.3074	.3385
15	.4124	**.4821**	.5577	.6055		60	.2108	**.2500**	.2948	.3248
						65	.2027	**.2404**	.2837	.3126
16	.4000	**.4683**	.5426	.5897		70	.1954	**.2319**	.2737	.3017
17	.3887	**.4555**	.5285	.5751		75	.1888	**.2242**	.2647	.2919
18	.3783	**.4438**	.5155	.5614						
19	.3687	**.4329**	.5034	.5487		80	.1829	**.2172**	.2565	.2830
20	.3598	**.4227**	.4921	.5368		85	.1775	**.2108**	.2491	.2748
						90	.1726	**.2050**	.2422	.2673
21	.3515	**.4132**	.4815	.5256		95	.1680	**.1996**	.2359	.2604
22	.3438	**.4044**	.4716	.5151		100	.1638	**.1946**	.2301	.2540
23	.3365	**.3961**	.4622	.5052						
24	.3297	**.3882**	.4534	.4958		120	.1496	**.1779**	.2104	.2324
25	.3233	**.3809**	.4451	.4869		140	.1386	**.1648**	.1951	.2155
						160	.1297	**.1543**	.1827	.2019
26	.3172	**.3739**	.4372	.4785		180	.1223	**.1455**	.1723	.1905
27	.3115	**.3673**	.4297	.4705		200	.1161	**.1381**	.1636	.1809
28	.3061	**.3610**	.4226	.4629						
29	.3009	**.3550**	.4158	.4556		250	.1039	**.1236**	.1465	.1620
30	.2960	**.3494**	.4093	.4487		300	.0948	**.1129**	.1338	.1480
						350	.0878	**.1046**	.1240	.1371
31	.2913	**.3440**	.4031	.4421		400	.0822	**.0978**	.1160	.1283
32	.2869	**.3388**	.3973	.4357		450	.0775	**.0922**	.1094	.1210
33	.2826	**.3338**	.3916	.4297						
34	.2785	**.3291**	.3862	.4238		500	.0735	**.0875**	.1038	.1149
35	.2746	**.3246**	.3810	.4182		600	.0671	**.0799**	.0948	.1049
						700	.0621	**.0740**	.0878	.0972
36	.2709	**.3202**	.3760	.4128		800	.0581	**.0692**	.0821	.0909
37	.2673	**.3160**	.3712	.4076		900	.0548	**.0653**	.0774	.0857
38	.2638	**.3120**	.3665	.4026		1000	.0520	**.0619**	.0735	.0813

Calculated via Microsoft Excel 2004

TABLE 5 Transformation of *r* to Fisher's *z*

	.000	.001	.002	.003	.004	.005	.006	.007	.008	.009
.00	.000	.001	.002	.003	.004	.005	.006	.007	.008	.009
.01	.010	.011	.012	.013	.014	.015	.016	.017	.018	.019
.02	.020	.021	.022	.023	.024	.025	.026	.027	.028	.029
.03	.030	.031	.032	.033	.034	.035	.036	.037	.038	.039
.04	.040	.041	.042	.043	.044	.045	.046	.047	.048	.049
.05	.050	.051	.052	.053	.054	.055	.056	.057	.058	.059
.06	.060	.061	.062	.063	.064	.065	.066	.067	.068	.069
.07	.070	.071	.072	.073	.074	.075	.076	.077	.078	.079
.08	.080	.081	.082	.083	.084	.085	.086	.087	.088	.089
.09	.090	.091	.092	.093	.094	.095	.096	.097	.098	.099
.10	.100	.101	.102	.103	.104	.105	.106	.107	.108	.109
.11	.110	.111	.112	.113	.114	.116	.117	.118	.119	.120
.12	.121	.122	.123	.124	.125	.126	.127	.128	.129	.130
.13	.131	.132	.133	.134	.135	.136	.137	.138	.139	.140
.14	.141	.142	.143	.144	.145	.146	.147	.148	.149	.150
.15	.151	.152	.153	.154	.155	.156	.157	.158	.159	.160
.16	.161	.162	.163	.164	.165	.167	.168	.169	.170	.171
.17	.172	.173	.174	.175	.176	.177	.178	.179	.180	.181
.18	.182	.183	.184	.185	.186	.187	.188	.189	.190	.191
.19	.192	.193	.194	.195	.196	.198	.199	.200	.201	.202
.20	.203	.204	.205	.206	.207	.208	.209	.210	.211	.212
.21	.213	.214	.215	.216	.217	.218	.219	.221	.222	.223
.22	.224	.225	.226	.227	.228	.229	.230	.231	.232	.233
.23	.234	.235	.236	.237	.238	.239	.241	.242	.243	.244
.24	.245	.246	.247	.248	.249	.250	.251	.252	.253	.254
.25	.255	.256	.258	.259	.260	.261	.262	.263	.264	.265
.26	.266	.267	.268	.269	.270	.271	.273	.274	.275	.276
.27	.277	.278	.279	.280	.281	.282	.283	.284	.286	.287
.28	.288	.289	.290	.291	.292	.293	.294	.295	.296	.297
.29	.299	.300	.301	.302	.303	.304	.305	.306	.307	.308
.30	.310	.311	.312	.313	.314	.315	.316	.317	.318	.319
.31	.321	.322	.323	.324	.325	.326	.327	.328	.329	.331
.32	.332	.333	.334	.335	.336	.337	.338	.339	.341	.342
.33	.343	.344	.345	.346	.347	.348	.350	.351	.352	.353
.34	.354	.355	.356	.357	.359	.360	.361	.362	.363	.364
.35	.365	.367	.368	.369	.370	.371	.372	.373	.375	.376
.36	.377	.378	.379	.380	.381	.383	.384	.385	.386	.387
.37	.388	.390	.391	.392	.393	.394	.395	.397	.398	.399
.38	.400	.401	.402	.404	.405	.406	.407	.408	.409	.411
.39	.412	.413	.414	.415	.417	.418	.419	.420	.421	.422
.40	.424	.425	.426	.427	.428	.430	.431	.432	.433	.434
.41	.436	.437	.438	.439	.440	.442	.443	.444	.445	.446
.42	.448	.449	.450	.451	.453	.454	.455	.456	.457	.459
.43	.460	.461	.462	.464	.465	.466	.467	.469	.470	.471
.44	.472	.473	.475	.476	.477	.478	.480	.481	.482	.483
.45	.485	.486	.487	.488	.490	.491	.492	.494	.495	.496
.46	.497	.499	.500	.501	.502	.504	.505	.506	.508	.509
.47	.510	.511	.513	.514	.515	.517	.518	.519	.520	.522
.48	.523	.524	.526	.527	.528	.530	.531	.532	.533	.535
.49	.536	.537	.539	.540	.541	.543	.544	.545	.547	.548
.50	.549	.551	.552	.553	.555	.556	.557	.559	.56	.561
.51	.563	.564	.565	.567	.568	.570	.571	.572	.574	.575
.52	.576	.578	.579	.580	.582	.583	.585	.586	.587	.589
.53	.590	.592	.593	.594	.596	.597	.599	.600	.601	.603
.54	.604	.606	.607	.608	.610	.611	.613	.614	.616	.617
.55	.618	.620	.621	.623	.624	.626	.627	.628	.630	.631
.56	.633	.634	.636	.637	.639	.640	.642	.643	.645	.646
.57	.648	.649	.650	.652	.653	.655	.656	.658	.659	.661
.58	.662	.664	.665	.667	.669	.670	.672	.673	.675	.676
.59	.678	.679	.681	.682	.684	.685	.687	.688	.690	.692

Continued

TABLE 5   Transformation of *r* to Fisher's *z*—cont'd

	.000	.001	.002	.003	.004	.005	.006	.007	.008	.009
.60	.693	.695	.696	.698	.699	.701	.703	.704	.706	.707
.61	.709	.711	.712	.714	.715	.717	.719	.720	.722	.723
.62	.725	.727	.728	.730	.732	.733	.735	.736	.738	.740
.63	.741	.743	.745	.746	.748	.750	.751	.753	.755	.756
.64	.758	.760	.762	.763	.765	.767	.768	.770	.772	.774
.65	.775	.777	.779	.781	.782	.784	.786	.788	.789	.791
.66	.793	.795	.796	.798	.800	.802	.804	.805	.807	.809
.67	.811	.813	.814	.816	.818	.820	.822	.824	.825	.827
.68	.829	.831	.833	.835	.837	.838	.840	.842	.844	.846
.69	.848	.850	.852	.854	.856	.858	.860	.861	.863	.865
.70	.867	.869	.871	.873	.875	.877	.879	.881	.883	.885
.71	.887	.889	.891	.893	.895	.897	.899	.901	.904	.906
.72	.908	.910	.912	.914	.916	.918	.920	.922	.924	.927
.73	.929	.931	.933	.935	.937	.940	.942	.944	.946	.948
.74	.950	.953	.955	.957	.959	.962	.964	.966	.968	.971
.75	.973	.975	.978	.980	.982	.984	.987	.989	.991	.994
.76	.996	.999	1.001	1.003	1.006	1.008	1.011	1.013	1.015	1.018
.77	1.020	1.023	1.025	1.028	1.030	1.033	1.035	1.038	1.040	1.043
.78	1.045	1.048	1.050	1.053	1.056	1.058	1.061	1.064	1.066	1.069
.79	1.071	1.074	1.077	1.079	1.082	1.085	1.088	1.090	1.093	1.096
.80	1.099	1.101	1.104	1.107	1.110	1.113	1.116	1.118	1.121	1.124
.81	1.127	1.130	1.133	1.136	1.139	1.142	1.145	1.148	1.151	1.154
.82	1.157	1.160	1.163	1.166	1.169	1.172	1.175	1.179	1.182	1.185
.83	1.188	1.191	1.195	1.198	1.201	1.204	1.208	1.211	1.214	1.218
.84	1.221	1.225	1.228	1.231	1.235	1.238	1.242	1.245	1.249	1.253
.85	1.256	1.260	1.263	1.267	1.271	1.274	1.278	1.282	1.286	1.290
.86	1.293	1.297	1.301	1.305	1.309	1.313	1.317	1.321	1.325	1.329
.87	1.333	1.337	1.341	1.346	1.350	1.354	1.358	1.363	1.367	1.371
.88	1.376	1.380	1.385	1.389	1.394	1.398	1.403	1.408	1.412	1.417
.89	1.422	1.427	1.432	1.437	1.442	1.447	1.452	1.457	1.462	1.467
.90	1.472	1.478	1.483	1.488	1.494	1.499	1.505	1.510	1.516	1.522
.91	1.528	1.533	1.539	1.545	1.551	1.557	1.564	1.570	1.576	1.583
.92	1.589	1.596	1.602	1.609	1.616	1.623	1.630	1.637	1.644	1.651
.93	1.658	1.666	1.673	1.681	1.689	1.697	1.705	1.713	1.721	1.730
.94	1.738	1.747	1.756	1.764	1.774	1.783	1.792	1.802	1.812	1.822
.95	1.832	1.842	1.853	1.863	1.874	1.886	1.897	1.909	1.921	1.933
.96	1.946	1.959	1.972	1.986	2.000	2.014	2.029	2.044	2.060	2.076
.97	2.092	2.110	2.127	2.146	2.165	2.185	2.205	2.227	2.249	2.273
.98	2.298	2.323	2.351	2.380	2.410	2.443	2.477	2.515	2.555	2.599
.99	2.647	2.700	2.759	2.826	2.903	2.994	3.106	3.250	3.453	3.800

Calculated via Microsoft Excel 2004

TABLE **6** **Transformation of Fisher's *z* to *r***

	.00	.01	.02	.03	.04	.05	.06	.07	.08	.09
.00	.000	.010	.020	.030	.040	.050	.060	.070	.080	.090
.10	.100	.110	.119	.129	.139	.149	.159	.168	.178	.188
.20	.197	.207	.217	.226	.235	.245	.254	.264	.273	.282
.30	.291	.300	.310	.319	.327	.336	.345	.354	.363	.371
.40	.380	.388	.397	.405	.414	.422	.430	.438	.446	.454
.50	.462	.470	.478	.485	.493	.501	.508	.515	.523	.530
.60	.537	.544	.551	.558	.565	.572	.578	.585	.592	.598
.70	.604	.611	.617	.623	.629	.635	.641	.647	.653	.658
.80	.664	.670	.675	.680	.686	.691	.696	.701	.706	.711
.90	.716	.721	.726	.731	.735	.740	.744	.749	.753	.757
1.00	.762	.766	.770	.774	.778	.782	.786	.789	.793	.797
1.10	.800	.804	.808	.811	.814	.818	.821	.824	.827	.831
1.20	.834	.837	.840	.843	.845	.848	.851	.854	.856	.859
1.30	.862	.864	.867	.869	.872	.874	.876	.879	.881	.883
1.40	.885	.887	.890	.892	.894	.896	.898	.900	.901	.903
1.50	.905	.907	.909	.910	.912	.914	.915	.917	.919	.920
1.60	.922	.923	.925	.926	.927	.929	.930	.932	.933	.934
1.70	.935	.937	.938	.939	.940	.941	.943	.944	.945	.946
1.80	.947	.948	.949	.950	.951	.952	.953	.954	.954	.955
1.90	.956	.957	.958	.959	.960	.960	.961	.962	.963	.963
2.00	.964	.965	.965	.966	.967	.967	.968	.969	.969	.970
2.10	.970	.971	.972	.972	.973	.973	.974	.974	.975	.975
2.20	.976	.976	.977	.977	.978	.978	.978	.979	.979	.980
2.30	.980	.980	.981	.981	.982	.982	.982	.983	.983	.983
2.40	.984	.984	.984	.985	.985	.985	.986	.986	.986	.986
2.50	.987	.987	.987	.987	.988	.988	.988	.988	.989	.989
2.60	.989	.989	.989	.990	.990	.990	.990	.990	.991	.991
2.70	.991	.991	.991	.992	.992	.992	.992	.992	.992	.992
2.80	.993	.993	.993	.993	.993	.993	.993	.994	.994	.994
2.90	.994	.994	.994	.994	.994	.995	.995	.995	.995	.995
3.00	.995	.995	.995	.995	.995	.996	.996	.996	.996	.996
3.10	.996	.996	.996	.996	.996	.996	.996	.996	.997	.997
3.20	.997	.997	.997	.997	.997	.997	.997	.997	.997	.997
3.30	.997	.997	.997	.997	.997	.998	.998	.998	.998	.998
3.40	.998	.998	.998	.998	.998	.998	.998	.998	.998	.998
3.50	.998	.998	.998	.998	.998	.998	.998	.998	.998	.998
3.60	.999	.999	.999	.999	.999	.999	.999	.999	.999	.999
3.70	.999	.999	.999	.999	.999	.999	.999	.999	.999	.999
3.80	.999	.999	.999	.999	.999	.999	.999	.999	.999	.999

Calculated via Microsoft Excel 2004

TABLE 7   Power for a Given *N* and a Given Observed or Hypothesized Correlation Value, $\alpha = .05$, Two-Tailed

N	\\ OBSERVED *r* VALUE OR HYPOTHESIZED ρ																		
	.05	.10	.15	.20	.25	.30	.35	.40	.45	.50	.55	.60	.65	.70	.75	.80	.85	.90	.95
5	.02	.03	.04	.04	.05	.06	.07	.08	.10	.11	.13	.16	.19	.23	.27	.34	.42	.54	.73
6	.03	.03	.04	.05	.06	.07	.09	.11	.13	.15	.18	.22	.26	.32	.39	.47	.58	.72	.88
7	.03	.03	.04	.06	.07	.08	.10	.13	.16	.19	.23	.28	.34	.41	.49	.59	.70	.83	.95
8	.03	.04	.05	.06	.08	.10	.12	.15	.19	.23	.28	.34	.41	.49	.58	.69	.80	.90	.98
9	.04	.04	.05	.07	.09	.11	.14	.17	.21	.26	.32	.39	.47	.56	.66	.76	.86	.95	
10	.03	.04	.05	.07	.09	.12	.16	.20	.24	.30	.37	.44	.53	.63	.73	.82	.91	.97	
11	.03	.04	.06	.08	.10	.13	.17	.22	.27	.34	.41	.50	.59	.68	.78	.87	.94	.98	
12	.03	.04	.06	.08	.11	.15	.19	.24	.30	.37	.45	.54	.64	.73	.83	.90	.96		
13	.03	.05	.06	.09	.12	.16	.21	.26	.33	.41	.49	.59	.68	.78	.86	.93	.97		
14	.03	.05	.07	.09	.13	.17	.22	.28	.36	.44	.53	.63	.72	.82	.89	.95	.98		
15	.03	.05	.07	.10	.14	.18	.24	.31	.38	.47	.57	.67	.76	.85	.92	.96			
16	.03	.05	.07	.10	.14	.19	.26	.33	.41	.50	.60	.70	.79	.87	.93	.97			
17	.03	.05	.08	.11	.15	.21	.27	.35	.44	.53	.63	.73	.82	.90	.95	.98			
18	.03	.05	.08	.12	.16	.22	.29	.37	.46	.56	.66	.76	.85	.91	.96	.98			
19	.03	.05	.08	.12	.17	.23	.30	.39	.49	.59	.69	.79	.87	.93	.97				
20	.03	.06	.09	.13	.18	.24	.32	.41	.51	.61	.72	.81	.89	.94	.97				
21	.04	.06	.09	.13	.19	.25	.34	.43	.53	.64	.74	.83	.90	.95	.98				
22	.04	.06	.09	.14	.19	.27	.35	.45	.56	.66	.76	.85	.92	.96	.98				
23	.04	.06	.09	.14	.20	.28	.37	.47	.58	.69	.78	.87	.93	.97					
24	.04	.06	.10	.15	.21	.29	.38	.49	.60	.71	.80	.88	.94	.97					
25	.04	.06	.10	.15	.22	.30	.40	.51	.62	.73	.82	.90	.95	.98					
26	.04	.06	.10	.16	.23	.31	.41	.52	.64	.74	.84	.91	.96	.98					
27	.04	.07	.11	.16	.23	.32	.43	.54	.66	.76	.85	.92	.96	.98					
28	.04	.07	.11	.17	.24	.34	.44	.56	.67	.78	.87	.93	.97						
29	.04	.07	.11	.17	.25	.35	.46	.57	.69	.79	.88	.94	.97						
30	.04	.07	.12	.18	.26	.36	.47	.59	.71	.81	.89	.94	.98						
32	.04	.07	.12	.19	.27	.38	.50	.62	.74	.84	.91	.96	.98						
34	.04	.08	.13	.20	.29	.40	.52	.65	.76	.86	.93	.97							
36	.04	.08	.13	.21	.31	.42	.55	.68	.79	.88	.94	.97							
38	.04	.08	.14	.22	.32	.44	.58	.70	.81	.90	.95	.98							
40	.04	.08	.14	.23	.34	.46	.60	.73	.83	.91	.96	.98							
42	.04	.09	.15	.24	.35	.48	.62	.75	.85	.92	.97								
44	.05	.09	.16	.25	.37	.50	.64	.77	.87	.94	.97								
46	.05	.09	.16	.26	.38	.52	.66	.79	.88	.94	.98								
48	.05	.09	.17	.27	.40	.54	.68	.81	.90	.95	.98								
50	.05	.10	.17	.28	.41	.56	.70	.82	.91	.96	.98								
55	.05	.10	.19	.30	.45	.60	.75	.86	.93	.97									
60	.05	.11	.20	.33	.48	.64	.78	.89	.95	.98									
65	.05	.12	.22	.35	.52	.68	.82	.91	.96										
70	.06	.12	.23	.38	.55	.71	.84	.93	.97										

NOTE: If cell is blank, power is greater than .99.
Beta (β) = probability of a Type II error = 1 − power

TABLE **7** **Power for a Given *N* and a Given Observed or Hypothesized Correlation Value, $\alpha = .05$, Two-Tailed—cont'd**

N	\.05	\.10	\.15	\.20	\.25	\.30	\.35	\.40	\.45	\.50	\.55	\.60	\.65	\.70	\.75	\.80	\.85	\.90	\.95
75	.06	.13	.24	.40	.58	.74	.87	.94	.98										
80	.06	.14	.26	.42	.61	.77	.89	.96	.98										
85	.06	.14	.27	.45	.63	.80	.91	.96											
90	.06	.15	.29	.47	.66	.82	.92	.97											
95	.06	.15	.30	.49	.68	.84	.93	.98											
100	.07	.16	.31	.51	.71	.86	.94	.98											
110	.07	.17	.34	.55	.75	.89	.96												
120	.07	.19	.37	.59	.78	.91	.97												
130	.08	.20	.39	.62	.82	.93	.98												
140	.08	.21	.42	.66	.84	.95	.98												
150	.08	.22	.44	.69	.87	.96													
160	.09	.24	.47	.71	.89	.97													
170	.09	.25	.49	.74	.90	.97													
180	.09	.26	.52	.76	.92	.98													
190	.10	.27	.54	.79	.93	.98													
200	.10	.29	.56	.81	.94														
220	.11	.31	.60	.84	.96														
240	.11	.33	.64	.87	.97														
260	.12	.36	.67	.90	.98														
280	.12	.38	.71	.92	.98														
300	.13	.40	.74	.93															
400	.16	.51	.85	.98															
500	.19	.60	.92																
600	.23	.68	.95																
700	.26	.75	.97																
800	.29	.80	.98																
900	.32	.85																	
1000	.35	.88																	
1500	.49	.97																	
2000	.60																		
3000	.78																		
4000	.88																		
5000	.94																		
6000	.97																		
7000	.98																		
8000																			

NOTE: If cell is blank, power is greater than .99.

Beta (β) = probability of a Type II error = 1 – power

Calculated via nQuery Advisor, 5.0

TABLE 8   *N* Needed for a Correlation Coefficient ($\alpha = .05$, Two-Tailed) at Different Levels of ρ and Different Levels of Power

ρ	POWER					
	.75	.80	.85	.90	.95	.99
.025	11,100	12,560	14,360	16,810	20,790	29,390
.050	2776	3139	3590	4200	5194	7341
.075	1234	1395	1595	1865	2306	3258
.100	694	784	896	1048	1295	1829
.125	444	502	573	670	827	1168
.150	308	348	398	464	573	809
.175	226	256	292	341	420	592
.200	173	195	223	260	321	451
.225	137	154	176	205	252	355
.250	111	125	142	166	204	286
.275	92	103	117	136	168	235
.300	77	86	98	114	140	196
.325	65	73	83	97	119	166
.350	56	63	72	83	102	142
.375	49	55	62	72	88	123
.400	43	48	54	63	77	107
.425	38	42	48	55	67	94
.450	34	38	43	49	60	83
.475	30	34	38	44	53	73
.500	27	30	34	39	47	65
.525	25	27	31	35	42	58
.550	22	25	28	32	38	52
.575	20	22	25	29	35	47
.600	19	20	23	26	31	43
.625	17	19	21	24	28	38
.650	16	17	19	22	26	35
.675	14	15	17	20	23	32
.700	13	14	16	18	21	29
.725	12	13	15	16	20	26
.750	11	12	13	15	18	24
.775	10	11	12	14	16	21
.800	9	10	11	13	15	19
.825	9	9	10	11	13	17
.850	8	9	9	10	12	16
.875	7	8	9	9	11	14
.900	7	7	8	8	10	12
.925	6	6	7	8	9	11
.950	5	6	6	7	7	9
.975	5	5	5	5	6	7

NOTE: β = probability of making a Type II error = 1 − power.
Calculations via Power Calculator available at http://calculators.stat.ucla.edu/powercalc/

TABLE 9   Critical Values of t When $\mu_1 = \mu_2$

	Level of Significance (α), One-Tailed Test						Level of Significance (α), One-Tailed Test			
	.05	.025	.01	.005			.05	.025	.01	.005
	Level of Significance (α), Two-Tailed Test						Level of Significance (α), Two-Tailed Test			
df	.10	.05	.02	.01		df	.10	.05	.02	.01
1	6.3138	12.7062	31.8205	63.6567		41	1.6829	2.0195	2.4208	2.7012
2	2.9200	4.3027	6.9646	9.9248		42	1.6820	2.0181	2.4185	2.6981
3	2.3534	3.1824	4.5407	5.8409		43	1.6811	2.0167	2.4163	2.6951
4	2.1318	2.7764	3.7469	4.6041		44	1.6802	2.0154	2.4141	2.6923
5	2.0150	2.5706	3.3649	4.0321		45	1.6794	2.0141	2.4121	2.6896
6	1.9432	2.4469	3.1427	3.7074		46	1.6787	2.0129	2.4102	2.6870
7	1.8946	2.3646	2.9980	3.4995		47	1.6779	2.0117	2.4083	2.6846
8	1.8595	2.3060	2.8965	3.3554		48	1.6772	2.0106	2.4066	2.6822
9	1.8331	2.2622	2.8214	3.2498		49	1.6766	2.0096	2.4049	2.6800
10	1.8125	2.2281	2.7638	3.1693		50	1.6759	2.0086	2.4033	2.6778
11	1.7959	2.2010	2.7181	3.1058		55	1.6730	2.0040	2.3961	2.6682
12	1.7823	2.1788	2.6810	3.0545		60	1.6706	2.0003	2.3901	2.6603
13	1.7709	2.1604	2.6503	3.0123		65	1.6686	1.9971	2.3851	2.6536
14	1.7613	2.1448	2.6245	2.9768		70	1.6669	1.9944	2.3808	2.6479
15	1.7531	2.1314	2.6025	2.9467		75	1.6654	1.9921	2.3771	2.6430
16	1.7459	2.1199	2.5835	2.9208		80	1.6641	1.9901	2.3739	2.6387
17	1.7396	2.1098	2.5669	2.8982		85	1.6630	1.9883	2.3710	2.6349
18	1.7341	2.1009	2.5524	2.8784		90	1.6620	1.9867	2.3685	2.6316
19	1.7291	2.0930	2.5395	2.8609		95	1.6611	1.9853	2.3662	2.6286
20	1.7247	2.0860	2.5280	2.8453		100	1.6602	1.9840	2.3642	2.6259
21	1.7207	2.0796	2.5176	2.8314		120	1.6577	1.9799	2.3578	2.6174
22	1.7171	2.0739	2.5083	2.8188		140	1.6558	1.9771	2.3533	2.6114
23	1.7139	2.0687	2.4999	2.8073		160	1.6544	1.9749	2.3499	2.6069
24	1.7109	2.0639	2.4922	2.7969		180	1.6534	1.9732	2.3472	2.6034
25	1.7081	2.0595	2.4851	2.7874		200	1.6525	1.9719	2.3451	2.6006
26	1.7056	2.0555	2.4786	2.7787		250	1.6510	1.9695	2.3414	2.5956
27	1.7033	2.0518	2.4727	2.7707		300	1.6499	1.9679	2.3388	2.5923
28	1.7011	2.0484	2.4671	2.7633		350	1.6492	1.9668	2.3370	2.5899
29	1.6991	2.0452	2.4620	2.7564		400	1.6487	1.9659	2.3357	2.5882
30	1.6973	2.0423	2.4573	2.7500		450	1.6482	1.9652	2.3347	2.5868
31	1.6955	2.0395	2.4528	2.7440		500	1.6479	1.9647	2.3338	2.5857
32	1.6939	2.0369	2.4487	2.7385		600	1.6474	1.9639	2.3326	2.5840
33	1.6924	2.0345	2.4448	2.7333		700	1.6470	1.9634	2.3317	2.5829
34	1.6909	2.0322	2.4411	2.7284		800	1.6468	1.9629	2.3310	2.5820
35	1.6896	2.0301	2.4377	2.7238		900	1.6465	1.9626	2.3305	2.5813
36	1.6883	2.0281	2.4345	2.7195		1000	1.6464	1.9623	2.3301	2.5808
37	1.6871	2.0262	2.4314	2.7154		Infinity	1.6449	1.9600	2.3263	2.5758
38	1.6860	2.0244	2.4286	2.7116						
39	1.6849	2.0227	2.4258	2.7079						
40	1.6839	2.0211	2.4233	2.7045						

Calculated via Microsoft Excel 2004

TABLE **10** **Critical Values of F ($\alpha = .05$) When All μs Are Equal**

DENOMINATOR DEGREES OF FREEDOM	NUMERATOR DEGREES OF FREEDOM 1	2	3	4	5	6	7	8
1	161.448	199.500	215.707	224.583	230.162	233.986	236.768	238.883
2	18.5128	19.0000	19.1643	19.2468	19.2964	19.3295	19.3532	19.3710
3	10.1280	9.5521	9.2766	9.1172	9.0135	8.9406	8.8867	8.8452
4	7.7086	6.9443	6.5914	6.3882	6.2561	6.1631	6.0942	6.0410
5	6.6079	5.7861	5.4095	5.1922	5.0503	4.9503	4.8759	4.8183
6	5.9874	5.1433	4.7571	4.5337	4.3874	4.2839	4.2067	4.1468
7	5.5914	4.7374	4.3468	4.1203	3.9715	3.8660	3.7870	3.7257
8	5.3177	4.4590	4.0662	3.8379	3.6875	3.5806	3.5005	3.4381
9	5.1174	4.2565	3.8625	3.6331	3.4817	3.3738	3.2927	3.2296
10	4.9646	4.1028	3.7083	3.4780	3.3258	3.2172	3.1355	3.0717
11	4.8443	3.9823	3.5874	3.3567	3.2039	3.0946	3.0123	2.9480
12	4.7472	3.8853	3.4903	3.2592	3.1059	2.9961	2.9134	2.8486
13	4.6672	3.8056	3.4105	3.1791	3.0254	2.9153	2.8321	2.7669
14	4.6001	3.7389	3.3439	3.1122	2.9582	2.8477	2.7642	2.6987
15	4.5431	3.6823	3.2874	3.0556	2.9013	2.7905	2.7066	2.6408
16	4.4940	3.6337	3.2389	3.0069	2.8524	2.7413	2.6572	2.5911
17	4.4513	3.5915	3.1968	2.9647	2.8100	2.6987	2.6143	2.5480
18	4.4139	3.5546	3.1599	2.9277	2.7729	2.6613	2.5767	2.5102
19	4.3807	3.5219	3.1274	2.8951	2.7401	2.6283	2.5435	2.4768
20	4.3512	3.4928	3.0984	2.8661	2.7109	2.5990	2.5140	2.4471
21	4.3248	3.4668	3.0725	2.8401	2.6848	2.5727	2.4876	2.4205
22	4.3009	3.4434	3.0491	2.8167	2.6613	2.5491	2.4638	2.3965
23	4.2793	3.4221	3.0280	2.7955	2.6400	2.5277	2.4422	2.3748
24	4.2597	3.4028	3.0088	2.7763	2.6207	2.5082	2.4226	2.3551
25	4.2417	3.3852	2.9912	2.7587	2.6030	2.4904	2.4047	2.3371
26	4.2252	3.3690	2.9752	2.7426	2.5868	2.4741	2.3883	2.3205
27	4.2100	3.3541	2.9604	2.7278	2.5719	2.4591	2.3732	2.3053
28	4.1960	3.3404	2.9467	2.7141	2.5581	2.4453	2.3593	2.2913
29	4.1830	3.3277	2.9340	2.7014	2.5454	2.4324	2.3463	2.2783
30	4.1709	3.3158	2.9223	2.6896	2.5336	2.4205	2.3343	2.2662
31	4.1596	3.3048	2.9113	2.6787	2.5225	2.4094	2.3232	2.2549
32	4.1491	3.2945	2.9011	2.6684	2.5123	2.3991	2.3127	2.2444
33	4.1393	3.2849	2.8916	2.6589	2.5026	2.3894	2.3030	2.2346
34	4.1300	3.2759	2.8826	2.6499	2.4936	2.3803	2.2938	2.2253
35	4.1213	3.2674	2.8742	2.6415	2.4851	2.3718	2.2852	2.2167
36	4.1132	3.2594	2.8663	2.6335	2.4772	2.3638	2.2771	2.2085
37	4.1055	3.2519	2.8588	2.6261	2.4696	2.3562	2.2695	2.2008
38	4.0982	3.2448	2.8517	2.6190	2.4625	2.3490	2.2623	2.1936
39	4.0913	3.2381	2.8451	2.6123	2.4558	2.3423	2.2555	2.1867
40	4.0847	3.2317	2.8387	2.6060	2.4495	2.3359	2.2490	2.1802
41	4.0785	3.2257	2.8327	2.6000	2.4434	2.3298	2.2429	2.1740
42	4.0727	3.2199	2.8270	2.5943	2.4377	2.3240	2.2371	2.1681
43	4.0670	3.2145	2.8216	2.5888	2.4322	2.3185	2.2315	2.1625
44	4.0617	3.2093	2.8165	2.5837	2.4270	2.3133	2.2263	2.1572
45	4.0566	3.2043	2.8115	2.5787	2.4221	2.3083	2.2212	2.1521
46	4.0517	3.1996	2.8068	2.5740	2.4174	2.3035	2.2164	2.1473
47	4.0471	3.1951	2.8024	2.5695	2.4128	2.2990	2.2118	2.1427
48	4.0427	3.1907	2.7981	2.5652	2.4085	2.2946	2.2074	2.1382
49	4.0384	3.1866	2.7939	2.5611	2.4044	2.2904	2.2032	2.1340
50	4.0343	3.1826	2.7900	2.5572	2.4004	2.2864	2.1992	2.1299
55	4.0162	3.1650	2.7725	2.5397	2.3828	2.2687	2.1813	2.1119
60	4.0012	3.1504	2.7581	2.5252	2.3683	2.2541	2.1665	2.0970
65	3.9886	3.1381	2.7459	2.5130	2.3560	2.2417	2.1541	2.0844
70	3.9778	3.1277	2.7355	2.5027	2.3456	2.2312	2.1435	2.0737
75	3.9685	3.1186	2.7266	2.4937	2.3366	2.2221	2.1343	2.0644
80	3.9604	3.1108	2.7188	2.4859	2.3287	2.2142	2.1263	2.0564
85	3.9532	3.1038	2.7119	2.4790	2.3218	2.2072	2.1193	2.0493
90	3.9469	3.0977	2.7058	2.4729	2.3157	2.2011	2.1131	2.0430
95	3.9412	3.0922	2.7004	2.4675	2.3102	2.1955	2.1075	2.0374
100	3.9361	3.0873	2.6955	2.4626	2.3053	2.1906	2.1025	2.0323
120	3.9201	3.0718	2.6802	2.4472	2.2899	2.1750	2.0868	2.0164
140	3.9087	3.0608	2.6693	2.4363	2.2789	2.1639	2.0756	2.0051
160	3.9002	3.0525	2.6611	2.4282	2.2707	2.1557	2.0672	1.9967
180	3.8936	3.0461	2.6548	2.4218	2.2643	2.1492	2.0608	1.9901
200	3.8884	3.0411	2.6498	2.4168	2.2592	2.1441	2.0556	1.9849
250	3.8789	3.0319	2.6407	2.4078	2.2501	2.1350	2.0463	1.9756
300	3.8726	3.0258	2.6347	2.4017	2.2441	2.1289	2.0402	1.9693
350	3.8682	3.0215	2.6304	2.3975	2.2398	2.1245	2.0358	1.9649
400	3.8648	3.0183	2.6272	2.3942	2.2366	2.1212	2.0325	1.9616
450	3.8622	3.0158	2.6247	2.3918	2.2340	2.1187	2.0299	1.9590
500	3.8601	3.0138	2.6227	2.3898	2.2320	2.1167	2.0279	1.9569
600	3.8570	3.0107	2.6198	2.3868	2.2290	2.1137	2.0248	1.9538
700	3.8548	3.0086	2.6176	2.3847	2.2269	2.1115	2.0226	1.9516
800	3.8531	3.0070	2.6160	2.3831	2.2253	2.1099	2.0210	1.9500
900	3.8518	3.0057	2.6148	2.3818	2.2240	2.1086	2.0197	1.9487
1000	3.8508	3.0047	2.6138	2.3808	2.2231	2.1076	2.0187	1.9476

Calculated via Microsoft Excel 2004

			NUMERATOR DEGREES OF FREEDOM					
9	**10**	**11**	**12**	**13**	**14**	**15**	**16**
240.543	241.882	242.983	243.906	244.690	245.364	245.950	246.464
19.3848	19.3959	19.4050	19.4125	19.4189	19.4244	19.4291	19.4333
8.8123	8.7855	8.7633	8.7446	8.7287	8.7149	8.7029	8.6923
5.9988	5.9644	5.9358	5.9117	5.8911	5.8733	5.8578	5.8441
4.7725	4.7351	4.7040	4.6777	4.6552	4.6358	4.6188	4.6038
4.0990	4.0600	4.0274	3.9999	3.9764	3.9559	3.9381	3.9223
3.6767	3.6365	3.6030	3.5747	3.5503	3.5292	3.5107	3.4944
3.3881	3.3472	3.3130	3.2839	3.2590	3.2374	3.2184	3.2016
3.1789	3.1373	3.1025	3.0729	3.0475	3.0255	3.0061	2.9890
3.0204	2.9782	2.9430	2.9130	2.8872	2.8647	2.8450	2.8276
2.8962	2.8536	2.8179	2.7876	2.7614	2.7386	2.7186	2.7009
2.7964	2.7534	2.7173	2.6866	2.6602	2.6371	2.6169	2.5989
2.7144	2.6710	2.6347	2.6037	2.5769	2.5536	2.5331	2.5149
2.6458	2.6022	2.5655	2.5342	2.5073	2.4837	2.4630	2.4446
2.5876	2.5437	2.5068	2.4753	2.4481	2.4244	2.4034	2.3849
2.5377	2.4935	2.4564	2.4247	2.3973	2.3733	2.3522	2.3335
2.4943	2.4499	2.4126	2.3807	2.3531	2.3290	2.3077	2.2888
2.4563	2.4117	2.3742	2.3421	2.3143	2.2900	2.2686	2.2496
2.4227	2.3779	2.3402	2.3080	2.2800	2.2556	2.2341	2.2149
2.3928	2.3479	2.3100	2.2776	2.2495	2.2250	2.2033	2.1840
2.3660	2.3210	2.2829	2.2504	2.2222	2.1975	2.1757	2.1563
2.3419	2.2967	2.2585	2.2258	2.1975	2.1727	2.1508	2.1313
2.3201	2.2747	2.2364	2.2036	2.1752	2.1502	2.1282	2.1086
2.3002	2.2547	2.2163	2.1834	2.1548	2.1298	2.1077	2.0880
2.2821	2.2365	2.1979	2.1649	2.1362	2.1111	2.0889	2.0691
2.2655	2.2197	2.1811	2.1479	2.1192	2.0939	2.0716	2.0518
2.2501	2.2043	2.1655	2.1323	2.1035	2.0781	2.0558	2.0358
2.2360	2.1900	2.1512	2.1179	2.0889	2.0635	2.0411	2.0210
2.2229	2.1768	2.1379	2.1045	2.0755	2.0500	2.0275	2.0073
2.2107	2.1646	2.1256	2.0921	2.0630	2.0374	2.0148	1.9946
2.1994	2.1532	2.1141	2.0805	2.0513	2.0257	2.0030	1.9828
2.1888	2.1425	2.1033	2.0697	2.0404	2.0147	1.9920	1.9717
2.1789	2.1325	2.0933	2.0595	2.0302	2.0045	1.9817	1.9613
2.1696	2.1231	2.0838	2.0500	2.0207	1.9949	1.9720	1.9516
2.1608	2.1143	2.0750	2.0411	2.0117	1.9858	1.9629	1.9424
2.1526	2.1061	2.0666	2.0327	2.0032	1.9773	1.9543	1.9338
2.1449	2.0982	2.0587	2.0248	1.9952	1.9692	1.9462	1.9256
2.1375	2.0909	2.0513	2.0173	1.9877	1.9616	1.9386	1.9179
2.1306	2.0839	2.0443	2.0102	1.9805	1.9545	1.9313	1.9107
2.1240	2.0772	2.0376	2.0035	1.9738	1.9476	1.9245	1.9037
2.1178	2.0710	2.0312	1.9971	1.9673	1.9412	1.9179	1.8972
2.1119	2.0650	2.0252	1.9910	1.9612	1.9350	1.9118	1.8910
2.1062	2.0593	2.0195	1.9852	1.9554	1.9292	1.9059	1.8850
2.1009	2.0539	2.0140	1.9797	1.9499	1.9236	1.9002	1.8794
2.0958	2.0487	2.0088	1.9745	1.9446	1.9182	1.8949	1.8740
2.0909	2.0438	2.0039	1.9695	1.9395	1.9132	1.8898	1.8688
2.0862	2.0391	1.9991	1.9647	1.9347	1.9083	1.8849	1.8639
2.0817	2.0346	1.9946	1.9601	1.9301	1.9037	1.8802	1.8592
2.0775	2.0303	1.9902	1.9557	1.9257	1.8992	1.8757	1.8546
2.0734	2.0261	1.9861	1.9515	1.9214	1.8949	1.8714	1.8503
2.0552	2.0078	1.9675	1.9329	1.9026	1.8760	1.8523	1.8311
2.0401	1.9926	1.9522	1.9174	1.8870	1.8602	1.8364	1.8151
2.0274	1.9798	1.9393	1.9044	1.8739	1.8470	1.8231	1.8017
2.0166	1.9689	1.9283	1.8932	1.8627	1.8357	1.8117	1.7902
2.0073	1.9594	1.9188	1.8836	1.8530	1.8259	1.8018	1.7802
1.9991	1.9512	1.9105	1.8753	1.8445	1.8174	1.7932	1.7716
1.9919	1.9440	1.9031	1.8679	1.8371	1.8099	1.7856	1.7639
1.9856	1.9376	1.8967	1.8613	1.8305	1.8032	1.7789	1.7571
1.9799	1.9318	1.8909	1.8555	1.8246	1.7973	1.7729	1.7511
1.9748	1.9267	1.8857	1.8503	1.8193	1.7919	1.7675	1.7456
1.9588	1.9105	1.8693	1.8337	1.8026	1.7750	1.7505	1.7285
1.9473	1.8989	1.8576	1.8219	1.7907	1.7630	1.7384	1.7162
1.9388	1.8903	1.8489	1.8131	1.7818	1.7540	1.7293	1.7071
1.9322	1.8836	1.8422	1.8063	1.7749	1.7471	1.7223	1.7000
1.9269	1.8783	1.8368	1.8008	1.7694	1.7415	1.7166	1.6943
1.9174	1.8687	1.8271	1.7910	1.7595	1.7315	1.7065	1.6841
1.9112	1.8623	1.8206	1.7845	1.7529	1.7249	1.6998	1.6773
1.9067	1.8578	1.8161	1.7799	1.7482	1.7201	1.6950	1.6725
1.9033	1.8544	1.8126	1.7764	1.7447	1.7166	1.6914	1.6688
1.9007	1.8517	1.8099	1.7737	1.7419	1.7138	1.6887	1.6660
1.8986	1.8496	1.8078	1.7715	1.7398	1.7116	1.6864	1.6638
1.8955	1.8465	1.8046	1.7683	1.7365	1.7083	1.6831	1.6604
1.8932	1.8442	1.8023	1.7660	1.7341	1.7059	1.6807	1.6580
1.8916	1.8425	1.8006	1.7643	1.7324	1.7041	1.6789	1.6562
1.8903	1.8412	1.7993	1.7629	1.7310	1.7028	1.6775	1.6548
1.8892	1.8402	1.7982	1.7618	1.7299	1.7017	1.6764	1.6536

TABLE **11**   **Power for Dependent-Samples *t* Test/Repeated Measures ANOVA ($\alpha = .05$, Two-Tailed)**

n	.1	.2	.3	.4	.5	.6	.7	.8	.9	1.0	1.1	1.2
3	.05	.05	.06	.07	.08	.09	.11	.13	.15	.17	.20	.23
4	.05	.05	.07	.08	.11	.13	.16	.20	.24	.28	.33	.38
5	.05	.06	.08	.10	.14	.18	.22	.28	.33	.40	.46	.53
6	.05	.06	.09	.12	.17	.22	.28	.35	.43	.50	.58	.65
7	.05	.07	.10	.14	.20	.26	.34	.42	.51	.60	.68	.75
8	.05	.07	.11	.16	.23	.31	.40	.49	.59	.68	.76	.82
9	.05	.08	.12	.18	.26	.35	.45	.55	.65	.74	.82	.88
10	.05	.08	.13	.20	.29	.39	.50	.61	.71	.80	.87	.92
11	.06	.09	.14	.22	.32	.43	.55	.66	.76	.84	.90	.94
12	.06	.09	.15	.24	.35	.47	.59	.71	.80	.88	.93	.96
13	.06	.10	.16	.26	.38	.51	.64	.75	.84	.91	.95	.97
14	.06	.10	.18	.28	.41	.54	.67	.79	.87	.93	.96	.98
15	.06	.11	.19	.30	.43	.58	.71	.82	.89	.94	.97	
16	.06	.11	.20	.32	.46	.61	.74	.84	.91	.96	.98	
17	.06	.12	.21	.34	.49	.64	.77	.87	.93	.97	.98	
18	.06	.12	.22	.36	.51	.67	.79	.89	.94	.97		
19	.06	.13	.23	.37	.54	.69	.82	.90	.95	.98		
20	.07	.13	.24	.39	.56	.72	.84	.92	.96	.98		
21	.07	.14	.25	.41	.58	.74	.86	.93	.97			
22	.07	.14	.26	.43	.60	.76	.87	.94	.98			
23	.07	.15	.28	.45	.63	.78	.89	.95	.98			
24	.07	.15	.29	.46	.65	.80	.90	.96	.98			
25	.07	.16	.30	.48	.66	.82	.91	.96				
26	.07	.16	.31	.50	.68	.83	.92	.97				
27	.07	.17	.32	.51	.70	.85	.93	.97				
28	.08	.17	.33	.53	.72	.86	.94	.98				
29	.08	.18	.34	.54	.73	.87	.95	.98				
30	.08	.18	.35	.56	.75	.88	.95	.98				
32	.08	.19	.37	.59	.78	.90	.96					
34	.08	.20	.39	.61	.80	.92	.97					
36	.08	.21	.41	.64	.83	.93	.98					
38	.09	.22	.43	.67	.85	.94	.98					
40	.09	.23	.45	.69	.86	.95						
42	.09	.24	.47	.71	.88	.96						
44	.09	.25	.49	.73	.90	.97						
46	.10	.26	.51	.75	.91	.97						
48	.10	.27	.53	.77	.92	.98						
50	.10	.28	.54	.79	.93	.98						
55	.11	.30	.58	.82	.95							
60	.11	.33	.62	.86	.96							
65	.12	.35	.66	.88	.97							
70	.13	.37	.69	.90	.98							
75	.13	.40	.72	.92	.98							
80	.14	.42	.75	.94								
85	.14	.44	.78	.95								
90	.15	.46	.80	.96								
95	.16	.48	.82	.97								
100	.16	.50	.84	.97								
110	.18	.54	.87	.98								
120	.19	.58	.90									
130	.20	.61	.92									
140	.21	.65	.94									
150	.22	.68	.95									
160	.24	.71	.96									
170	.25	.73	.97									
180	.26	.76	.97									
190	.27	.78	.98									
200	.29	.80	.98									
220	.31	.83										
240	.33	.86										
260	.36	.89										
280	.38	.91										
300	.40	.93										
400	.51	.97										
500	.60											
600	.68											
700	.75											
800	.80											
900	.85											
1000	.88											
1500	.97											
2000												

NOTE: Probability of Type II error $= \beta = 1 - $ power
If cell is blank, power is greater than .99.
Calculated via nQuery Advisor, 5.0

						EFFECT SIZE (D)						
1.3	1.4	1.5	1.6	1.7	1.8	1.9	2.0	2.1	2.2	2.3	2.4	2.5
.25	.28	.31	.34	.37	.40	.43	.47	.50	.53	.56	.59	.61
.43	.48	.53	.58	.62	.67	.71	.75	.79	.82	.85	.87	.89
.59	.65	.71	.76	.80	.84	.88	.90	.93	.94	.96	.97	.98
.72	.78	.83	.87	.90	.93	.95	.97	.98	.98			
.81	.86	.90	.93	.95	.97	.98						
.88	.92	.95	.97	.98								
.92	.95	.97	.98									
.95	.97	.98										
.97	.98											
.98												

TABLE **12** **Sample Size (*n*) Needed for Power of .80 and .95 for Dependent-Samples *t* Test (or Two-Samples Repeated Measures ANOVA),** $\alpha = .05$, **Two-Tailed**

	POWER	
d	.80	.95
.05	3142	5200
.10	787	1302
.15	351	580
.20	199	327
.25	128	210
.30	90	147
.35	67	109
.40	52	84
.45	41	67
.50	34	54
.55	28	45
.60	24	39
.65	21	33
.70	19	29
.75	16	26
.80	15	23
.85	13	21
.90	12	19
.95	11	17
1.00	10	16
1.05	10	14
1.10	9	13
1.15	9	12
1.20	8	12
1.25	8	11
1.30	7	10
1.35	7	10
1.40	7	9
1.45	6	9
1.50	6	8
1.55	6	8
1.60	6	8
1.65	6	8
1.70	5	7
1.75	5	7
1.80	5	7
1.85	5	7
1.90	5	6
1.95	5	6
2.00	5	6

NOTE: *d* = effect size (calculated via Equation 11.6); *n* = sample size per cell
Probability of Type II error = $\beta = 1 -$ power
Calculated via nQuery Advisor, 5.0

TABLE 13 Critical Values of Chi-Square (χ^2)

df	ALPHA (α) LEVEL				
	.10	.05	.025	.01	.001
1	2.7055	3.8415	5.0239	6.6349	10.8276
2	4.6052	5.9915	7.3778	9.2103	13.8155
3	6.2514	7.8147	9.3484	11.3449	16.2662
4	7.7794	9.4877	11.1433	13.2767	18.4668
5	9.2364	11.0705	12.8325	15.0863	20.5150
6	10.6446	12.5916	14.4494	16.8119	22.4577
7	12.0170	14.0671	16.0128	18.4753	24.3219
8	13.3616	15.5073	17.5345	20.0902	26.1245
9	14.6837	16.9190	19.0228	21.6660	27.8772
10	15.9872	18.3070	20.4832	23.2093	29.5883
11	17.2750	19.6751	21.9200	24.7250	31.2641
12	18.5493	21.0261	23.3367	26.2170	32.9095
13	19.8119	22.3620	24.7356	27.6882	34.5282
14	21.0641	23.6848	26.1189	29.1412	36.1233
15	22.3071	24.9958	27.4884	30.5779	37.6973
16	23.5418	26.2962	28.8454	31.9999	39.2524
17	24.7690	27.5871	30.1910	33.4087	40.7902
18	25.9894	28.8693	31.5264	34.8053	42.3124
19	27.2036	30.1435	32.8523	36.1909	43.8202
20	28.4120	31.4104	34.1696	37.5662	45.3147
21	29.6151	32.6706	35.4789	38.9322	46.7970
22	30.8133	33.9244	36.7807	40.2894	48.2679
23	32.0069	35.1725	38.0756	41.6384	49.7282
24	33.1962	36.4150	39.3641	42.9798	51.1786
25	34.3816	37.6525	40.6465	44.3141	52.6197
26	35.5632	38.8851	41.9232	45.6417	54.0520
27	36.7412	40.1133	43.1945	46.9629	55.4760
28	37.9159	41.3371	44.4608	48.2782	56.8923
29	39.0875	42.5570	45.7223	49.5879	58.3012
30	40.2560	43.7730	46.9792	50.8922	59.7031
31	41.4217	44.9853	48.2319	52.1914	61.0983
32	42.5847	46.1943	49.4804	53.4858	62.4872
33	43.7452	47.3999	50.7251	54.7755	63.8701
34	44.9032	48.6024	51.9660	56.0609	65.2472
35	46.0588	49.8018	53.2033	57.3421	66.6188
36	47.2122	50.9985	54.4373	58.6192	67.9852
37	48.3634	52.1923	55.6680	59.8925	69.3465
38	49.5126	53.3835	56.8955	61.1621	70.7029
39	50.6598	54.5722	58.1201	62.4281	72.0547
40	51.8051	55.7585	59.3417	63.6907	73.4020
41	52.9485	56.9424	60.5606	64.9501	74.7449
42	54.0902	58.1240	61.7768	66.2062	76.0838
43	55.2302	59.3035	62.9904	67.4593	77.4186
44	56.3685	60.4809	64.2015	68.7095	78.7495
45	57.5053	61.6562	65.4102	69.9568	80.0767

Calculated via Microsoft Excel 2004

ANSWERS TO REVIEW EXERCISES

CHAPTER 1

Review Exercises

1. NOIR questions
   a. The numbers are entirely arbitrary and are equivalent to names for the different types of weather. So, all the numbers indicate is difference/sameness: **Nominal**
   b. The numbers tell difference and direction of the difference. Each firing of a neuron is equivalent, so there is equality of units. There is also a real zero point: **Ratio**
   c. The numbers tell difference and direction, but there is no equality of units: **Ordinal**
   d. The numbers tell difference and direction, but there is no equality of units: **Ordinal**
   e. Difference, direction, equality of units, and a real zero point: **Ratio**
   f. Difference, direction, equality of units, and an arbitrary zero point: **Interval**
2. Regarding the college dean who was comparing liberal arts students to professional students...
   a. This is a hard question. The averages are **statistics;** they are means for samples. He may be using the statistics to make inferences about populations (see the next answer), but he is using statistics, not parameters.
   b. He is using the numbers to make inferences about the population, so he is using **inferential** statistics.
   c. Since she finds the same result consistently, we conclude it reflects a real difference between the populations: it is a **statistically significant** result. However, I don't think a 1 IQ-point difference has much practical meaning, so the results are **not practically significant.**
   d. Since the results vary each time, it is unlikely that they reflect a real difference between the populations; the results are **not statistically significant.** Inconsistent results can't be trusted and applied, so the results **can't be practically significant.**
3. The first set of rounding questions involves rounding to two more places than the original data.
   a. The original data are integers (i.e., no decimal places), so the final answer should have two decimal places: $18 \div 17 = $ **1.06**
   b. $18.12 \div 17.76 = $ starting with two decimal places. Final answer should have four: **1.0203**

c. Though the numbers here are the same as in the question just above, I've added two more decimal places, so the final answer should now have six: **1.020270**
   d. $425 \div 3 = $ **141.67**
   The next set involves rounding to two decimal places:
   e. **55.55.** This one was already at two decimal places.
   f. $55.0055 = $ **55.01**
   g. $55.555 = $ **55.56.** Remember, round to even if the unrounded number is equidistant from the two options.
   h. $99.995 = $ **100.00**
   i. $99.9905 = $ **99.99**
   The next set involves the number of decimal places to carry, and rounding as one goes vs. rounding at the end. I'll be honest: I find rounding as one goes awkward to do. It is much easier to leave all the decimal places in your calculator and carry them all. However, to make the point that carrying two more decimal places than you plan to end up with leads to a reasonable approximation of the real answer, I put this question in here.
   j. Carrying all decimal places = **14.03**
   Carrying four decimal places = **14.03**
   Carrying two decimal places = **14.05**
   k. Carrying all decimal places = **8.35**
   Carrying four decimal places = **8.35**
   Carrying two decimal places = **8.30**
4. Independent vs. dependent variable questions
   a. Dependent variable = amount of abrasion
   b. Independent variable = group assignment (aspirin vs. placebo vs. nothing)
   c. Independent variable = paint under the eye (yes vs. no)
   d. Dependent variable = intelligence as measured by an IQ test
   e. Independent variable = amount of sleep (5 hr vs. 8 hr)
5. This question tested whether you know how to deal with ties when rank-ordering a data set. If you are a bicyclist, you might recognize these names as past and present Tour de France racers. I just made up the data, so I couldn't resist putting Lance Armstrong up at the top. And, I never liked Bernard Hinault after what

he did to Greg Lemond in 1985, so I put him at the bottom. (Hey, if you can't settle scores in your own stats text, what's the point of writing one?)

1	Armstrong
2	Ullrich
3	Indurain
4	Zabel
5.5	Delgado
5.5	Lemond
7.5	Roche
7.5	Hamilton

9.5	Pantani
9.5	Hincapie
11	Heras
12	Leipheimer
13	Anquetil
14.5	Fignon
14.5	McEwen
17	Coppi
17	Merckx
17	Riis
19	Garin
20	Hinault

CHAPTER 2

Review Exercises

1. Number of usable chairs is a **ratio**-level variable. (There's a real zero point, equal intervals, direction, and difference.)

   Number of usable chairs is a **discrete** variable since there are no in-between values (i.e., you can't have 1.43 usable chairs in a classroom).

2. Here's the stem-and-leaf display for the number of chairs. Don't forget a title!

Stem-and-leaf display for number of usable chairs in classrooms at College X

12	0
11	
10	0
9	
8	
7	5
6	0002
5	0002344588
4	00002344555556
3	00334555667889
2	0034444568888889
1	02788
0	7

I'd describe the data as **unimodal** and **positively skewed.** Again, unless peakedness is extreme, I'm hard-pressed to comment on it.

3.

Grouped frequency distribution for usable chairs in classrooms

X	m	f	f_c	%	$\%_c$
115-124	119.5	1	67	1.49	100.00
105-114	109.5	0	66	.00	98.51
95-104	99.5	1	66	1.49	98.51
85-94	89.5	0	65	.00	97.01
75-84	79.5	1	65	1.49	97.01

Continued in next column

X	m	f	f_c	%	$\%_c$
65-74	69.5	0	64	.00	95.52
55-64	59.5	7	64	10.45	95.52
45-54	49.5	13	57	19.40	85.07
35-44	39.5	17	44	25.37	65.67
25-34	29.5	14	27	20.90	40.30
15-24	19.5	10	13	14.93	19.40
5-14	9.5	3	3	4.48	4.48

NOTE: X = number of usable chairs
   m = interval midpoint
   f = frequency
   f_c = cumulative frequency
   % = percentage
   $\%_c$ = cumulative percentage

4. Since number of chairs is a discrete variable, the graph should be a bar graph.

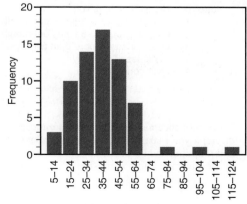

Number of chairs per classroom

Regarding the shape, I'd describe it as positively skewed and unimodal. This is the same conclusion I reached for the stem-and-leaf display.

5. The lowest interval was 5-14, and the highest was 115-124. The data are discrete, so the real limits are the same as the apparent limits.

6. The predictor variable is speed, and the criterion variable is death rate. Both are being measured at the ratio level.

7. The data are ordinal, and the intervals are unequal in terms of the number of days of overconsumption they represent. In addition, the underlying variable, days, is discrete. So, I've made a bar graph. (I would listen to you seriously if you argued that we could consider the underlying variable as "time" and should consider that a continuous variable, in which case a histogram or frequency polygon becomes an option.)

days?" Thus a bar graph makes the most sense to me. However, as noted above, I can see conceptualizing the underlying variable as time, not days, and construing time as a continuous variable. If you do so, it opens the door to histograms and frequency polygons.

In addition, you need to think about what it is that you want the graph to communicate. I think that the objective is to give an overview of alcohol overconsumption by these students, so I think the graph should be based on a grouped frequency distribution.

However, there is a problem in making a grouped frequency distribution for these data since there are 31 values of X (the number of days of overconsumption ranges from 0 to 30). The number 31 is prime and can't be divided into equally sized intervals. I chose to set $i = 5$ and kept the students with zero days of overconsumption in an interval by themselves.

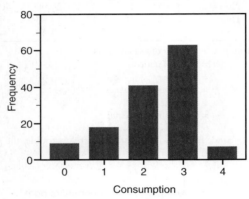

Alcohol overconsumption by 138 male college students

Note: 0 = No overconsumption
1 = Over consume 1–3 times per month
2 = Over consume 4–8 times per month
3 = Over consume more than twice per week, less than daily
4 = Over consume daily

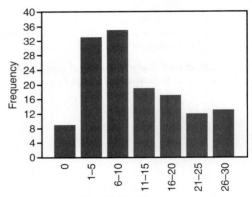

Number of days of alcohol overconsumption by 138 male college students

8. How you conceptualize the data determines the type of graph you make. The data represent days of overconsumption, and I think of this as discrete, in answer to the question "how many days?" not "how much

9. a. The thermometer appears to measure to the nearest tenth of a degree, so the person's temperature falls in the range from 100.25 to 100.35.
   b. This is a discrete variable, so seven kids = seven kids.
   c. The person's IQ falls in the range from 114.5 to 115.5.
   d. From 299,500,000 to 300,500,000 people live in the United States.
   e. Discrete variable: Three televisions = three televisions.

CHAPTER 3

Review Exercises

1. Shape of distribution questions
   a. I would expect that few women get married before age 16, that most get married for the first time in their late teens or early to mid 20s, and that through the late 20s and into the 30s women will continue to get married for the first time. Thus, I would expect the distribution to be limited in how low it goes and to tail off to the right, to be positively skewed.
   b. Where the ball lands in a roulette wheel should be random, meaning that in the long run, it will land in each number an equal number of times. Hence, I would expect that this distribution would be flat.
   c. I would expect that the length of the thigh bone in adult men would be normally distributed, just as height is normally distributed. That is, most thigh bones would be around the average, with the number being longer or shorter tailing off symmetrically.
   d. I expect that the length of the thigh bone is normally distributed for men and that it is normally distributed for women. However, since men are in general taller than women, and since length of the thigh bone is one of the contributors to height, I would expect that men would have longer thigh bones than women. As a result, I would expect the combined distribution to be bimodal with one peak at the average length for men and the other at the average length for women.
2. The temperature for noon could be taken as early as 11:45 AM (or as late as 12:15 PM).
3. Once again I've given you a table that contains only frequency information. In order to calculate percentile rank you need to make a more complete table. Here it is:

X	f	f_c	$\%$	$\%_c$
45-49	9	264	3.41	100.00
40-44	11	255	4.17	96.59
35-39	19	244	7.20	92.42
30-34	21	225	7.95	85.23
25-29	24	204	9.09	77.27
20-24	38	180	14.39	68.18
15-19	44	142	16.67	53.79
10-14	59	98	22.35	37.12
5-9	28	39	10.61	14.77
0-4	11	11	4.17	4.17

Did you estimate first? 38 is in the range from 34.5 to 39.5, or from PRs 85.23 to 92.42. 38 is 70% of the way into the range, which is ≈ 7 PR units wide. This means I added ≈ 5 PR units to the bottom of the range, ending up with an estimate of ≈ 90.

The percentile rank associated with eating 38 grams of fiber is as follows:

$$PR = \left(\frac{38.0000 - 34.5000}{5.0000} \right) 7.1970 + 85.2273$$
$$= 5.0379 + 85.2273$$
$$= 90.2652 = 90.27$$

4. How much fiber does a person at in the middle of the distribution (the 50th percentile, what we'll soon learn is called the median) consume?

   Let's estimate first: a PR of 50 is in the ≈ 17 PR unit wide interval from PR 37.12 to 52.79; it is about ¾ of the way into the interval. The raw score interval associated is 5 units wide and starts at 14.5. 14.5 + 3.75 = 18.25.

$$X = \left(\frac{\left(\frac{50.0000}{100} \right) 264 - 98}{44} \right) 5.000 + 14.5000$$
$$= 3.8636 + 14.5000$$
$$= 18.3636 = 18.36$$

Oh yes, you needed to compare the "average" amount of fiber consumed, the amount consumed by a person at PR 50 to the recommended amount for daily consumption of 25 grams. The "average" person in Dr. Amiama's study is consuming less fiber than he or she should.

5. This is a challenging question. The real upper limit is easy: 4.50. OK, but what about the real lower limit? If you believe in symmetry you would put the real lower limit at −.5. However, that doesn't make much sense, since a person can't consume less than 0 grams of fiber a day. So, I'd leave the real lower limit at .00.
6. Dr. Amiama is simply doing a descriptive study; she is not manipulating anything or examining the relationship between two variables. All she is doing is measuring fiber consumption. So, fiber consumption is her dependent variable, and there is no independent variable.

CHAPTER 4

Review Exercises

1. On the January day the range (inclusive) was 12° (from 21° to 32°); on the June day the range was 22° (from 56° to 77°). Thus there appears to be more variability in June.

   However, the range only takes into account the two extreme temperatures for a day. Both the IQR and the standard deviation take more information into account. I calculated $\hat{s}$ for both months and found that the standard deviation for January was 4.27 and for June it was 8.12. Thus there was more variability for the day in June than there was for the one in January.

   Why did I calculate $\hat{s}$ and not s to answer this question? Because though the data were for a sample, the question was asking about variability for the whole day. Thus it made sense to estimate the amount of variability in the population from which the sample came.

   Would we find more variability in June than in January for the interquartile range? Yes. The IQR for January is 8 points wide (from 22.50 to 30.50) and for June it is 15.50 points wide (from 59.50 to 75.00).

2. The data are ratio level, so a mean is an appropriate measure of central tendency: 150/25 = 6.00.

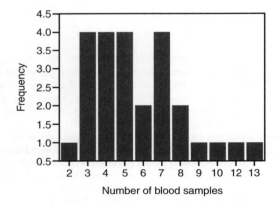

Number of blood samples

   Though the graph suggests that these data may be positively skewed, the skewness is not so great that I would consider the distribution skewed. However,

since you don't know yet how to evaluate skewness, I wouldn't be upset if you calculated the median for these discrete data via Equation 4.2. (It equals 5.38.)

   The population to which the phlebotomist wishes to generalize her results would almost certainly be admissions to her hospital, not to all hospital patients in the world.

   We haven't yet learned a way to use a sample measure of central tendency to estimate a population value from a sample value. Her sample was a random sample, so it likely is representative of the population; so my best guess is that μ is probably reasonably close to M. You'll learn how to estimate μ from M in Chapter 6.

3. You need to complete the table in order to calculate the median (PR 50) and the IQR:

Interval	Frequency	Cumulative Frequency
70-79	12	79
60-69	14	67
50-59	18	53
40-49	16	35
30-39	11	19
20-29	8	8

$$Mdn = \left(\frac{\frac{79}{2} - 35}{18}\right)10.0000 + 49.5000$$

$$= 2.5000 + 49.5000$$

$$= 52.0000 = 52.00$$

$$PR_{25} = \left(\frac{.25(79) - 19}{16}\right)10.0000 + 39.5000$$

$$= .4688 + 39.5000$$

$$= 39.9688 = 39.97$$

$$PR_{75} = \left(\frac{.75(79) - 53}{14}\right)10.0000 + 59.5000$$

$$= 4.4643 + 59.5000$$

$$= 63.9643 = 63.96$$

Though I prefer to report the *IQR* as a range, in this instance from 39.97 to 63.96, it can also be reported as the single value of **24.00**.

4. The table needs to be completed in order to calculate a mean:

Interval	Midpoint	Frequency	Midpoint × frequency
70-79	74.5	12	894.0000
60-69	64.5	14	903.0000
50-59	54.5	18	981.0000
40-49	44.5	16	712.0000
30-39	34.5	11	379.5000
20-29	24.5	8	196.0000
			$\Sigma = 4065.5000$

$$M = \frac{4065.5000}{79} = 51.4620 = 51.46$$

Remember, that is just our *estimate* of the mean since it is based on assuming that the value assigned to each case is its interval midpoint.

5. By Equation 4.10:

$$\hat{s} = \sqrt{\frac{(s^2)N}{N-1}} = \sqrt{\frac{(12.44^2)45}{44}} = 12.5806 = 12.58$$

6. The easiest way to work this problem is to make a small table. It doesn't matter if the scores are arrayed in rank order.

	X	$X - M$	$(X - M)^2$
	34	−16.1250	260.0156
	65	14.8750	221.2656
	56	5.8750	34.5156
	45	−5.1250	26.2656
	55	4.8750	23.7656
	49	−1.1250	1.2656
	38	−12.1250	147.0156
	59	8.8750	78.7656
Σ	401.0000	.0000	792.8748

a. $M = \dfrac{401.000}{8} = 50.1250 = 50.12$

b. To figure out s you need to figure out s^2, which is $\dfrac{792.8748}{8} = 99.1094 = 99.11$. s is then calculated via $\sqrt{99.1094} = 9.9554 = 9.96$

c. $\hat{s}^2 = \dfrac{792.8748}{7} = 113.2678 = 113.27$

d. We can't calculate σ, but we can estimate it via $\hat{s}$. So: $\hat{s}^2 = \sqrt{113.2678} = 10.6427 = 10.64$

e. By definition, the sum of the deviation scores is 0. If you calculate it, you will find that this is true.

f. The inclusive range is 32.00, the distance from 65.5000 to 33.5000.

g. There is no mode since each score occurs once.

7. Rounding like a statistician means that once we've reached half a unit of measurement, in this case half a year, we move to the next higher unit. So, as long as Skip is less than half a year old he is, in integer years, 0. Once he's a day older than half a year, a statistician would consider him 1 year old. (Don't worry, I've avoided the situation when he is exactly halfway between 2 years.)

a. 0 years old
b. 1 year old
c. 1 year old
d. 1 year old
e. 1 year old
f. 2 years old
g. 0 years old
h. −1 year old

CHAPTER 5

Review Exercises

1. Both variables are measured at the **ratio** level.
2. Did you draw and estimate first?

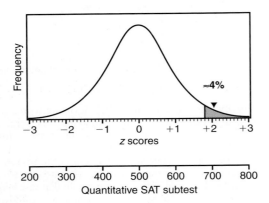

Only **3.59%** of people should do better than Buffy on this test. (Her z score, by the bye, was 1.80.)

3. Skip's score, as a z, would have to be above .44 to earn the $100. In IQ-score units, he needs to score above **106.60.**

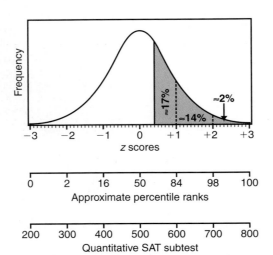

4. Spending the $1000 makes more sense for Desdemona than it does for Clothilde. Adding 1% of the normal dis-

tribution will change Clothilde's score, as a *PR*, from 57.93 to 58.93, and Desdemona's from 98.61 to 99.61. This 1% *PR* change will change Clothilde's score from 520 to 523, a 3-point change, whereas it will change Desdemona's score from 720 to 766, a 46-point change! Why? Remember that the area under the curve gets less and less as one moves further away from the mean. Thus the *PR* bite that is taken out of the distribution, in z score units, increases as one moves away from the mean.

5. From −.50 to +.25, **29.02%** of the scores should fall. (Remember, add the areas 19.15% and 9.87%.) Between 1.80 and 2.20, **2.20%** of scores will fall. (Subtract 46.41% from 48.61%.)

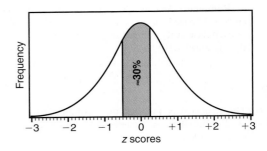

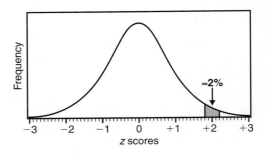

6. If vos Savant's IQ really were 228, that would put it 8.53 standard deviations above the mean. Our estimation techniques put 100% of observations within three standard deviations of the mean, and vos Savant's purported IQ is still more than 5.5 standard deviations further out. In fact, I can't find a z score table that goes to 8.53. The most extreme z score for which I can find a value is a z score of 8.17, and the

percent of cases under the normal distribution that have a score higher than this is **.000000000000011%.** The last time I checked, there were almost 6.5 billion people in the world. Taking .000000000000011% of 6.5 billion gets you ≈.0000007. In other words, if intelligence is normally distributed, there should be about .0000007 people in the whole world who have IQs higher than 223. Somehow I doubt that Marilyn really has an IQ of 228.

In her defense it is estimated that her adult IQ would be, if measured using more modern techniques, a more realistic 180, a mere 5.33 standard deviations above the mean. If this is the case then about .000005% of the world is smarter than she is. In human terms, that means that there are about 320 people, out of 6.5 billion, who should be smarter than Marilyn.

7. The radiographer's new imaging technique will find an additional **.1242%** more tumors (via 49.9892% – 49.865%) but will still leave **.0108%** tumors unfound (via 50.00% – 49.9892% or via Column C in Appendix Table 1).

8. The mean for this sample is 16.2000, and the standard deviation is 4.4677. A score 3.5 standard deviations above the mean has a value of **31.8370.**

9. The z scores associated with the middle 75% of scores are ± **1.15.**

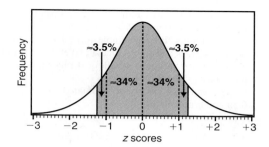

10. The z scores associated with the extreme 1% of scores are ± **2.58.** (Yes, I already asked you this question in Group Practice 5.3, #6. Did you remember from that answer that I said that 2.58 was a better answer than 2.57?)

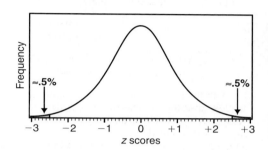

CHAPTER 6

Review Exercises

1. In order to determine whether the sample is normally distributed, we need to calculate skewness and kurtosis and then put confidence intervals around them. I've saved you from the onerous task of calculating skewness and kurtosis so far, but no longer...

   Calculating skewness and kurtosis involves calculating z scores, which means knowing the mean (9.8750) and the standard deviation (2.7128). The z scores are raised to the third and fourth powers to calculate skewness (Equation 6.4a) and kurtosis (Equation 6.4b).

Data	z	z^3	z^4
7	−1.0598	−1.1903	1.2615
12	.7833	.4806	.3765
9	−.3225	−.0335	.0108
16	2.2578	11.5095	25.9861

Continued in next column

Data	z	z^3	z^4
8	−.6912	−.3302	.2283
8	−.6912	−.3302	.2283
10	.0461	.0001	.0000
9	−.3225	−.0335	.0108
	Σ	10.0725	28.1023

I calculate skewness and kurtosis as follows:

$$Skewness = \frac{10.0725}{8} = 1.2591$$

$$Kurtosis = \frac{28.1023}{8} - 3 = 3.5128 - 3 = .5128$$

By the bye, if you use SPSS to calculate skewness and kurtosis for these data, you will get different answers (1.57 and 2.48). Their value for skewness is in my ballpark, but their value for kurtosis is very different. SPSS uses more complex formulae, ones that have correction factors in order to estimate population values. I like my simple formulae. Though, to be honest, it is a pain to calculate skewness and kurtosis by hand and most people just rely on computer programs.

The standard errors are estimated via Equations 6.5a and b as follows:

$$SE_{Skewness} = \sqrt{\frac{6}{8}} = .8660 = .8660$$

$$SE_{Kurtosis} = \sqrt{\frac{24}{8}} = 1.7321 = 1.7321$$

The 95% confidence intervals are then calculated via Equations 6.6a and b as follows:

$$95\% \ CI_{Skewness} = 1.2591 \pm 1.96(.8660)$$
$$= 1.2591 \pm 1.6974$$

$$95\% \ CI_{Kurtosis} = .5128 \pm 1.96 \ (1.7321)$$
$$= .5128 \pm 3.3949$$

With the *95% CI* for skewness ranging from −.44 to 2.96 and for kurtosis from −2.88 to 3.91, it **is** reasonable to conclude that the population is likely normally distributed.

2. This question is meant to make you think about the point of a confidence interval: making an inference about a *population* from a sample. In this case, the results of an election, we have the population value, the proportion in the population that voted for the winning candidate. Thus whatever the confidence interval tells us is irrelevant, since we already have the population value. Candidate L is the loser, plain and simple, no matter what the confidence interval says *could* have happened.

3. This question should make you think about the factors that determine the width of a confidence interval. There are three: how confident you want to be, *σ*, and *N*. Buffy and Skip both are calculating 95% confidence intervals, and both draw samples from a population where *σ* = 12.34, so they don't differ on these two variables. They do differ on *N*. You could go ahead and calculate the confidence intervals, or you could, in the words of Winnie the Pooh, "Think, think, think." A confidence interval depends on σ_M, and the denominator for this is *N*: as *N* gets larger, σ_M gets smaller. Thus, **Buffy,** with the smaller *N* has the wider *CI*.

By the bye, the information about means is irrelevant for determining the width of a confidence interval. I just threw it in there as a red herring and to enable me to make the point that a mean has no impact on confidence interval width.

4. In this question, Buffy's and Skip's samples differ in *N*, *σ*, and how sure they want to be, so we can't figure out which one has a wider CI just by thinking. In order to tell which has the wider CI there is no option but calculation.

$$Buffy's \ CI = M \pm 1.65 \left(\frac{8.00}{\sqrt{50}}\right)$$
$$= M \pm 1.65(1.1313)$$
$$= M \pm 1.8666 = M \pm 1.87$$

$$Skip's \ CI = M \pm 1.96 \left(\frac{9.50}{\sqrt{80}}\right)$$
$$= M \pm 1.96(1.0621)$$
$$= M \pm 2.0817 = M \pm 2.08$$

Skip's CI is wider.

5. This question involves figuring out what sample size one must have in order to have a confidence interval of a certain width. The relevant formula is Equation 6.3, which we plug in as follows. (Remember to convert the percentage (2%) to a proportion (.02).)

$$N = \left(\frac{.5000}{.02/1.96}\right)^2 = 2401.0000 = 2401$$

N = **2401** is the answer if one carries all decimal places. (If one rounds to four decimal places as one goes, the answer turns out to be 2403.)

6. This question has a lot of parts and has the objective of making you think about what *N* is used for what equation, and what the difference is between a population and a sampling distribution.

As a first step, it is a good idea to figure out what the samples are that make up the sampling distribution. (Oh yes, I didn't mention it because I assume that you know this by now, but we sample *with* replacement for sampling distributions.)

You should end up with 21 samples:

108,108	108,116	108,120	108,120	108,124	108,132
116,116	116,120	116,120	116,124	116,132	
120,120	120,120	120,124	120,132		
120,120	120,124	120,132			
124,124	124,132				
132,132					

Part I:

Here's a graph of the systolic BP for the population ($N = 6$)

```
                                        X
 X                        X             X                       X
108   110   112   114   116   118   120   122   124   126   128   130   132
```

and for the sampling distribution ($N = 21$)

```
                                        X
                                        X
                                        X
                  X     X     X     X   X     X     X
 X          X     X     X     X     X   X     X     X                       X
108   110   112   114   116   118   120   122   124   126   128   130   132
```

The graph for the population has the highest frequency at the center but is not particularly normal in shape. The sampling distribution looks more normal. (Skewness for both the population and the sampling distribution are zero; kurtosis for the population is −.54, and for the sampling distribution it is −.13.)

Why is the sampling distribution more normal? Because the central limit theorem says that the sampling distribution will be normally distributed, as long as N is large, even if the population is not normally distributed. N is not large here— it equals 2—but even so, the sampling distribution is starting to approximate a normal distribution.

Part II:

Though it is a pain to calculate because there are 21 cases in the sample, s, the standard deviation of the sampling distribution, is 5.5205.

To calculate σ_M I need N (2 in this instance) and σ. Since I have the whole population of the town, all six of them, this is one of those rare instances where σ can be calculated: 7.3030

Thus, I calculate $\sigma_M = \dfrac{7.3030}{\sqrt{2}} = 5.1640$

σ_M is an *estimate* of the standard deviation of the sampling distribution, but in this case we have already calculated the *actual* value (5.5205) of the standard deviation of the sampling distribution.

Though the two values (5.52 and 5.16) are close, they are not the same. Why? Because the calculation of σ_M is based on the central limit theorem, and the central limit theorem holds true when N (the size of the sample) is large. N, which in this case is 2, is not large. So, 5.5205 is the actual standard deviation of the sampling distribution and is more accurate than the estimate of the standard deviation of the sampling distribution (which is also known of as σ_M). Presumably, if N were large, ≥50, then there would be less difference between the actual standard deviation of the sampling distribution (s) and the *estimation* of the standard deviation of the sampling distribution via σ_M.

7. With a confidence interval we can't be sure that our calculated interval actually contains μ, since we might have obtained a nonrepresentative sample from the population. Similarly, we can't be sure that our sample of Martians, even though N is >50, is representative of Martians. So, we can't know for sure that the conclusion we make about the population of Martians, based on this sample of Martians, is accurate. As always, the best bet is replication—sending another probe and obtaining another sample. If both samples yield the same conclusions, then our faith in the accuracy of the results should improve.

8. The smaller the standard error of the mean, the narrower the confidence interval. Narrower *CI*s are better since there is a smaller range within which we believe a population value falls. In other words, with a narrow confidence interval, our prediction is more exact.

However, narrower *CI*s don't necessarily mean that we have more confidence that the mean falls in that range. If N is small we can have a very wide 95% *CI*, and if N is large we can have a very narrow 95% *CI*. In both cases we are equally sure, 95% sure, that we have captured the population value.

9. Given the information that you have about this sample, is it reasonable to conclude that ≈84% of cases fall below a z score of 1? Well, thanks to what we know about the area under the normal curve, if the population is normally distributed, then it is reasonable to conclude that 84% of the cases fall below a z score of 1.

   The question then becomes, how do we determine if it is reasonable to conclude that the population is normally distributed? We can conclude that it is reasonably likely that the population is normally distributed if the confidence intervals for skewness and kurtosis both capture zero.

   You have been given that skewness = −1.4546 and that kurtosis = .9873. From Equations 6.5a and b you can calculate their standard errors:

   $$SE_{Skewness} = \sqrt{\frac{6}{66}} = .3015$$

   $$SE_{Kurtosis} = \sqrt{\frac{24}{66}} = .6030$$

   The 95% CI for skewness is then −1.4546 ± 1.96(.3015), or from −2.05 to −.86.

   The 95% CI for kurtosis is then .9873 ± 1.96(.6030), or from −.19 to 2.17.

   Since the 95% CI for skewness does not capture zero, it is reasonable to conclude that the population is negatively skewed, that it is not normally distributed. Therefore, it is **not** reasonable to conclude that ≈84% of the cases fall below a z score of 1 in the population.

10. This question is making sure that you understand that a confidence interval can be set at any width you want by changing the value that the standard error of the mean is being multiplied by. (Remember the z score table and how the value of ±1.96 marks off the middle 95% of the area under the normal curve?) Roughly, within one standard deviation of the mean 68% of the area under the normal curve falls, so a 68% confidence interval would be roughly $M ± 1 \ \sigma_M$. Thus, the 68% confidence interval is 45.00 ± 4.00, or from 41.00 to 49.00.

11. The important thing to note here is that N is small, so Equation 6.2b should be used to estimate the confidence interval. Via Equation 6.1, I calculate σ_M as

    $$\frac{1.50}{\sqrt{17}} = .3638.$$ Plugging this into Equation 6.2b yields:

    15.00 ± 2.1199(.3638) = 15.00 ± .7712. Thus the 95% confidence interval ranges from 14.23 to 15.77.

CHAPTER 7

Review Exercises

1. **T = what test are we doing and why.** We're doing a Pearson r because we are asking about the relationship between two interval- or ratio-level variables, between severity of illness (APACHE score) and length of stay in the intensive care unit (ICU).

   I'm going to treat the APACHE score as my predictor variable (X) and the number of ICU days as my criterion variable (Y) because it makes sense to me that someone might be interested in predicting how long people will remain in the ICU based on how sick they were when they entered it.

   A = Assumptions? OK to go on? These are the five assumptions for r_p: random samples, interval- or ratio-level variables, normality, linearity, and homoscedasticity. Random samples was violated, but the Pearson r is robust to this (though we'll need to be concerned about generalizability). Number of ICU days is ratio; APACHE score is, as the question says, interval. All the CIs for skewness and kurtosis capture zero, so it is reasonable to conclude that each variable may be normally distributed in the population. Below is the scatterplot, which supports the assumptions of linearity and homoscedasticity. So, we can proceed with the test.

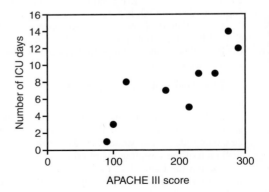

H = Hypotheses

$$H_0: \rho_{xy} = 0$$
$$H_1: \rho_{xy} \neq 0$$

The null hypothesis says that the linear relationship between X and Y in the population is zero. Even if $\rho = 0$, our $r_{observed}$ may not exactly equal zero, though the deviation of $r_{observed}$ from zero should be small enough that it can be accounted for by sampling error.

The alternative hypothesis says that there is a linear relationship between X and Y in the population. As a result, the observed deviation of $r_{observed}$ from zero will be too large to be accounted for by sampling error if $\rho = 0$. Rather, it reflects the reality that ρ_{xy} is not zero.

D = Decision rule. Using a two-tailed test with α set at .05 and $df = 7$, our critical value of $r = .6664$. If $|r_{observed}| \geq .6664$ we shall reject the null hypothesis, be forced to accept the alternative hypothesis, report that the probability of $r_{observed}$ is < .05 when the null hypothesis is true, find that the linear relationship between X and Y is statistically different from zero, conclude that there is probably a linear relationship between X and Y in the population, and worry about Type I error.

If $|r_{observed}| < .6664$, then we shall fail to reject H_0, will report the probability of $r_{observed}$ as > .05 when the null hypothesis is true, find that the degree of linear relationship between X and Y is not statistically different from zero, conclude that there is not sufficient evidence to conclude that there is a linear relationship between X and Y in the population, and worry about Type II error.

C = Calculation. I didn't give you means (or standard deviations), so you needed to calculate them. These descriptive statistics for the APACHE are 195.0000 (71.9182), and for the number of ICU days they are 7.5556 (3.8905). Based on these, here is a table showing the conversion of the raw scores to z scores and the cross-products of the z scores:

X	Y	z_x	z_y	$z_x z_y$
90	1	−1.4600	−1.6850	2.4601
290	12	1.3209	1.1424	1.5090
100	3	−1.3209	−1.1710	1.5468
275	14	1.1124	1.6564	1.8426
120	8	−1.0429	.1142	−.1191
255	9	.8343	.3713	.3098
180	7	−.2086	−.1428	.0298
230	9	.4867	.3713	.1807
215	5	.2781	−.6569	−.1827
				$\Sigma = 7.5770$

$$r = \frac{7.5770}{9} = .8419 = .84$$

This observed r falls in the rare zone, so we conclude, in APA format: $r\,(7) = .84, p < .05$. We have rejected the null hypothesis and have concluded that there is a probably, in the population, a linear relationship between APACHE score and ICU length of stay.

To what population can the results be generalized? To patients who entered the ICU in this hospital during this one month period. Are you comfortable generalizing to patients who enter the ICU during other months? To ICU patients at other small, community hospitals? Might there not be something unique about this month or this hospital? I'm not comfortable generalizing beyond this sample.

2. **Test:** We are doing an as-yet-unspecified difference test because we are investigating the relationship between one interval- or ratio-level variable (number of days of alcohol consumption) and one nominal level variable (return to school yes or no). We haven't learned what the assumptions are for this test or how to calculate it, so I have to stop here.

In any event, to what population could the results of this study be generalized? It was a random sample from one college. Are you comfortable generalizing the results to other first year students at other colleges? I'm comfortable generalizing to first year students at that school.

(This question should serve as a reminder that I am, sometimes, a bit devious. That is, I provided enough information here that you could have gone on and, erroneously, calculated a Pearson r. Carpenters have a saying, "Measure twice, cut once.")

3. **Test:** I am going to conduct a Pearson r because we are examining the relationship between two interval- or ratio-level variables, between visual ability and eye-hand coordination.

I'm going to treat visual ability as my predictor variable (X) and number of balls caught as my criterion variable (Y).

Assumptions: These are the five assumptions for a Pearson product moment correlation coefficient: random samples, interval- or ratio-level variables, normality, linearity, and homoscedasticity. The participants in this study were a "sample" of children, but I don't know how this sample was obtained. I am going to assume that it was not a random sample from the entire population of elementary school children or even a random sample from the children at a single school. Thus, this assumption was violated. The violation of the assumption of a random sample is not problematic, and we can still go ahead and calculate a Pearson r. Both variables are interval- or ratio-level variables, so the assumption of interval- or ratio-level variables was not violated. The 95% confidence intervals for skewness and kurtosis for both variables capture zero, so it is reasonable to conclude that both variables may be normally distributed in the population. (By the bye, I used SPSS to calculate skewness and kurtosis values.)

The scatterplot for these data is on page 560.

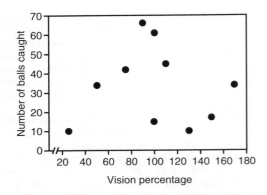

There is no apparent nonlinear relationship, so I shall accept the linearity assumption as not having been violated. I am not as sure about the homoscedasticity assumption, since there appears to be more spread of Y around X in the middle of the distribution (with a small sample size this is hard to tell). Since it is not clear to me that this assumption has been violated, I am going to proceed with calculating the correlation.

Hypotheses:

$$H_0: \rho_{xy} = 0$$
$$H_1: \rho_{xy} \neq 0$$

The null hypothesis states that there is no linear relationship, in the population, between visual acuity and eye-hand coordination. Though ρ is expected to be zero, $r_{obsserved}$ may turn out to be slightly off zero. The deviation from zero, however, should be small enough that it can be explained by sampling error.

The alternative hypothesis states that there is a linear relationship, in the population, between visual acuity and eye-hand coordination. Thus, the observed r should reflect this relationship and should be far enough away from zero that its deviation from zero can't reasonably be explained by sampling error from a population where $\rho = 0$.

Decision rule: Using a two-tailed test with alpha set at .05 and 8 degrees of freedom, the critical value of r is .6319.

If the absolute value of my calculated value of r is greater than or equal to the critical value, then I shall reject the null hypothesis, be forced to accept the alternative hypothesis, report that this result occurs less than 5% of the time when the null hypothesis is true (i.e., report $p < .05$), find the linear relationship between X and Y to be statistically different from zero, conclude that there is probably a linear relationship between visual acuity and eye-hand coordination in the population, and worry about Type I error.

If the absolute value of my calculated value of r is less than the critical value, then I shall fail to reject the null hypothesis. I'll report that this is a common result when the null hypothesis is true—that it occurs more than 5% of the time (i.e., $p > .05$)—and I'll say that the linear relationship between X and Y is not statistically different from zero, conclude that there is not sufficient evidence to believe that there is a nonzero linear relationship between visual acuity and eye-hand coordination in the population, and worry about Type II error.

Calculation: This time I provided the means and standard deviations. Based on them, here is a table showing raw scores converted to z scores and the cross-products of the z scores:

X	Y	z_x	z_y	$z_x z_y$
25	10	−1.8058	−1.2106	2.1861
170	34	1.6854	.0310	.0522
130	10	.7223	−1.2106	−.8744
50	34	−1.2039	.0310	−.0373
150	17	1.2039	−.8484	−1.0214
100	61	.0000	1.4278	.0000
90	66	−.2408	1.6865	−.4061
75	42	−.6019	.4449	−.2678
110	45	.2408	.6001	.1445
100	15	.0000	−.9519	.0000

The sum of the cross-products of the z scores is $-.2242$, and $r = \dfrac{-.2242}{10} = -.0224 = -.02$. As $r_{observed}$ falls in the common zone, this is what I report: $\boldsymbol{r\ (8) = -.02,\ p > .05}$.

To what population can the results be generalized? The sample wasn't random. Are you comfortable generalizing to all the students at the school? To students at other schools? I think generalizability is very limited. I'm not comfortable generalizing beyond the sample.

4. In order to understand the two types of errors that statisticians and researchers can make, Type I and Type II error, you have to understand the logic of hypothesis testing. If a statistician were trying to decide if a coin were fair, he or she would make two opposing assumptions. One, which we'll call the null hypothesis, says that the coin is fair. The other, which we'll call the alternative hypothesis, says that the coin is not fair. Both of these can't be true; and if one is true, then the other can't be true.

What the statistician does is obtain a sample of tosses from the coin and compares the observed outcome to the outcome that he or she would expect from a fair coin. (This is what would be expected if the null hypothesis were true.) If the sample yields roughly equal numbers of heads and tails, which is what we would expect from a fair coin, then the statistician says that the null hypothesis is probably true. If the sample yields a disproportionate number of heads or tails, then the statistician says that the alternative hypothesis is probably true because a fair coin shouldn't generate this disproportion.

However, isn't it possible for a fair coin to turn up heads, say, 10 times in a row? This isn't very likely, but it could happen. If the statistician had the bad luck to have this happen, then he or she would say that the coin was not fair when it really was. This is an error, and statisticians have come up with a name for it: Type I error. In statisticians' language, Type I error occurs when one incorrectly rejects the null hypothesis.

There is another error that could occur. Just as a fair coin could give an odd sample, so could an unfair coin. That is, it is possible that an unfair coin could yield a sample of tosses that have roughly equal numbers of heads and tails. If this happened the statistician would conclude that the coin was fair, and he or she would be in error. This type of error is called Type II error. In statistician's language, Type II error occurs when the null hypothesis is incorrectly accepted.

5. Positive correlations: *(These are just examples; yours should be different!)*

    Number of books in the house and score on the verbal section of the SAT

    Physical attractiveness of women and number of times they are asked for their phone number by men

    Negative correlations: *(These are just examples; yours should be different!)*

    Age of person and comfort level with modern technology

    Age of car and number of safety features on the car

    Zero correlations: *(These are just examples; yours should be different!)*

    Intelligence and number of times ice cream is eaten per year

    For cities, percentage of population that owns dogs and number of games of bingo offered on a Tuesday night

6. In Figure 7.12 I have marked off the bottom and top 2.5% of correlations for the 1000 samples of size $N = 6$ that I drew from a population. The values associated with these cutoff points were $-.75$ and $.83$. The r_{cv} for a two-tailed Pearson r with $df = 4$ and $\alpha = .05$ is $\pm.8114$. The values of $-.75$ and $.83$ are close to r_{cv} but not exactly the same. They differ because r_{cv} is based on the infinitely large theoretical sampling distribution, the sampling distribution that would occur if every possible repeated, random sample (with replacement) were drawn from the population. One set of critical values—the one in the table of critical values of r at the back of the book, $\pm.8114$—is the theoretical set of critical values, and the other, $-.75$ and $.83$ are the critical values observed from 1000 samples. We would expect them to be close, which they are, but not the same.

7. This question is checking to make sure that you remember how to use the z score table at the back of the book.

    Having a blood pressure of 55 or lower means that one has a blood pressure that is two or more standard deviations below the mean. In the population, 2.28% have scores this low or lower. This now becomes an algebra problem: $50 = .0228\ (X)$. Solving for X gives us $X = 2192.98$. And, since we can't have fractional people, we end up concluding that our cardiovascular researcher would need to screen **2193** people in order to end up with 50 who met her criteria.

8. $H_0: \rho_{xy} = 0$
   $H_1: \rho_{xy} \neq 0$
   The null hypothesis says that there is no linear relationship between X and Y in the population. However, when we draw a sample from the population and calculate r_{xy}, we'll find that r_{xy} almost certainly doesn't exactly equal zero. Why does r differ from zero? Because of sampling error.

    The alternative hypothesis says that there really is a linear relationship between X and Y. Thus when we draw a sample from the population, our sample will reflect that reality and r_{xy} will be different from zero, different enough that sampling error from a population where $\rho = 0$ is not a credible explanation for the discrepancy.

    The sample that the respiratory therapist used consisted of healthy college students. Probably this was not a random sample from the population of healthy college students, but was a group of students from one college who agreed, for some reason, to participate in this research. Thus the results can be generalized to a young, healthy, intelligent population. In addition, the sample is probably geographically limited, since many colleges draw their students from a specific region, and it probably is relatively wealthy, since college is expensive. To the extent that these factors (age, health, intelligence, geography, wealth, etc.) influence the relationship between exercise and oxygen saturation, generalizability is limited.

9. This is a one-tailed test! Xerxes decision rule is based on a critical value of r of $.4973$. Thus, if $r_{xy} \geq .4973$, he'll reject the null hypothesis, be forced to accept the alternative hypothesis, call his correlation statistically different from zero, report $p < .05$, conclude that there is probably a positive linear relationship between the two variables in the population, and worry about having made a Type I error.

    If $r_{xy} < .4973$, he'll fail to reject the null hypothesis, report that the correlation does not appear to be statistically different from zero, report $p > .05$, conclude that there is no reason to conclude that there is a positive relationship between the variables in the population and worry about having made a Type II error.

    On page 562 is the sampling distribution with the rare and common zones marked off.

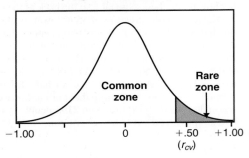

Sampling distribution of *r*, *df* = 10

Common zone

Rare zone

−1.00   0   +.50 +1.00
                        (r_{cv})

10. She has a sample of schools where the program was implemented and a sample where it wasn't. She's comparing results from two samples to see if there is a difference between them. This requires a difference test.

11. This researcher has one sample of cases and is measuring two variables on each to see if there is a relationship between the two variables. Thus, this is a **relationship test.** *(And, if you want to get specific, since both variables are ratio-level, it should be a Pearson r.)*

CHAPTER 8

Review Exercises

1. $r = .3714$, $N = 2512$, $r_{cv} = .0619$

    95% CI = .336 to .405

    $r^2 = .1379 = .14$

    BESD:

	↑ GPA	↓ GPA
↑ **SAT**	68.57 ($\approx$69)	31.43 ($\approx$31)
↓ **SAT**	31.43 ($\approx$31)	68.57 ($\approx$69)

    There's no information about means and standard deviations, so we can't predict Y'.

    Interpretation:

    "I examined the linear relationship, for a random sample of college-bound high-school seniors from the United States, between their combined SAT score and their first year GPA. I found a positive, or direct, relationship that was statistically different from zero (r (2510) = .37, $p < .05$). According to the results of this study, the higher the SAT score, the better the first year GPA.

    "The relationship appears to be a strong and meaningful one. Because I had a random sample of college-bound high-school seniors I can generalize to this population. By calculating the confidence interval for the correlation, I conclude that the real value of the correlation coefficient in this population has a 95% chance of falling in the range from .34 to .40. Though a correlation of .34 may not sound that large, it indicates a strong effect in general. If the correlation between SAT and GPA were .34, then a person with an above-average SAT score would have a 67% chance of having an above-average GPA. This is in contrast to a person with a below-average GPA who would have only a 33% chance of having an above-average GPA.

Thus, being conservative and assuming that the relationship between the two variables is lower than I observed, having a high SAT score more than doubles a person's chance of having a high GPA.

"Of course, there is a chance that the conclusion that there is a relationship between SAT and GPA is in error and that there really is no relationship in the larger population. Though there is a 5% chance of this having happened, I am not, given the large and random sample, overly concerned that my conclusion is in error. Nevertheless, it is always a wise idea to replicate a study, and so I recommend that this study be replicated in order to increase confidence in the results."

2. $r_{xy} = .8419$, $N = 9$, $M_X = 195.000$, $s_X = 71.9182$, $M_Y = 7.5556$, and $s_Y = 3.8905$.

    95% CI = .405 to .966

    $r^2 = .7088$

    BESD:

	↑ days	↓ days
↑ **APACHE**	$\approx$92	$\approx$8
↓ **APACHE**	$\approx$8	$\approx$92

    If APACHE = 231, $Y' = 9.1954$

    $\hat{s}_{Y-Y'} = 3.8905 \times .5396 \times 1.1339 \times 1.0672 = 2.5404$

    95% PI = $9.1954 \pm (2.3646 \times 2.5404)$
    $= 3.1884$ to 15.2024

    $\beta = .24$. If power = .80, $N = 9$; $N = 13$ for power = .95

    Interpretation:

    Note that though power was almost adequate and the sample size was OK, I'm recommending a much larger sample size. An N of 9 just makes me uncom-

fortable for important decisions, so I found a way, using the low end of the CI, to propose a larger N.

The researcher examined the linear relationship between severity of illness (APACHE scores) on intensive care unit (ICU) entry and length of stay in the ICU for all the ICU patients admitted during a given month to a small rural hospital. She found a positive, direct relationship that was statistically different from zero and which showed that people who had more severe illnesses stayed longer in the ICU (r (7) = .84, p < .05). The sample size for the present study was small, resulting in a 95% confidence interval for the value of the correlation in the population that was fairly broad, ranging from .41 to .97. Even so, the correlation seems meaningful since a correlation of .41 means that a person with a more severe illness of above average severity has a 70% chance of an above average ICU stay compared with only a 30% chance of an above average ICU stay for a person with a below average severity of illness.

There are a couple of cautions regarding the current study. First, there is a 5% chance that the conclusion is in error, that there really is no relationship between illness severity and ICU length of stay. To reduce concern over this error having occurred, I recommend replicating this study with a larger sample size. To be specific, given the possibility that the population value of the correlation is as low as .41, I recommend redoing the study with at least 48 subjects.

My second concern regards the nature of the sample. The sample consists of ICU patients from a single month at a single rural hospital. Thus, the extent to which these results would generalize to the larger population of ICU patients in other hospitals, cities, and countries is unknown. I advise, when replicating the study, to make sure that the sample is representative of the population to which the researcher wants to generalize.

Finally, one wants to be cautious in applying these results to any single ICU patient in an attempt to predict, based on his or her APACHE score, how long he or she will remain in the ICU. If a person has an APACHE score of 231, then it is predicted that his or her ICU stay will be a little over 9 days. However, because of variability and error in prediction, the predicted ICU stay falls in the range from 3 to 15 days. Though this study says that in general higher APACHE scores are related to longer ICU stays, this will not always be true for individual patients.

3. r_{xy} = −.0224, N = 10, M_X =100.0000, s_x = 41.5331, M_Y = 33.4000, s_Y = 19.3298.

95% CI = −.641 to .617

β = .97 (Using r = .05 in the power table.) If r = .025, N for power of .80 = 12,560; for power of .95, N = 20,790. If ρ = .05 and power = .80, then N = 3139.

Interpretation:

"A researcher examined the linear relationship between visual ability and eye-hand coordination in 10 elementary-school children by comparing their eyesight to the number of balls, out of 50, that they were able to catch. He found that the relationship between the two variables was not statistically different from zero (r (8) = −.02, p > .05). That is, there is no evidence from this study that a child's visual abilities have any impact on his or her ball catching ability.

"There are a couple of limitations to this study that should be mentioned. First, there is a chance that this conclusion is in error, that there really is a relationship between vision and eye-hand coordination. The sample size in the present study was small, and if such a relationship did exist at a very low level, say if the level of the correlation were .05, there would be only a 3% chance of finding a significant relationship with 10 participants. However, having enough subjects to have an 80% chance of finding such a small relationship is a daunting task, since one would need to have over 3000 subjects.

"A second concern involves the sample used in the current study. All the children came from the school where the researcher teaches, which limits generalizability greatly. I recommend obtaining a sample that is representative of whatever population it is to which the researcher wants to generalize.

"It is counterintuitive that visual skill is unrelated to eye-hand coordination. If there is a relationship between visual ability and eye-hand coordination, this study gives little guidance as to the direction or strength of the correlation. The small sample size means that the confidence interval within which I estimate the population value of the correlation falls is quite wide and ranges from a strong positive relationship (better visual abilities predict better eye-hand coordination) to a zero relationship (there is no correlation between the two variables) to a strong negative relationship (those with better visual skills have worse eye-hand coordination). Because it makes sense to me that there is a relationship, and I suspect a direct one, I recommend replicating this study with a larger, and representative, sample. In addition, perhaps a more sensitive measure than the number of balls caught can be used to measure eye-hand coordination."

4. Using Appendix Table 8 (the power table), I see that for a two-tailed test with α set at .05, I would need 38 cases in order to have an 80% chance of rejecting the null hypothesis if ρ were really .45. If I wanted to have a 95% chance of rejecting the null hypothesis under these conditions, I would need 60 cases.

Making α smaller, moving it from .05 to .01, say, has the effect of making the rare zone smaller, making it harder to reject the null hypothesis. Since power is the likelihood of rejecting the null hypothesis, power is smaller when $\alpha = .01$ compared to when $\alpha = .05$, if everything else is held constant. Thus, to have the same likelihood of being able to reject the null hypothesis when $\alpha = .01$ as when $\alpha = .05$, something else has to change. That something else is sample size. So, if I move α from .05 to .01 and want to keep my power the same, I'll need to increase my sample size. However, the power tables in the Appendix don't tell us by how much.

5. Since the scale weighs to the nearest half pound, Desdemona's starting weight was in the range from 135.25 to 135.75. Two weeks later, her weight was in the range from 130.75 to 131.25. Thus, the most weight she could have lost was 5 pounds (135.75-130.75) and the least was 4 pounds (135.25-131.25).

6. The dependent variable is whether the bandage is still in place. The independent variable is whether the arm is bent or straight while applying the bandage.

7. Given $M = 100$ and $s = 25$, the z score for a score of 70 is −1.2000. Looking in Table 1, we find that scores this low or lower occur 11.51% of the time. Thus, surgeons can expect a bad surgical outcome, in terms of quality of life, 11.51% of the time.

CHAPTER 9

Review Exercises

1. This question gives information about a sample statistic and asks what we know about a population parameter. In other words, this question is asking you to calculate a confidence interval.

However, in order to do so we first need to figure out what M is! If their mean score has a percentile rank of 91, then, via Appendix Table 1 we know that their mean score, as a z score, was 1.34. This converts, via Equation 5.2, to an IQ score of 120.1000.* I'm going to choose to calculate a 95% confidence interval and will use Equation 6.2b to do so:

$$95\% \ CI = 120.1000 \pm 2.0281(2.4660)$$
$$= 120.1000 \pm 5.0013$$
$$= 115.0987 \text{ to } 125.1013$$

Thus, the 95% confidence interval for the mean intelligence of the population of United States Senators ranges from 115.10 to 125.10.

2. The critical value of t is larger, farther away from zero, for a two-tailed test than for a one-tailed test. For example, with a sample size of infinity and with α set at .05, t_{cv} for a one-tailed test is 1.6449 and for a two-tailed test it is 1.9600. This means that the rare zone is larger for a one-tailed test than for a two-tailed test; it is easier to reject H_0 with a one-tailed test than with a two-tailed test as long as the difference between means is in the expected direction.

3. **Test:** The test we are doing is an independent-samples t test since we are comparing the means of two independent samples.

Assumptions: We have independent samples and an interval-level measure, so those assumptions are not violated. We don't have random samples, so that assumption was violated. We can proceed; we'll just

---

*(1.34 × 15.0000) + 100.0000 = 120.1000

have to be circumspect in the interpretation. Via my calculations of the confidence intervals for skewness and kurtosis, each variable is likely normally distributed. Also, one $\hat{s}$ is not twice the other, so the homogeneity of variance assumption is not violated. On another positive note, the sample sizes are large and equal. We can proceed with the test.

Hypotheses:

$$H_0: \ \mu_1 = \mu_2$$
$$H_1: \ \mu_1 \neq \mu_2$$

The null hypothesis says that the two population means are the same, that the two populations are really one population. Even so, when two samples are drawn from this one population, the sample means won't be exactly the same because of sampling error. They should, however, be close enough to each other that the difference can be accounted for by sampling error.

The alternative hypothesis says that the two populations really are different. As a result, the two sample means will be different. They should be different enough that the difference is too large to be accounted for by sampling error for two means drawn from the same population.

Decision rule: I'm willing to make a Type I error 5% of the time, and I have nondirectional hypotheses, so I am going to set α at .05, two-tailed. My degrees of freedom are 48, so $t_{cv} = 2.0106$. If $|t_{observed}| \geq 2.0106$, then I'll reject the null hypothesis and conclude that there is a statistically significant difference between the two sample means, that the two populations probably have different means. If $|t_{observed}| < 2.0106$, I'll fail to reject H_0 and conclude that I have no reason to question the belief that the two populations have the same mean.

Using the rule-of-thumb method of calculating sample size, Equation 9.9, and treating the adoptive group as the control group (because $\hat{s}$ is bigger for them), I find that I need 19 cases per group in order to have power > .80. Since I have 25 cases per group, I appear to have sufficient power to proceed.

Calculations: Via Equation 9.3, this is how I calculate $\hat{s}_{M_1-M_2}$:

$$\sqrt{\left[\frac{(25-1)74.6168 + (25-1)118.5660}{25+25-2}\right]\left[\frac{25+25}{25\times25}\right]}$$

$$= \sqrt{[96.5914][.0800]} = 2.7798$$

(Note that I've kept separate the information I'll need to calculate the pooled standard deviation used in calculating d.)

Thus $t = \dfrac{61.4400 - 51.3200}{2.7798} = \dfrac{10.1200}{2.7798}$

$$= 3.6405 = 3.64$$

In APA format, this is reported as follows: $t(48) = 3.64$, $p < .05$.

Interpretation: The difference is statistically significant, with adoptive mothers scoring higher in terms of mental health than nonadoptive mothers. I'll calculate all of the options for interpretation and then select the ones I want to use for interpretation. As always, remember that interpretation is subjective, so you may choose to emphasize something different from me.

Observed		Low end of *CI*	High end of *CI*
Difference between means	10.1200	4.5309	15.7091
Observed *t* value	3.6405	1.6299	5.6512
Effect size (d)	1.0297	.4610	1.5984
% adoptive moms with higher score than average nonadoptive mom	84.85	67.72	94.52
ω^2	.1968	.0321	.3822
$\hat{r}$	.4436		
r_{pb}	.4652	.217*	.658*
BESD (% adoptive moms above average in mental health)	$\approx$73	$\approx$61	$\approx$83
Power	.91	.28	> .99
N via Table 8, $\alpha = .05$, two-tailed for power = .80 / .95	38 / 60	195 / 321	17 / 26

*Calculated via formula for *95% CI* for *p* from Chapter 8.

Here's my interpretation:

"I analyzed the data from a study that compared the mental health of adoptive and nonadoptive mothers to see the impact of the screening procedures that are used to qualify parents for adoptions. The participants were samples of convenience, and all were first-time mothers with a child less than 2 years of age. The results showed that the mental health of adoptive mothers ($M = 61.44$, $\hat{s} = 8.64$) was statistically higher than the mental health of nonadoptive mothers ($M = 51.32$, $\hat{s} = 10.89$) using an independent-samples *t* test ($t(48) = 3.64$, $p < .05$).

"I think that this over 10-point difference in scores on a measure of mental health indicates a substantially higher level of mental health for adoptive mothers than for nonadoptive ones. Converting this into an effect size shows that the average adoptive mother has a score on the mental health scale that is higher than about 85% of the nonadoptive mothers. Of course, the size of the mean difference between the

population of adoptive mothers and the population of nonadoptive mothers may be larger or smaller: the 95% confidence interval shows that the 'real' difference between the two populations probably falls in the range from about 5 to 15 points.

"There are, of course, limitations to the present study. One is that there is a 5% chance that these results are in error, that there really is no difference between the mental health level of adoptive and nonadoptive parents. One way to determine if this is so would be to replicate the study, and I recommend doing so. A second concern arises from the two samples used in this study. They were samples of convenience, not random samples, and so the results of the present study cannot be generalized to the larger general populations of adoptive and nonadoptive mothers. Similarly, the results cannot be generalized to fathers or to mothers with more than one child. Though it would be difficult to do so, I recommend trying to obtain more representative samples of these two populations when replicating this study. In addition, when the study is replicated, I recommend having a somewhat larger sample size to get a better estimate of the difference between the two populations.

"Though there are limitations to the present study, as there are to all studies, the current results suggest that adoptive mothers score higher on a measure of mental health than do nonadoptive mothers. Based on the present study, it seems that the screening procedures that are used when people want to form their families via adoption result in the selection of parents who have higher levels of mental health."

4. a. **Factorial multiple samples difference test:** a difference question with two grouping variables (Lamaze yes/no and partner present yes/no) and an interval-level dependent variable, that is, a 2×2 matrix with four samples or cells

   b. **Chi-square test of association (or chi-square difference test):** two nominal-level variables, concep-

tualized either as (i) a relationship test (chi-square test of association) or (ii) a two independent-samples difference test (chi-square difference test)

   c. **Pearson product moment correlation coefficient:** relationship question with two interval-level variables in one sample

   d. **Mann Whitney U:** difference test comparing two independent groups (more fit vs. less fit) on an ordinal-level dependent variable

   e. **Chi-square goodness-of-fit test** (comparing a sample to a population on a nominal-level variable)

   f. **Dependent-samples t test:** difference test, two dependent samples, ratio-level dependent variable

   g. It is always important to recognize one's limitations. Though there is such a relationship test, and it is called multiple regression, we haven't learned a test that can combine three variables to predict one variable. So, the correct answer is, "I don't know what the appropriate statistical test is."

CHAPTER 10

Review Exercises

1. **Test:** Comparing the means of four independent groups: one-way ANOVA
   Assumptions:
   - Independent samples (random assignment, not violated)
   - Interval- or ratio-level data (ratio level, not violated)
   - Random samples (not a random sample from the population of people with severe spider phobia, so violated, but OK to proceed)
   - Normality (I told you to assume this was not violated)
   - Homogeneity of variance (no standard deviation twice another, not violated)

   Hypotheses:

   $$H_0: \mu_1 = \mu_2 = \mu_3 = \mu_4$$
   $$H_1: \text{Not all } \mu\text{s are equal}$$

   The null hypothesis says that each of the four populations has the same mean, that, in essence, the four populations are really just one population. Thus, the four samples are samples from the same population and the four sample means should be close enough to each other that sampling error can explain any discrepancies.

   The alternative hypothesis says that at least two of the four populations have different means. As a result, at least two of the sample means will be far enough away from each other that their difference is too large

to be explained as sampling error for two means drawn from the same population.

Decision rule: Set α at .05 because I am willing to make a Type I error 5% of the time. F_{cv} (3, 8) = 4.0662. If $F_{observed} \geq 4.0662$, then reject H_0. If $F_{observed} < 4.0662$, then fail to reject H_0.

In order to decide if sample size is adequate... I would hope for at least a moderate effect of treatment. Cohen (1988)* calls it a moderate effect if $r = .30$. If $\rho = .30$, then the N required to have power of .80 is 86. For four samples, this works out to about 22 cases per group, and I have only 3. The study is underpowered.

Alternatively, one could use Equation 9.9 to find the n required to have power of .80 for an independent-samples t test using the two means furthest apart and the larger of the two standard deviations as $\hat{s}_c$. Under those conditions, n works out to be five. Even with five, the study is still underpowered.

Since the rule-of-thumb results are based on data, not pure speculation, I tend to trust them more. I'd recommend gaining two more cases per sample before proceeding.

Calculations: Grand mean = 28.0000.

---

*Cohen, J. (1988). *Statistical power analysis for the behavioral sciences.* Hillsdale, NJ: Lawrence Erlbaum Associates.

$SS_{between} = 3(31.3333 - 28)^2 + 3(27.6667 - 28)^2 +$
$\quad 3(29.6667 - 28)^2 + 3(23.3333 - 28)^2 = 107.3333$

$SS_{within} = (36 - 31.3333)^2 + (28 - 31.3333)^2 +$
$\quad (30 - 31.3333)^2 + (31 - 27.6667)^2 +$
$\quad (28 - 27.6667)^2 + (24 - 27.6667)^2 +$
$\quad (27 - 29.6667)^2 + (29 - 29.6667)^2 +$
$\quad (33 - 29.6667)^2 + (21 - 23.3333)^2 +$
$\quad (27 - 23.3333)^2 + (22 - 23.3333)^2 = 98.6667$

SS_{total} via Dirty Harry shortcut $= 107.3333 + 98.6667$
$\quad\quad\quad\quad\quad\quad\quad\quad\quad = 206.0000$

SS_{total} via formula $= (36 - 28)^2 + (28 - 28)^2 +$
$\quad (30 - 28)^2 + (31 - 28)^2 + (28 - 28)^2 +$
$\quad (24 - 28)^2 + (27 - 28)^2 + (29 - 28)^2 +$
$\quad (33 - 28)^2 + (21 - 28)^2 + (27 - 28)^2 +$
$\quad (22 - 28)^2 = 206.0000$

ANOVA summary table for evaluation of treatments for spider phobia

Source	SS	df	MS	F
Between	107.33	3	35.78	2.91
Within	98.67	8	12.33	
Total	206.00	11		

APA format: $F(3, 8) = 2.91$, $p > .05$. We have failed to reject the null hypothesis, and there is no reason to conclude that any of the population means differ from each other.

Interpretation: I failed to reject H_0, and so will conclude that there is no statistically significant difference between different treatments for spider phobia in terms of how closely a person is willing to approach a spider. I need to worry about Type II error, and need to calculate ω^2 to convert it to $\hat{r}$, so I can use that to approximate β. I'll also calculate the 95% confidence intervals, so I can get some sense of how large the effect might be.

$$\omega^2 = \frac{107.3333 - (3)12.3333}{206.0000 + 12.3333} = .3221$$

$$\hat{r} = \sqrt{.3221} = .5675 = .57$$

NOTE: This seems like a large effect, and it may bother you that the results were not statistically significant. If so, you're worried about Type II error.

Based on ρ of .55, power is .45, and β is .55; there's a 55% chance we made a Type II error. To have power set at .80, I would need a total of 25 cases, ≈ 6 per group. For power = .95, I would need 38 cases total, 9 to 10 per group. Since this is a clinical study and I am concerned about the costs of making a Type II error, I am going to want power set at .95.

For calculating 95% confidence intervals for the difference between two means, since the ns are all the same, we can just calculate the denominator term, the standard error of the difference, once:

$$2.3060\sqrt{12.3333\left(\frac{1}{3} + \frac{1}{3}\right)} = 6.6123$$

Hence the absolute values of the 95% confidence intervals are the following:

Control vs. education:	−2.95 to 10.28
Control vs. modeling:	−4.95 to 8.28
Control vs. relaxation:	1.39 to 14.61
Education vs. modeling:	−4.61 to 8.61
Education vs. relaxation:	−2.28 to 10.95
Modeling vs. relaxation:	−.28 to 12.95

Note that one of the confidence intervals, the worst outcome vs. the best outcome (control group vs. relaxation group), does not capture zero. Do not interpret this as indicating a statistically significant difference between the two groups! The rules that we agreed to when we chose analysis of variance said that we would only consider differences statistically significant if the overall F were statistically significant.

What the confidence intervals tell me are that there are some potentially large differences between the effectiveness of the different treatments for spider phobias, that some—for example, modeling vs. relaxation—could lead to one group getting more than a foot closer to a spider. Coupled with the fact that the study was underpowered, I will recommend replicating this study with a larger sample size since I believe that some of these treatments may turn out to be better than others.

So, here is my interpretation:

"A psychologist investigated the effectiveness of three different treatments for people with phobias by comparing them to each other and to a no-treatment control group. Twelve patients with severe spider phobias were randomly assigned to one of four groups: a no-treatment control group, an education group in which they learned about spiders, a modeling group in which a therapist modeled spider handling, or a relaxation group in which relaxation skills were learned. After therapy was completed, its effectiveness was measured by seeing how closely the patient would approach a large spider that was placed 36″ away. The smaller the distance, the closer the patient got to the spider and the more effective the treatment was. The means [and standard deviations] for the four groups were, in descending order, control group (31.33 [4.16]), modeling group (29.67 [3.06]), education group (27.67 [3.51]), and relaxation group (23.33 [3.21]).

"The results of the one-way analysis of variance that was used to analyze the data showed that there were no statistically significant differences between any of the groups: $F(3, 8) = 2.91$, $p > .05$. Thus there was not sufficient evidence in this study to conclude that any treatment was better than no treatment or that any one treatment was better than any other treatment.

"There is a reasonable chance, however, that the conclusions of the present study are in error, since the sample size was too small to provide the study with adequate statistical power. In fact, there is close to a 50% chance that the conclusions of this study are in error. Thus I recommend that the study be replicated with a sample size large enough to yield only a 5% chance of making this type of error, about 9 to 10 cases in each group. Until this is done, it is unreasonable to draw any conclusions about the (in)effectiveness of any of the treatments for spider phobia. In addition, when the study is replicated, I hope that more details are provided about the source of the participants so that some sense of the population to which the results can be generalized can be obtained."

2. **Test:** Comparing three different independent groups in terms of an interval-level variable: one-way ANOVA
   Assumptions:
   - Independent samples (no apparent connection between samples so probably not violated)
   - Interval- or ratio-level data (interval level, not violated)
   - Random samples (all cases from one sixth-grade classroom, not a random sample of sixth-graders, so violated; but OK to proceed)
   - Normality (I told you to assume this is OK)
   - Homogeneity of variance (no standard deviation twice another, not violated)

   Hypotheses:

   $$H_0: \mu_1 = \mu_2 = \mu_3$$
   $$H_1: \text{Not all } \mu\text{s are equal}$$

The null hypothesis says that each of the three populations has the same mean: that, in essence, the three populations are really one population. Thus, the three samples are samples from the same population, and the sample means should be close enough to each other that sampling error can explain any discrepancies.

The alternative hypothesis says that at least two of the three populations have different means. As a result, at least two of the sample means will be far enough away from each other that their difference is too large to be explained as sampling error for two means drawn from the same population.

   Decision rule: There are 3 groups and 13 cases, so the degrees of freedom are $df_{between} = 2$, $df_{within} = 10$, and $df_{total} = 12$. I am willing to make a Type I error 5% of the time, so $F_{cv}(2, 10) = 4.1028$.

If $F_{observed} \geq 4.1028$, then I'll reject H_0 and conclude that there is a statistically significant difference between at least two of the means. If $F_{observed} < 4.1028$, I'll fail to reject the null hypothesis and conclude that there is not sufficient evidence to conclude that any of the samples come from populations with different means.

I think that whatever change a school district would make in the teaching of reading would be made because the new method shows at least a moderate improvement, a medium effect size, over the old method. According to Cohen (1988), a medium effect is equivalent to an r of .30, and the sample size required to have an 80% chance of finding such an effect is 86. Given three groups, this is almost 30 cases per sample. This suggests that my study is underpowered.

Using Equation 9.9 to find the n required for an independent-samples t test if I were comparing the two samples that are the farthest apart (the control group and the advanced reading group), I find a recommended N of two. This suggests that my study has adequate power. I'm going to tend to believe that I have adequate power because the conclusion from Equation 9.9 is based on my actual data, not speculation in a vacuum. (And why is the n so low from Equation 9.9? Because the standard deviation, the within-group variability, is so small.) Power may be adequate, but I won't be comfortable drawing very strong conclusions from such small sample sizes.

Calculations: The grand mean is 6.7308. (Because all the samples don't have the same n, you can't simply average the three grand means. Either add up all the scores and divide by N to find M_{Grand}, or weight each mean by its respective n, add up these three products, and divide by N.)

$$SS_{between} = 4(6.475 - 6.7308)^2 + 5(7 - 6.7308)^2 + 4(6.65 - 6.7308)^2 = .6502$$

$$SS_{within} = (6.5 - 6.475)^2 + (6.3 - 6.475)^2 + (6.6 - 6.475)^2 + (6.5 - 6.475)^2 + (7.1 - 7)^2 + (6.8 - 7)^2 + (7 - 7)^2 + (6.9 - 7)^2 + (7.2 - 7)^2 + (6.6 - 6.65)^2 + (6.8 - 6.65)^2 + (6.5 - 6.65)^2 + (6.7 - 6.65)^2 = .1975$$

SS_{total} via the Dirty Harry shortcut = .6502 + .1975
$$= .8477$$

Alternatively, $SS_{total} = (6.5 - 6.7308)^2 +$
$(6.3 - 6.7308)^2 + (6.6 - 6.7308)^2 +$
$(6.5 - 6.7308)^2 + (7.1 - 6.7308^2 +$
$(6.8 - 6.7308)^2 + (7 - 6.7308)^2 +$
$(6.9 - 6.7308)^2 + (7.2 - 6.7308)^2 +$
$(6.6 - 6.7308)^2 + (6.8 - 6.7308)^2 +$
$(6.5 - 6.7308)^2 + (6.7 - 6.7308)^2 = .8477$

Here's the ANOVA summary table:

ANOVA summary table for sixth-grade writing test scores

Source	SS	df	MS	F
Between	.65	2	.32	16.46
Within	.20	10	.02	
Total	.85	12		

In APA format: $F(2, 10) = 16.46$, $p < .05$. $F_{observed}$ fell in the rare zone, so we reject the null hypothesis and conclude that it is reasonable to conclude that at least two of the population means differ from each other.

Interpretation: Since there is a statistically significant difference, we have a lot of interpretation to do. We need to compute ω^2 and $\hat{r}$, confidence intervals and post-hoc tests, power, and sample size.

$$\omega^2 = \frac{.6502 - (2).0198}{.8477 + .0198} = .7039 = .70$$

$$\hat{r} = \sqrt{.7039} = .8390 = .84$$

$t_{Protectedcv} = 2.2281$

The ns for the groups bounce around a bit, so doing post-hoc tests is a bit more tedious.

$$t_{1vs2} = \frac{7.0000 - 6.4750}{\sqrt{.0198\left(\frac{1}{4} + \frac{1}{5}\right)}} = \frac{.5250}{.0944}$$

$$= 5.5614 = 5.57$$

$$t_{1vs3} = \frac{6.6500 - 6.4750}{\sqrt{.0198\left(\frac{1}{4} + \frac{1}{4}\right)}} = \frac{.1750}{.0995}$$

$$= 1.7588 = 1.76$$

$$t_{2vs3} = \frac{7.0000 - 6.6500}{\sqrt{.0198\left(\frac{1}{4} + \frac{1}{5}\right)}} = \frac{.3500}{.0944}$$

$$= 3.7076 = 3.71$$

95% CI_{1vs2} = .5250 ± 2.2281(.0944) = .5250 ± .2103 = from .31 to .74

95% CI_{1vs3} = .1750 ± 2.2281(.0995) = .1750 ± .2217 = from −.05 to .40

95% CI_{2vs3} = .3500 ± 2.2281(.0944) = .3500 ± .2103 = from .14 to .56

Power ≈ .93

N necessary is 9 if power = .80 and 13 if power = .95

Interpretation: "I analyzed the data from a study in which an education researcher tested two ways of improving writing in sixth-grade students. Thirteen students were assigned to three different groups: (1) a control group that received the standard sixth-grade writing curriculum, (2) an experimental group, the reading group, that was given advanced *reading* material in hopes that this would indirectly foster advanced *writing* skills, and (3) an experimental group, the writing group, that was directly taught advanced writing skills. At the end of the year, each student took a writing test that provided a grade-level score for his or her writing ability.

"The highest score was achieved by the reading group ($M = 7.00$, $\hat{s} = .16$), followed by the writing group ($M = 6.65$, $\hat{s} = .13$), and the control group ($M = 6.48$, $\hat{s} = .13$). The one-way analysis of variance that I used to analyze the data showed that there was a statistically significant difference between the groups ($F(2, 10) = 16.46$, $p < .05$). Using a post-hoc test, I found that the reading group performed significantly better than the control group and the writing group but that the writing group did not perform statistically better than the control group. In other words, reading more advanced material seems to lead to more advanced writing skills whereas teaching advanced writing directly does not statistically seem to benefit students.

"The advantages for learning to write by reading advanced material seem substantial, with type of instruction received explaining (or predicting) about 70% of the variability in the end-of-year writing-test score. By calculating the 95% confidence interval I was able to find the range within which the mean difference for the larger populations likely falls. Thus I concluded that reading advanced material leads to writing skills that are from about 30% to 75% of a school year more advanced than what the regular instruction would result in, and from about 15% to 55% of a school year more advanced than when writing is taught directly.

"Though the results seem compelling and suggest that the most effective way to teach writing is indirectly, by exposing students to challenging reading material, there are several limitations to this study that must be noted. All of the limitations could be addressed in replications of the study, and I strongly suggest that this be done before revamping a school district's writing curriculum on the basis of the results of the current study. First, all the students came from one school, in one school district, in one city. To the extent that this school/district/city differs from other schools/districts/cities in some way that could affect writing ability—for example, socioeconomic status—then the results may be unique to the specific school/district/city studied. Second, students were not randomly assigned to the three different types of instruction, and thus it is possible that the students in the different groups already differed in writing abilities before the school year began. Third, though the sample size was adequate given the large size of the effect, I would recommend increasing sample size in subsequent studies. With a larger sample size it is possible that the difference between the writing group and the control group, which did not show a statistically significant improvement in writing skills by writing being taught directly, would rise to the level of statistical significance. In any event, larger sample sizes from a variety of schools would lead to better estimates of the effectiveness of this writing curriculum as well as help elucidate other factors that may influence the program's effectiveness. A replication would also address the fact that there is a 5% chance that the conclusions of the present study are in error.

"In conclusion, the current results certainly suggest that an effective way to improve students' writing abilities is an indirect approach, by challenging them with advanced reading material, but further research is needed before implementing this technique."

(I feel compelled to mention that I just made these data up, so don't go around quoting me that the best way to teach writing is via reading.)

3. Comparing the results from a sample to a population value on a nominal-level variable (elm yes vs. elm no): **chi-square goodness-of-fit test**

4. Three independent samples (small, medium, and large trees) being compared on a ratio-level variable: **one-way ANOVA**

5. Three dependent samples (each person cooks on each of three different applicances) being compared on an ordinal-level variable (rating of hamburger tastiness): **Friedman two-way ANOVA by ranks**

6. Three dependent samples (same retirees being surveyed at three points in time) being compared on a nominal-level variable (interest in Florida, yes/no): **Cochran's Q test**

7. Two independent samples (internship yes/no) being compared on an interval-level variable: **independent-samples *t* test**

CHAPTER 11

Review Exercises

1. a. Research question: Does surgery A or surgery B have more of an impact on back pain depending on whether there is an apparent physical cause for the back pain?

      Statistical test: Four independent groups formed on the basis of two independent or grouping variables (with/without apparent physical cause for pain and type of surgery) and an interval-level dependent variable: **factorial analysis of variance.**

   b. Research question: What is the long-term impact of the family dinner hour during first grade on high-school graduation?

      Statistical test: One grouping variable, three independent samples being assessed on a nominal-level dependent variable: **chi-square difference test.**

   c. Research question: What is the relationship between familial college attendance and high-school GPA?

      Statistical test: One grouping variable, three independent samples being compared on a ratio-level dependent variable: **one-way ANOVA.**

   d. Research question: What is the relationship between lung capacity and ability to endure exercise?

      Statistical test: One sample on which two ratio-level variables are being measured: **Pearson product moment correlation coefficient.**

   e. Research question: Controlling for age, gender, and IQ, does length of time one has been in the United States have an impact on one's income?

      Statistical test: One grouping variable, three dependent samples being compared on a ratio-level dependent variable: **repeated-measures ANOVA.**

2. Here's a table with marginal and grand means:

Perception of Racism in the United States as a Function of Type of Employment and Area of Origin

	European Descent	African Descent	Mexican Descent	
Blue-collar	12	24	22	19.33
White-collar	10	28	26	21.33
	11.00	26.00	24.00	20.33

It looks to me as if, in general, workers of European descent perceive the United States as being less racist than do workers of African or Mexican descent. In addition, there may be an interaction between worker status (white- vs. blue-collar) and region of descent: whereas perceived racism is lower for

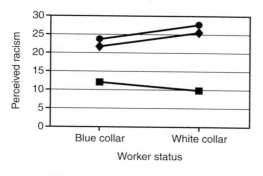

Perception of racism in the United States as a function of type of employment and area of origin

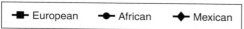

European-descent white-collar workers than it is for European-descent blue-collar workers, it increases for white-collar workers, compared to blue-collar workers, who are of African or Mexican descent.

Be aware: it is possible to make the graph differently by putting the area of origin on the *X* axis and having separate lines for blue- and white-collar workers, and I've done so. The graph still shows a slight interaction, and you can still see that workers of European descent perceive less racism than do workers of African or Mexican descent. I think that this stands out more with the first graph, but the second graph is acceptable too.

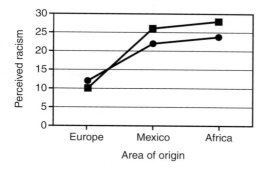

Perception of racism in the United States as a function of type of employment and area of origin

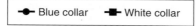

3. **Test:** Comparing the means of four dependent samples: repeated-measures ANOVA
   Assumptions:
   - Dependent samples: not violated
   - Interval- or ratio-level data: not violated
   - Random samples: no information given, so assume violated. OK to proceed as long as address issues of generalizability in interpretation
   - Normality: not violated (calculate 95% confidence intervals for each group for skewness and kurtosis)
   - Sphericity: not violated (assessed by comparing standard deviations)

   Hypotheses:

   $$H_0: \mu_1 = \mu_2 = \mu_3 = \mu_4$$
   $$H_1: \text{Not all population means are equal}$$

   Null hypothesis in English: There is no difference in outcome depending on which type of treatment one receives. The differences observed between the four sample means should be small and can be attributed to sampling error for four samples drawn from the same population.

   Alternative hypothesis in English: At least one of the four treatments is more (or less) effective than at least one of the others. Thus, at least one sample mean will differ from at least one of the other three. This difference will be too large to be explained away as sampling error for the differences between two means drawn from the same population.

   Decision rule:
   I'm willing to make a Type I error 5% of the time. F_{cv} (3, 24) = 3.0088. If $F_{observed} \geq 3.0088$, then it falls in the rare zone and reject H_0. If $F_{observed} < 3.0088$, then it falls in the common zone and fail to reject H_0.

   We don't know how to calculate power or sample size for a repeated measures ANOVA, so I can't speculate about the adequacy of the sample size on the basis of power. You might guess, however, that I am not going to be too excited about drawing strong conclusions about the treatment of GERD on the basis of a grand total of 36 patients.

   Calculations:

ANOVA summary table for gastroesophageal reflux disease treatment outcome data

Source	SS	df	MS	F
Subjects	1051.56	8	131.44	
Treatment	784.97	3	261.66	15.32*
Residual	409.78	24	17.07	
Total	2246.31	35		

Note: * = $p < .05$

APA format: F (3, 24) = 15.32, $p < .05$.

Interpretation:

$$\omega^2 = \frac{784.9722 - (4-1)17.0741}{2246.3056 + 17.0741} = \frac{733.7499}{2263.3797}$$

$$= .3242 = .32$$

$$LSD = 2.0639\sqrt{\frac{2(17.0741)}{9}} = 2.0639 \times 1.9479 = 4.0203$$

	$|M_1 - M_2|$	Statistically significant?	95% CI
Diet vs. medication	5.33	yes	1.31 to 9.35
Diet vs. acupuncture	5.22	yes	1.20 to 9.24
Diet vs. waiting list	6.44	yes	2.42 to 10.46
Medication vs. acupuncture	10.56	yes	6.54 to 14.58
Medication vs. waiting list	11.78	yes	7.76 to 15.80
Acupuncture vs. waiting list	1.22	no	−2.80 to 5.24

"I analyzed the data from a study conducted by a gastroenterologist in which she evaluated the effectiveness of three different treatments for gastroesophageal reflux disease (diet, medication, and acupuncture) by comparing them to a waiting-list control group. Thirty-six participants were matched in terms of symptom severity and then randomly assigned to one of the four treatment or control groups. After 8 weeks of treatment, symptom severity level was assessed on a scale that ranged from 0 (no symptoms) to 50 (extremely debilitating symptoms). Using repeated measures analysis of variance, I found that there were significant differences in outcome among the four groups (F (3, 24) = 15.32, $p < .05$). In ascending order of symptomatology, the outcomes were: medication ($M = 28.22$, $\hat{s} = 6.50$), diet ($M = 33.56$, $\hat{s} = 9.28$), acupuncture ($M = 38.78$, $\hat{s} = 4.73$), and waiting list control ($M = 40.00$, $\hat{s} = 5.66$).

"Overall, type of treatment given accounted for 32% of the variability in outcome, showing a substantial effect of treatment. To get a better idea of which treatment was most effective, I used the Fisher LSD post-hoc test. This showed that medication worked statistically significantly better than diet and that diet worked statistically significantly better than acupuncture, but that there was no statistically significant improvement in outcome for acupuncture over the waiting-list control group. Thus, if one is suffering

from gastroesophageal reflux disease, the results of the current study suggest that medication is the most effective treatment, but that dietary changes lead to a significant improvement over doing nothing as well.

"One of the limitations of the current study is that all the participants came from the gastroenterologist's practice. To the extent that there is something unique about her practice or the city where this study took place (e.g., level of socioeconomic status, baseline health status), then the conclusions of this study cannot be generalized beyond this physician's practice. There is a 5% chance that the conclusions of this study are in error and treatment has no differential impact. To increase confidence in these results, I suggest that the study be replicated. When the study is replicated, I recommend using a larger sample size from a variety of cities and gastroenterology practices to increase the generalizability of the results."

4. **Test:** The means of two dependent samples could be compared using a dependent-samples t test, but I am going to use a repeated-measures ANOVA instead, since it will give me an better measure of the size of the effect of the grouping variable.

Assumptions:
- Dependent samples: not violated
- Interval- or ratio-level data: not violated
- Random samples: violated, but OK to proceed as long as address limits to generalizability in interpretation
- Normality: not violated (calculate 95% confidence intervals for skewness and kurtosis for both samples)
- Homogeneity of variance: not violated since one $\hat{s}$ is not twice the other

Hypotheses:

$$H_0: \mu_1 = \mu_2$$
$$H_1: \mu_1 \neq \mu_2$$

Null hypothesis in English: There is no change over time in college in the political beliefs of these young adults. Thus, the difference in the means at T1 and T2 is small and can be explained as sampling error for two means drawn from the same population.

Alternative hypothesis in English: There is a change over time in college in the political beliefs of these young adults. This change will be reflected in the two sample means, and the difference between the two sample means will be larger than can be accounted for as a sampling error induced difference between two means from the same population.

Decision rule:
I'm willing to make a Type I error 5% of the time. Thus, F_{cv} (1, 24) = 4.2597. If $F_{observed} \geq 4.2597$, we'll reject H_0; if $F_{observed} < 4.2597$, we'll fail to reject H_0.

$$d = \frac{1.2800}{2.4583} = .5207 = .52$$

Looking up $d = .50$ and $n = 25$ in Appendix Table 11, I see that power = .66. Thus, if the null hypothesis is true there is a 34% chance of making a Type II error. This is higher than the accepted minimum standard of having only a 20% chance for making a Type II error. This study is underpowered. According to Appendix Table 12, I should be following 34 cases, not the 25 I am following. Thus, I recommend redoing the study with a sample size of at least 34.

This study takes over 4 years to complete, since students are followed from high school through college. I think it is unlikely that the researcher will heed my advice, find 9 more cases, and redo the study.

Calculations:

ANOVA summary table for data on political beliefs of children of conservative parents

Source	SS	df	MS	F
Subjects	4832.28	24		
Treatment	20.48	1	20.48	6.78*
Residual	72.52	24	3.02	
Total	4925.28	49		

Note: * = $p < .05$

Results in APA format: $F(1, 24) = 6.78$, $p < .05$

Interpretation:
I already calculated d, above, as .5207 and found that power = .66. To have an 80% chance of rejecting H_0 if it should be rejected, there should have been 34 cases, not 25. To have a 95% chance of rejecting H_0, there should be 54 cases, not 25.

$$\omega^2 = \frac{20.4800 - (2-1)3.0217}{4925.2800 + 3.0217} = \frac{17.4583}{4928.3017}$$

$$= .0035 = .004$$

$$95\% \ CI = |61.7600 - 60.4800| \pm 2.0639 \sqrt{\frac{2(3.0217)}{25}}$$

$$= 1.2800 \pm 2.0639(.4917) = 1.2800 \pm 1.0148$$

$$= \text{ranges from .27 to 2.29}$$

"I analyzed the data from a study in which a political scientist explored how the political beliefs of the children of conservative parents changed during their college careers. He administered the Political Belief Inventory at the end of high school and then again at the end of college to 25 children of conservative parents. Scores on the Political Belief Inventory can range from 0 (ultraliberal) to 75 (ultraconservative). At the end of high school, the average score of the students was very conservative ($M = 61.76$, $\hat{s} = 9.45$), and after college it was 1.28 points lower ($M = 60.48$, $\hat{s} = 10.72$). This change over time in the direction of becoming more liberal was statistically significant ($F(1, 24) = 6.78$, $p < .05$).

"Though these young adults became statistically more liberal during college, the change does not seem like a meaningful one since the effect of time, moving from Time 1 at the end of high school to Time 2 at the end of college, accounted for less than 1% of the variability in political beliefs. The students were only marginally less conservative after college than they had been before. According to this study, conservative parents do not have to worry that college will 'liberalize' their children.

"As with all studies, this one has limitations. First, there is a 5% chance that the conclusion is in error and there is no change in political beliefs over college. To allay this concern, I recommend the study be replicated. Though the study did yield results that were statistically significant, it had fewer subjects than it should and was, as statisticians would say, underpowered. If this study is replicated, at least 34 cases, not 25, should be followed; better would be to have a sample size of 54. In addition, the present sample consisted of children of parents who were identified as politically conservative and who were large donors to conservative causes. The current results may not generalize beyond this restricted population. If the study is replicated and if that is not the population of interest, I recommend obtaining a more representative sample. Further, it would be of interest to obtain information about the colleges attended by these students. If all the students in the present study, for example, attended conservative, religious universities, then it is not surprising that little liberalization occurred during their college years."

CHAPTER 12

Review Exercises

1. a. To find power, we first need to convert χ^2 into r via

    Equation 12.6: $\sqrt{\frac{4.52}{57}} = .2816 = .28$. Then, looking at the intersection of $N = 55$ and $r = .25$ in Appendix Table 7, we find power = .45; there is a 55% chance of Type II error.

    b. To find the N required to have a 95% chance of rejecting the null hypothesis, we look at the intersection of $r = .275$ and power = .95 in Appendix Table 8 and find $N = 168$. For power of .80, N equals 103.

2. a. $r = \sqrt{\frac{3.80}{37}} = .3205 = .32$. Power, for $N = 36$ (the

value closest to 37) = .42. We had a 58% chance of making a Type II error.

b. Required $N = 140$ for power of .95 and 86 for power of .80.

c. Though in part a we calculated $r = .32$, the best estimate is that the value of the correlation in the population is zero since we have failed to reject the null hypothesis.*

d. Following through on the same logic that there is no reason to believe there is a relationship, it is possible to conclude that RR probably equals 1.00, that the risk of a bad outcome for the control group is the same as the risk of a bad outcome for the treatment group. Otherwise, we don't have enough information to calculate a risk ratio.

3. a. Research question: Does the full moon have an impact on whether admissions to emergency rooms are for psychiatric or medical emergencies?

Statistical test: I have one group of cases, people admitted to emergency rooms, for which I am asking a question about a relationship between two variables. Both of my variables, type of admission and whether admitted during a full-moon day or not, are nominal-level variables: the test is the **chi-square test of association.** (Alternatively, you could conceptualize this as two independent samples of cases, one admitted for psychiatric reasons and the other for medical reasons, being measured on a nominal-level dependent variable, and end up with a **chi-square difference test.** Remember, both the chi-square difference test and the chi-square test of association are the same test, a **chi-square test for contingency tables.**)

b. Research question: Does a gel foot cushion reduce fatigue?

Statistical test: One grouping variable, three independent samples of cases being measured on an interval-level dependent variable: **one-way ANOVA.**

c. Research question: Is there a relationship between astrological sign and intelligence?

Statistical test: One grouping variable, 12 independent samples of cases being measured on an ordinal-level scale: **Kruskal-Wallis one-way ANOVA by ranks.**

d. Research question: Do those who get flu shots differ from those who don't in terms of how much risk they take with their health?

Statistical test: Two independent samples, those with and those without flu shots, being measured on an interval-level dependent variable: **independent-samples t test.**

---

*Some instructors will prefer the conclusion that the value of the correlation is .32, reasoning that we do have information from the sample about the size of the correlation between the two variables and it is better to extrapolate from existing data.

e. Research question: Is there a relationship between high school class rank and on-time college graduation?

Statistical test: One sample with two variables, one measured on a nominal level (on-time college graduation yes/no) and the other on an ordinal level (HS rank). Treat this, as directed in Chapter 6, as a **difference test.** (What difference test? I'll explain that in the next chapter, but here's a preview. Treat the nominal variable as a grouping variable, so we now have two independent samples: on-time graduates vs. not-on-time graduates. Treat the other variable, high school rank, as an ordinal-level dependent variable. As a result, we'll end up at the Mann Whitney U.)

4. **Test:** Can a graphologist predict gender from samples of handwriting? I have two independent samples, one from males and one from females, that are being classified on a nominal-level variable (gender): chi-square difference test

Assumptions:
- Nominal-level dependent variable: not violated
- Independent samples: not violated
- Random samples: violated but robust to violations
- Adequate expected frequencies: not violated
- No nonrobust assumptions were violated, so OK to proceed

Hypotheses:

H_0: Actual gender and predicted gender are independent of each other

H_1: Actual gender and predicted gender are not independent of each other

The null hypothesis says that there is no relationship, in the population, between what gender a person is and what gender the graphologist predicts the person to be. That is, the graphologist cannot accurately predict a person's gender from the person's handwriting. Even so, when we take a sample from the population and measure both of these variables, we don't expect there to be exactly a zero relationship between a person's actual gender and his or her predicted gender. However, the level of relationship found in the sample should be small enough that it can be explained as a deviation from zero that is due to sampling error.

The alternative hypothesis says that, in the population, there is a relationship between a person's gender and his or her predicted gender. (Note that this does not necessarily mean that the graphologist accurately predicts gender. The relationship could be such that that the graphologist consistently, but "accurately," mispredicts gender. That is, if he claims that the person is female, then it is likely that the person is male.) This level of relationship that is in the population should be found in a sample taken from the population. The observed relationship found in the sample between predicted and actual gender should be far enough away from a zero relationship that explaining the deviation as being due to sampling error is untenable.

Decision rule:

I'm willing to make a Type I error, to find that there is a relationship between the two variables when there isn't, 5% of the time. There is 1 degree of freedom (see Equation 12.1), so $\chi^2_{cv} = 3.8415$. If $\chi^2_{observed} \geq 3.8415$, then I'll reject H_0 and conclude that there is probably a relationship between actual gender and predicted gender. If $\chi^2_{observed} < 3.8415$, then I'll fail to reject H_0 and conclude that there is insufficient evidence to believe there is a relationship between actual and predicted gender.

It is appropriate at this stage to decide if one's sample size is adequate. I think that for graphology to be useful at predicting personality, the size of the effect should be at least moderate. Using Cohen's typology, a moderate effect is a correlation of .30. Looking at Appendix Table 8, I see that to have power of .80 when $r = .30$, that one should have 86 cases. Since this study has 98, I feel confident going in that if the effect is as large as I think it should be, I have enough cases to have a reasonable chance of finding it.

Calculations:

Using Equation 12.2, I calculate the expected frequency for the top, left cell (male/male) as $f_{expected} = \frac{51 \times 49}{98} = 25.5$. I'll use that, and the marginal frequencies, to calculate the other cell frequencies. Here's my table of expected frequencies:

	Predicts male	Predicts female	
Actually male	25.50	25.50	51
Actually female	23.50	23.50	47
	49	49	98

Via Equation 12.3:

$$\chi^2 = \frac{(29 - 25.50)^2}{25.50} + \frac{(22 - 25.50)^2}{25.50} +$$

$$\frac{(20 - 23.50)^2}{23.50} + \frac{(27 - 23.50)^2}{23.50}$$

$$= .4804 + .4804 + .5213 + .5213$$

$$= 2.0034$$

$$= 2.00$$

$$\chi^2 (1, N = 98) = 2.00, p > .05.$$

Interpretation:

Before starting the interpretation, let's think, using Table 12.12 as a guide, about how to proceed in this situation where I have failed to reject the null hypothesis. Having failed to reject H_0, I need to worry about the possibility of Type II error. To calculate this, and to determine if my sample size were adequate (given the actual observed size of the effect, not what I hoped it would be in advance), I am going to need to convert χ^2 into r. Also, though I am not sure that I am going to use it, I want to take a look at the 95% confidence interval for the difference between proportions. So, here are the necessary calculations for these.

$$\phi = r = \sqrt{\frac{2.0034}{98}} = .1430 = .14$$

Thus, power = .15, $\beta = .85$, and N, for power of .80, = 502. The likelihood of a Type II error is quite high.

Calculating the 95% confidence interval takes a little thought. I'm going to concentrate on the proportion of each sample that was predicted to be male. Since 29 of 51 males were predicted to be male, the proportion = .5686. (You can think of this as an accuracy rate, a hit rate.) The proportion of females that was predicted to be male was .4255. (You can think of this as an error rate, a miss rate.) Thus, the difference between proportions is .1431. If the handwriting expert were perfectly accurate at predicting gender, the difference would be 1.00. If he were perfectly inaccurate, it would be −1.00. And, if he was flipping a coin for each person, the difference between proportions should be 0.

Given this, we can now proceed to calculate the standard error for the difference between proportions via Equation 12.4:

$$s_{P_1 - P_2} = \sqrt{\frac{(.5686)(.4314)}{51} + \frac{(.4255)(.5745)}{47}}$$

$$= \sqrt{.0048 + .0052} = .1000$$

Via Equation 12.5, the 95% CI for the difference between proportions is as follows:

$$= .1431 \pm 1.96\,(.1000)$$

$$= .1431 \pm .1960$$

$$= \text{from} -.0529 \text{ to } .3391. \text{ You can think of this as}$$
indicating that, in the larger population, the handwriting expert may be a little inaccurate (−.05) or modestly accurate (.34). Note also that it is lopsided, that it barely captures zero on one side.

With all my calculations done, here is my interpretation:

"I conducted a study to see if a handwriting expert who claimed that he could predict facts about a person from his or her handwriting was able to do so. I took handwriting samples from 98 men and women, gave them to the handwriting expert, and asked him to classify each sample as coming from a man or a woman. Overall, he correctly classified 57% of the cases,* a rate that was not statistically different from what would be expected if he were unable to tell gender from handwriting (χ^2 (1, $N = 98$) = 2.00, $p >$ .05). Put simply, the expert was not statistically able accurately to predict a person's gender from his or her handwriting.

"Though a success rate of 57% does not sound far away from the 50% success rate that would be expected if a person flipped a coin to classify people as male or female, it is an improvement over 50%. To have an 80% chance of finding an effect this small to be statistically different from 50%, one would need to have close to 500 cases in one's study. As the present study had substantially fewer, it should be considered underpowered and inconclusive because it has a large chance, more than an 80% chance, that the conclusion is in error. If one wishes to continue with this research to determine if the small predictive ability exists, one would need a considerably larger sample size.

"In addition, the present study involved only one handwriting expert. It is possible that a different expert would have better (or worse) results. If one wishes to continue with this research, one may consider examining whether there are differences in prediction ability among handwriting experts.

"In conclusion, the present study offers no evidence that a handwriting expert can successfully predict a person's gender from the person's handwriting."

5. The researcher can't do the test she was planning because the expected frequencies in six of the cells are below 5. Here are the expected frequencies:

	A	B	Neutral	X	Y	
New	7	3	11	4.5	4.5	30
Standard	7	3	11	4.5	4.5	30
	14	6	22	9	9	60

The solution to this problem is to collapse cells. Both outcome A and B are positive outcomes, as Outcomes X and Y are negative outcomes. By collapsing the two positive and the two negative

---

*How did I get that 57%? Well 56 cases were correctly classified in terms of their gender, and there were 98 cases total, so 56 of 98 = 57%.

outcomes together, our observed frequencies now look like this:

	Positive	Neutral	Negative	
New	11	10	9	30
Standard	9	12	9	30
	20	22	18	60

and the expected frequencies are now all adequate:

	Positive	Neutral	Negative	
New	10	11	9	30
Standard	10	11	9	30
	20	22	18	60

6. a. *95% CI* for the difference between proportions:
Observed difference = .7568 − .5875 = .1693 (That is, almost 17% more of the experimental group than the control group has not started smoking cigarettes three years later.)

$$s_{P_1 - P_2} = \sqrt{\frac{(.7568)(.2432)}{74} + \frac{(.5875)(.4125)}{80}}$$
$$= \sqrt{.0025 + .0030} = .0742$$

95% CI = .1693 ± 1.96(.0742) = .1693 ± .1454 = from .02 to .31 (In the larger population the effect of the experimental treatment ranges, compared to the control group, from 2% fewer starting to smoke up to almost one third fewer kids starting to smoke.)

b. r (or ϕ) = $\sqrt{\dfrac{4.9720}{154}}$ = .1797. (The correlation between type of treatment received and outcome is .18.)

c. $d = \dfrac{2(.1797)}{\sqrt{1 - .1797^2}} = \dfrac{.3594}{.9837}$ = .3654 (I find d hard to interpret for chi-square. Using Cohen's 1988 rough guide, this effect is on the small to medium side.)

d. $RR = \dfrac{.4125}{.2432}$ = 1.6961. (A poor outcome (starting to smoke) is 1.70 times more likely for kids in the control group than in the experimental group, almost twice as likely. This seems to contradict d, which said that the effect was on the small side.

The *CI*, if you calculated it, ranges from 1.07 to 2.85.)

e. $NNT = \dfrac{1}{.7568 - .5875} = 5.9067$ (For every six kids to whom we give the experimental treatment, we are likely to end up with one less kid starting to smoke cigarettes. This also contradicts *d*. The *CI* for *NNT* ranges from 43 to 4.)

f. $\alpha = .05$ (Just testing to see if you were paying attention.)

g. $\beta = .56$ (This is relatively large, a 56% chance of Type II error. However, since we succeeded in rejecting the null hypothesis, we are not particularly worried about how likely the probability of a Type II error is.)

h. *N* required for power of .80 = 256; *N* = 420 for power = .95 (If we replicated this study, we'd like to have this many cases since the effect size is not very large.)

"This study investigated the effectiveness of a new ninth-grade health curriculum in preventing the onset of cigarette smoking. One hundred and fifty-four ninth-graders in a suburban district who were considered at risk to start smoking cigarettes were randomly divided into two groups. One group, the control group, received the standard health class curriculum about the dangers of smoking. The other group, the experimental group, received a new anti-smoking curriculum. Three years later the students were assessed, and it was found that 24% of the students who had received the experimental curriculum had started to smoke, compared to 41% of the students in the control group. This was a statistically significant difference between the two groups (χ^2 (1, *N* = 154) = 4.97, *p* < .05), indicating that the experimental new curriculum reduced the onset of smoking.

As with all studies, there is a chance that the conclusion is in error, and for the present study this is a 5% chance.

"Not only were the results statistically significant, but they seem practically meaningful as well. The risk of starting to smoke was 1.7 times higher in the control group than in the experimental group, and for every six students who received the new curriculum there was a net gain of one more nonsmoker.

"At the same time, I must point out that this study took place in only one school district, a suburban school district, and there may be something unique about this district that led to these results. Further, I am concerned that there may be a novelty effect, that the fact that the curriculum is new has led to these results. For these reasons, I recommend replication over time, in other settings, and with other teachers, to determine the robustness of the effect. For example, I calculated the 95% confidence interval for difference between the proportions of nonsmokers in the two groups and found that the size of the difference in the larger population likely falls in this range: from 2% more of the students who receive the new curriculum than the standard curriculum remaining nonsmokers, to as high as 31% more remaining nonsmokers. Replicating the study will help to clarify the size of the effect. To make sure that there are enough cases to have sufficient power to find the effect again, I recommend having about 250 students in the replication study.

"The bottom line is that the findings of the present study are certainly positive about the effectiveness of the new curriculum and suggest that it may be effective in reducing the onset of smoking among at-risk high school students. However, until further research is carried out, I do not suggest implementing this new curriculum on a larger scale."

CHAPTER 13

Review Exercises

1. There are three dependent samples being compared on a nominal-level dependent variable: **Cochran's Q test.**
2. There are four independent samples and two independent variables: **factorial multiple-samples difference test** (since the dependent variable is interval or ratio, we could be more specific and say factorial ANOVA).
3. There is one sample being compared to a population on a nominal-level dependent variable: **chi-square goodness-of-fit test.**
4. There are two independent samples being compared on a ratio-level dependent variable: **independent-samples *t* test.**
5. One grouping variable, three dependent samples, ordinal-level dependent variable: **Friedman two-way ANOVA by ranks.**
6. Test: There are four independent samples, two independent or grouping variables, and an ordinal-level dependent variable. The test to choose is a **factorial multiple-samples difference test.** We haven't learned how to calculate this sort of test, so we can stop here.
7. **Test:** Comparing the means of three independent samples: one-way ANOVA
   Assumptions:
   • Independent samples: not violated
   • Interval- or ratio-level data: not violated

- Random samples: not violated
- Normality: not violated
- Homogeneity of variance: not violated

Hypotheses:

H_0: $\mu_1 = \mu_2 = \mu_3$

H_1: Not all μs are equal

Decision rule:

If $F_{observed} \geq 3.3541$, reject H_0

If $F_{observed} < 3.3541$, fail to reject H_0

Applying the rule-of-thumb formula for sample size for an independent-samples t test to the two samples that are farthest apart, $n = 2$. Since I have 10 cases per group, I'm confident that my sample size is adequate.

Calculations:

The calculations are tedious by hand with 30 cases. Here's a table that shows how to calculate what is needed to find SS_{total} and SS_{within}:

		SS Total Calculations		SS within Calculations	
	X	X – Grand Mean	$(X$ – Grand Mean$)^2$	X – Group Mean	$(X$ – Group Mean$)^2$
Mon	2.31	−.2180	.0475	−.0760	.0058
Mon	2.27	−.2580	.0666	−.1160	.0135
Mon	2.37	−.1580	.0250	−.0160	.0003
Mon	2.37	−.1580	.0250	−.0160	.0003
Mon	2.39	−.1380	.0190	.0040	.0000
Mon	2.40	−.1280	.0164	.0140	.0002
Mon	2.42	−.1080	.0117	.0340	.0012
Mon	2.42	−.1080	.0117	.0340	.0012
Mon	2.43	−.0980	.0096	.0440	.0019
Mon	2.48	−.0480	.0023	.0940	.0088
Wed	2.31	−.2180	.0475	−.1340	.0180
Wed	2.38	−.1480	.0219	−.0640	.0041
Wed	2.40	−.1280	.0164	−.0440	.0019
Wed	2.41	−.1180	.0139	−.0340	.0012
Wed	2.42	−.1080	.0117	−.0240	.0006
Wed	2.45	−.0780	.0061	.0060	.0000
Wed	2.46	−.0680	.0046	.0160	.0003
Wed	2.49	−.0380	.0014	.0460	.0021
Wed	2.53	.0020	.0000	.0860	.0074
Wed	2.59	.0620	.0038	.1460	.0213
Fri	2.75	.2220	.0493	−.0040	.0000
Fri	2.63	.1020	.0104	−.1240	.0154
Fri	2.64	.1120	.0125	−.1140	.0130
Fri	2.64	.1120	.0125	−.1140	.0130
Fri	2.67	.1420	.0202	−.0840	.0071
Fri	2.69	.1620	.0262	−.0640	.0041
Fri	2.84	.3120	.0973	.0860	.0074
Fri	2.86	.3320	.1102	.1060	.0112
Fri	2.90	.3720	.1384	.1460	.0213
Fri	2.92	.3920	.1537	.1660	.0276

$$SS_{total} = (.0475 + .0666 + .0250 + .0250 + .0190 +$$
$$.0164 + .0117 + .0117 + .0096 + .0023) +$$
$$(.0475 + .0219 + .0164 + .0139 + .0117 +$$
$$.0061 + .0046 + .0014 + .0000 + .0038) +$$
$$(.0493 + .0104 + .0125 + .0125 + .0202 +$$
$$.0262 + .0973 + .1102 + .1384 + .1537)$$
$$= .9928$$

$$SS_{between} = 10(2.3860 - 2.5280)^2 + 10(2.4440 -$$
$$2.5280)^2 + 10(2.7540 - 2.5280)^2$$
$$= .2016 + .0706 + .5108$$
$$= .7830$$

$SS_{within} = SS_{total} - SS_{between}$ (I'm taking the Dirty Harry shortcut here rather than go through the tedium of calculating SS_{within} for 30 cases.)

$$= .9928 - .7830$$
$$= .2098$$

ANOVA summary table for crossword puzzle data

Source	SS	df	MS	F
Between	.7830	2	.3915	
Within	.2098	27	.0078	50.1923*
Total	.9928	29		

Note: * = $p < .05$

Note: I am filling this table out to four decimal places, not two, to make calculating below easier.

APA format: $F(2, 27) = 50.19$, $p < .05$

Interpretation:
The null hypothesis was rejected, so it will be reasonable to calculate ω^2, convert this to $\hat{r}$ to check power and sample size, calculate an *LSD* value for post-hoc tests, and calculate 95% confidence intervals.

$$\omega^2 = \frac{.7830 - (2).0078}{.9928 + .0078} = \frac{.7674}{1.0006} = .7669$$

$$\hat{r} = \sqrt{.7669} = .8757$$

Power > .99

N for power of .80 = 8, for power of .95 = 11

$$LSD = 2.0518\sqrt{.0078\left(\frac{1}{10} + \frac{1}{10}\right)}$$
$$= 2.0518\sqrt{.00156}$$
$$= 2.0518 \times .0395$$
$$= .0810$$

Significant differences: Monday vs. Friday, Wednesday vs. Friday

95% CIs:
Mon vs. Wed: .0580 ± .0810 = from −.02 to .14
Mon vs. Fri: .3680 ± .0810 = from .29 to .45
Wed vs. Fri: .3100 ± .0810 = from .23 to .39

"I conducted a study in which I compared the length of answers for *New York Times* crossword puzzles of three levels of difficulty: easy, medium, and hard. From the past 10 years, I obtained random samples of Monday puzzles (easy), Wednesday puzzles (medium), and Friday puzzles (hard), and calculated the average number of letters per answer for each level of puzzle. The mean letter lengths (and standard deviations) for the easy, medium, and hard puzzles were, respectively, 2.39 (.06), 2.44 (.08), and 2.75 (.12). The overall difference in the lengths of the answers was a statistically significant one by a one-way analysis of variance ($F(2, 27) = 50.19$, $p < .05$).

"Though there is a 5% chance that this conclusion is erroneous, these results indicate that different difficulty level *New York Times* puzzles have different answer lengths. In fact, difficulty level of the puzzle explains most of the variability, 77% to be exact, that occurs in answer length. Inspections of the means shows that answer length increases with puzzle difficulty. Though in general harder puzzles have answers that are longer, a post-hoc comparison of means shows that there is no statistically significant difference in the length of answers for Monday and Wednesday puzzles. Friday puzzles, however, have answers that are statistically longer than Monday or Wednesday puzzles. Thus, it seems that hard puzzles have answers that are longer than easy or medium puzzles. The difference does not seem dramatic as the average answer to a hard puzzle is only a third of a letter longer than an average answer to an easy puzzle.

"Generalizability of the results is limited, technically, only to puzzles from *The New York Times* and only to puzzles from the past 10 years. Though I believe that the results—that a puzzle with longer answers is a harder puzzle—would hold true for puzzles from other sources and for other years, I recommend replication in other populations to be sure. Replication would also serve to address the possibility that my random sample was not representative of the larger population of *New York Times* puzzles and that the conclusions of this study are in error."

8. **Test:** Comparing the means of two, independent samples: independent-samples *t* test
Assumptions:
• Independent samples: not violated
• Interval- or ratio-level data: not violated
• Random samples: violated, but OK to proceed as long as discuss limitations to generalizability
• Normality: not violated
• Homogeneity of variance: not violated
Hypotheses:

$$H_0: \mu_1 = \mu_2$$
$$H_1: \mu_1 \neq \mu_2$$

The null hypothesis says that the length of time to be symptom-free is the same for the populations of people who receive the experimental treatment or a placebo treatment for the common cold. Any observed difference between the means of samples from the two populations is small enough that it can be explained as sampling error between two samples drawn from the same population.

The alternative hypothesis says that there is a difference in time to be symptom-free for people with colds who are treated with the experimental treatment vs. a placebo treatment. The difference is a real one, and it will be reflected in the means of a sample of people from the experimental population vs. a sample of people from the placebo population. The difference is too large to be explained by sampling error.

Decision rule:
The researcher is willing to make a Type I error 5% of the time, so he sets α at .05. His null hypothesis is nondirectional, so he'll use a two-tailed test. With 20 degrees of freedom, the critical value of *t* is 2.0860.

If $t_{observed} \geq 2.0860$, then he'll reject H_0. If $t_{observed} < 2.0860$, he'll fail to reject H_0.

This is also the point to consider whether the sample size is adequate. Via the rule of thumb formula:

$$n = \frac{16}{\left(\dfrac{27.0000 - 19.4000}{7.1678}\right)^2} = \frac{16}{1.1242}$$

$$= 14.2323 = 15$$

Thus, given the sample means and the standard deviation of the control group, and if he is willing to have a 20% chance of a Type II error and a 5% chance of a Type I error, then he should have about 15 cases per sample. Since he has 10 cases in the control group and 12 cases in the experimental group, the researcher should be concerned that the study is underpowered. He should obtain about 10 more cases, 6 for the control group and 4 for the experimental group, before analyzing the data.

Calculations:

$\hat{s}_{M_1 - M_2}$

$$= \sqrt{\left[\frac{(12-1)5.1522^2 + (10-1)7.1678^2}{12 + 10 - 2}\right]\left[\frac{12 + 10}{12 \times 10}\right]}$$

$$= \sqrt{\left[\frac{291.9968 + 462.3962}{20}\right]\left[\frac{22}{120}\right]}$$

$$= \sqrt{\left[37.7196\right]\left[.1833\right]}$$

$$= \sqrt{6.9140}$$

$$= 2.6294$$

$$t = \frac{27.0000 - 19.4000}{2.6294} = \frac{7.6000}{2.6294} = 2.8904$$

In APA format: $t (20) = 2.89$, $p < .05$

Interpretation:
The null hypothesis was rejected, so he will want to calculate the 95% confidence interval for the difference between population means, d, and ω^2, turn t into r, and calculate power.

95% $CI = (27.0000 - 19.4000) \pm 2.0860(2.6294)$
$= 7.6000 \pm 5.4849$
$= $ from 2.1151 to 13.0849

$\hat{s}_{pooled} = \sqrt{37.7196} = 6.1416$

$d = \dfrac{7.6000}{6.1416} = 1.2375$

$\omega^2 = \dfrac{2.8904^2}{2.8904^2 + 20 + 1} = \dfrac{7.3544}{29.3544} = .2505$

$r_{pb} = \sqrt{\dfrac{2.8904^2}{2.8904^2 + 20}} = \sqrt{\dfrac{8.3544}{28.3544}}$

$= \sqrt{.2946} = .5428$

Power = .66

N needed = 27 (for $\alpha = .05$ and $\beta = .20$) and 42 (for $\alpha = .05$ and $\beta = .05$)

NOTE: Don't forget that interpretation is a human endeavor and you need to keep alert. Inspection of the means shows that the treatment leads to a *worse* outcome.

"I analyzed the data from a study in which a medical researcher tested a new treatment for the common cold by comparing it to a placebo. Twenty-two people with colds were randomly assigned to receive either the experimental treatment or a placebo treatment. After receiving treatment, the number of hours that elapsed until the person felt symptom-free were tallied. A statistically significant effect of treatment was found (t (20) = 2.89, $p < .05$), but unfortunately it indicated that people who received the new treatment took a statistically longer time, almost an additional third of a day, to be symptom-free. Put more simply, the current study suggests that the new treatment worked worse than did the placebo.

"People receiving the placebo treatment reported being symptom-free, on average, in 19.4 hours ($\hat{s} = 5.15$) and people receiving the experimental treatment reported being symptom-free in 27.0 hours ($\hat{s} = 7.17$). The results of this study suggest that the size of the effect, in the larger population, is such that people receiving the new treatment will have symptoms for from 2 to 13 hours longer than do people who receive a placebo treatment. The new treatment appears to have no benefit over a placebo treatment, and it actually appears to slow down recovery from a cold.

"Though there is a 5% chance that this conclusion is wrong, the results of the present study certainly suggest that it is not worthwhile to pursue this new treatment as a treatment for the common cold. However, at the same time I want to note that this study was a bit underpowered (i.e., it would have been better to have about 30 cases, not just 22) and that how the participants in the present study were obtained is not clear. If other studies with this new treatment have shown it to have some benefit, I suggest gathering more information about how the participants in the present study were obtained to decide if there was something unique about this sample that led to these results. However, failing any other evidence that suggests this new treatment has any benefit, I believe that further research into its efficacy as a treatment for the common cold is not warranted."

Index

Page numbers followed by f refer to figures;
those followed by t refer to tables.

581

INDEX

585

INDEX

Predictions
  with independent-samples *t* test,
      percentage of variance predicted in,
      336-338
  with linear regression, 263-273
  with one-way ANOVA, percentage of
      variance predicted in, 383-387
  with Pearson product moment correlation
      coefficient, 263-273, 291, 292
  and binomial effect size display,
      255-262
  percentage of variance predicted in,
      252-255
  with repeated-measures ANOVA, percentage
      of variance predicted in, 422-424
Predictor variable, 11, 12, 182, 231
  in binomial effect size display, 255
  in chi-square tests, 463
  definition of, 11
Pre-post samples, 302
Probability calculations, 135-136, 136f, 144,
      209-212
  conjunctional, 211, 470-471
Proportion compared to percentage, 126
Protected *t* test, 388-396

R

Random error, 149-151, 150f-151f
  definition of, 149
  variability from, 365, 366
Random numbers table, 146t, 146-147, 531t
Random sample, 5-6, 6t, 143-176. *See also*
      Sample.
Range, 99-100, 109
  calculation of, 99
  definition of, 99
  interquartile, 100-102, 102t, 109
Ranking
  in ordinal measurements, 16-19, 17t, 18t
  percentile rank in, 79-86, 100-102, 132-135
  tie scores in, 17-18, 18t
    and median calculations, 94
    and percentile rank, 83

Rare zone in sampling distribution
  in chi-square tests, 467, 469, 469f
  in independent-samples *t* test, 318-319,
      320-321, 321f
  in one-way ANOVA, 372, 374, 375, 375f,
      398, 399f
  in Pearson product moment correlation
      coefficient, 217, 218-219, 220, 226,
      227t, 231-232
  in repeated-measures ANOVA, 418, 419,
      419f, 421, 443
Ratio measurement level, 15, 20-22, 36
  central tendency measures in, 91, 96
  definition of, 20
  equality of units in, 21-22, 23
  histogram display in, 63
  independent-samples *t* test in, 303t, 307,
      311
    assumptions for, 311
  one-way ANOVA in, 364t, 369
  Pearson product moment correlation
      coefficient in, 185, 188, 193-194,
      198, 231, 277
  questions for identification of, 22-24
  range in, 99
  real zero points in, 20-21, 23
  relationship to continuous and discrete
      numbers, 52, 53
  repeated-measures ANOVA in, 416, 434,
      448-449
  Spearman rank order correlation coefficient
      in, 185-186, 231
  variability measures in, 107
Raw scores, 78-86
  definition of, 79
  percentile rank converted to, 84-86, 86
  percentile rank estimated from, 81f, 81-82,
      86
  transformed to percentile rank, 79-84, 86
  transformed to *z* score, 115-117, 140, 267
  z score converted to, 117-119
Real limits for interval, 55-58
  calculation of, 55, 57
  definition of, 55
  in percentile rank, 81-82, 84, 85
Regression, linear, 263-274. *See also* Linear
      regression.
Relationship tests, 179-292
  chi-square test as, 186, 186f, 188, 231, 460,
      462-463, 503, 512
    assumptions in, 466
    indications for, 186f, 188, 231, 464, 514

Relationship tests—cont'd
      interpretation of, 475-494
      null and alternative hypothesis in, 466
  in one sample, 462, 514
  compared to difference tests, 181-183, 185,
      186, 188-189, 231, 299, 512-513
  definition of, 181
  multiple sample, 516
  number of cases and sample size in, 183,
      184f, 185
  one sample, 513-514
    chi-square test in, 462, 514
  Pearson product moment correlation
      coefficient in, 185, 186f, 187-232
  predictor and predicted (criterion) variables
      in, 182, 231
  selection of, 185-187, 186f
  Spearman rank order correlation coefficient
      in, 185-186, 186f
  two sample, 515
Relative benefit ratio, 486
Relative risk ratio, 460, 484-488, 500-501, 504
  calculation of, 485
  confidence intervals for, 486-488
  definition of, 484
  and number needed to treat, 489-490,
      490t
Repeated measures analysis of variance, 305,
      406, 414-453
  assumptions for, 416-417
    in two dependent samples, 434,
      448-449
  calculations in, 420-421
    in two dependent samples, 435, 450
  column effect in, 415, 433
  compared to dependent samples *t* test,
      429-453
  confidence intervals for, 425-426, 427, 446,
      453
    in two dependent samples, 434,
      436-437, 443, 451
  decision rules for, 418-420
    in two dependent samples, 435,
      449-450
  degrees of freedom in, 418, 419, 419t,
      421t, 430, 435, 449
  effect size in, 436-441, 450, 453
    and *d* values, 438-441, 445, 445t, 544t
  F ratio in, 417, 418-420
    calculation of, 420-421
    critical values for, 419, 420, 435, 449
    omnibus or overall, 422, 424

INDEX

Variance—cont'd

    compared to standard deviation, 107

    factorial analysis of, 304-305, 406, 407-413. *See also* Factorial analysis of variance.

    homogeneity assumption for, 416, 417

        in independent-samples *t* test, 311, 313, 314

        in one-way ANOVA, 370, 371

        in repeated-measures ANOVA, 434, 448-449

    in independent-samples *t* tests, 313, 314

        homogeneity assumption for, 311, 313, 314

        percentage of variance predicted in, 336-338

        population variance in, 327, 332, 333

    in individual differences, 364-365, 366

    one-way analysis of, 304, 359-401. *See also* One way analysis of variance.

    percentage of variance predicted

        in independent-samples *t* test, 336-338

Variance—cont'd

    in one-way ANOVA, 383-387

    in Pearson product moment correlation efficient, 252-255

    in repeated-measures ANOVA, 422-424, 437-438

    in population, 103-104, 105-106, 157

        in independent-samples *t* test, 327, 332, 333

        mean square in, 377, 380

    repeated-measures analysis of, 305, 406, 414-453. *See also* Repeated measures analysis of variance.

    in sample, 103, 105-106

        formula for, 380

    within-group variability, 364, 365, 366, 368

        sum of squares in, 377, 379

        summary table on, 380-382

W

What test when. *See* selection of test.

Y

Yates' correction for continuity in chi-square tests, 465

Z

z scores, 114-136, 158

    definition of, 115

    extreme values in, 135, 135f

    negative values in, 115, 127f, 127-128, 140

    normal distribution in, 118, 120, 123-136, 323

        estimates and table information for, 125-136, 528t-531t

    and Pearson product moment correlation coefficient, 228-230, 232

    raw score transformed to, 115-117, 140, 267

    transformed to raw score, 117-119

Zero points, 17

    arbitrary, in interval measurements, 20

    in Pearson product moment correlation coefficients

        and results not statistically different from zero, 274-289, 291

        and results statistically different from zero, 243-246, 291

        and scatterplot for zero correlation, 209, 209f

    real, 23-24

        in ratio measurements, 20-21, 23